# METAL IONS
# AND BACTERIA

# METAL IONS AND BACTERIA

Edited by

## Terrance J. Beveridge
Department of Microbiology
College of Biological Science
University of Guelph
Guelph, Ontario, Canada

## Ronald J. Doyle
Department of Microbiology and Immunology
Health Science Center
University of Louisville
Louisville, Kentucky

WILEY

A WILEY-INTERSCIENCE PUBLICATION

**JOHN WILEY & SONS**

New York • Chichester • Brisbane • Toronto • Singapore

*Library of Congress Cataloging in Publication Data:*

Metal ions and bacteria / edited by Terrance J. Beveridge, Ronald J.
   Doyle
      p.   cm.
      "A Wiley-Interscience publication."

   Includes bibliographies and index.
   ISBN 0-471-62918-9
   1. Metals—Physiological effect.   2. Microorganisms—Physiology.
I. Beveridge, Terrance J.   II. Doyle, Ronald J.

   QR92.M45M47   1989                                88-28189
   589.9′019214—dc19                                 CIP

Printed in the United States of America

10  9  8  7  6  5  4  3  2  1

# CONTRIBUTORS

**Terrance J. Beveridge,** Department of Microbiology, University of Guelph, Guelph, Ontario, Canada

**Corale L. Brierley,** VistaTech Partnership, Ltd., Salt Lake City, Utah

**James A. Brierley,** Wheat Ridge, Colorado

**Yvonne E. Collins,** Department of Biology, New York University, New York, New York

**Charles D. Cox,** Department of Microbiology, University of Iowa, Iowa City, Iowa

**Michael S. Davidson,** Orange County Water District, Fountain Valley, California

**Ronald J. Doyle,** Department of Microbiology and Immunology, Health Science Center, University of Louisville, Louisville, Kentucky

**F. Grant Ferris,** Nora Husky Research Corp., Calgary, Alberta, Canada

**William S. Fyfe,** Department of Geology, University of Western Ontario, London, Ontario, Canada

**Gill G. Geesey,** Department of Microbiology, California State University, Long Beach, California

**Larry Jang,** Department of Chemical Engineering, California State University, Long Beach, California

**Richard A. Laddaga,** Department of Biological Sciences, Bowling Green State University, Bowling Green, Ohio

**Robert E. Marquis,** Department of Microbiology and Immunology, University of Rochester, Rochester, New York

**Tapan K. Misra,** Department of Microbiology and Immunology, University of Illinois College of Medicine, Chicago, Illinois

**Charles R. Myers,** Center for Great Lakes Studies, University of Wisconsin-Milwaukee, Milwaukee, Wisconsin

**Kenneth H. Nealson,** Department of Biology and Center for Great Lakes Studies, University of Wisconsin-Milwaukee, Milwaukee, Wisconsin

**J. B. Neilands,** Department of Biochemistry, University of California, Berkeley, California

**William H. Orme-Johnson,** Department of Chemistry, Massachusetts Institute of Technology, Cambridge, Massachusetts

**Reinhardt A. Rosson,** Center for Great Lakes Studies, University of Wisconsin-Milwaukee, Milwaukee, Wisconsin

**William Shotyk,** Department of Geology, University of Western Ontario, London, Ontario, Canada

**Simon Silver,** Department of Microbiology and Immunology, University of Illinois College of Medicine, Chicago, Illinois

**G. Dennis Sprott,** Division of Biological Sciences, National Research Council of Canada, Ottawa, Ontario, Canada

**Gunter Stotzky,** Department of Biology, New York University, New York, New York

**Lawrence P. Wackett,** Department of Biochemistry, Gray Freshwater Biological Institute, University of Minnesota, Navarre, Minnesota

**Christopher T. Walsh,** Department of Biological Chemistry and Molecular Pharmacology, Harvard Medical School, Boston, Massachusetts

# ■■■■■ PREFACE

The impetus for this book came from the overwhelming response that an American Society for Microbiology symposium on Bacterial Interactions with Metallic Ions received during the Society's annual meeting in 1986. It was evident that there was an awareness of the importance of metal–microbe interactions and that the field was growing both in stature and in numbers of active researchers. That symposium could cover only a small portion of the relevant topics, and it became apparent that even by increasing the spectrum of topics for this book, a single book could not be all-inclusive.

We have made little attempt to expand the subject to the realm of eukaryotic microorganisms and clearly, molds, yeasts, algae, and some protozoans are important vehicles for the microbial cycling of metals. This is not an oversight, but merely an attempt to keep the book within reasonable bounds. Yvonne Collins and Guenther Stotzky, Joe Neilands, and Corale Brierley, Jim Brierley, and Mike Davidson have been kind enough to give brief discussions of eukaryotic microorganisms in Chapters 2, 5, and 12. Obviously, too, not all topics on bacteria–metal interactions could be covered within the boundaries of a single book. The subjects that are included in *Metal Ions and Bacteria* are those we believe to be most relevant and interesting. Although this book is not meant to be all-inclusive, it does cover a wide variety of aspects, some of which seem initially to be quite unrelated to the others except for that single, tenuous string of metallic ions that keeps these bacteria in their gilded cages.

Books such as this depend entirely on the quality of the contributions. We owe much to our authors, especially those who withstood the "slings and arrows" suffered from the whims of Ron Doyle and myself, and to our publisher, whose patience was instrumental.

T.J.B.
R.J.D.

*Guelph, Ontario, Canada*
*Louisville, Kentucky*
*January 1989*

# CONTENTS

ix

# METAL IONS
# AND BACTERIA

# CHAPTER 1

# Metal Ions and Bacteria

TERRANCE J. BEVERIDGE

Department of Microbiology
University of Guelph
Guelph, Ontario, Canada

## Contents

## 1.1   THE ARCHEAN EARTH

Astronomers tell us that the accretion and maturation of planets within the solar system was a grindingly slow process. Current estimates suggest the solar system was first initiated about 4.6 Ga (Ga = giga anna, $10^9$ years) ago and that the accretion of the Earth was complete about 0.1 Ga after this date (1). Obviously, both events are of paramount importance to us, for the ultimate result was the concentration of the ingredients of which our present habitat consists. It has taken about 4.5 Ga for the Earth to evolve into its current geological format and throughout this time span tremendous changes have occurred. The kinetic energy of impactation during global accretion resulted in a rather homogeneous mixture of metallic iron and silicates. Cooling of this magma both concentrated and separated various elements and their minerals into defined locations within our globe so that, at present, a solid silicaceous crust floats upon a series of molten layers suspended over an iron-rich core.

Certainly the initial phases of the cooling (the Hadean period, 4.5–3.9 Ga) instigated severe global surface alterations as the crust evolved. As the magma cooled, it contracted and split, causing local upwellings. At the same time, subduction buried and remelted large regions of the early crust. The scale of these events was tremendous and they occurred over the briefest periods on the geological time scale. The Earth's surface was in a constant flux between melt and solidification as it strove to relinquish a proportion of the heat of accretion. It was a tumultuous but important period because the fundamental character of the Earth's surface was imprinted at this time. Crustal elements and their eventual minerals were being stirred in the caldron and their zonal distribution throughout the lithosphere was underway. Iron-rich melt was descending to form the metal core. The geological record of the early Hadean is hazy because no terrestrial rocks survived these tremulous times, but we suspect meteorite impactation also contributed to the ingredient mix and the total energy to be dispersed. Our earliest records rely on the Isua supracrustal belt of western Greenland, which is no older than 3.8 Ga, and imply that water-laid, silicic sediments were being deposited to form the continental crust (2).

Together with this Hadean crust formation, tremendous outgassing occurred, forming the primitive atmosphere. There are several ideas about the makeup of this atmosphere, and they range from suggesting the prebiotic atmosphere was strongly reducing, mildly reducing, to nonreducing; most authorities agree it was anoxic. It is not my intention to enter the debate about the composition of the Hadean atmosphere and its contributions to the formulation of life. Instead, I retreat to the Isua Greenland rock, which indicates that at least $H_2O$ and $CO_2$ were present in the atmosphere by the late Hadean (3). Unfortunately, because this rock has undergone a series of severe metamorphisms through time, it is impossible to establish whether or not biological carbon fixation was in evidence (4), but obviously outgassed $H_2O$ had accounted for large crustal accumulations of water by this time. We believe this rock to be a subaqueous, volcanic-exhalative sequence (5).

This is our starting point for Chapter 1. By the late Hadean, a solid crust had formed on the Earth that was predominantly silicaceous but contained an ample mix of other materials; metals in abundance were coordinated throughout the matrices. Overlaying the crust was an anoxic atmosphere laden with water vapor. The atmosphere's reducing power and its ability to relinquish the water as rain contributed to the weathering of rock, the so-lubilization of metal salts, and the accumulation of brine in the oceans. This is the delicious soup our earliest life forms inherited.

## 1.2   THE AGE AND UBIQUITY OF BACTERIA

The evidence is clear that prokaryotic life evolved first on this planet and that it was present during the late Archean and Proterozoic periods. This evidence stems from abundant observations of so-called microfossils found in ancient, organic-rich cherts and the detection of distinctly biological residues in a range of ancient sediments, cherts, and shales (6–10).

Ancient stromatolites (Fig. 1.1), because of their laminated structure, first evoked the idea of a biological origin (8) and are believed to be the mineralized remnants of filamentous bacteria similar to cyanobacteria. Certainly there are many morphological similarities between these microfossils and present-day bacterial biofilms (cf. Figs. 1.2 and 1.3). The most convincing argument for middle Archean life is found in stromatolitic cherts of the Western Australia Warrawoona Group (6). These indicate that bacteria inhabited this surficial environment at least 3.5 Ga ago, and, the complexity of their cellular remains is persuasive evidence that simpler life predates this period.

One of the difficulties in the interpretation of microfossils is that the exact mechanism of their preservation is unclear. Unlike you and me, bacteria have no internal mineralized skeleton to resist the ravages of time after death; they are made entirely of soft tissue (11). Yet they have in their walls some of the most resilient biopolymers known. Eubacteria use peptidoglycan to form a rigid murein sacculus that gives the cell its shape and form (12). Archaebacteria rely, instead, on pseudomurein, complex heteropolysaccharides, or protein for their rigid framework (12, 13). In either case, these external corsets of bacteria resist all but the most harsh degradative chemical treatments, and are the best candidates for instigating and retaining cellular form as microfossils through geological time. At the same time, recent evidence suggests that the very affinity of bacterial walls for heavy metals (e.g., Fe) inhibits constituent wall autolysins, thereby ensuring the maintenance of shape (14). These surfaces sorb metallic ions from solution and initiate mineral formation (15). Low-temperature diagenesis simulations of metal-loaded cells suggest that mineralization occurs first at the bacterial surface and progresses throughout the cytoplasm (16) until the entire cell consists of a series of loosely connected crystallites that mimic the shape of the cell (Fig. 1.4). In situ observations on a variety of natural settings indicate that this could be a common feature in sediments and soils (17–19). It is probable that bacteria are not unique in this regard because a variety of eukaryotic microorganisms also have some ability to sorb metals onto their surfaces (e.g., Ref. 20), but of all life-forms, bacteria inhabit the greatest diversity of habitats and have the greatest capacity to sorb metals from solution (on

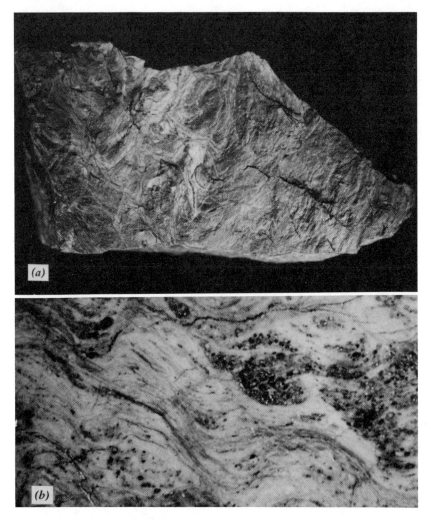

**Figure 1.1**  Picture of a piece of the Gunflint Chert (*a*) from the Northern Superior region in Canada. Note the laminations, which are attributable to the layers of cyanobacteria-like organisms that composed this ancient stromatolite. A close-up (*b*) reveals how distinct the layers of the bacterial mat are.

a biomass to dry weight metals basis) (21). Their importance in reworking the distribution of crustal metals stems not only from their antiquity but also from their ubiquity.

   Today, bacteria are found throughout nature; they form a major proportion of the Earth's global biomass. They inhabit the land and the seas, our driest deserts and saltiest brines, and some of the hottest and coldest climes. Some require molecular oxygen for respiration, some can be poisoned by

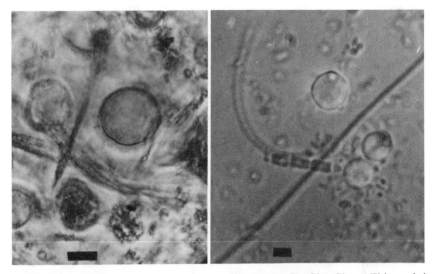

**Figure 1.2**  Bright-field micrograph of a section of the Gunflint Chert. This rock is filled with the crystallized remains of filamentous and spherical bacteria. Although these microfossils are from an ancient stromatolite, they bear striking resemblance to the bacteria seen in Figure 1.3. Bar = 10 μm. Reprinted with permission of the author and the National Research Council of Canada (Ref. 56).

**Figure 1.3**  Phase micrograph of a biofilm from a stream in Southern Ontario. Bar = 10 μm. Reprinted with permission of the author and the National Research Council of Canada (Ref. 56).

only a few molecules of oxygen, and others lie somewhere in between these two atmospheric extremes. Some can hibernate until unsuitable conditions improve (e.g., endospores, cysts, and ultramicrocells). The diversity of the microbial environment is clear evidence of mutation and natural selection on a grand scale. In fact, we believe it is due to an unwitting conspiracy between ancient prokaryotes and the primitive earth that we owe our present congenial environment. Earth's surface has been terraformed and maintained within its present narrow limits for life by its microbiota; these are the true monitors of life.

## 1.3   THE AVAILABILITY OF METALLIC IONS BOTH THEN AND NOW

Certainly the availability of water was important not only for the generation of life, but also for the mobilization of metals by the solubilization of their constituent salts. As now, the oceans represented the largest reservoir for solubilized metals during the Precambrian. Today, except near local belts

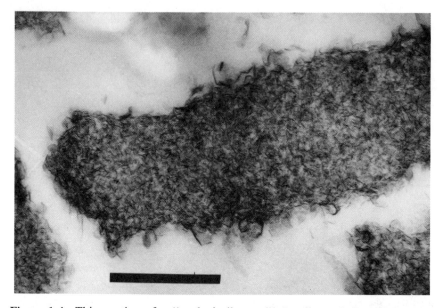

**Figure 1.4** Thin section of a "geologically aged" *Bacillus subtilis* cell that was previously loaded with uranyl ion and incubated with fine-grain quartz and calcite during a low-temperature diagenesis experiment as outlined in Ref. 16. Note that although the cell is a mass of uranium phosphate microcrysts, the general shape of the cell is retained. This cell is well on its way to becoming a bona fide microfossil. Bar = 500 nm.

of submarine volcanic activity, the ocean floor is in steady equilibrium with its overlying waters so that mean water composition and temperature differ only slightly from place to place. Within reasonable limits, this has been true since the middle of the Proterozoic so that the amount of salt in the seas has been maintained at a constant level of about 3.4%. Clearly most of this was in the form of sodium, magnesium, calcium, potassium, chloride, phosphate, and sulfate salts, but a wide range of other constituents were also involved (Table 1.1).

Previous to the Proterozoic, the composition of oceanic water probably differed in several important respects. Hydrothermal venting was more vigorous, as was leaching from mafic and ultramafic rocks, and this must have increased magnesium, chromium, cobalt, manganese, nickel, copper, precious metal and, particularly, iron concentrations (C. Meyer, personal communication). Because atmospheric oxygen levels were low during the Archean and early Proterozoic, the oceans would have been deplete of oxygen and most ionic iron would have been $Fe^{2+}$. Consequently, less sulfate would be available; what was not removed by barite and anhydrite would likely be reduced to sulfide and precipitated by excess ferrous ion (C. Meyer, personal communication). During this period, too, active hydrothermal activity would

**TABLE 1.1    The Composition of Present-Day Seawater**

| Element | Concentration ($\mu$mol/L$^{-1}$) | Element | Concentration ($\mu$mol/L$^{-1}$) |
|---|---|---|---|
| Ag | $4 \times 10^{-4}$ | Mg | $5.31 \times 10^{4}$ |
| Al | 0.07 | Mn | $3.6 \times 10^{-3}$ |
| As | 0.05 | Mo | 0.10 |
| Au | $2 \times 10^{-4}$ | N | 35.7 |
| B[a] | 410.7 | Na | $4.68 \times 10^{5}$ |
| Ba | 0.146 | Nd | $2 \times 10^{-5}$ |
| Br[a] | 838.6 | Ni | 0.03 |
| C[a] | $2.33 \times 10^{3}$ | P | 1.94 |
| Ca | $1.03 \times 10^{4}$ | Pb | $1 \times 10^{-4}$ |
| Cd | $9 \times 10^{-4}$ | Pr | $4 \times 10^{-6}$ |
| Ce | $7 \times 10^{-6}$ | Rb | 1.40 |
| Cl[a] | $5.303 \times 10^{5}$ | S[a] | $2.83 \times 10^{4}$ |
| Co | $9 \times 10^{-4}$ | Sb | $2.0 \times 10^{-3}$ |
| Cr | $5.8 \times 10^{-3}$ | Sc | $1 \times 10^{-5}$ |
| Cs | $3.0 \times 10^{-3}$ | Se | $2.5 \times 10^{-3}$ |
| Cu | $7.8 \times 10^{-3}$ | Si | 71.4 |
| Er | $5 \times 10^{-6}$ | Sm | $3 \times 10^{-6}$ |
| Eu | $7 \times 10^{-7}$ | Sn | $8 \times 10^{-5}$ |
| F | 68.4 | Sr | 90.9 |
| Fe | 0.04 | Tb | $6 \times 10^{-7}$ |
| Ga | $4 \times 10^{-4}$ | Th | $4 \times 10^{-5}$ |
| Gd | $5 \times 10^{-6}$ | Ti | $2.09 \times 10^{-2}$ |
| Hg | $2 \times 10^{-4}$ | Tm | $1 \times 10^{-6}$ |
| Ho | $1 \times 10^{-6}$ | U | $1.35 \times 10^{-2}$ |
| I[a] | 0.47 | V | $4.90 \times 10^{-2}$ |
| K | $9.74 \times 10^{3}$ | W | $5 \times 10^{-4}$ |
| La | $2 \times 10^{-5}$ | Yb | $5 \times 10^{-6}$ |
| Li | 26.1 | Zn | $7.54 \times 10^{-2}$ |
| Lu | $1 \times 10^{-6}$ | Zr | $3 \times 10^{-4}$ |

*Source:* Adapted from M. Whitfield, The world ocean; mechanism or machination?, Interdisciplinary Sci. Rev., 6, 11–35 (1981).

[a] Principal anionic components.

have increased the temperature of the oceans and given them the capacity to dissolve and retain more metals in solution.

Other than these aspects, it is unlikely that the composition of our oceans has been profoundly different during their early history. Yet in an evolutionary sense, this is the "soup" from which we are derived. It is an attractive idea to believe that the kinds and levels of inorganic salts in our present cells are derived from this brine that the earliest life forms found themselves to be in. It is obvious that the presence of an element is a necessary prerequisite to the evolutionary development of an essential metabolism based on that single ingredient, and that initial environmental concentrations had something to do with the choice of element. No element is commonly found to be essential for life if its abundance is less than about 2 nmol in the ocean (22).

For bacteria, metal ions are required for a range of metabolic activities and structural arrangements. For example, magnesium is used for assembling ribosomes and becomes an essential component part of the finished structure. It is also used to stabilize the polar head groups of the phospholipids that are incorporated into membranes. Ion gradients across the plasma (cytoplasmic) membrane of bacteria rely on the active uptake of potassium at the expense of sodium. An extreme example of this occurs with *Halobacterium salinarium* which, when grown on medium containing $4M$ NaCl and $0.03\ M$ KCl, concentrates the level of internal potassium to $4.6\ M$ and reduces that of sodium to $1.4\ M$. G. D. Sprott gives a more detailed account of membrane gradients in Chapter 3 of this book.

It is the abundant elements within the ocean that bacteria prefer to work with. Rare heavy metal ions are only occasionally used; more frequently they are toxic. It is interesting that the binding strength of metallic ions to biological molecules is related to crustal abundance of the metal; in general the rarer the metal, the stronger the binding constant (J. R. Watterson, personal communication). It is quite possible that heavy metal toxicity is an adaptive result of this relationship. Toxic heavy metals, in general, have low abundances and bind irreversibly to essential biological components, such as enzymes, thereby inactivating them. The strength of this binding can also be used to advantage by some bacteria because certain, unique metalloenzymes require low-abundance metals as cofactors for their activation. This is discussed in detail in Chapter 6.


## 1.4   THE STRUCTURE OF BACTERIA

### 1.4.1   Internal Structures

To understand properly bacteria and how they interact with metal ions, it is necessary to reacquaint ourselves with their physical structure. All present-day bacteria have one characteristic in common and that is their small size. A single bacterium typically has a volume of about 1.5–2.0 $\mu m^3$, which houses all of the machinery for transcription, translation, energy production, growth, and division. There is not much room for the segregation of various metabolic processes into separate, cytoplasmic organelles; bacteria such as *Escherichia coli* possess a rather unassuming cytoplasm. The single chromosome (and extrachromosomal elements) is spread throughout the cytoplasm, and appears to be in contact both with randomly arranged ribosomes and with the inner face of the plasma membrane (Fig. 1.5). That area of the cell that contains the nucleoplasm is a considerable portion of

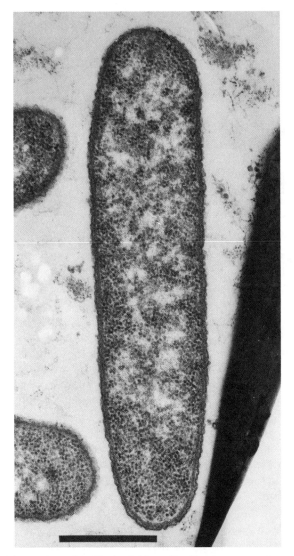

**Figure 1.5**   Thin section of an *Escherichia coli* cell to represent the general structure of a bacterium. The light regions concentrated toward the cell center and disposed throughout the cytoplasm compose the nucleoid. The dark particles in the cytoplasm are ribosomes and linear clusters of ribosomes along the plasma membrane are polysomes. Bar = 500 nm.

the cytoplasm and is called the nucleoid. Frequently, ribosomes are arranged into polysomes along the plasma membrane and these, we believe, are responsible for the synthesis of polypeptides destined for the cell wall, other external layers, or the external milieu. Depending on the nutritional status of the cell, internal deposits such as poly-β-hydroxybutyrate, polyphosphate, glycogen, or sulfur granules can be found (11). Some bacteria require extra membrane for their particular metabolic life styles. This is arranged as plasma membrane infoldings into internal vesicles or concentric lamellae that underlie the membrane and is frequently found in photosynthetic bacteria (both aerobic and anaerobic varieties), nitrifiers, and methylotrophs (23). This arrangement increases the deployment of membrane-bound enzymes as well as the interfacial character of the cytoplasm, both of which aid catalysis.

It is not my intention to pursue the internal structure of bacteria in detail and I refer the reader to Refs. 11 and 23 for more detail. Yet one internal granule is of particular importance to this book and this is the magnetosome (24). Magnetosomes are tiny, membrane-bound crystals of magnetite ($Fe_3O_4$), which are in the single magnetic domain size range (40–50 nm). They are aligned in chains along the longitudinal cell axis within the cytoplasm (Fig. 1.6) and impart a permanent magnetic dipole moment parallel to the axis. This allows these bacteria to align themselves with the earth's geomagnetic field and, eventually, distinguish "up" from "down." Our best studied magnetotactic bacterium, *Aquaspirillum magnetotacticum,* is able to find its way in sediments down to optimal microaerophilic levels. It is debatable whether or not these levels have a natural redox potential that ensures that the iron couple is in the reduced state, but laboratory growth implies that it is $Fe^{2+}$ that is taken up by the bacterium. Somehow, the cell concentrates iron some 20,000–40,000-fold over the extracellular condition and forms it into well-ordered $Fe_3O_4$ hexagonal prisms of (011) faces truncated by specific low index planes (25). Other magnetotactic bacteria exhibit different magnetosome shapes (24).

Little is known about the mechanism of iron uptake in *A. magnetotacticum,* or how iron is aligned into discrete crystals of magnetite. Some crystals possess amorphous hydrated iron(III) oxide phases in association with magnetite, and it is possible that these domains are a transient state existing before crystallization forms the mature magnetite of the magnetosome. Intuitively, it is easiest to imagine that this energetically difficult task of concentrating iron and directing its correct crystallization would be best performed by an intracellular membrane. Recently, distinct evidence of a lipid–protein bilayer surrounding the magnetite has become available (26). In fact, iron depletion of cultures causes readsorption of the magnetite and results in empty magnetosome membrane vesicles (Fig. 1.7). The isolation of these membranes may illuminate the mechanisms involved in bacteriomagnetite synthesis.

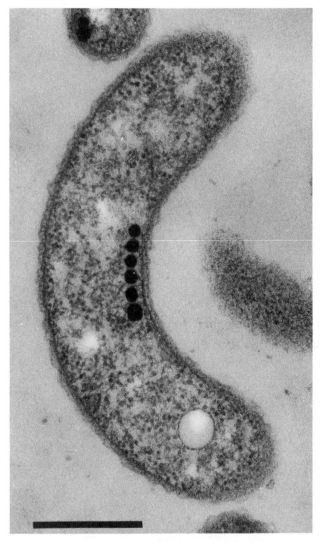

**Figure 1.6**  Thin section of the magnetotactic bacterium, *Aquaspirillum magneto-tacticum,* showing the linear placement of the magnetosomes which contain crystals of magnetite ($Fe_3O_4$) along the long axis of the cell. Bar = 500 nm.

## 1.4.2  External Structures

There are a variety of external structures that decorate the surface of the protoplast. Most important for this chapter are the enveloping layers; these are the cell wall and any superficial layer that resides above it. These include capsules, slime layers, sheaths, and S-layers. Pili (fimbriae), spinae, flagella,

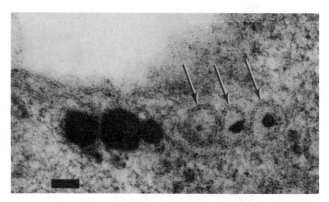

**Figure 1.7**    Thin section of a portion of *A. magnetotacticum* after iron depletion for several generations. Three empty magnetosomes can be seen and the bilayer format of their membrane is clearly revealed (arrows). Bar = 50 nm. Figures 1.6 and 1.7 both represent research done in the author's laboratory in collaboration with Y. Gorby and R. Blakemore of the Department of Microbiology, University of New Hampshire.

and division sites (septa) are not discussed here; I refer you to Refs. 11 and 23 for more details on these structures.

Eubacterial walls have two fundamental designs which can be distinguished by the Gram stain, those that are Gram-positive and those that are Gram-negative (12, 27). On a structural basis, I have previously defined the cell envelope to consist of the plasma membrane plus all external layers that reside on its surface (28). The wall includes the periplasm and the physical layers that entrap it (28).

**1.4.2.1  *Eubacterial Gram-Positive Walls.*** For Gram-positive eubacteria, this physical layer is a rather amorphous matrix about 25 nm thick, which is composed primarily of one or two constituents. The new technique of freeze-substitution reveals the outer surface to be decorated with delicate fibrils (Fig. 1.8). Peptidoglycan is the rigid component to which secondary polymers (such as teichoic or teichuronic acids) are attached, and consists of strands of repeating $\beta(1 \rightarrow 4)$-linked *N*-acetylglucosamine and *N*-acetylmuramic acid. These strands are covalently bonded together by short peptide stems that emanate from the muramic acid residues. The linkage unit and degree of linkage depend on the taxonomic identity of the bacterium (29). The entire peptidoglycan framework is covalently bonded together to form the murein sacculus and represents one of the most resilient structures made by bacteria. Strong chemical perturbants are required to break it apart after cell death and, unless lytic enzymes such as autolysins or those from neighboring microorganisms are present, the sacculus will remain intact for long periods of time in the environment.

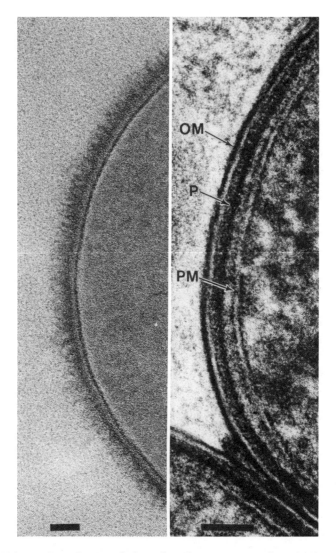

**Figure 1.8**   Thin section of a *B. subtilis* cell wall as representative of a freeze-substituted Gram-positive eubacterial variety. Bar = 25 nm.

**Figure 1.9**   Thin section of an *E. coli* wall as representative of a Gram-negative format. Because this is a freeze-substitution, a periplasmic gel (P) that contains the peptidoglycan is situated between the outer membrane (OM) and the plasma membrane (PM). Bar = 25 nm.

Frequently, secondary polymers are attached to the peptidoglycan in Gram-positive walls. For example, *Bacillus subtilis* possesses either teichoic acids (a glycerol- or ribitol-based polymer joined together by phosphodiester linkages to form a flexible, linear strand) or teichuronic acids (uronic acid-based polymers), which are bonded to a variable number of peptidoglycan muramic acid residues. The type of secondary polymer is under physiological control and depends on the levels of phosphate and magnesium in the growth medium (30). Gram-positive walls can possess a wide range of more minor constituents; the reader is referred to Ref. 28 and Chapter 9 for more details.

A combination of free carboxyl and phosphoryl groups within the wall dfabric of Gram-positive walls usually imparts an overall electronegative charge density to them. In most isolated *Bacillus* walls this charge is symmetrically displayed over both inner and outer surfaces (T. Beveridge and R. Doyle, unpublished observations), but *B. subtilis* 168 walls concentrate the charge to the outer surface (31) and distribute it to discrete, localized regions (32). The electronegative character of Gram-positive walls makes them potent structures for the binding of metallic ions (33–37). A more detailed account of this subject is found in Chapter 9.

***1.4.2.2  Eubacterial Gram-Negative Walls.*** Gram-negative eubacterial walls are more complex in both chemical and structural (Fig. 1.9) terms than their Gram-positive counterparts. They consist of an external outer membrane that overlies a thin layer of peptidoglycan (28). Freeze-substitution preserves the periplasm efficiently and reveals a "periplasmic gel" between the outer and inner membranes (Fig. 1.9). The outer membrane consists of protein, phospholipid, and lipopolysaccharide arranged in an exact format. Almost all of the lipopolysaccharide is appropriated to the external face of the membrane, whereas the phospholipid (in *E. coli* this is mostly phosphatidylethanolamine) aligns along the inner face (38). Protein is distributed throughout the membrane and can be oriented on either surface or can span it completely. Most of the protein in the outer membranes of the Enterobacteriaceae exists as high levels of 3- or 4-polypeptide species (38). One of these polypeptides, the lipoprotein, is a small α-helix consisting of 58 amino acids and possesses three fatty acid residues at its C-terminus. This effectively produces a molecule with an apolar end (which is destined for the hydrophobic domain of the outer membrane) and a polar end that, we believe, extends down below the lower leaflet. One out of every three lipoproteins in *E. coli* is covalently bonded to the peptidoglycan layer; the other two are not but are each associated with the bound variety to make a trimer. Accordingly, these lipoprotein complexes form an actual chemical union between the outer membrane and the underlying peptidoglycan and effectively cement the two wall layers together.

Another important outer membrane polypeptide is the matrix or porin protein. In *E. coli* this protein consists of two chemical varieties whose levels are modulated by the osmolarity of the external milieu; each is a different gene product. The OmpF polypeptide is slightly larger and more basic than the OmpC polypeptide, but each has the same function within the outer membrane. They are intrinsic proteins that are closely associated with lipoprotein and lipopolysaccharide and form small, hydrophilic channels that span the bilayer. Hydrophilic molecules with molecular weights of about 600–1000 can percolate through these channels, but larger molecules are excluded; it is a sieving mechanism. Presumably, metallic ions would be free to diffuse through these channels and reach the underlying periplasm. In fact, because of the preponderance of electronegative amino acids at the channel mouth, small cations would be encouraged to pass (39). Certainly for some inorganic ions there are more specific routes. For example, the PhoE protein of *E. coli* and protein P of *Pseudomonas aeruginosa* are used to siphon phosphate through the membrane (38, 39). In addition, many bacteria have a crucial metabolic need for iron and have developed siderophore systems for use under iron limitation to trap and concentrate environmental iron for the cell. The organo–iron complex uses specific receptors and ports of entry into the cell (e.g., the *fhu* system for ferrichrome uptake in *E. coli*); these systems are more fully outlined in Chapter 5.

By its physicochemical nature, the outer membrane of Gram-negative bacteria must orient its lipids so that the hydrophilic, polar head groups align themselves along each of the bilayer's faces; their hydrophobic acyl groups point toward the bilayer's interior. Consequently, each face has reactive chemical groups available that interact with and bind metal (40). Magnesium and calcium form an integral component part of the membrane and are required for the correct packing order of the lipid constituents (41). Because lipopolysaccharide possesses more phosphoryl groups than phospholipid, these metals are especially important for its retention in the outer membrane (42, 43). The importance of metallic ions for the outer membrane is more fully explained in Chapter 10.

The peptidoglycan is usually of the Alγ type in Gram-negatives and therefore resembles that of *B. subtilis,* except there is less of it per cell. Accordingly, the peptidoglycan of Gram-negative bacteria has similar but fewer reactive sites for metal binding than Gram-positive walls (44). It is also shielded from the external milieu by the outer membrane.

### 1.4.2.3  *S-Layers.*  S-layers are proteinaceous (or glycoproteinaceous) paracrystalline arrays that are sometimes found on top of bacterial walls (Fig. 1.10) (28, 45). They grow as self-assembly products and two types of bonding are required for them to coat the bacterial cell; subunit–subunit interaction binds the protein (or glycoprotein) into a planar array and subunit–wall interaction cements the array on to the wall surface. For both these reactions to occur, calcium or magnesium is sometimes an essential ingredient (e.g., *Aquaspirillum* and *Sporosarcina* spp.) (28, 46). The specificity is quite exact because an S-layer that requires $Ca^{2+}$ will not assemble if $Mg^{2+}$ is added (although $Sr^{2+}$ will substitute). Obviously, for these ion-specific arrays, the

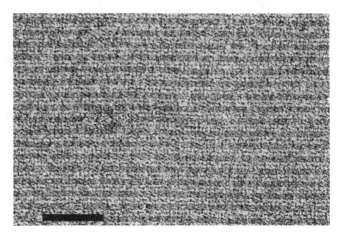

**Figure 1.10** Negative stain of the S-layer from *Aquaspirillum putridiconchylium* which requires $Ca^{2+}$ for its assembly on the outer membrane surface of the bacterium. Bar = 50 nm.

metal is important for salt linkage, polypeptide folding, or both. For some reason, S-layers are frequently found on bacteria in their natural environment, but are often lost during laboratory subculture. Presumably, these are expensive structures for the bacteria to maintain (they can account for over 25% of the total cellular protein) and are often not expressed without environmental pressure.

*1.4.2.4 Capsules and Sheaths.* Capsules are highly hydrated structures and suffer severely from desiccation during electron microscopy. For this reason, it has been difficult to examine, exactly, their native structure by this technique. Various stabilizing agents have been added to them (e.g., specific antibodies, ruthenium red, Alcian Blue) but they all either add to their substance or condense them by salt linkage (28). Possibly our best method, so far, for maintaining their native structure is freeze-substitution, but even then some condensation of the polymeric network has occurred (Fig. 1.11).

Most bacterial capsules are built up from repetitive sequences of sugar residues or their derivatives and are therefore referred to as glycocalyces (28, 47). Yet some entirely proteinaceous capsules also exist [e.g., that of *B. licheniformis* 9945A (28)], so this term cannot be used in all cases.

Because capsules are mostly water, they are thixotropic and alternate between gel and liquid phases depending on their free energy load (23). This water also makes them freely exchangeable with metallic ions in their vicinity. Our own experience with these structures suggests that multivalent cations are preferred by carboxylate-containing capsules and that salt linkage

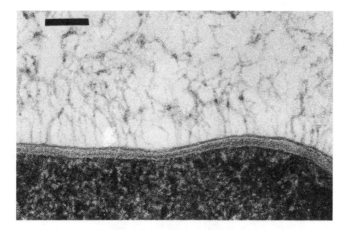

**Figure 1.11**   Thin section of a capsule on *E. coli* K30 prepared by the freeze-substitution technique. Bar = 100 nm. Reprinted with permission of the author and the American Society for Microbiology.

has a preservative effect (R. McLean and T. Beveridge, unpublished data). Chapter 11 discusses this aspect for a wide range of capsule types.

   *Leptothrix* and *Sphaerotilus* possess sheaths and are two genera noted for their interaction with manganese and iron, respectively. They possess one of the most complex surfaces found in eubacteria. For example, *Leptothrix discophora* possesses a Gram-negative wall to which a capsule is attached (Fig. 1.12). The cells grow as chains and are surrounded by a fibrous sheath. During growth, in the presence of dilute levels of manganese, the sheath becomes encrusted with manganese oxide (arrows in Fig. 1.12). This and related reactions are outlined in Chapter 13.

### 1.4.2.5  *Archaebacterial Walls.*

I have saved a brief discussion of archaebacterial walls to the last of this section. This is because our knowledge of them is not as encompassing as it is for the eubacterial variety, and an understanding of their interactions with environmental metals is still in its infancy. So far we recognize that there is tremendous diversity of wall structure and chemistry; there does not seem to be a simple common denominator (13). For example, *Methanobacterium* spp. possess a polymeric network within their walls similar to that of peptidoglycan, but the muramic acid is replaced by $N$-acetyl-L-talosaminuronic acid; the network is called "pseudomurein" (13). Three genera, *Methanococcus*, *Sulfolobus*, and *Thermoproteus*, possess quite unusual walls in that they are so simplistic; they consist of a single S-layer (Fig. 1.13 and Refs. 13, 48) that somehow is able to withstand internal turgor pressure, maintain shape, accommodate flagella insertion, and contribute to the division process. One archaebacterium, *Thermoplasma*, has no wall. At the other extreme reside *Methanospirillum*

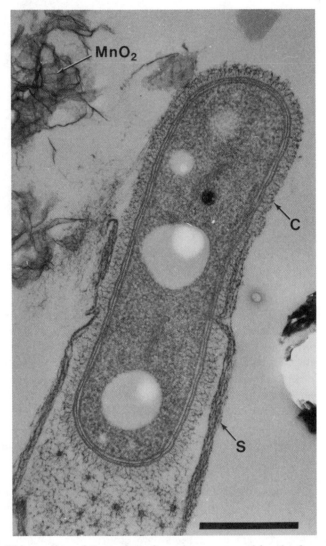

**Figure 1.12**  Thin section of *Leptothrix discophora* prepared by the freeze-substitution method and showing a capsule surrounding the cell (C), which is confined within the sheath (S). The arrow points toward mineralized $MnO_2$. Bar = 500 nm. This work was in collaboration with W. Ghiorse, Department of Microbiology, Cornell University and is reprinted with the permission of the American Society for Microbiology.

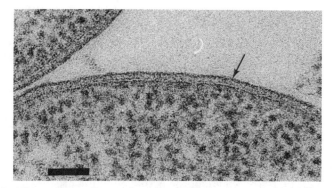

**Figure 1.13**   Thin section of a portion of a *Methanococcus voltae* cell to show the simple format of this type of archaebacterial wall. The arrow points towards the S-layer. Bar = 100 nm. This work was done in collaboration with K. Jarrell, Department of Microbiology and Immunology, Queen's University and S. Koval, Department of Microbiology and Immunology, the University of Western Ontario.

and *Methanothrix,* which possess multiple surface layers including a wall and a proteinaceous sheath reminiscent of eubacterial S-layers (49, 50).

Very little is known about how archaebacterial surfaces interact with metallic ions. Very recent information suggests that the sheaths of *Methanothrix concilii* bind nickel and cobalt very well (G. Patel and G. D. Sprott, personal communication). Perhaps, this is not so surprising, because metalloenzymes requiring $Ni^{2+}$ play an important role in the metabolism of these bacteria (see Chapter 6).

## 1.5   ACTIVE CONCENTRATION OF METALS

It is an established fact that all living cells concentrate certain types of metallic ions, and bacteria are no exception. Chemical gradients across plasma membranes are a necessity of life and $Na^+/K^+$ gradients are ubiquitous (Chapter 3). Yet of all life forms, bacteria have the greatest tolerance to unusually high saline conditions and can cope with saturated solutions of salt (e.g., *Halobacterium* spp. and Walsby's square bacterium, which are both archaebacteria). Without discriminatory active uptake and exclusion systems, these bacteria could not possibly survive.

At the same time, bacteria are resistant to a variety of toxic heavy metals. Several of these metals are actively transported into the cell by preexisting uptake systems. Here they should prove toxic but instead are either chemically neutralized or quickly exported from the cell again. The basis for this active heavy metal resistance is the expression of factors encoded by special plasmids (Chapter 4). Another form of resistance is passive, and is due to chemical complexation of the heavy metal at the bacterial surface; this is explained in Section 1.6.

Not all heavy metals prove toxic to bacteria. It is not unusual that small quantities of distinct metallic species are actually required as cofactors or as component parts of metalloenzymes (Chapter 6). In fact, four nickel-containing enzymes (two hydrogenases, a methyl coenzyme M reductase, and a CO dehydrogenase) are the basis for $CO_2/H_2/CH_4$ metabolism in methanogens such as *M. thermoautotrophicum*. For these bacteria, very specific concentrating mechanisms for the metal must be required.

Possibly the most tangible form of active heavy metal concentration is that of iron in magnetotactic bacteria, discussed in an earlier section. Unfortunately, little is known about the actual pumping process other than that external Fe(II) eventually is mineralized to magnetite within the boundaries of the magnetosome, although hydrous ferric oxide precursors are thought to be involved (51). Ancient magnetite, attributable to bacterial magnetosomes, has been detected in marine sediments (52); at least these bacterial minerals are able to withstand the test of time.

Another apparent concentrating device is found with the iron- and manganese-depositing bacteria (53). These bacteria accumulate large quantities of iron and manganese oxides within their sheaths (Fig. 1.14 and Chapter 13). Until recently, it was debatable whether or not this was a passive or active process. Now, at least with *Leptothrix discophora,* an active process seems likely because a manganese-oxidizing protein has been isolated from the sheath (54, 55). Old remnants of sheath from which the cells have departed are so encrusted with $MnO_2$ that the biological constituents can no longer be identified (Fig. 1.14). Obviously, too, ferromanganese concretions on the floors of deep seas and lakes also have a bacterial contribution that relies on the oxidative powers of certain cells (Chapter 13).

## 1.6  PASSIVE METAL INTERACTIONS

Bacteria depend entirely on diffusion gradients for their nourishment and for the dispersal of their waste products (56). Not even tenacious microbes that inhabit the "varnishes" of rocks in our driest deserts can circumvent this dependence (57). A living, growing prokaryote requires an aqueous milieu. Obviously, this means that bacteria are continuously surrounded by a "brine" of various ions (both organic and inorganic) at various concentrations. Halophilic bacteria can cope with saturated salt solutions, marine varieties with about 3.5% salt, and terrestrial bacteria with more dilute solutions. It is safe to say that absolutely pure (high resistance) water is extremely rare in natural environments (freezing isotherms of water easily show this), and in fact, pure water would inhibit bacterial life.

Bacteria have adopted a variety of strategies to cope with their dependence on water and its various soluble components. One of the strategies

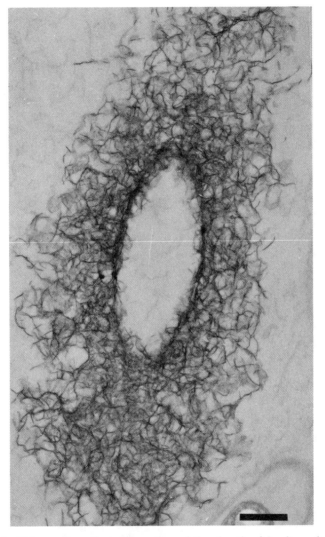

**Figure 1.14**  Thin section of an old portion of the sheath of *L. discophora* that no longer contains a cell. This sheath is so encrusted with $MnO_2$ that the biological constituents can no longer be seen. Bar = 500 nm.

is to assemble a surface that grapples successfully with the bacterium's local environment. The broad choice is to engineer an interface that is hydrophobic or one that is hydrophilic. Needless to say, the former is rarely encountered and is used only for special application (58). For example, a bacterium that cannot manufacture an emulsifying agent and whose sole carbon source is an insoluble hydrocarbon (e.g., hexadecane), must somehow revamp its outer membrane to be compatible with the hydrophobic hydro-

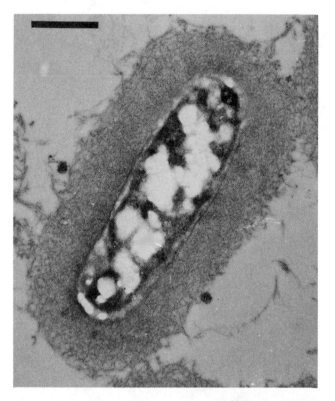

**Figure 1.15** Thin section of an *Alcaligenes faecalis* cell that produces curdelin, a polyglucose, as its capsule. This capsule should therefore consist of a neutrally charged polymer and yet the heavy metals of the strain have bound to it. Bar = 500 nm. This culture was supplied to the author by J. Fein, Weston Research Centre, Toronto.

carbon droplets so that it can adhere and feed. Under these conditions, *P. aeruginosa* reworks its lipopolysaccharide to a more hydrophobic variety (58).

Most bacterial surfaces are hydrophilic (28) and therefore wettable. This statement encompasses all of the surface layers we have so far discussed. Capsules are almost entirely water and all but a few are composed of constituents possessing available reactive chemical groups (28; Chapter 11). Even so-called neutral capsules such as curdelin, a polyglucose polymer from *Alcaligenes faecalis,* must contain some reactive substituents for it can be stained for electron microscopy (i.e., uranyl and lead ions are adsorbed; Fig. 1.15).

S-layers are composed of proteins or glycoproteins whose molecular weight ranges from about 24,000 to 150,000 and possess a full variety of amino acids with the exception of cysteine and methionine, which occur only at low levels (28, 45, 46). Depending on pH, carboxyl and amine functions provide most chemical reactivity and are presumably important in polypeptide folding. Metallic ions can be involved as the folding evolves and a planar array, attached to the wall surface, is assembled (46). The resultant conformation of the protein forces most polar residues toward the interior of the subunit, yet the subunit meshwork provides a regular series of water-filled channels [similar to but larger than porin channels (38)] that allow the passage of a variety of solutes (59); polar residues must coat the channels. At least one S-layer, that of *Sporosarcina ureae,* is capable of interacting with and mineralizing heavy metal (15).

Gram-positive walls are thoroughly discussed in Chapter 9, and suffice to say that with the exception of some mycobacterial/corynebacterial/nocardial varieties that possess unique unwettable, long-chain, β-hydroxy, branched fatty acids [e.g., mycolic, corynemycolenic and corynemycolic acids (12, 28)], these walls are typically hydrophilic and possess a net electronegative charge. Similarly, for Gram-negative walls, the constituents of both the outer membrane and peptidoglycan layers are arranged so as to interact with the aqueous milieu in a hydrophilic manner (28; Chapter 10).

Thus bacterial surfaces of all structural varieties are good interfaces for the reaction with and binding of surrounding metallic ions. These are passive but important bacteria–metal interactions; soluble metal abounds and interfacial reactive groups on bacteria are plentiful. Consequently, bacterial surfaces, by their very nature, are continuously in some salt form or another. In fact, important wall polymers such as teichoic acids of bacilli or lipopolysaccharides of coliforms require $Mg^{2+}$ and $Ca^{2+}$, respectively, as an integral wall cement (41, 43, 60).

At the same time, analytical observations of these surfaces subjected to saturating concentrations of metal solutions show that much more metal can be bound than the available chemical groups would indicate (33, 35, 40). Electron microscopy clearly established that metal precipitates within and on the walls are common, and a two-step mechanism to account for this observation was invoked (33). First, metal ions interact in a stoichiometric manner with accessible reactive wall groups. Next, these sites nucleate the growth of a mineral precipitate. For *B. subtilis,* carboxyl groups seem most important (34, 36), whereas lipopolysaccharide phosphoryl groups in *E. coli* have been implicated (15, 40, 41).

Even dormant cells, such as endospores, are highly interactive with select metallic ions during their formation and germination (Chapter 8). Even though mature endospores have a reduced free-water content, soluble metals are capable of interacting with their exosporium, spore coat, and (less frequently) cortex. Some metals, such as gold [Au(III)] are capable of penetrating as far as the core (Fig. 1.16).

In situ observations of bacteria and their biofilms in soils and sediments frequently show the cells to be encased in a mineralized coat (Refs. 17–19 and Fig. 1.17). The implications are fantastic and may show a further im-

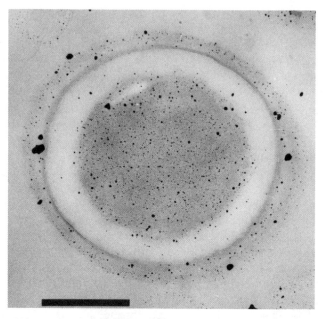

**Figure 1.16**  Thin section of a *Clostridium botulinum* spore that was suspended in 5 m*M* AuCl₃ for 10 min at room temperature and washed of unsorbed gold. The section is unstained except for the gold, which can be seen to have penetrated right to the core. Bar = 500 nm. This work was done as an undergraduate project by C. Atkinson in the author's laboratory.

portant aspect of bacteria in nature, the biogeoprocessing of soluble salts in our environment! It is possible that bacteria, by their very surface physicochemistry, can instigate and direct the production of distinct minerals. Certainly, too, in an energetic sense, they can accomplish this over a short time frame that purely geochemical mechanisms could not make possible. To determine the global extent of this phenomenon and its importance to recycling of environmental metals is a pressing necessity and will be one of the most important aspects of microbe-metal interactions in the years to come.

## 1.7  METALS ARE IMPORTANT TO BACTERIA

I hope that this chapter fulfills at least two important functions for the reader. For the first, I have attempted to outline broadly the topics dealt with in detail in other chapters. It is not, I hope, simply "setting the stage" for these chapters, but rather melding them together in a way to offer the reader a very real perspective of what is to come. Second and more importantly, I

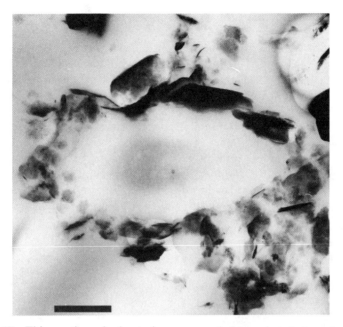

**Figure 1.17**   Thin section of a bacterium surrounded by mineral deposits found in an in situ sediment sample from the Irvine Creek in Southern Ontario. Bar = 500 nm.

hope that the reader gains a sense of the excitement generated by this emerging branch of microbiological science.

Certainly metals are important to bacteria; they may be essential components of a life-promoting process (e.g., $Na^+/K^+$ gradients across plasma membranes or metal constituents of metalloenzymes), or they may be toxic agents that are encountered in the environment. Over the ages, bacteria have evolved systems to use some metals as vital constituents and have learned to grapple with others as toxins. Metals are a part of their lives. Over the last few decades, humankind has learned to use bacteria as essential biological agents for the mining (leaching) of low-grade ores. More recently, bacteria hold promise for the immobilization of toxic metals from industrial and mining wastes (61; Chapter 12). Maybe more important for you and me, they may be the most important life form for the biological cycling of metals on a global scale (Chapter 14).

## ACKNOWLEDGMENTS

Many of the global aspects of bacterial cycling of metals over the ages stems from discussions with W. S. Fyfe, Department of Geology, the University of Western Ontario, and J. R. Watterson, Branch of Exploration Geochemistry, U.S. Geological Survey, Denver, Colorado; to them both I express my gratitude. While writing this chapter, I learned of and was saddened by the death of C. Meyers, Sedona, Arizona, whose expertise was in ore development, and who explained to me how and why the metal load of the Proterozoic differed from present-day. To these colleagues, I dedicate the chapter.

The literature on metal–microbe interactions is voluminous and it was impossible to cite all literature. I apologize to those I have neglected; my ample use of reviews as references will make actual research data easy to trace. The work that is outlined from my own laboratory has been made possible by operating grants from the Natural Science and Engineering Research Council of Canada and the Medical Research Council of Canada.

## REFERENCES

1. D. J. Stevenson. "The nature of the Earth prior to the oldest known rock record: The Hadean Earth," Chapter 2 in J. W. Schopf, Ed., *Earth's Earliest Biosphere: Its Origin and Evolution,* Princeton University Press, Princeton, NJ, 1983, pp. 32–40.

2. S. Moorbath. The oldest rocks and the growth of the continents, Sci. Am. *236,* 92–104 (1977).

3. S. Chang, D. DesMarais, R. Mack, S. L. Miller, and G. E. Strathearn. "Prebiotic organic syntheses and the origin of life," Chapter 4 in J. W. Schopf, Ed., *Earth's Earliest Biosphere: Its Origin and Evolution.* Princeton University Press, Princeton, NJ, 1983, p. 92.

4. M. Schidlowski, J. M. Hayes, and I. R. Kaplan. "Isotopic inferences of ancient biochemistries: Carbon, sulfur, hydrogen, and nitrogen," Chapter 7 in J. W. Schopf, Ed., *Earth's Earliest Biosphere: Its Origin and Evolution,* Princeton University Press, Princeton, NJ, 1983, p. 162.

5. M. R. Walter, H. J. Hofman, and J. W. Schopf. "Geographic and geologic data for processed rock samples," Appendix I in J. W. Schopf, Ed., *Earth's Earliest Biosphere: Its Origin and Evolution,* Princeton University Press, Princeton, NJ, 1983, p. 407.

6. M. R. Walter. "Archean stromatolites: Evidence of the Earth's earliest benthos," Chapter 8 in J. W. Schopf, Ed., *Earth's Earliest Biosphere: Its Origin and Evolution,* Princeton University Press, Princeton, NJ, 1983, pp. 187–213.

7. J. W. Schopf and M. R. Walker. "Archean microfossils: New evidence of ancient microbes," Chapter 9 in J. W. Schopf, Ed., *Earth's Earliest Biosphere: Its Origin and Evolution,* Princeton University Press, Princeton, NJ, 1983, pp. 214–239.

8. E. S. Barghoorn and S. A. Tyler. Microorganisms from the Gunflint chert, Science, *147,* 563–577 (1965).

9. G. Eglinton, P. M. Scott, T. Belsky, A. L. Burlingame, and M. Calvin. Hydrocarbons of biological origin from a one-billion-year-old sediment, Science, *145,* 263–264 (1964).

10. J. D. Saxby. Metal-organic chemistry of the geochemical cycle, Rev. Pure Appl. Chem., *19,* 131–150 (1969).

11. P. J. Krell and T. J. Beveridge. "The structure of bacteria and molecular biology of viruses," Chapter 2 in G. H. Bourne, K. W. Jeon, and M. Friedlander, Eds., *Cytology and Cell Physiology,* 4th ed., Int. Rev. Cytol. Suppl. 17, Academic, New York, 1987, pp. 15–88.

12. T. J. Beveridge. "Wall ultrastructure: How little we know," Chapter 1 in P. Actor, L. Daneo-Moore, M. L. Higgins, M. R. J. Salton, and G. D. Shockman, Eds., *Antibiotic Inhibition of Bacterial Cell Surface Assembly and Function.* Am. Society for Microbiology, Washington, DC, 1988, pp. 3–20.

13. O. Kandler and H. König. "Cell envelopes of Archaebacteria," in C. R. Woese and R. S. Wolfe, Eds., *The Bacteria,* Vol. VIII, Academic, New York, 1985, pp. 413–457.

14. F. G. Ferris, W. S. Fyfe, and T. J. Beveridge. Metallic ion binding by *Bacillus subtilis*: Implications for the fossilization of microorganisms, Geology, *16,* 149–152 (1988).

15. T. J. Beveridge. Mechanisms of the binding of metallic ions to bacterial walls and the possible impact on microbial ecology, in M. J. Klug and C. A. Reddy, Eds., *Current Perspectives in Microbial Ecology.* American Society for Microbiology, Washington, DC, 1984, pp. 601–607.

16. T. J. Beveridge, J. D. Meloche, W. S. Fyfe, and R. G. E. Murray. Diagenesis of metals chemically complexed to bacteria: Laboratory formation of metal phosphates, sulfides, and organic condensates in artificial sediments, Appl. Environ. Microbiol., *45,* 1094–1108 (1983).

17. F. G. Ferris, T. J. Beveridge, and W. S. Fyfe. Iron-silica crystallite nucleation by bacteria in a geothermal sediment, Nature (London), *320,* 609–611 (1986).

18. F. G. Ferris, W. S. Fyfe, and T. J. Beveridge. Manganese oxide deposition in a hot spring microbial mat, Geomicrobiol. J., *5,* 33–42 (1986).

19. F. G. Ferris, W. S. Fyfe, and T. J. Beveridge. Bacteria as nucleation sites for authigenic minerals in a metal-contaminated lake sediment, Chem. Geol., *63,* 225–232 (1987).

20. G. M. Gadd. "Fungal responses towards heavy metals," Chapter 4 in R. A. Herbert and G. A. Codd, Eds., *Microbes in Extreme Environments,* Society of General Microbiology, Academic, London, 1986, pp. 83–110.

21. T. J. Beveridge and W. S. Fyfe. Metal fixation by bacterial cell walls, Can. J. Earth Sci., *22,* 1893–1898 (1985).

22. J. H. McClendon. Elemental abundance as a factor in the origins of mineral nutrient requirements, J. Mol. Evol., *8,* 175–195 (1976).

23. T. J. Beveridge. "The structure of bacteria," in E. R. Leadbetter and J. S. Poindexter, Eds., *Bacteria in Nature: A Treatise on the Interaction of Bacteria and their Habitats,* Plenum, New York (in press).

24. R. P. Blakemore. Magnetotactic bacteria, Ann. Rev. Microbiol., *36,* 217–238 (1982).

25. S. Mann, R. B. Frankel, and R. P. Blakemore. Structure, morphology and crystal growth of bacterial magnetite, Nature (London), *310,* 405–407 (1984).

26. Y. A. Gorby, T. J. Beveridge, and R. P. Blakemore. Characterization of the bacterial magnetosome membrane, J. Bacteriol., *170*, 834–841 (1988).

27. T. J. Beveridge and J. A. Davies. Cellular responses of *Bacillus subtilis* and *Escherichia coli* to the Gram stain, J. Bacteriol., *156*, 846–858 (1983).

28. T. J. Beveridge. Ultrastructure, chemistry, and function of bacterial walls, Int. Rev. Cytol., *72*, 229–317 (1981).

29. K. H. Schleifer and O. Kandler. Peptidoglycan types of bacterial cell walls and their taxonomic implications, Bacteriol. Rev., *36*, 407–477 (1972).

30. A. R. Archibald. The structure, biosynthesis and function of teichoic acid, Adv. Microb. Physiol., *11*, 53–95 (1974).

31. E. M. Sonnenfeld, T. J. Beveridge, A. Koch, and R. J. Doyle. Asymmetric distribution of charge on the cell wall of *Bacillus subtilis*, J. Bacteriol., *163*, 1167–1171 (1985).

32. E. M. Sonnenfeld, T. J. Beveridge, and R. J. Doyle. Discontinuity of charge on cell wall poles of *Bacillus subtilis*, Can. J. Microbiol., *31*, 875–877 (1985).

33. T. J. Beveridge and R. G. E. Murray. Uptake and retention of metals by cell walls of *Bacillus subtilis*, J. Bacteriol., *127*, 1502–1518 (1976).

34. T. J. Beveridge and R. G. E. Murray. Sites of metal deposition in the cell wall of *Bacillus subtilis*, J. Bacteriol., *141*, 876–887 (1980).

35. T. J. Beveridge, C. F. Forsberg, and R. J. Doyle. Major sites of metal binding in *Bacillus licheniformis* walls, J. Bacteriol., *150*, 1438–1448 (1982).

36. R. J. Doyle, T. A. Matthews, and U. N. Streips. Chemical basis for selectivity of metal ions by the *Bacillus subtilis* cell wall, J. Bacteriol., *143*, 471–480 (1980).

37. R. E. Marquis, K. Mayzel, and E. L. Carstensen. Cation exchange in cell walls of gram-positive bacteria, Can. J. Microbiol., *22*, 975–982 (1976).

38. B. Lugtenberg and L. van Alphen. Molecular architecture and functioning of the outer membrane of *Escherichia coli* and other gram-negative bacteria, Biochim. Biophys. Acta, *737*, 51–115 (1983).

39. R. E. W. Hancock. "Model membrane studies of porin function," Chapter 8 in M. Inouye, Ed., *Bacterial Outer Membranes as Model Systems*, Wiley, New York, 1987, pp. 187–225.

40. B. Hoyle and T. J. Beveridge. Binding of metallic ions to the outer membrane of *Escherichia coli*, Appl. Environ. Microbiol., *46*, 749–752 (1983).

41. F. G. Ferris and T. J. Beveridge. Physicochemical roles of soluble metal cations in the outer membrane of *Escherichia coli* K-12, Can. J. Microbiol., *32*, 594–601 (1986).

42. L. Leive. The barrier function of the gram-negative envelope, Ann. N.Y. Acad. Sci., *235*, 109–127 (1974).

43. F. G. Ferris and T. J. Beveridge. Binding of a paramagnetic metal cation to *Escherichia coli* K-12 outer membrane vesicles, FEMS Microbiol. Lett., *24*, 43–46 (1984).

44. B. D. Hoyle and T. J. Beveridge. Metal binding by the peptidoglycan sacculus of *Escherichia coli* K-12, Can. J. Microbiol., *30*, 204–211 (1984).

45. U. B. Sleytr and P. Messner. Crystalline surface layers on bacteria, Ann. Rev. Microbiol., *37*, 311–339 (1983).

46. S. F. Koval and R. G. E. Murray. The superficial protein arrays on bacteria, Microbiol. Sci., *3*, 357–361 (1986).

47. J. W. Costerton, R. T. Irvin, and K.-J. Cheng. The bacterial glycocalyx in nature and disease, Ann. Rev. Microbiol., *35*, 299–324 (1981).

48. U. B. Sleytr, P. Messner, M. Sára, and D. Pum. Crystalline envelope layers on archaebacteria, Syst. Appl. Microbiol., *7*, 310–313 (1986).

49. M. Stewart, T. J. Beveridge, and G. D. Sprott. Crystalline order to high resolution in the sheath of *Methanospirillum hungatei*: a cross-beta structure, J. Mol. Biol., *183*, 509–515 (1985).

50. T. J. Beveridge, G. B. Patel, B. J. Harris, and G. D. Sprott. The ultrastructure of *Methanothrix concilii*, a mesophilic aceticlastic methanogen, Can. J. Microbiol., *32*, 703–710 (1986).

51. R. B. Frankel, G. C. Papaefthymiou, R. P. Blakemore, and W. O'Brien. $Fe_3O_4$ precipitation in magnetotactic bacteria, Biochim. Biophys. Acta, *763*, 157–159 (1983).

52. N. Peterson, T. von Dobeneck, and H. Vali. Fossil bacterial magnetite in deep-sea sediments from the South Atlantic Ocean, Nature (London), *320*, 611–615 (1986).

53. W. C. Ghiorse. Biology of iron- and manganese-depositing bacteria, Ann. Rev. Microbiol., *38*, 515–550 (1984).

54. F. C. Boogerd and J. P. M. deVrind. Manganese oxidation by *Leptothrix discophora*, J. Bacteriol., *169*, 489–494 (1987).

55. L. F. Adams and W. C. Ghiorse. Characterization of extra-cellular $Mn^{2+}$-oxidizing activity and isolation of an $Mn^{2+}$-oxidizing protein from *Leptothrix discophora* SS-1. J. Bacteriol. *169*, 1279–1285 (1987).

56. T. J. Beveridge. The bacterial surface: general considerations towards design and function, Can. J. Microbiol. *34*, 363–372.

57. E. I. Friedmann and R. Ocampo-Friedmann. "Endolithic microorganisms in extreme dry environments: Analysis of a lithobiontic microbial habitat," in M. J. Klug and C. A. Reddy, Eds., *Current Perspectives in Microbial Ecology*, American Society for Microbiology, Washington, DC, 1984, p. 182.

58. C. B. Miguez, T. J. Beveridge, and J. M. Ingram. Lipopolysaccharide changes and cytoplasmic polyphosphate granule accumulation in *Pseudomonas aeruginosa* during growth on hexadecane, Can. J. Microbiol., *32*, 248–253 (1986).

59. M. Sára and U. B. Sleytr. Molecular sieving through S-layers of *Bacillus stearothermophilus* strains, J. Bacteriol., *169*, 4092–4098 (1987).

60. P. A. Lambert, I. C. Hancock, and J. Baddiley. The interaction of magnesium ions with teichoic acid, Biochem. J., *149*, 519–524 (1975).

61. S. R. Hutchins, M. S. Davidson, J. A. Brierley, and C. L. Brierley. Microorganisms in reclamation of metals, Ann. Rev. Microbiol., *40*, 311–336 (1986).

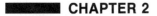 **CHAPTER 2**

# Factors Affecting the Toxicity of Heavy Metals to Microbes

YVONNE E. COLLINS and GUENTHER STOTZKY

Department of Biology
New York University
New York, New York

## Contents

## 2.1   INTRODUCTION

Metals usually occur geologically as ores in mineral deposits that are physically or chemically processed to yield a purer form of the metal. Metals are introduced into the environment during mining and refining of ores and from other sources, such as the combustion of fossil fuels, industrial processes, spraying of pesticides, and disposal of industrial and domestic wastes. Metals have been mined and used extensively by human beings; however, the rapid expansion of industry and increases in domestic activities have caused a concomitant increase in the quantities of metals being released to the environment. The natural recycling of some metals in biogeochemical cycles has been disrupted as a result of the large quantities of metals and pollutants that are currently entering the natural environment (1–8).

For example, copper and zinc salts are used extensively as pesticides and, therefore, are introduced into the environment during the spraying of crops. Copper is also used in electrical, plumbing, and heating equipment and in alloys with other metals. Cadmium is used in industrial processes, for example, to protect iron from rusting, for electroplating, in batteries, and as a color pigment in plastics and paints (9). Nickel is used in the production of steel and in alloys that are used in coins and household utensils (10). Lead is utilized in the production of batteries, cable sheathing, pigments, and alloys. Organolead compounds, such as tetramethyllead and tetraethyllead, are used as antiknock additives in gasoline (11). Mercury compounds are used in electrical equipment, paints, thermometers, and fungicides, and as preservatives in pharmaceuticals and cosmetics (12).

## 2.2   DEFINITION AND CLASSIFICATION OF "HEAVY METALS"

Elements whose compounds form positive ions (i.e., cations) when in solution and whose oxides form hydroxides rather than acids with water are termed "metals." Metals with a specific gravity greater than 5 have been termed "heavy metals" (13). However, this definition, which is based solely on a physical parameter, is not a suitable criterion for the classification of these metals, as it includes metals with widely different chemical and biological properties. Many metals with a specific gravity above 5 are lanthanides (atomic number $Z = 57-71$) and actinides ($Z = 89-103$), which are usually not considered to be "heavy metals."

Lewis acids are atoms, molecules, or ions that have at least one vacant orbital that can accommodate a pair of electrons. Pearson (14–18) classified metals according to the principle of "hard" and "soft" acids and bases (HSAB theory) (Table 2.1). Hard acids (e.g., $Na^+$, $Mg^{2+}$) have small atoms and a high positive charge, and they do not contain unshared pairs of electrons in their valence shell. These properties result in high electronegativity and low polarizability. Hard acids have an inert gas type ($d^0$) electron con-

**TABLE 2.1  Classification of Metal Ions and Other Lewis Acids into Hard and Soft Acids**[a]

| Hard Acids (Class A) | Soft Acids (Class B) |
|---|---|
| Small size, low polarizability, high positive oxidation state | Large size, high polarizability, low electronegativity |
| Most A-metal cations have outer shell of 8 electrons | Filled outer orbitals. Most B-metal cations have an outer shell of 18 electrons |
| $H^+$, $Li^+$, $Na^+$, $K^+$ | $Cu^+$, $Ag^+$, $Au^+$, $Hg^+$ |
| $Be^{2+}$, $Mg^{2+}$, $Ca^{2+}$, $Sr^{2+}$ | $Pd^{2+}$, $Cd^{2+}$, $Hg^{2+}$, $CH_3Hg^+$ |
| $Al^{3+}$, $Sc^{3+}$, $La^{3+}$, $Cr^{3+}$ $Co^{3+}$, $Fe^{3+}$, $As^{3+}$ | $Tl^{3+}$, $Au^{3+}$ |
| $Si^{4+}$, $Ti^{4+}$, $Zr^{4+}$, $Th^{4+}$, $Pu^{4+}$ $UO_2^{2+}$, $VO^{2+}$ | |
| $BF_3$, $BCl_3$, $B(OR)_3$ $SO_3$, $RSO_2^+$, $RPO_2^+$ $I^{7+}$, $I^{5+}$, $Cl^{7+}$ $CO_2$, $RCO^+$, $R_3C^+$ | All metal atoms, bulk metals $I_2$, $Br_2$, ION $I^+$, $Sr^+$, $HO^+$ |

Borderline

$Fe^{2+}$, $Co^{2+}$, $Ni^{2+}$, $Cu^{2+}$
$Zn^{2+}$, $Pb^{2+}$, $Bi^{2+}$
$B(CH_3)_2$, $SO_2$, $NO^+$

| *Ligand Atom Preference:* | *Ligand Atom Preference:* |
|---|---|
| $N \gg P$ | $P \gg N$ |
| $C \gg S$ | $S \gg O$ |
| $F \gg Cl$ | $I \gg Br > Cl > F$ |

*Qualitative Generalization:*
Preference by hard acids

←——————————————

F, O, N = Cl, Br, I, S = C

——————————————→

Preference by soft acids

*Source:* Ref. 324.

[a] A Lewis acid is an atom, molecule, or ion that has at least one vacant orbital that can accommodate a pair of electrons.

figuration, are spherical in symmetry, and have electron shells that do not readily undergo deformation when influenced by the electric fields produced by adjacent charged ions (i.e., they are hard spheres). Water is more strongly attracted to hard acids than is ammonia or cyanide, and chloro or iodo complexes are unstable and tend to occur more readily in acid solutions where competition with $OH^-$ is minimal. Hard acids participate in electrostatic bonding with ligands.

Soft acids have large atoms and a low positive charge, and they contain unshared pairs of electrons ($p$ or $d$ electrons) in their valence shell. Therefore, soft acids (e.g., $Hg^{2+}$) have low electronegativity and high polarizability. Soft acids have electron shells that are more easily deformable (i.e., they are soft spheres). Soft acids bind ammonia more strongly than water, bind cyanide rather than $OH^-$, and form stable chloro or iodo complexes. Both transition metal cations and soft acids form insoluble sulfides and soluble complexes with $S^{2-}$ and $HS^-$. Soft acids participate in covalent bonding with ligands, and electrostatic bonding is relatively unimportant. When the donor atoms of the most common bases are arranged in order of increasing electronegativity, the following order is obtained: F > O > Cl, N > Br > I, S, Se, C > P, As (15). Soft acids form more stable complexes with the right-hand members of this series, whereas hard acids form more stable complexes with the left-hand members of the series. The general rule is that hard acids bind to hard bases and soft acids bind to soft bases. Some metals do not fit into either category and were classified by Pearson (14–18) as borderline.

Nieboer and Richardson (19) proposed another system of classification of metals, using the terminology of Ahrland et al. (20). This system is based on equilibrium constants that describe the formation of metal ion–ligand complexes. Metal ions are separated into three categories: Class A, Class B, and borderline ions (Fig. 2.1). Class A metal ions have the following preference sequence for ligands: F > Cl > Br > I; for metal-binding donor atoms in ligands, the preference sequences are O > S > Se, N > As, O > N > S. Class B metal ions have the opposite preference sequences: I > Br > Cl > F, Se $\simeq$ S > O, As > N, S > N > O. Borderline metal ions form an intermediate group and bind to any of these ligands and metal-binding donor atoms without any preference sequence.

Although the distinction between Class A and borderline ions is very sharp, the separation between Class B and borderline ions is not as distinct. The Class B character increases among the borderline ions in the following order: $Pb^{2+}$ > $Cu^{2+}$ > $Cd^{2+}$ > $Co^{2+}$ $\simeq$ $Fe^{2+}$ > $Ni^{2+}$ > $Zn^{2+}$ > $Mn^{2+}$. The position of Class A, Class B, and borderline metal and metalloid ions in the periodic table is shown in Fig. 2.1 (19). Class A ions are found on the left side of the periodic table (except $Al^{3+}$) and include the alkali metals, alkaline earth metals, lanthanides, and actinides. Class B ions form a small triangular shape with $Ir^{3+}$ and $Bi^{3+}$ at the base and $Cu^+$ at the apex of the triangle ($Cu^{2+}$ is a borderline ion). The borderline ions consist of the first

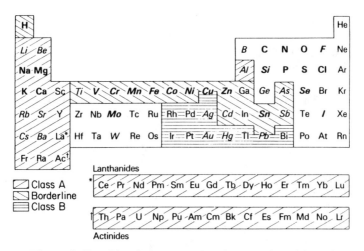

**Figure 2.1** The periodic table of elements, showing the disposition of the Class A, Class B, and borderline metals and metalloid ions (Ref. 19).

row of transition metals, in their common oxidation states, and also include $Ga^{3+}$, $In^{3+}$, $Cd^{2+}$, $Sn^{2+}$, and $Pb^{2+}$. The metalloid ions, $As^{3+}$ and $Sb^{3+}$, and $H^+$ are also considered to be borderline ions.

The classification of metals into Class A, Class B, and borderline as proposed by Nieboer and Richardson is similar to Pearson's HSAB theory. The classification of hard and soft acids and bases of Pearson, however, includes the Class A metal ions of Nieboer and Richardson plus $Cr^{3+}$, $Mn^{3+}$, $Fe^{3+}$, $Co^{3+}$, $UO_2^{2+}$, and $VO^{2+}$. The soft acids of Pearson's classification include all the Class B metal cations in the classification of Nieboer and Richardson, except $Zn^{2+}$, $Pb^{2+}$, and $Bi^{3+}$, which are classified by Pearson as borderline metal ions.

The classification of metal ions into hard and soft acids and bases or Class A, Class B, and borderline can be used to categorize the interactions of metals with microorganisms. Many metal ions (e.g., $Ca^{2+}$, $Mg^{2+}$) essential to microorganisms are usually hard acids and Class A metals. For example, $Mg^{2+}$ is required for the assembly and stability of the plasma membrane of bacteria (21); for the integrity of the outer membrane of the cell wall of Gram-negative bacteria (22–24); and for the stabilization of intracellular structures, especially RNA and DNA, and macromolecules involved in the production and use of ATP, as $Mg^{2+}$ is a counterion for the negatively charged phosphate moieties in these molecules (19). Metal ions are required for the integrity of bacterial cell walls and for the attachment of their superficial layers (25–27, 30). Cations, especially $Ca^{2+}$ and $Mg^{2+}$, have been found in the ash of some wall constituents (e.g., murein) of *Klebsiella pneumoniae* (28) and a marine pseudomonad (29). $Ca^{2+}$ has also been shown to be necessary for the assembly of the regularly structured (RS) superficial protein layer of *Aquaspirillum serpens* VHA (27).

Other metals (e.g., $Zn^{2+}$, $Cu^{2+}$) required in trace concentrations by microbes (micronutrients) are classified as borderline in the schema of Nieboer and Richardson (19). Some metals, especially the Class B metals (e.g., $Hg^{2+}$, $Cd^{2+}$), are considered to be pollutants, as they are not necessary for biological functions and are toxic. The toxic characteristics of Class B ions are illustrated by $Hg^{2+}$, which forms methylated derivatives that are stable in aqueous solution. Methylated forms of Class A ions are not stable in aqueous solution and decompose on contact with water, and with certain exceptions (e.g., $Co^{2+}$), methylated derivatives of borderline ions are also unstable in aqueous solution. Methylated derivatives of $Hg^{2+}$ and inorganic $Hg^{2+}$ have a high affinity for –SH and –S–S– groups (31), which are ubiquitous in living organisms (e.g., in enzymes and other proteins). Therefore the toxic effects of $Hg^{2+}$ are the result of the ability of $Hg^{2+}$ to bind to these important functional groups of biological molecules. Methylated forms of $Hg^{2+}$ have been shown also to bind to the nitrogen of nucleotide bases in RNA and DNA, and they could interfere with the functioning of these nucleic acids (31). Other heavy metals (e.g., $Pb^{2+}$, $Cd^{2+}$) can also bind to ligands, such as phosphate and the cysteinyl and histidyl groups of proteins, and can therefore have deleterious effects on membrane structure and function, in addition to being enzyme inhibitors.

The chemical reactivity of a heavy metal, as measured by the physicochemical parameter of softness, correlates well with the $LD_{50}$ (the lethal dose that kills 50% of a population) of the metal ions (32–37). Jones and Vaughn (38) suggested that the HSAB theory can be used to correlate metal ion toxicity and the relative effectiveness of therapeutic chelating agents with parameters used to characterize "hardness" and "softness."

The mechanisms of metal ion toxicity can be divided into three main categories, according to whether the metal ions (1) block essential functional groups of biological molecules, (2) displace an essential metal ion in biomolecules, or (3) modify the active conformation of biomolecules. Class B ions tend to displace borderline ions in metalloenzymes. In aquatic systems, some Class B metals (e.g., $Hg^{2+}$, $Tl^{3+}$) form water-stable organometallic cations that are highly lipid soluble and therefore readily cross biological membranes and accumulate in cells, where they exert toxic effects. The mutagenicity and carcinogenicity of $Ni^{2+}$ may result from the ability of $Ni^{2+}$ to substitute for $Mg^{2+}$ bound to the phosphate moieties of DNA and nucleotides (39, 40).

Richardson et al. (41) showed that lichens adsorbed both Class A and Class B ions and that Class A (e.g., $Ca^{2+}$) and borderline ions with Class A characteristics (e.g., $Ni^{2+}$, $Zn^{2+}$) protected the lichens from the damaging effects of $SO_2$. However, the adsorption of borderline ions with Class B characteristics (i.e., ions that form covalent bonds, such as $Cu^{2+}$) had the opposite effect and enhanced the damage caused by $SO_2$ (42).

Essential metal ions (e.g., $Na^+$, $Mg^{2+}$) tend to form bonds that are ionic in nature, as their electron shells are nondeformable, whereas toxic metal ions (e.g., $Hg^{2+}$, $Cd^{2+}$), as a result of having more easily deformable electron shells, form bonds that are covalent in nature. Hard acids also have lower stability constants with ligands. Regardless of the ligand involved, the order of stability of complexes with divalent metal ions is Pd > Cu > Ni > Co > Zn > Cd > Fe > Mn > Mg (43). For example, Crist et al. (44) showed that the strength of adsorption of metals on algal cell walls was in the order Cu > Sr > Zn > Mg > Na, suggesting a trend from covalent to ionic bonding.

Soft acids form more stable complexes with cellular components than hard acids when they replace essential ions in cells, thereby interfering with the normal physiological functions of the cell and causing toxic effects. The substitution of a hard acid for another in a ligand may not have such serious consequences on cell functions as when a hard acid is replaced by a soft acid or a borderline ion. Not only do soft acids and borderline ions tend to form tighter bonds with ligands (e.g., carboxylate groups in cell wall acids) than hard acids, but borderline cations have a high affinity for both oxygen- and nitrogen-containing ligands and can also bind to sulfhydryl groups. The presence of these ions at certain sites in the cell will disrupt the normal functions and the integrity of membrane and cellular components (e.g., metalloenzymes and DNA).

Changes in the toxicity of metals occur with changes in pH. For example, the toxicity of Cu increases as pH increases, whereas the toxicity of Ni decreases (1, 45). Such variations in toxicity may be the result of the effects of pH on physicochemical parameters, such as metal hydrolysis (and the increased adsorption that is associated with hydrolysis) and the electric field strength of ligands (changes in the electric field strength of a ligand will affect which cations will be preferentially adsorbed). Although the ionic strength of the medium may remain constant, changes in the cationic composition of the environment of the cell can alter the expression of surface ionogenic sites. Such changes in cell surface properties may be important in the carcinogenicity and mutagenicity of eukaryotic cells (46).

Class A cations have a greater preference for oxygen-containing ligands than for nitrogen- and sulfur-containing ligands, whereas the sequence for Class B cations is sulfur- > nitrogen- > oxygen-containing ligands. Borderline ions have both Class A and Class B properties and have a high affinity for oxygen-, nitrogen-, and sulfur-containing ligands. As each metal may bind to a different ligand in the cell, toxicity may vary with pH, for the affinity of a metal for a ligand may vary as the result of the effect of pH on metal hydrolysis.

## 2.3 EFFECTS OF HEAVY METALS ON MICROORGANISMS

There have been numerous reviews on the effects of metals on microorganisms (1, 2, 6, 47–56) that have dealt mainly with in vitro studies of the biochemical and physiological mechanisms whereby metals exert their effects on microorganisms. Babich and Stotzky (45, 57) reviewed the effects of $Cd^{2+}$ and $Ni^{2+}$ on microorganisms, and Failla (58) reviewed zinc metabolism in microorganisms. The ecological aspects of microbial responses to heavy metals was reviewed by Duxbury (59), and the effects of various gaseous and heavy metal pollutants on microorganisms were reviewed by Babich and Stotzky (2) and Stotzky and Babich (51). Babich and Stotzky (3, 4) also reviewed the toxicity of heavy metals to microbe-mediated ecological processes and the potential application of the effects of physico-chemical environmental factors on toxicity to risk assessment and regulatory policies. The "ecological dose" (EcD) concept and its potential application to evaluating the toxicity of heavy metals and other pollutants to microbe-mediated ecological processes was developed by Babich and Stotzky (3, 4) and Babich et al. (60, 61). Biotic and abiotic environmental factors affect the toxicity of heavy metal pollutants to microbes (1, 3, 6, 7, 8, 45, 48, 50, 51, 62, 63), their mutagenicity and clastogenicity (40), and the utility of microbial assays for evaluating the toxicity and mutagenicity of chemical pollutants (5).

Heavy metals influence microorganisms by affecting their growth, morphology, and biochemical activities. The examples in Table 2.2 illustrate only some of the effects of heavy metals on microorganisms. Additional and older data can be found in the review articles mentioned previously (e.g., 1, 2, 4–6, 45, 50, 54, 55).

## 2.4   INTERACTIONS OF MICROBIAL CELL WALLS WITH METALS

### 2.4.1   Bacteria

The phosphodiester groups of the teichoic acid polymer and the carboxyl groups of peptidoglycan are potent metal coordinators in Gram-positive bacteria (64–70) (see Chapters 1 and 9). The amount of metal bound to Gram-positive cell walls often exceeds the stoichiometric values based on the available reactive groups in the wall, suggesting that metal deposition in these walls occurs as a two-step process. The initial interaction between the soluble metal species and the reactive chemical group, which is stoichiometric, provides nucleation sites around which there is secondary deposition of more metal, thereby forming large deposits. Electron-scattering profiles of thin-sectioned, unstained walls of *Bacillus subtilis* reacted with soluble metal showed discrete granules of metal associated with the wall fabric, which may have represented deposits at discrete nucleation sites (70).

It has been suggested that the cell walls of many bacteria are analogous to an open, low-density ion exchange system (71, 72). However, in some bacteria, for example, *B. subtilis*, the ion exchange system is more condensed and has a higher density. Bacteria readily exchange cations adsorbed on the cell wall with cations in the ambient environment. In *Arthrobacter*

**TABLE 2.2   Examples of Effects of Heavy Metals on Microorganisms**

Example and Reference

EFFECT: GROWTH INHIBITION

**Filamentous Fungi**

100 ppm Ni reduced growth of *Asteromyces cruciatus, Dendryphiella salina, Pleospora vagens,* and *Dreschlera halodes* in nutrient-enriched seawater (Ref. 2)

100 ppm Cd inhibited growth of *Botrytris cinerea, Penicillium vermiculatum,* and *Fomes annosus*; 1000 ppm Cd inhibited *Aspergillus niger, Scopulariopsis brevicaulis,* and *Phycomyces blakesleeanus* (Ref. 140)

110 ppm Pb inhibited *Chaetomium* sp. and *Pestalotiopsis* sp.; 275 ppm Pb inhibited *Pleurophomella* sp. and *Gnomonia platani* (Ref. 276)

10 m$M$ Zn inhibited *Fusarium solani, Cunninghamella echinulata, A. niger,* and *Trichoderma viride* (Ref. 57)

50 ppm Pb reduced growth of *Rhizoctonia solani* and *Aspergillus giganteus*; 110 ppm that of *F. solani, T. viride,* and *C. echinulata*; and 500 ppm that of *B. cinerea* and *Penicillium brefeldianum* (Ref. 167)

**Yeasts**

0.15 m$M$ Hg, 0.10 m$M$ Ag, 0.01 m$M$ Cd, 0.33 m$M$ Ni, and 0.16 m$M$ Cu inhibited growth of *Saccharomyces cerevisiae* by 50% (Ref. 111)

100 ppm Ni inhibited *Ansenula anomala* and reduced growth of *Rhodotorula glutins, Rhodotorula colostrii,* and *Torula utilis* (Ref. 277)

1, 5, and 10 ppm Ni reduced growth of *Torulopsis glabrata, Rhodotorula rubra,* and *Cryptococcus terreus,* respectively; *T. glabrata* and *C. terreus* were totally inhibited by 20 ppm and *R. rubra* by 30–40 ppm Ni (Ref. 2)

**Bacteria**

5–10 ppm Cd lengthened the lag phase of *Agrobacterium tumefaciens* from 3 to 6 h (Ref. 140)

$4 \times 10^{-4}$ $M$ Ni extended the lag phase of *Arthrobacter marinus* sp. nov. from 3 to 72 h (Ref. 278)

5 ppm Hg extended the lag phase of a *Vibrio* sp. from 3 to 72 h; 15 ppm Hg extended that of *Bacillus* sp. from 3 to 41 h; and 20 ppm Hg extended that of *Citrobacter* sp. from 3 to 70 h (Ref. 279)

Cd, Zn, Cu, Hg, and Ni decreased growth of *Escherichia coli* (Ref. 280)

$10^{-2}$ $M$ Ni completely inhibited growth of *Pseudomonas tabaci*; $10^{-3}$ $M$ Ni partially inhibited (Ref. 281)

Zn and Cd (100, 500, and 1000 μ$M$) inhibited *Streptococcus faecalis* (Ref. 282)

**TABLE 2.2** (*continued*)

---

Example and Reference

---

**EFFECT: GROWTH INHIBITION**

55–910 µM Mn decreased growth of *Leptothrix discophora* (strain SS-1) (Ref. 283)

10–12 ppm $Cr^{6+}$ inhibited growth of soil bacteria; 1 and 10–12 ppm $Cr^{6+}$ affected Gram-negative bacteria more than Gram-positive bacteria (Ref. 284)

Th, Fe, and Cu inhibited *S. faecalis* (Ref. 239)

Hg, Cd, Cu, Ni, and Zn inhibited soil bacteria in vitro (Ref. 285)

50% of 58 species of bacteria were intolerant of 5 ppm Cd but tolerant of concentrations <5 ppm (Ref. 286)

$10^{-8}$ M methyl mercuric acetate had a bacteriostatic effect on *Rhodopseudomonas capsulata* (Ref. 287)

**Algae**

0.15–20 ppm Hg inhibited the growth of a marine diatom, *Nitzschia acicularis* (Ref. 288)

0.05 ppm Cu reduced the growth of *Spirulina platensis* by 60% (Ref. 289)

Cu and Cd inhibited the growth of the green alga *Scenedesmus obliquus* LH (Ref. 120)

Cu, Zn, and Pb were toxic to the growth of a freshwater green alga, *Scenedesmus quadricauda*; the sequence of toxicity was Cu > Zn > Pb (Ref. 290)

**EFFECT: SPORULATION**

**Fungi**

1 and 10 ppm Cd inhibited sporulation in *A. niger, T. viride,* and *Rhizopus stolonifer* (Ref. 140)

$Cr^{6+}$ was more toxic than $Cr^{3+}$ to spore germination of *R. stolonifer,* an *Oospora* sp., *T. viride, P. vermiculatum,* and *Aspergillus giganteus* (Ref. 163)

1 ppm Ni inhibited sporulation by *A. niger, A. giganteus,* and *Gliocladium* sp. (Ref. 2)

**EFFECT: ADHESION**

**Bacteria**

100 µM Zn impaired adherence of *S. faecalis* to human buccal cells at low cell densities; however, at high cell densities the presence of Zn increased adherence; 50 µM Cd in the growth medium caused a steady increase in adhesion as the density of bacteria increased over a narrow range; a plateau was attained at relatively low cell densities (Ref. 282)

**TABLE 2.2** (*continued*)

Example and Reference

EFFECT: MORPHOLOGICAL CHANGES

**Bacteria**

$4 \times 10^{-4}$ $M$ NiCl$_2$ induced formation of abnormally long and frequently swollen cells (megalomorphs) in *A. marinus* sp. nov. (Ref. 278)

2 ppm Pb caused induction of coccoid-shaped cells, abnormal cross walls, and formation of protoplasts in *Bacillus subtilis* (Ref. 291)

Hg induced formation of irregular and multiple septa in a *Bacillus* sp. (Ref. 279)

Exposure to Pb produced ultrastructural changes (e.g., disaggregated ribosomal particles from membranes) in *Micrococcus luteus* (Ref. 292)

**Fungi**

39.3 $\mu M$ Cu resulted in the development of a blue color in the mycelium and cell walls of *Cunninghamella blakesleeana* (Ref. 99)

9 m$M$ Cu induced the formation in *C. blakesleeana* of larger hyphae with rough, granular surfaces and thicker cell walls and abnormal and compressed cytoplasm (Ref. 100)

50 ppm Ni produced extensive branching and shortening of the hyphae of *R. stolonifer* (Ref. 148)

10 ppm Cd caused modification of mitochondria and respiratory deficiency in yeast cells (Ref. 293)

50 ppm Zn inhibited trap formation by the nematode-trapping fungus *Monacrosporium endermathum* (Ref. 294)

**Algae**

Exposure to 100 ppm Ni for 4 h caused a decrease in the size and volume of the cells, a reduction in the number of lipid inclusions per cell, the formation of intracellular membranous whorls, an increase in the surface area of thylakoids, and a reduction in the volume of intrathylakoidal spaces of the cyanobacterium, *Cyanobacterium boryanum* (Ref. 295)

Exposure to 0.05–0.125 ppm Ni for 12 days caused a decrease in the number of vegetative cells per filament and an absence of heterocysts in filaments of the cyanobacterium *Anabaena inequalis*; exposure to Ni for 7 days caused a loss in the cellular contents of apical cells and bleaching of the pigment in vegetative cells (Ref. 296)

Exposure to 0.001 ppm Cd caused the formation of straight chains of cells in the freshwater diatom *Tabellaria flocculosa* (Ref. 297)

**TABLE 2.2**   (*continued*)

Example and Reference

EFFECT: MORPHOLOGICAL CHANGES

$10^{-4}$ $M$ Cu produced large multinucleate cells with thickened cell walls in the green alga *Ankistrodesmus braunii* (Ref. 298)

Tetraethyl Pb induced the production of giant, multinucleate cells in the alga *Porterioochromonas malhamensis* (Ref. 299)

300–600 µg $L^{-1}$ Pb caused the formation of large, swollen, and rounded cells that were clumped together; there was a lack of colony formation and of sheaths and spines around the cells of *S. quadricauda* (Ref. 290)

Cd in the growth medium of *Euglena gracilis* caused the production of cells that contained mitochondria with numerous myelin-like structures, chloroplasts that were altered in shape and had thylakoid rearrangements, and an increase in the number of osmophilic plastoglobuli. Respiratory processes may be the initial target of Cd toxicity in *E. gracilis* (Ref. 300)

Cd decreased chlorophyll content per cell in *Chlorella stigmatophora* (Ref. 301)

EFFECT: BIOCHEMICAL ACTIVITIES

**Bacteria**

Cu, Hg, and Ag inhibited the rate of respiration of a mutant strain of *Bacillus megaterium* with a small capsule to a greater extent than the encapsulated parent strain (ATCC 19213), indicating that these heavy metals were bound to the capsule of the parent strain (Ref. 133)

Cd, Zn, Cu, Hg, and Ni caused a reduction in the synthesis of RNA and protein in *E. coli* (Ref. 280)

Cells of *P. tabaci* contained higher internal concentrations of Ni when grown in $10^{-3}$ $M$ Ni (toxic) than in $10^{-4}$ $M$ Ni (nontoxic) (Ref. 281)

**Fungi**

39.3 µ$M$ Cu altered the nitrate reductive pathway, resulting in the accumulation of nitrite; increased the phosphorus and decreased the hexosamine content of the cell walls of *C. blakesleeana*; cell walls from Cu-containing cultures contained hydroxyproline (normally absent); 59.4 µ$M$ Co increased the phosphorus and citrulline content of the cell walls (Ref. 99)

9 m$M$ Cu decreased Mg and increased sulfur content of mycelia of *C. blakesleeana*; the protein composition of Cu-grown cell walls was different from that of control or Co-grown cultures (Ref. 100)

Low concentrations ($<0.5 \times 10^{-5}$ $M$) of U inhibited fermentation of glucose, mannose, and fructose by yeast, but $1 \times 10^{-5}$ $M$ was necessary to inhibit the enzyme, invertase, which is located in the cell membrane (Ref. 110)

**TABLE 2.2**  (*continued*)

Example and Reference

**EFFECT: BIOCHEMICAL ACTIVITIES**

Ni inhibited fermentation in *S. cerevisiae,* as a result of the inhibition of alcohol dehydrogenase (Ref. 113)

160 ppm Ni reduced the rate of fermentation of a mixed rumen microbiota by 50% (Ref. 302)

0.05 *M* Ni reduced photosynthesis of the lichens *Stereocaulon paschale* and *Umbilicaria muhlenbergii* (Ref. 303)

The uptake of Cu and Pb by *U. muhlenbergii* caused an efflux of K from the thallus. The efflux of K was unaffected by Ca, Mg, Sr, and Zn. A larger efflux of K occurred with the uptake of higher concentrations of Cu (Ref. 42)

Cu greatly reduced $^{14}$C-fixation (from $NaH^{14}CO_3$) by *U. muhlenbergii*; Ni, Pb, and Cu increased the release of photosynthate from the lichen. Pb, Cu, Zn, as well as $SO_2$, caused a reduction in the amount $^{14}$C incorporated into ribitol, sucrose, and other sugars during photosynthesis. The adsorption of Ca, Ni, and Pb reversed the shift from ribitol production to the production of sucrose and other sugars induced by $SO_2$. Ca, Mg, Sr, Zn, and Ni (Class A metal ions or borderline ions with Class A characteristics) did not affect $^{14}$C fixation (Ref. 41)

5 min exposure to 50 μ*M* Ni caused a reduction in the synthesis of ATP and the inhibition of DNA replication, transcription, and translation, which was correlated with an inhibition of some enzymes of the tricarboxylic acid cycle (glutamate, succinate, α-ketoglutarate, and isocitrate dehydrogenases) (Ref. 304)

**Algae**

0.18 m*M* Ni inhibited photosynthesis and 0.03 m*M* Ni inhibited flagellar regeneration in *Chlamydomonas reinhardtii* (Ref. 305)

Cu inhibited photosynthesis (but to a lesser extent than growth) in *S. platensis* (Ref. 289)

Al and Cu inhibited alkaline phosphatase activity in *S. quadricauda* (Ref. 182)

$10^{-10}$ *M* Cu inhibited photosynthesis by the cyanobacterium *Oscillatoria theibauti*; 1 ppm Cd inhibited photosynthesis and 2 ppm Cd inhibited $N_2$ fixation in the cyanobacterium *Anabaena spiroides* (Ref. 307)

10 ppm Ni inhibited photosynthesis and 20 ppm Ni inhibited $N_2$ fixation in *A. inequalis* (Ref. 296)

100 ppb Hg inhibited photosynthesis and $N_2$ fixation *A. inequalis* (Ref. 308)

15–18 ppm Pb reduced photosynthesis in *C. reinhardtii* (Ref. 309)

**TABLE 2.2**    (*continued*)

Example and Reference

**EFFECT: BIOCHEMICAL ACTIVITIES**

5 ppb Cu reduced photosynthesis in the marine dinoflagellate *Scrippsiella faeronse* (Ref. 310)

100 $\mu$g L$^{-1}$ Cu, 250 $\mu$g L$^{-1}$ Zn, and 2700 $\mu$g L$^{-1}$ Pb inhibited photosynthesis in *S. quadricauda* (Ref. 290)

Low concentrations of some metals induced DNA lesions (e.g., strand breaks and cross-links) or induced sister chromatid exchanges. Relatively nontoxic concentrations of Ni and Cr induced multiple types of DNA lesions (Ref. 311)

**Protozoa**

2.5 mg L$^{-1}$ Ni inhibited ciliary movement in *Paramecium caudatum* (Ref. 306)

**EFFECT: STIMULATORY EFFECTS OF HEAVY METALS ON MICROBES**

**Bacteria**

5–10 ppm Cd stimulated growth of *E. coli* and *S. faecalis* (Ref. 83)

Trace amounts of Ni were necessary for the formation of the enzyme carbon monoxide dehydrogenase in *Clostridium pasteurianum* (Ref. 312)

Ni was required as a component of $F_{430}$, the prosthetic group of coenzyme reductase in *Methanobacterium thermoautotrophicum* (Refs. 313–317)

Ni was required for growth of *Xanthobacter autotrophicus, Pseudomonas flava,* an *Arthrobacter* sp., *Hydrogenomonas* sp., and *Alcaligenes* (formerly *Hydrogenomonas*) *eutrophus,* in which the uptake of Ni was energy dependent (Refs. 318–320)

**Algae**

3 ppb Ni produced greater cell yields of a *Chlorella* sp. than cultures not exposed to Ni (Ref. 321)

100 $\mu$g L$^{-1}$ Cu stimulated the growth of *S. quadricauda* (Ref. 290)

25 ppb Hg stimulated photosynthesis and $N_2$ fixation by *A. inequalis* (Ref. 308)

0.005–125 ppm Ni and 0.005–0.025 ppm Pb stimulated $N_2$ fixation by the cyanobacterium *Nostoc mucorum* (Ref. 322)

Ni was an absolute growth requirement for a cyanobacterium, *Oscillatoria* sp., isolated from a marine mud (Ref. 323) *globiformis*, the affinity displacement series for cations was H > Fe > Al > Mn > Ba > Ca > Mg > K > $NH_4^+$ > Na (73); and in *Bacillus megaterium* and *Micrococcus lysodeikticus*, the series was H $\gg$ La $\gg$ Cd > Sr > Ca > Mg > K > Na > Li (69).

The cell walls of Gram-positive bacteria make up 10–40% of the dry weight of the cell, depending on the species and the growth conditions. The walls consist of a matrix (20–30 nm thick) containing cross-linked and noncross-linked peptidoglycan strands to which teichoic acids or teichuronic acids are covalently linked. The cell wall of Gram-negative bacteria is chemically and structurally more complex than that of Gram-positive bacteria, and the peptidoglycan layer makes up only approximately 2–10% of the dry weight of the cell and is only 3 nm thick (74). However, in Gram-negative cell walls, an additional layer, termed the outer membrane (OM), is located above the peptidoglycan layer.

The membranous structure of the Gram-negative cell wall results in a more complex interaction with metals. Hoyle and Beveridge (75) demonstrated the binding of metals (i.e., Na, Ca, Mg, Sr, Ni, Mn, Pb, and Fe) by the OM of *Escherichia coli* K-12. Approximately 50% of the bound metal was usually present in the OM, except for Mn and Sr. Pb aggregated on the hydrophilic side of the bilayer, perhaps as a result of a charge asymmetry across the OM. Mg and Ca are important components of the OM, and metal chelators, such as ethylenediaminetetraacetic acid (EDTA), can remove the outer membrane, thereby releasing protein–lipopolysaccharide and protein–phospholipid complexes (76, 77). After EDTA treatment, the cells become more permeable to a variety of metabolites (76, 78) and more sensitive to antibiotics (79).

Studies with *Pseudomonas aeruginosa* PAO1 (77, 80, 81) have shown that divalent metals, especially Mg, maintain the OM structure and help to bind the major macromolecular constituents. However, Mg was not absolutely required for the maintenance of membrane integrity, as the integrity was still maintained when *P. aeruginosa* was grown in a Mg-deficient medium. However, in a marine pseudomonad, *Alteromonas haloplanktis*, Mg was an absolute requirement for the stability of the peptidoglycan layer (29).

The peptidoglycan layer of Gram-negative cell walls also contains sites with which metals can interact, and the types of reactive sites in the peptidoglycan of *E. coli* are identical with those of *B. subtilis*, as the structure of the peptidoglycan is similar, even though the degree of cross-linking is different (74). However, the amounts of metal chelated by Gram-negative cell walls were less than those chelated by Gram-positive cell walls, presumably because the peptidoglycan layer is thinner in Gram-negative bacteria and does not contain teichoic acid, a potent chelator of metals.

Although the cell walls of living bacteria have been shown to adsorb cations (70, 73, 74, 82, 83), dead bacterial cells can also adsorb metals. Dead cells adsorbed more Cd from a medium than did live bacteria, clay (montmorillonite), or sand (84, 85), and the method by which the cells were killed, that is, by physical (γ-radiation) or chemical means (ethanol, formaldehyde, or propylene oxide), had an effect on the amount of Cd adsorbed.

*Pseudomonas aeruginosa* accumulated U intracellularly very rapidly (< 10 sec), and environmental factors, such as pH and temperature, had no effect on the accumulation of U. Visible deposits of U were detected in 44% of the population of *P. aeruginosa* cells by electron microscopy (86).

The Cd-binding sites on the cell wall of a Cd-sensitive marine pseudomonad were mainly ionic materials, such as polygalacturonic acids, and to a lesser extent nonionic polymers, such as dextrans (87). The amount of soluble Pb removed from solution and interacting with cells of *Micrococcus luteus* was related to the concentration of negative charges on the cell surface. The transfer of Pb was initiated by the surface charge, which caused a concomitant shift in the solubility equilibrium of Pb and affected the translocation of Pb from the surface into the cells. It was suggested that other organisms may have a similar type of metal translocation system (88).

The accumulation of U by 10 species of bacteria, 13 actinomycetes, 11 yeasts, and 18 filamentous fungi followed the order actinomycetes > bacteria > yeasts > fungi. Two species of actinomycetes, *Actinomyces levoris* and *Streptomyces viridochromogenes*, rapidly accumulated extremely high levels of U, and the uptake was affected by pH and the concentration of carbonate ions but not by temperature and metabolic inhibitors. The accumulation of U by these actinomycetes apparently depended on physicochemical adsorption at the cell surface, and U was bound to the surface by ligands, which could be substituted by EDTA (89).

Ge and other nonessential metals were accumulated in the cell envelope of *Pseudomonas putida* grown in a medium supplemented with organic substrates (acetate or catechol) that were able to bind Ge (90). The accumulation of Ge by *P. putida* from a medium supplemented with catechol or catechol plus acetate was biphasic. A low level of accumulation, corresponding to the value obtained in the presence of acetate alone, was followed by a further increase to a high saturation level. The second phase of Ge accumulation corresponded with the linear degradation of catechol, and it was suggested that catechol facilitates the transport of Ge into cells of *P. putida* through the nonspecific uptake of a Ge–catechol complex. The catechol transport system in *P. putida* is inducible (91).

The nucleation of crystalline metal phosphates, metal sulfides, and polymeric metal–complex organic residues occurred on metal-loaded cells (i.e., cells with metals bound to the cell walls) of *B. subtilis* when mixed with a synthetic sediment and placed under laboratory conditions to simulate sediment diagenesis at low temperatures (92). The loss of specific groups of molecules in the cell wall can affect the metal-binding ability of the wall. For example, the loss of specific molecules from the core region of the lipopolysaccharide (LPS) of a rough mutant strain (D21f2) of *E. coli* resulted in a more open structure that allowed the binding of both larger cations and more monovalent cations (93).

High-resolution phosphorus nuclear magnetic resonance ($^{31}$P-NMR) spectra revealed high affinity interactions between $Eu^{3+}$, a paramagnetic cation, and all the phosphoryl groups in the LPS of *E. coli* K-12, suggesting that the high affinity of LPS for divalent metallic ions results primarily from the phosphoryl substituents, not from the free carboxyl groups. Small, electron-dense precipitates, presumably stable, neutrally charged, and water-insoluble coordination complexes of phosphoryl groups of the constituent molecules of the OM and $Eu^{3+}$, were found associated with the OM vesicles of *E. coli* K-12 (94).

The cell wall of *B. subtilis* appears to be partially differentiated, and cell wall poles seem to represent localized areas of high electronegativity (95). The negative charges, contributed by phosphate and carboxyl groups, were responsible for the binding of cationized ferritin (CF) by the walls of *B. subtilis*, which was asymmetric as the result of the orientation of teichoic acid and muramylpeptides toward the outside of the wall, above the plane of the glycan strands (96).

The exopolymers from adherent cells of a bacterium from a freshwater sediment had $Cu^{2+}$-binding activity. Crude, cell-free, exopolymer preparations containing protein and polysaccharide components bound up to 37 nmol Cu mg$^{-1}$ dry weight, and a highly purified exopolysaccharide preparation bound up to 253 nmol Cu mg$^{-1}$ carbohydrate (97). Extracellular polymers from *Klebsiella aerogenes* bound Cu, Cd, Co, and Ni, and the log conditional stability constant ($K_i$) values were 7.69, 5.16, 5.48, and 5.49, respectively (98). Adsorption of Ni ceased when the complexation capacity of the polymers was reached, whereas the uptake of Cu, Cd, and Co continued, suggesting that there was more than one binding site for these three metals. Ni was associated with the soluble form of the polymers and Cu and Cd with the colloidal fraction. A more detailed account of the interactions between metals and extracellular polymers can be found in Chapter 11.

## 2.4.2 Fungi

The cell wall composition of *Cunninghamella blakesleeana* was altered in the presence of Cu and Co (99). Both the mycelium and the cell walls became blue when the fungus was grown in toxic concentrations of Cu (2.5 µg mL$^{-1}$). Isolated cell walls contained higher concentrations of Cu and Co than the mycelia. When grown in the presence of Cu, the phosphate content of the mycelium was less than when grown in the presence of Co, which was the same as in the control mycelium. However, the isolated cell walls from cultures grown in the presence of Cu or Co contained higher concentrations of phosphate than the control walls. The cell walls from fungus grown in the presence of Cu also contained less hexosamine and alkali-soluble neutral sugar, but more protein, than the walls from the control and Co-grown cultures, and chitin and chitosan were present in equal amounts. Both the Co cell walls and the control cell walls contained the same amount of hexosamine; however, 88% of the hexosamine in the Co cell walls was present as chitosan, whereas the control cell walls contained 60% chitosan. The affinity of chitinase for the Cu cell walls was greater than for the Co and control cell walls. The cell walls from Cu-grown cultures were more easily hydrolyzed by chitinase than were the other cell walls, and the differential rates of hydrolysis were not related to differences in melanin content. The amino acid composition of the cell walls was also different, in that there was a high concentration of hydroxyproline, which is usually absent in the cell walls of fungi, in the Cu cell walls but none in the control and Co cell walls, whereas the Co cell walls had an abnormally high citrulline content. More DNA was bound by control cell walls than by Cu and Co cell walls. The changes in the chemical composition and structure of the walls of the fungus grown in the presence of Cu or Co resulted in alterations in the metal-binding capacity of the cell walls (100).

Cell walls from Co-grown cultures of *C. blakesleeana* bound more Cu and Co than Cu-grown or control cell walls. The quantitative binding of other metals also differed: for control cell walls, Zn > Fe > Mn > Cd > Ca > Ni > Cu > Ag > Co; for Cu cell walls, Zn > Fe > Mn > Cu > Ni > Cd > Ag > Ca > Co; and for Co cell walls, Fe > Zn > Cu > Mn > Cd > Ag > Ca > Ni > Co. In the presence of Mn, Ni, and Ca, the cell walls bound less Zn than in the presence of Zn alone. The binding of Cu depended on temperature and pH, whereas the binding of Co was independent of temperature and pH. As the binding of Co was inhibited by Cu but the binding of Cu was not inhibited by Co, it was suggested that there are two binding sites on the cell walls of *C. blakesleeana*; one binding site that is common for both Co and Cu but with a higher affinity for Co, and another site that binds Cu exclusively. The binding of Co was totally suppressed in the presence of Cd but not of Cu, and the cell walls did not bind Mg. Elution of metal-loaded cell walls with 5 m$M$ EDTA did not diminish their metal binding ability, because metals could rebind to these cell walls to the same or greater extent as the original walls. However, elution with HCl reduced the binding capacity (101).

*Rhizopus stolonifer* and *C. blakesleeana* were "trained" to tolerate elevated concentrations of Cu (102). The trained mycelia also acquired tolerance to elevated levels of Cd, Co, Ni, and Pb. The fungi could be "untrained" by serial transfers to Cu-free media, which reduced their tolerance to Cu and the other metals to the level of the original cultures. There was no evidence of induction of mutations or of the selection of resistant cells, indicating that physiological adaptation to Cu was involved. However, tolerance or intolerance to Cu could be imprinted on the sporangiospores. Extracellular metabolites that could complex with, exclude, or detoxify Cu were not produced by the trained mycelia, which removed more Cu from solution than mycelia from nontrained parentals, suggesting that Cu tolerance may have been the result of either the binding of Cu to the cell wall or of intracellular mechanisms that detoxified Cu.

The mycelium of *Penicillium digitatum* accumulated $U^{6+}$ from aqueous solutions of uranyl chloride. The amount of U adsorbed was increased by killing the mycelium with boiling water, alcohols, dimethyl sulfoxide, or potassium hydroxide, but killing with formaldehyde did not increase the uptake. Isolated wall-related biopolymers (i.e., chitin, cellulose, cellulose derivatives) were able to adsorb U (103). The selectivity sequence for the binding of cations to the mycelium of *P. digitatum* was Fe, Ni, Zn > Cu > Pb, $UO_2 \gg MoO_4$. Uptake and binding of Ni, Zn, Cd, and Pb by the mycelium were pH sensitive, whereas those of Cu and $UO_2$ were pH insensitive (104). Biomass obtained from *Rhizopus arrhizus* did not adsorb monovalent metal ions (i.e., Na) but adsorbed divalent cations (i.e., La, Cu, Zn), and uptake of divalent cations increased as their ionic radius increased (105).

*Penicillium* sp. adsorbed Pb from solutions of $Pb(NO_3)_2$, and although uptake of Pb was more rapid after heat treatment of the mycelium, the maximum amount of Pb bound remained unchanged. Chromate ($CrO_4^{2-}$) was not adsorbed by the mycelial preparations without preincubation in $Pb(NO_3)_2$, suggesting that the binding of divalent cations to the net negatively charged fungal cell wall changed the net charge of the wall to positive (106). The uptake of Cu by protoplasts of *Penicillum ochro-chloron* is apparently energy dependent, and both protoplasts and mycelia tolerated Cu over a pH range of 3.0–5.5 but were sensitive at pH 6.0, where the uptake of Cu was approximately 10 times greater than at lower pH values. The influx of Cu showed saturation kinetics, with half maximal influx at an external Cu concentration of 390 $\mu M$ and a maximum influx rate of 22 nmol $h^{-1}$ $10^7$ cells$^{-1}$ at pH 3.0. However, saturation kinetics were not observed at pH 6.0 (107).

The amount of Cd and Hg translocated into the fruiting bodies of some higher fungi varied with species: the fruiting bodies of *Pleurotus flabellatus* accumulated 75 and 38.5% of applied Cd and Hg, respectively, in contrast to *Pleurotus sajor-caju*, which accumulated only 3.7% Cd and 3.63% Hg. More Hg than Cd was translocated into the fruiting bodies of four (*Agaricus bisporus, Pleurotus ostreatus, Flamulina velutipes*, and *Agrocybe aegerita*) of six species (these four plus *P. flabellatus* and *P. sajor-caju*), indicating that the translocation system was both species- and metal-specific (108). Based on equilibrium studies, the mass balance for the exchange of Ni for Sr, Sr for Tl, and Sr for H was consistent with a cation exchange mechanism for metal uptake by the lichen, *Umbilicaria muhlenbergii* (109).

*Saccharomyces cerevisiae* accumulated U extracellularly, and the rate and extent of accumulation was affected by pH and some anions and cations. The rate of uptake of U was increased by pretreatment of the yeast with 1% $HgCl_2$ and 10% formaldehyde. Uranium that was bound to the yeast could be removed chemically, and it was suggested that the cells of *S. cerevisiae* could be reused as biosorbents (86).

Yeasts adsorbed U very rapidly when exposed to low concentrations of $UO_2^{2+}$ ($0.5 \times 10^{-5}$ $M$), and at higher concentrations, a maximal uptake of

$1 \times 10^{-3} \, M \, kg^{-1}$ cells was obtained. The binding of U to the yeasts was reversible, and U could be displaced by several cations. The cytoplasmic membranes of the yeasts appear to have two different sites for U (as well as for Mn): one binding site consists of the phosphoryl groups of the cell membrane, and the binding of U to this site causes inhibition of the fermentation of glucose, mannose, and fructose; the other binding site is the carboxyl groups of invertase, a membrane-bound enzyme (110).

S. *cerevisiae* also binds and accumulates other metal cations, and the adsorption of Hg, Ag, Cd, Al, Ni, Cu, and Pb depends on cell concentration. For example, more Hg was bound at low than at high cell concentrations (111). The cell membrane of yeasts can be damaged by adsorbed metals, resulting in the leakage of K and cellular anions to the medium: complete leakage of K was caused by Hg; Cu, at twice the Hg concentration, had a smaller effect; and Zn and Pb had no measurable effect (112).

A system that transports Mg and Mn was also responsible for the transport of other metal ions into a nonexchangeable pool in yeasts; the affinity of the system was Mg, Co, Zn > Mn > Ni > Ca > Sr. Uptake was reduced at pH levels below 5.0, but a $H^+$ exchange system did not seem to be involved, as two $K^+$ or two $Na^+$ were secreted for each divalent cation absorbed (113).

The accumulation of Zn by starved cells of *Candida utilis* occurred by two different processes: the first process was rapid, independent of energy, pH, and temperature, and represented the binding of Zn to the cell surface; the second process was slower, depended on energy, pH, and temperature, and accumulated greater quantities of Zn than did the binding process. The uptake of Zn was inhibited by Cd but not by Ca, Cr, Mn, Co, or Cu. Cells of *C. utilis* accumulated Zn only during the lag phase and the latter half of the exponential growth phase and contained a protein fraction resembling the metallothionein of animal cells (114). S. *cerevisiae* also accumulated Co and Cd by two processes: a metabolism-independent process (i.e., binding to the cell surface) and a metabolism-dependent process. The accumulation of Co and Cd was accompanied by the loss of K from the cells. Co and Cd appeared to be accumulated via a cation uptake system (that may also be involved in the accumulation of other cations), which showed a limited specificity that was related to the ionic radius of the cations (115).

### 2.4.3  Algae

The accumulation of Zn and Cd by *Chlorella kessleri* was pH dependent, whereas the accumulation of Cr, Hg, and As was pH independent in the range from pH 3 to 8: in neutral media, the accumulation of these metals was in the order Cr > Hg > Zn > Cd > As (arsenate) > methylarsonic acid > dimethylarsinic acid (116). A green microalga, *Stichococcus bacillaris*, at a constant biomass of 1 g dry weight $L^{-1}$, removed 60–80% of Cd from solutions containing 4 mg Cd $L^{-1}$. The extent of Cd removal depended on the density of the algal suspension, and 96% of the Cd in solutions containing 0.5 and 4 mg Cd L$^{-1}$ was removed by four sequential batches of algae at a density of 1 g dry weight L$^{-1}$ (117).

The concentrations of Cu, Cd, and U were higher in the soluble intra-cellular fraction of a *Chlorella* sp., with only 3–5% in the cell wall. Copper ions were present in both high- and low-molecular-weight intracellular frac-tions, whereas Cd and U were present only in the high-molecular-weight intracellular fraction, indicating that in *Chlorella*, different substances within the cell combine with different heavy metals (118).

*Chlorella pyrenoidosa* grown in a medium with low levels of Mn incor-porated both Cd and Mn at a faster rate than cells grown in a medium with high levels of Mn. Cells previously exposed to Cd incorporated Cd and Mn at a faster rate, indicating that Cd and Mn may share a common transport system in *C. pyrenoidosa* (119).

The strength of adsorption of ions on algal cell walls was in the order Cu > Sr > Zn > Mg > Na, suggesting a trend from probable covalent to ionic bonding. Ionic bonding was demonstrated directly by the addition of Na, which decreased the adsorption of positively charged metallic ion complexes and increased that of negatively charged ones (44). *Scenedesmus obliquus* LH accelerated and increased the removal of Cu and Cd from growth media when compared with precipitation and formation of colloidal hydroxides in the controls without algae or light (120).

The adsorption of Cd on three unicellular green algae, *Chlorella vulgaris, Ankistrodesmus braunii*, and *Eremosphaera viridis*, showed a fast and a slow phase of adsorption. Approximately 80% of the Cd was adsorbed during the fast phase, and the slow phase had a marked influence only on the amount of Cd adsorbed on *E. viridis*. Cd was adsorbed mainly on the cell wall, and the binding sites seemed to be acidic groups (121).

The cell wall of *Nitella flexilis*, a freshwater alga, adsorbed Cu selectively, as the result of the stronger chelation of Cu than of other metallic ions by the cell wall. The selectivity sequence in cation exchange studies was Cu ≫ Zn > Ca. The cell wall of *N. flexilis* appears to reflect a two-site model, based on the nature of the ligands. The first group of sites (amines) reacts exothermically, whereas the second group of sites (hydroxylic–carboxylic), which has a lower affinity, reacts endothermically (122). The Cu ions appear to form inner-sphere coordination complexes with these sites, resulting in lower rotational mobilities and lower activity coefficients of the Cu ions, as they are immobilized close to the negative charges in the Stern layer. The Cu ions in the diffuse layer are more mobile and have activity coefficients close to 1 at higher equivalent fractions (123).

*Chlorella regularis* absorbed Mo rapidly during the first 2 h after exposure, but then uptake occurred more slowly. Temperature, pH, and the presence of metabolic inhibitors did not affect the uptake of Mo. The amount of Mo absorbed (μg Mo g$^{-1}$ dry weight) increased as the concentration of Mo in the solution increased but decreased with increasing concentrations of algae.

Pretreatment of the cells with heat increased the accumulation of Mo, and more Mo was accumulated from freshwater than from seawater. The biological reduction of $Mo^{6+}$ to $Mo^{5+}$ or $Mo^{3+}$ occurred intracellularly. The efficiency of Mo accumulation by green algae was species specific: *Scenedesmus chlorelloides > Chlamydomonas reinhardtii > C. regularis > Scenedesmus bijuga > Chlamydomonas angulosa > S. obliquus* (124).

Uranium (as $UO_2^{2+}$) was selectively accumulated by *C. regularis*, and both living and dead cells accumulated higher concentrations of U and Cu than of other heavy metals (i.e., Ni, Co, Cd) (125). Heavy metal adsorption by living cells of *C. regularis* followed the order U ≫ Cu ≫ Zn ≳ Ba ≈ Mn ≳ Co ≈ Cd ≳ Ni ≈ Sr; for heat-killed cells, the order was U ≫ Cu ≫ Mn ≳ Ba ≳ Zn > Co ≳ Cd ≳ Ni ≳ Sr. It was suggested that heavy metal ions bind to proteins both in the cell wall and inside the cells of *C. regularis*. The uptake of Cd was reduced as a result of competition by U and Cu. The acid-extractable components were mainly responsible for the binding of Cu and Cd, but they were only slightly involved in the binding of U.

## 2.5   TRANSPORT OF METAL IONS INTO MICROORGANISMS

The transport of metal ions into microorganisms can occur by one of the following mechanisms: (1) essential nutrient ions, for example, $Mg^{2+}$, $Ca^{2+}$, $Mn^{2+}$, transported via carriers; (2) specific transport of metals complexed with specifically exuded low-molecular-weight ligands, for example, the iron-transporting compounds (siderophores or ferrichromes) produced by some microorganisms (126, 127) (see Chapter 5); and (3) nonspecific transport of metal ions complexed with substrates that serve as carrier molecules through a transport system specific for these substrates, for example, the transport of Ge into cells of *P. putida* through the nonspecific uptake of a Ge–catechol complex by an inducible catechol transport system (91).

Metal ions can also be passively immobilized in the cell envelope, as the result of the binding of the ions to charged groups in the cell wall (67, 68, 70, 92, 94, 128–131), and they can also become immobilized, albeit less firmly, within capsules and slime layers by adsorption (89, 132, 133) (see Chapter 11). Soil bacteria may obtain essential minerals by exchanging $H^+$ for exchangeable cations present on clay particles (73, 82, 134).

Heavy metals accumulated by bacteria may become concentrated and be passed to other organisms in a food chain (i.e., biomagnification). For example, tubificid worms fed bacterial cultures containing heavy metals had an increased concentration of metals (135). Lead and Cd adsorbed by bacteria and fungi had an inhibitory effect on the reproduction rate of two nematodes, *Mesorhabditus monohystera* and *Aplenchus avenae*, that preyed on these microbes (136).

## 2.6  PHYSICOCHEMICAL FACTORS THAT AFFECT THE TOXICITY OF HEAVY METALS TO MICROBES

### 2.6.1  pH

The pH of an environment can affect the toxicity of heavy metals to microbes by affecting (1) the physiological state and biochemical activities of microbes and, hence, their reaction to toxic substances, and (2) the chemical speciation of heavy metals, which affects their mobility and ability to bind to cell surfaces.

Heavy metals ($M^{2+}$) form multiple hydroxylated species as the pH of the solution increases (137–139):

$$M^{2+} \xrightarrow{\ [OH^-]\ } MOH^+ \xrightarrow{\ [OH^-]\ } M(OH)_2$$

$$\xrightarrow{\ [OH^-]\ } M(OH)_3{}^- \xrightarrow{\ [OH^-]\ } M(OH)_4{}^{2-}$$

However, the pH at which these hydroxylated species form varies for each metal. Different hydroxylated forms of the same metal have different toxicities (1, 6, 50, 51, 63, 140–142), and the speciation form affects the adsorption of a metal to a charged surface (143).

As the pH of the medium is lowered and the concentration of $H^+$ increases, the $H^+$ can compete with heavy metal cations for ionogenic sites on the surface of cells. The charge of these ionogenic groups is also influenced by pH, and therefore the affinity of the cell surface for metal ions will also be affected by changes in ambient pH.

The speciation form of organic ligands is also affected by pH, and therefore the complexation of metals with organic compounds depends on pH (144). Some metals (e.g., Cu, Pb, Ni) when complexed with organic compounds are generally less toxic than the free forms of the metals (1, 145).

Cd was more toxic to *M. luteus*, *Staphylococcus aureus*, and *Clostridium perfringens* when the pH was increased from acidic to alkaline levels (pH 5–9) (146). Similar results were obtained with *Alcaligenes faecalis*, *Bacillus cereus*, *Aspergillus niger* (140), and *C. pyrenoidosa* (147). Fungi (*Penicillium vermiculatum*, *Penicillium asperum*, *A. niger*, and *Cunninghamella echinulata*) were more tolerant of Cd when grown in a naturally acidic soil (pH 5.1) than when grown in a naturally alkaline soil (pH 7.8) (57). The increased Cd toxicity at higher pH values may be the result of formation of the monovalent cation, $CdOH^+$, which may penetrate microbial cells more easily than the divalent form ($Cd^{2+}$) and consequently be more toxic. Furthermore, as the pH is increased, fewer $H^+$ are available for competition with Cd, and thus more Cd ions are taken up (1).

Conversely, the toxicity of Ni to microbes decreases as the pH increases. Ni was less toxic to bacteria, actinomycetes, yeasts, and filamentous fungi between pH 5.5 and 8.5 (148, 149) than at lower pH values. Fungi grew more slowly in a naturally acidic soil (pH 4.9) amended with 1000 ppm Ni than in the same soil adjusted to pH 7.1 (150). The survival of *Serratia marcescens* and *Nocardia corallina* in the presence of 75 ppm Ni was greater in a natural lake water with a pH of 6.8 than in the same water adjusted to pH 5.3 (45, 149). However, Ni occurs as the divalent cation ($Ni^{2+}$) to approximately pH 8.5 (151), and therefore increases in pH do not appear to reduce the toxicity of Ni by the formation of hydroxylated species.

Increasing the pH from 3.5 to 4.7 caused an increase in the toxicity of Cu to the fungus *Aureobasidium pullulans*, which was related to an increase in the uptake of Cu (152). Increasing the pH from 5 to 8 caused an increase in the toxic effects of Cu on growth (153) and photosynthesis (154) of *C. pyrenoidosa*. The toxicity of Cu to spores of *Fusarium lycopersici* increased with increasing pH (155). An energy-dependent influx of Cu occurred in the protoplasts of *P. ochro-chloron*, and both protoplasts and hyphae tolerated Cu from pH 3.0 to 5.5 but were sensitive at pH 6.0, where the uptake of Cu was approximately 10 times greater than at lower pH values (107). The uptake of Cu ($10^{-5}$ M) and Pb ($10^{-6}$ M) by a blue-green alga, *Nostoc muscorum*, increased as the pH increased from 4 to 7 but decreased at pH values above 7 (156).

The effects of pH on the toxicity of Zn to microorganisms appear to vary with the type of organism. For example, the toxicity of Zn to fungi increased as the pH was increased from 5.5 to 7.5, but further increases in pH to 9.5 did not enhance the toxicity (50). Increasing the pH from 4 to 8 increased the toxicity of Zn to Zn-resistant and Zn-sensitive populations of a freshwater alga, *Hormidium rivulare* (157, 158). However, the toxicity of Zn to growth of *C. vulgaris* decreased as the pH was increased from 4 to 8 (159).

The effects of pH on the toxicity of Hg also varied with different organisms. The toxicity of Hg to an *Achyla* sp. and a *Saprolegnia* sp. was not affected when the pH was increased from acidic to alkaline levels (50). However, Hg was more toxic to the spores and mycelium of *F. lycopersici* at alkaline levels (155). Conversely, methyl Hg was more toxic to the growth and photosynthesis of *Ankistrodesmus* sp. at pH 4 than at pH 8 (160).

The adsorption of Zn and Cd by the green alga, *C. kessleri*, was pH dependent, whereas the accumulation of Hg, Cr, As, methylarsonic acid, and dimethylarsinic acid was pH independent within the range of pH 3–8. The order of accumulation at pH 7 was Cr > Hg > Zn > Cd > As > methylarsonic acid > dimethylarsinic acid (116).

Similar results were obtained with *S. obliquus*: adsorption of Zn and Cd was pH dependent, whereas adsorption of Hg was pH independent. The amount of metal accumulated was not affected by the presence of other metals but was reduced by substances that formed negatively charged complexes with the metals (161). The maximum amount of Cd that could be adsorbed on the cells of a microalga, *S. bacillaris*, was 11.7 mg $g^{-1}$ dry weight at pH 7, 6.2 mg $g^{-1}$ dry weight at pH 6, and 1.4 mg $g^{-1}$ dry weight at pH 4 (162).

Metal adsorption on algal cell walls displaces $H^+$, and the ratios for $H^+$ displaced : $M^{2+}$ adsorbed at pH 4.5 were 1.2 for Cu, 0.66 for Zn, 0.59 for Mg, and 0.30 for Sr; Na was not adsorbed (44).

## 2.6.2 Oxidation–Reduction Potential

The oxidation–reduction potential $(E_h)$ of an environment can affect the availability and toxicity of heavy metals. Reducing environments have a negative $E_h$, whereas oxidizing environments have a positive $E_h$. Heavy metals that are deposited into an environment with a negative $E_h$ may combine with $S^{2-}$ to form insoluble sulfide salts that are unavailable for uptake by microbes and therefore are not toxic. The $E_h$ also affects the valence state of metals; for example, Cr can exist as $Cr^{3+}$ or $Cr^{6+}$, depending on the $E_h$ of the environment. $Cr^{6+}$ was more toxic than $Cr^{3+}$ to mycelial growth and spore germination of *R. stolonifer*, an *Oospora* sp., *Trichoderma viride*, *P. vermiculatum*, and *Aspergillus giganteus* (163).

## 2.6.3 Inorganic Anions

The inorganic anionic composition of an environment influences the speciation and hence the toxicity of heavy metals to microbes. Heavy metals form coordination complexes with inorganic anions (e.g., $OH^-$, $Cl^-$), and most heavy metals have coordination numbers from 1 to 4. Increasing the concentration of a monovalent anionic ligand $(L^-)$ in the presence of a divalent metal $(M^{2+})$ leads to the formation of the following (138, 139):

$$M^{2+} \xrightarrow{[L^-]} ML^+ \xrightarrow{[L^-]} ML_2 \xrightarrow{[L^-]} ML_3^- \xrightarrow{[L^-]} ML_4^{2-}$$

The different speciation forms of a heavy metal that occur in the presence of increasing concentrations of an anionic ligand can exert different toxicities to microbes. For example, *Agrobacterium tumefaciens*, *Erwinia herbicola*, marine species of *Acinetobacter* and *Aeromonas*, and the bacteriophages, φ11M15 of *S. aureus* and P1 of *E. coli*, were able to tolerate Hg better when Hg was present as mixtures of $HgCl_3^-/HgCl_4^{2-}$ than as $Hg^{2+}$ (142).

Increasing the concentration of $Cl^-$ decreased the toxicity of Cd to *A. niger*, *R. stolonifer*, *Aspergillus conoides*, and an *Oospora* sp. (164). The uptake and consequently the toxicity of Cd to the estuarine alga, *Chlorella salina*, was reduced when the salinity was increased from 5 to 15 parts per thousand (165). Similar results were obtained with an unidentified marine bacterium when the salinity was increased from 13.5 to 45 parts per thousand (166). Reductions in toxicity that occurred at higher $Cl^-$ concentrations may have been related to the formation of negatively charged Cd–Cl coordination complexes, which would have lower affinities for net negatively charged cell surfaces than $Cd^{2+}$.

In contrast to Cd, Zn was more toxic to coliphages as $ZnCl_3^-/ZnCl_4^{2-}$ than as $Zn^{2+}$ (141), presumably as a result of the interaction between the positively charged tails of the coliphages (which are involved in recognizing sites on host cells) and the negatively charged speciation forms of the metal. The speciation of Ni is not affected by an increase in chlorinity, as Ni occurs as $Ni^{2+}$ in both seawater and freshwater (151). The toxicity of Ni to marine fungi (*Dendryphiella salina, Asteromyces cruciatus,* and *Dreschlera halodes*) was not affected by levels of $Cl^-$ that occur in seawater (50).

Other inorganic ions interact with heavy metals to form insoluble salts that are unavailable for uptake by microbes. For example, $CO_3^{2-}$ and $PO_4^{3-}$ decreased the toxicity of Pb and Ni to fungi (145, 167, 168), and $PO_4^{3-}$ reduced the toxicity of Zn to the algae *C. vulgaris* (159, 169), *H. rivulare* (158), *Plectonema boryanum* (169), and *Anacystis nidulans* (170), and of Pb to *C. reinhardtii* (171). $S^{2-}$ also forms insoluble salts with most heavy metals (49, 172).

At concentrations of Zn ($7.5 \times 10^{-8}$ and $1.5 \times 10^{-7}$ *M*) that were detrimental to algal growth and affected the lag, exponential, and stationary phases of growth, $PO_4^{3-}$ behaved as a yield-limiting nutrient; cell densities increased linearly as the concentration of $PO_4^{3-}$ was increased. Increasing the concentrations of Zn intensified the yield-limiting effect of $PO_4^{3-}$. In nature, elevated Zn concentrations could cause apparent $PO_4^{3-}$-limiting conditions (173). Sulfate reduced the uptake of Cu by the cyanobacterium, *Nostoc muscorum*, at pH values below 5.6 but enhanced the uptake of Pb at the same pH values (156).

### 2.6.4 Inorganic Cations

The presence of other cations in the environment can affect the toxicity of heavy metals to microbes, as a result of competition with the cationic forms of the heavy metals for anionic sites on cell surfaces. Magnesium especially can ameliorate the toxicity of some heavy metals to microbes. For example, increased levels of Mg decreased the toxicity of Ni to various filamentous fungi (50, 62, 168, 174), *B. megaterium, B. subtilis* (175, 176), *E. coli,* and a yeast, *Torula utilis* (177). The toxicity of Ni to coliphage T1 (178), *Caulobacter maris,* and marine fungi was less in seawater than in simulated estuarine water, as a result of the higher concentration of Mg in the seawater (45, 149, 174). Increasing levels of Mg also decreased the toxicity of Cd to *E. coli* (177) and *A. niger* (179) and of Zn to *E. coli* (177), *A. nidulans* (170), *H. rivulare* (158), and *Klebsiella pneumoniae* (180).

Increasing levels of Ca decreased the toxicity of Zn and Hg to *C. vulgaris* (159), of Cd to *A. niger* (181), and of Zn to *H. rivulare* (158) and *A. nidulans* (170). Zn reduced the toxicity of Ni to a species of *Achyla* (62) and of Cd to *A. niger* (179). The uptake of Cu and Pb by *N. muscorum* was reduced in the presence of Ca, as a result of the competition by Ca for sites on the cell surface (156).

There were both synergistic and antagonistic interactions between Pb and Cd on the reproduction of the nematodes *M. monohystera* and *A. avenae* (136). The presence of Al increased the toxicity of Cu to the growth of *Scenedesmus quadricauda*, as a result of the displacement of Cu from ligands and the subsequent increase in the concentration of Cu ions (182).

### 2.6.5  Water Hardness

Hardness in water is caused by the presence of dissolved alkaline earth ions (e.g., Ca, Mg) together with $HCO_3^-$ and $CO_3^{2-}$. Water hardness is usually expressed as an equivalent concentration of $CaCO_3$: water containing 0–75 mg $L^{-1}$ $CaCO_3$ is termed "soft" water; "moderately hard" water contains from 75 to 150 mg $L^{-1}$; "hard" water contains from 150 to 300 mg $L^{-1}$; and water with >300 mg $L^{-1}$ $CaCO_3$ is termed "very hard" water (183). In general, the toxicity of a heavy metal is reduced in hard water. For example, Ni was less toxic to fungi in hard than in soft water (149, 168), and survival of *Rhodotorula rubra* in lake water containing 10 ppm Ni and amended with 200 or 400 mg $L^{-1}$ $CaCO_3$ was greater after 35 days than in natural lake water wherein the background concentration of $CaCO_3$ was 34 mg $L^{-1}$. Ni was also less toxic to filamentous fungi in lake water amended with 400 mg $L^{-1}$ $CaCO_3$ (149). The effects of $CaCO_3$ in reducing the toxicity of Ni was attributed to $CO_3^{2-}$ (168). The toxicity of Cd to the filamentous fungi, *Beauvaria* sp., *A. giganteus, P. vermiculatum*, and *T. viride*, and of Pb to *R. stolonifer* and *Oospora* sp. were reduced in hard water (50).

### 2.6.6  Clay Minerals

Clay minerals affect the toxicity of heavy metals to microorganisms, as the charge-compensating cations that are adsorbed on clays can be exchanged by other cations, including those of heavy metals, present in the environment. The bioavailability of toxic heavy metals is reduced when these metals are adsorbed on clay minerals and consequently temporarily removed from solution (134). In general, clays with a high cation exchange capacity (CEC) are more effective than those with a lower CEC in reducing the toxicity of heavy metals to microbes. For example, the toxicity of 40 ppm Ni to a species of *Achyla* was reduced when the concentration of montmorillonite, with a CEC of about 98 milliequivalents (meq) 100 $g^{-1}$, was increased from 1 to 3%, whereas increasing the concentration of kaolinite, with a CEC of about 5.8 meq 100 $g^{-1}$, from 1 to 3% did not reduce the toxicity (45).

The presence of clay minerals in a synthetic medium also reduced the toxicity of Cd to fungi and bacteria (184). Montmorillonite was more effective than kaolinite, and this was correlated with the higher CEC of montmorillonite (141, 185). Montmorillonite also protected fungi against the toxicity of Cd when the clay was added to soil, whereas kaolinite was less effective (184). The toxicity of Pb to fungi was reduced by montmorillonite, attapulgite (palygorskite, with a CEC of about 38 meq 100 g$^{-1}$), and kaolinite, and the ability of these clay minerals to reduce the toxicity of Pb was again correlated with their CEC: (montmorillonite > attapulgite > kaolinite) (167).

The addition of clay minerals to soil reduced the toxicity of Ni to fungi: in the presence of montmorillonite, which was more effective than kaolinite at the same concentration, 750 ppm Ni was not toxic to *R. stolonifer* and a species of *Gliocladium*, and the toxicity to *Aspergillus flavipes, Aspergillus clavatus, P. vermiculatum*, and *T. viride* was reduced (150); in an acidic soil lacking montmorillonite, 500 ppm Ni was toxic to *Agrobacterium radiobacter* and *B. megaterium* and 1000 ppm Ni was toxic to *S. marcescens*, whereas in an alkaline soil containing montmorillonite, concentrations of Ni to 1000 ppm were not toxic to the same organisms (150). Clay minerals (montmorillonite more than kaolinite) also reduced the toxicity of Pb (186), Cd, and Zn (187, 188) to soil respiration. The survival of *S. marcescens* and *Bacillus cereus* in lake water containing 50 ppm Ni was increased when montmorillonite was present at a concentration of 1 mg L$^{-1}$ (50).

## 2.6.7   Organic Matter

The dissolved and particulate organic matter present in an ecosystem can influence the mobility and bioavailability of heavy metals and, thereby, their toxicity. The types of organic matter that influence the toxicity of heavy metals include synthetic chelators [e.g., ethylenediaminetetraacetic acid (EDTA) and nitrilotriacetic acid (NTA)], natural chelators (e.g., dicarboxylic and amino acids, humic acids, organic exudates from aquatic microbes and plant roots), and complex soluble organic substances (e.g., yeast extract, peptone, humic acids).

EDTA reduced the toxicity of Zn to photosynthesis of *Microcystis aeruginosa* (189); of Cu, Zn, Cd, and Pb to growth of *Ditylum brightwellii* (190); and of Ni to growth of *K. pneumoniae* (180) and an actinomycete (149); and reduced the mutagenicity of Cr$^{6+}$ to *B. subtilis* (191). NTA reduced the toxicity of Ni, Cu, Cd, and Zn to a variety of microbes (145, 189, 192).

Aspartic acid reduced the toxicity of Ni to fungi and bacteria (145, 180); cysteine reduced the toxicity of Pb to fungi (167) and of Hg to marine and terrestrial bacteria and to phage φ11M15 of *S. aureus* (1); and citrate reduced the toxicity of Ni to *K. pneumoniae* (180) and *N. rhodocrous* (145) and of Cu to *C. pyrenoidosa* (153) and to a cyanobacterium, *P. boryanum* (UTEX 594) (193), and decreased the uptake of Cu and Pb by *N. muscorum* (156). Organic exudates from *Anabaena cylindrica*, a freshwater cyanobacterium, and from *S. quadricauda*, a green alga, reduced the toxicity of Cu to *C. vulgaris* (194).

The ability of soluble organics to bind metals varies. For example, the sequence of binding of Hg was casamino acids ≫ proteose peptone > yeast extract ≫ tryptone > peptone; with Pb, the sequence was casamino acids ≫ yeast extract > tryptone > peptone > proteose peptone; with Cu, it was casamino acids $\gg$ yeast extract $>$ tryptone $>$ proteose peptone $\gg$ peptone; and with Cd, it was casamino acids $>$ proteose peptone $>$ tryptone $\gg$ yeast extract (peptone did not bind Cd) (195). Yeast extract and increasing levels of neopeptone reduced the toxicity of Pb to fungi (167). The toxicity of Ni to eubacteria, actinomycetes, and yeasts was reduced or eliminated in media containing 0.5% yeast extract, neopeptone, casamino acids, or tryptone, whereas the same concentrations of peptone or proteose peptone had little or no effect on toxicity. However, higher concentrations of peptone or proteose peptone also reduced the toxicity of Ni (145).

The interactions of heavy metals with soluble organic matter can be affected by environmental factors, such as pH (144). The effect of pH on the toxicity of Cd to fungi was influenced by the composition of the medium: at pH values between 7.5 and 9.5, 25 ppm Cd was less toxic to a *Saprolegnia* sp. in a medium containing neopeptone than in a medium containing peptone. Similar results were obtained with an *Achlya* sp.: the toxicity of Cd at pH 8.5–9.5 decreased in a medium containing neopeptone but increased when peptone was present. There were no differences between peptone and neopeptone in the toxicity of Cd to the *Saprolegnia* sp. when the pH was increased from 5.5 to 7.5 and to the *Achlya* sp. when the pH was increased from 5.5 to 8.5 (50).

Particulate organic matter (i.e., humic acids) incorporated into a synthetic medium protected *A. niger*, *A. giganteus*, *Fusarium solani*, *C. echinulata*, *T. viride*, and *Penicillium brefeldianum* against lethal or inhibitory concentrations of Pb (6, 167) and *A. flavus*, a *Saprolegnia* sp., and *C. blakesleeana* against inhibitory concentrations of Ni (62, 63). Soluble humic acids also reduced the toxicity of Zn, Pb, Cu, and Hg to a freshwater phytoplankton population (192). Particulate humic acid and aerobically composted sewage sludge reduced the toxicity of 20,000 ppm Pb to carbon mineralization in soil (186).

### 2.6.8 Temperature

Temperature affects the toxicity of heavy metals to microbes, presumably as a result of the effect of temperature on the physiological state of cells rather than on the chemical speciation or availability of metals. Increasing the temperature from 25 to 37°C did not affect the toxicity of Zn to the growth of *A. niger*. However, a $ZnCl^+/ZnCl_2/ZnCl_3^-$ mixture was more toxic at 25 than at 37°C (57). The lower toxicity at the higher temperature was attributed to an enhanced physiological state of the fungus, as both the rate of growth and spore production were higher at 37 than at 25°C when Zn was absent from the medium. When the temperature was raised from 23 to 33°C, *A. flavus* showed greater resistance to Ni at the higher temperature (62).

At temperatures above the optimum for growth, toxicity increases. For example, the resistance of a psychrophilic marine species of *Pseudomonas* to Ni (149), of *Paramecium tetraurelia* to Cu (196), and of *Scenedesmus acutis* to Hg (197) increased as the temperature was increased above the optimum.

## 2.7  RESISTANCE OF MICROORGANISMS TO TOXIC METALS

Microorganisms have developed several mechanisms to reduce the toxicity of metals in their environment (see Chapter 4). One mechanism is biomethylation; toxic metals, such as Hg, Pb, Tl, Pd, Pt, Au, Sn, and Cr, and metalloids, such as As and Se, can be methylated by microorganisms (198–200). Biomethylation can occur by two mechanisms: (1) the heavy metal displaces the methyl group from methyl vitamin $B_{12}$ by electrophilically attacking the Co–C bond; or (2) there is transfer of a methyl free radical to a metal complexed on the corrin ring of the vitamin $B_{12}$ molecule.

Volatilization as a detoxification mechanism is used by some microorganisms. For example, cells of *Thiobacillus ferrooxidans* tolerant of Hg volatilized elemental mercury ($Hg^0$) when grown in media containing $HgCl_2$, suggesting that this bacterium may be important in the natural cycling of Hg, as *T. ferrooxidans* is usually found in habitats containing high concentrations of heavy metals, including Hg (201). Trace amounts of volatile Cd were produced from inorganic Cd by a *Pseudomonas* sp. (202).

Some metal-resistant microorganisms have intracellular "traps" by which toxic metals are detoxified. A Ni-tolerant mutant of the cyanobacterium, *Synechococcus* sp., that tolerated $2.0 \times 10^{-4} M$ $NiSO_4$ contained large quantities of intracellular cyanophycin granules that strongly bound both Ni and Cu (199). A Cd-inducible metal-binding protein was isolated from Cd-exposed cells of *Synechococcus* sp., providing evidence for the presence of metallothionein in a procaryotic organism (203), and the partial purification of megamodulin, which also binds metals, from *E. coli* has been reported (204).

Some microorganisms precipitate toxic metals at the cell surface. Certain strains of a thermoacidophilic green alga, *Cyanidium caldarium*, precipitated toxic metals (e.g., Cu, Ni, Cr) extracellularly as metal sulfides (199). The cell walls of bacteria (67, 68, 205), fungi (99, 102, 206), and algae (89, 124) can bind toxic metals, which reduces their entry into the cytoplasm.

Cadmium resistance in *S. aureus* is determined by a plasmid (207), and an energy-dependent Cd efflux system, coded for by the plasmid, catalyzes the exchange of cellular Cd for external $H^+$ (208). At high concentrations of Cd, accumulation occurs via the plasmid-determined efflux system that converts the Cd–H exchange system into a Cd–Cd exchange system. When high external Cd concentrations are removed, the efflux system returns to its normal function of exchanging cellular Cd for $H^+$. Resistance to arsenate, arsenite, and antimony (III) in *S. aureus* and *E. coli* also occurs through energy-driven efflux pumps. Arsenate is transported from the cell by a phosphate-dependent mechanism, whereas arsenite is transported via a phosphate-independent pump (199).

Accumulation of $^{109}$Cd in Cd-sensitive cells of *B. subtilis* was via an active transport system for Mn, and the resistance of a Cd-resistant strain was the result of reduced $^{109}$Cd accumulation, although transport of $^{54}$Mn was unaffected. Uptake of $^{54}$Mn and $^{109}$Cd apparently occurred by the same mechanism, and cation specificity was involved (209). Cadmium uptake by another Cd-resistant strain of *B. subtilis* was also less than the uptake by a Cd-sensitive strain. The Cd resistance of the Cd-resistant strain was chromosomally encoded, and protection against increased concentrations of Cd did not affect the transport of Mn (210).

In *E. coli* K-12, $^{109}$Cd was accumulated via an energy-dependent and temperature-sensitive mechanism, and uptake of $^{109}$Cd was inhibited by Zn but not by Mn. The uptake of $^{54}$Mn was inhibited by $^{112}$Cd and Zn, suggesting that the accumulation of $^{54}$Mn occurred through a transport system separate from that for $^{109}$Cd, as Mn did not inhibit the uptake of $^{109}$Cd. The uptake of Mn was competitively inhibited by Co. The resistance of *E. coli* to Cd did not appear to be the result of energy-driven efflux systems, as in *S. aureus*, or by reduced uptake, as in Cd-resistant strains of *B. subtilis* (211). Resistance of Gram-negative bacteria to Cd may be the result of the production of metallothionein-like proteins (211–213).

The resistance to Cd and Hg of strains of *Bacillus* sp. isolated from a salt marsh and from Boston Harbor was chromosomally determined. Resistance to Cd in isolates from the salt marsh was the result of reduced Cd transport. Three of the Cd-resistant isolates from Boston Harbor showed influx but no efflux of Cd. No Cd-specific binding proteins were detected in the isolates from either the salt marsh or Boston Harbor. Therefore, it was suggested that resistant strains sequestered or chelated Cd. Resistance to Hg was the result of detoxification, that is, the transformation of $Hg^{2+}$ to volatile $Hg^0$ by mercuric reductase (214).

Bacterial populations from natural and metal-polluted soils could be divided into two subgroups, with one subgroup being more metal-tolerant than the other. The more metal-tolerant subgroup also exhibited multiple drug resistance and consisted primarily of Gram-negative bacteria. It was suggested that because Gram-negative bacteria are generally more tolerant of heavy metals than Gram-positive bacteria, Gram-negative bacteria may be able to function without plasmid-mediated metal tolerance in soils containing comparatively low levels of metal pollutants (215).

## 2.8  EFFECTS OF HEAVY METALS ON THE ELECTROKINETIC PROPERTIES OF MICROORGANISMS AND VIRUSES

The surface of most microbial cells is charged as the result of the presence of carboxyl, amino, and phosphodiester groups in the cell wall. At a certain pH, cells have a net zero charge (i.e., they do not move in an electrical field), which is the isoelectric point (p$I$). The p$I$ depends on the species. At pH values below the p$I$, the cells have a net positive charge, and at pH values above the p$I$, the cells are net negatively charged. Under physiological conditions, most microbial cells are net negatively charged.

The net surface charge and the p$I$ of cells can be determined by measuring their mobility in an electric field. The movement of a charged entity relative to a stationary liquid phase in an applied electric field is termed "electrophoresis." Microelectrophoresis [i.e., electrophoresis in suspension wherein the electrophoretic mobilities (EPM) of microscopically visible particles are measured directly with a microscope] has established that the p$I$ of most bacteria is between pH 2 and 4 (216–219).

The surface of a cell has an important role in the relation between the cell and its environment, as the cell surface is in direct contact with the ambient environment of the cell. The importance of the cell surface in microbial ecology, in the adhesion of microbes to surfaces, and in interactions between microorganisms and clay minerals and other particulates is well recognized (134, 220–225). The effects of the products of natural microbial populations on the electrokinetic potential of bacterial cells and clay minerals have been studied (226).

Studies of the EPM of microorganisms have provided valuable information on the effects of the physicochemical factors (e.g., pH, metals) of natural environments on the cell surface, the relation between microorganisms and their environment, and on how changes in the cell can affect their surface properties. Only a few examples of representative electrokinetic studies are given, but more extensive information may be obtained from other reviews (134, 216–223, 225).

The binding of metals on microorganisms alters their electrokinetic properties (226–231). The electrokinetic patterns of four species of bacteria (*B. subtilis*, *B. megaterium*, *P. aeruginosa*, and *A. radiobacter*), two species of yeasts (*S. cerevisiae*, *Candida albicans*), and two clay minerals (montmorillonite and kaolinite) differed in the presence of the chloride salts of both toxic (e.g., Cd, Cr, Cu, Hg, Pb, Ni, Zn) and nontoxic (e.g., Na, Mg) metals at the same ionic strength ($\mu$) (228). The cells were negatively charged at all pH values above their p$I$ in solutions of Na, Mg, Hg, and Pb at a $\mu$ of 3 $\times$ $10^{-4}$ (e.g., Fig. 2.2), but the charge of the bacteria, *S. cerevisiae*, and kaolinite changed from a net negative charge to a net positive charge (charge reversal) in the presence of Ni, Cu, Zn, Cd, and Cr at higher pH values (e.g., Fig. 2.3). The pH at which charge reversal occurred varied with each heavy metal and usually occurred at the pH at which the concentration of the uncomplexed metal cation ($M^{2+}$) decreased and the concentration of the monovalent hydroxylated cation ($MOH^{+}$) increased. Adsorption of the metals increased when the pH approached conditions for hydrolysis of the metals, and this increase in adsorption of the hydroxylated species appeared to be responsible for the charge reversal.

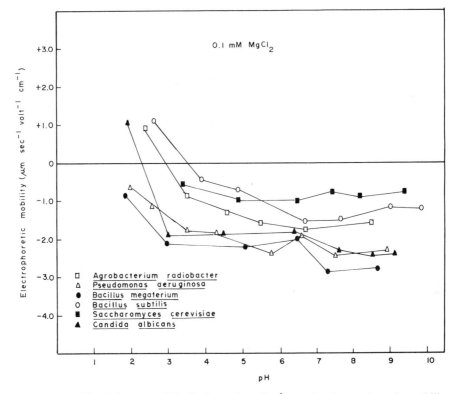

**Figure 2.2** The influence of $MgCl_2$ ($\mu = 3 \times 10^{-4}$) on the electrophoretic mobility of four species of bacteria and two species of yeasts.

Charge reversal occurred with Cu, Zn, and Ni, which are classified as borderline metals, and with Cr, a Class A metal, and Cd, a Class B metal (19). With Cu, the change from the divalent to the monovalent hydroxylated cation occurs between pH 5.5 and 8.0, and this was the pH range in which charge reversal occurred. With Zn, the concentration of divalent Zn decreases between pH 6.0 and 8.0, and charge reversal occurred within this range. With Ni, charge reversal occurred between pH 8.0 and 10.0, when the concentration of the divalent cation decreases and that of the monovalent hydroxylated cation increases. With Cd, the concentration of the monovalent hydroxylated cation increases in the pH range (8.4–9.3) in which charge reversal occurred.

Na and Mg did not cause charge reversal. In aqueous solutions, Na and Mg hydrolyze only at high pH values (>9.0), and because charge reversal is usually associated with the formation of the first hydrolysis products of the metal, Na and Mg would not cause charge reversal at the pH values (2–10) used in these experiments. The sign of the zeta ($\zeta$) potential of quartz was reversed from negative to positive at pH 10.9 and 9.9, in the presence of $1 \times 10^{-4}$ $M$ and $1 \times 10^{-3}$ $M$ $MgCl_2$, respectively (232).

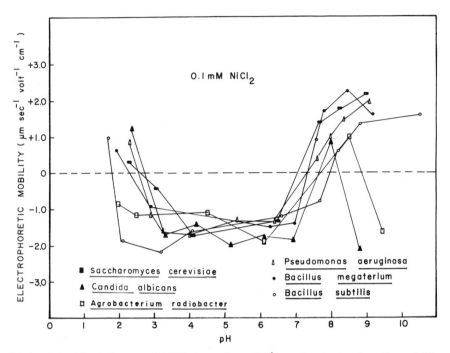

**Figure 2.3**   The influence of NiCl$_2$ ($\mu = 3 \times 10^{-4}$) on the electrophoretic mobility of four species of bacteria and two species of yeasts.

Charge reversal also did not occur with Pb and Hg, although the change from the divalent to the monovalent hydroxylated cation occurs between pH 5.0 and 7.0 with Pb and between pH 1.0 and 3.0 with Hg. Pb and Hg form negatively charged and uncharged chlorinated species in the presence of Cl$^-$ in the pH range used in these studies. The ability of Cl$^-$ to inhibit the adsorption of Hg and Pb and prevent the reversal of charge was probably the result of the formation of chloride complexes (e.g., HgCl$_3$$^-$/HgCl$_4$$^{2-}$; PbCl$_2$), that is, Cl$^-$ was preferred to OH$^-$ as a ligand. In contrast, metals such as Cu and Ni have a lower affinity for Cl$^-$ than for OH$^-$ in aqueous solutions. Metals that are less adsorbable in the presence of Cl$^-$ are the same metals for which chloride complexes predominate over hydroxo complexes in seawater (138, 139, 233, 234).

Although reversal of charge of the four species of bacteria and *S. cerevisiae* occurred in the presence of Cu, charge reversal did not occur in the presence of a mixture of Mg and Cu at the same total $\mu$ ($3 \times 10^{-4}$), indicating that the ability of Cu to bind to the cells was affected by the presence of Mg. In contrast, charge reversal occurred in the presence of both Ni and Mg and Ni but not of Mg alone, indicating that the ability of Ni to bind on the cells was not affected by Mg. Charge reversal also occurred in the presence of Cu and Ni.

Increasing the $\mu$ of Cu or Ni above $3 \times 10^{-4}$ also reversed the charge of the bacteria and *S. cerevisiae*, whereas charge reversal did not occur in solutions with a $\mu$ below $3 \times 10^{-4}$. Increasing the $\mu$ of Cu ($>3 \times 10^{-4}$) and Ni ($>1.5 \times 10^{-4}$) reversed the charge of the clays. The p$I$ of the cells was also affected by the heavy metals; in general, the p$I$ was shifted to pH values that were higher than in the presence of Na or Mg (228, 231).

There appear to be specific sites for metal cations in the cell wall of *B. subtilis*, as partial digestion of the cell wall with lysozyme reduced the ability of the wall to retain Mg but not Ca, Fe, or Ni, and modification of amine groups reduced the binding of Cu (in *B. subtilis*, Cu appears to bind to amines) (67, 68). Two types of binding sites appear to be present in the cell wall of *N. flexilis*: the first group of sites (amines) had a higher affinity for Cu than the second group of sites (hydroxylic–carboxylic) (122). Cu has the highest Class B character among the first-row divalent transition metal ions, which may account for the high affinity of Cu for amine groups.

Studies on the effects of monovalent and multivalent cations, at constant $\mu$, on the electrokinetic properties of cultured *Rana pipiens* kidney cells, normal human lymphoid and Burkitt lymphoma cells (46, 235), and guinea pig macrophages and lymphocytes (236, 237) indicated the presence of different binding sites on the surfaces of these cells. The effects of the cations were related to their physicochemical characteristics, such as their hydrated ionic radius, and the differential affinities of the various cations for negative sites on the cells. Microelectrophoresis was also used to study specific antibody adsorption by cells of *Streptococcus pyogenes* (219).

In aqueous solutions, cations show selectivity and specificity with respect to their preference for particular ligands. Both biological and nonbiological systems have selectivity patterns for the adsorption of monovalent and divalent cations. In some biological systems, there is a selectivity pattern for monovalent cations that is based on the size of their hydrated ionic radius (lyotropic series), for example, Cs > Rb > K > Na > Li; for divalent cations, the selectivity sequence, for example, Mg > Ca > Sr > Ba, is based on the size of their nonhydrated ionic radius (238). In *N. flexilis*, a selectivity sequence of $Cu^{2+} \gg Zn^{2+} > Ca^{2+}$ was observed (123).

The charge reversal of cells and clays that occurs as the result of the specific adsorption of some metals indicates a close binding of these metals on the surface (i.e., in the Stern layer). Such close binding of certain metals on sites in the cell wall may lead to perturbations in the cell surface, disrupt normal functioning of the cell, and cause toxic effects. Inasmuch as different metals probably bind to different sites on the cell, strong specific binding could enhance toxicity in some cases and decrease toxicity in others, at a particular pH, as a result of the replacement of essential metals (e.g., Mg) by toxic metals (e.g., Ni) and vice versa.

$Th^{4+}$ and hydrolyzed $Fe^{3+}$ at a $\mu$ of $1 \times 10^{-2}$ reversed the net electrical charge of *Streptococcus faecalis* from negative to positive, whereas $Ca^{2+}$, $Pb^{2+}$, $Cu^{2+}$, and $Cr^{3+}$, at the same $\mu$, only reduced the negative $\zeta$ potential.

The order of effectiveness in changing the sign of the $\zeta$ potential was $Th^{4+}$ $\simeq Fe^{3+} \gg Cr^{3+} \gg Cu^{2+} > Pb^{2+} > Ca^{2+}$ (239).

At pH values between 2 and 9, the net charge of the clay minerals kaolinite and montmorillonite remained negative regardless of the valency of the cations (mainly Class A or hard acids), at the same $\mu$, in the suspending medium (231). However, as the valency of the cations, both on the exchange complex of the clays and in the medium, was increased, the electronegativity of the clays decreased. The electronegativity of bacteria, above their p$I$, also decreased as the valency and concentration of the cations in the medium increased, and the p$I$ of the cells was shifted to higher pH values as the valency of the cations increased. For example, $Fe^{3+}$ and $Al^{3+}$ shifted the p$I$ of the cells from pH 2.5–3.5 to approximately pH 7.0.

Sorption between bacterial cells and montmorillonite or kaolinite homoionic to different cations was studied by measuring changes in particle size distribution with a Coulter Counter and by electron microscopy. Sorption between bacteria and clay minerals (227) and flocculation of the clays by microbial metabolites (243) occurred only in the presence of polyvalent cations, as the result of the reduction in the electrokinetic potentials of the bacteria and clays. Sorption also occurred when the cells were net positively charged (i.e., at pH values below their p$I$) and the clays remained net negatively charged. The amount of sorption increased as the valency of the cations increased. Suspension of the bacteria in dilute soil extracts (1:5 soil:water), dilute seawater (1:100 seawater:distilled water), various metabolites, or culture media containing organic constituents also resulted in reductions in the net negative charge of the cells and in shifts of the p$I$ to higher pH values. Reductions in the surface charge of either or both the clay and bacterial populations can result in the sorption between the particles, and such surface interactions can affect the activity, ecology, and population dynamics of microbes in environments containing clays or other surface-active particulates (134, 225).

The EPM and $\zeta$ potential of reovirus were found to depend on pH, $\mu$, and the nature and concentration of the electrolyte (241). The EPM toward the anode decreased with increasing electrolyte concentration. The effect of salts on the EPM was: $KCl \simeq NaCl$, $2\ NaCl \simeq Na_2SO_4$, $100\ NaCl \simeq CaCl_2 \simeq MgCl_2$, and $MgCl_2 \simeq MgSO_4$ (i.e., higher concentrations of $Na^+$ had the same effect on mobility as lower concentrations of $Ca^{2+}$ and $Mg^{2+}$, whereas $Ca^{2+}$ and $Mg^{2+}$ had the same effect at the same concentration, and the type of anion had no effect). The p$I$ of the virus was unaffected by phosphate but was elevated by $Ca^{2+}$ and acetate. In NaCl at pH 8.1, the reovirus was net negatively charged, but cationic flocculants, for example, $Al_2(SO_4)_3$ and polydiallyl-dimethylammonium chloride (PDADMA), neutralized or reversed the charge. The use of dark-field laser-illuminated microelectrophoresis showed that microelectrophoresis can be extended to viruses and that useful information on the electrokinetic and related surface properties of viruses can be obtained (242).

## 2.9 MECHANISMS OF ADSORPTION OF HYDROLYZED METAL IONS ON MINERAL AND CELLULAR SURFACES

The adsorption of metal ions on mineral and cell surfaces exhibits similarities (e.g., variations in adsorption with changes in pH, reversal of charge), which suggests that the theories for the mechanism of adsorption of hydrolyzed metal ions on mineral surfaces (244, 245) may also be used to explain the mechanism of adsorption of metal ions on cell surfaces. Metals can exist either as the "free" (i.e., uncomplexed) metal ion, for example, $Cu^{2+}$, or in a complexed form, for example, $CuOH^+$, $CuCO_3^0$ (246). However, the free metal ion may be coordinated with water molecules (e.g., $Cu(H_2O)_4^{2+}$ or $Cu(H_2O)_6^{2+}$) (247), and the formation of complexes may occur as a result of the replacement of $H_2O$ molecules by more preferred ligands (e.g., $OH^-$, $Cl^-$, NTA, EDTA) (246). The free metal ion may not be the dominant metal species, even in the absence of ligands, as indirect complex formation can occur. For example, hydroxo species, such as $M(OH)_n^{z-n}$, can be formed as a result of changes in pH. In aqueous solutions, metal (M) ions hydrolyze to form soluble metal complexes, according to the generalized equation

$$M_{aq}^{z+} + nH_2O \rightleftharpoons M(OH)_n^{z-n} + nH^+$$

where $z$ is the valence and $n$ is the number of ions.

The concentration of ligands and of soluble metal [if polynuclear complexes (e.g., $M_2(OH)_2^{(2n-2)+}$ complexes, such as $Al_8(OH)_{20}^{4+}$), are in fact important] determines the nature and distribution of the resulting hydroxo complexes. The adsorption of metal ions at solid/liquid interfaces is probably not primarily dependent on the concentration of the free metal ion but on the concentration of the hydroxo, sulfato, carbonato, and other complex species of the metal that are more strongly adsorbed (248).

Hydrolysis and metal uptake appear to be related, as adsorption of hydrolyzed metals onto solid oxides (249) and other surfaces (250) varies with the pH of the solution. At low pH values, little or no adsorption is usually observed (251), but as the pH is increased, an abrupt increase to maximum adsorption occurs over a narrow pH range (252). Although the exact pH at which this abrupt increase in adsorption occurs varies considerably for different metals (e.g., Fig. 2.4), it appears to be related to the p*$K$ of the first hydrolysis product of the metal (233), where *$K$ is the equilibrium constant for the above reaction when $n = 1$. The order of increasing p*$K$ values for metals corresponds to the order of the onset of increased adsorption of the metals as the pH of the solution becomes more alkaline: $Fe^{3+} > Hg^{2+} > Cu^{2+} > Co^{2+} > Cd^{2+}$. When the $\zeta$ potential of quartz in the presence of Ni and Co was compared with the distribution of the pH-dependent hydroxylated speciation forms of these metals, $Ni_{aq}^{2+}$ and $Co_{aq}^{2+}$ had little affinity for quartz surfaces, whereas $NiOH^+$ and $CoOH^+$ were the predom-

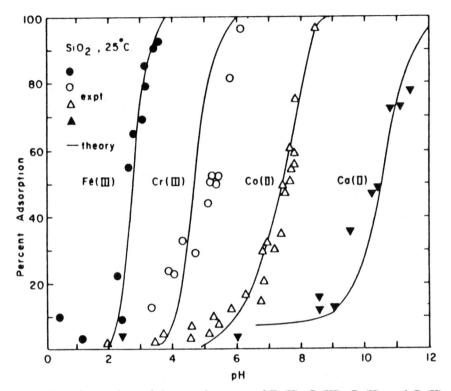

**Figure 2.4**  Comparison of the actual amount of Fe(II), Cr(III), Co(II), and Ca(II) adsorbed on SiO₂ as a function of pH with the amount adsorbed computed from a model theory. The concentrations of metals added were $1.2 \times 10^{-4}$, $2.0 \times 10^{-4}$, $1.2 \times 10^{-4}$, and $1.4 \times 10^{-4}$ $M$, respectively (With permission of the authors and the J. Colloid Interface Sci., Ref. 244).

inant ionic species adsorbed, supporting the concept that hydrolyzed metal ions are adsorbed more readily than the free ion (253).

Several qualitative reasons have been suggested to explain why the hydrolyzed form of a metal is adsorbed more than the free metal ion (254). The adsorption appears to be noncoulombic, because a di- or trivalent cation should be electrostatically preferred by a negatively charged surface over the corresponding hydroxo complexes that have a lower positive charge (246). Therefore, it has been suggested that specific interaction with the surface (i.e., adsorption into the Stern layer) occurs and that the presence of OH⁻ is the key factor in the enhanced removal of metal ions from aqueous solutions. Most ionic species containing OH⁻, regardless of their charge characteristics, exhibit a strong affinity for solid/liquid interfaces (251, 254).

The fact that OH⁻ is often the potential-determining ion on oxide surfaces suggests that OH⁻ is strongly bound on solid surfaces (254), possibly as the result of hydrogen bonding between oxygen atoms on the surface and such species as $NiOH^+$ and $CoOH^+$ (250, 253). Removal or rearrangement of the hydration sheath of the adsorbate probably precedes adsorption, and the replacement of a molecule of water of hydration by an $OH^-$ group on the central metal ion might reduce the amount of free energy required for adsorption (244, 245, 254). Furthermore, $MOH^+$ may be more hydrophobic than $M_{aq}^{2+}$ and thus may be more susceptible to the formation of bonds with specific surface sites (254).

However, as adsorption, hydrolysis, and precipitation of hydrolyzable metal ions occur over a narrow pH range (244, 245), the concept of the presence of monomeric hydroxo complexes as the determining factor in metal adsorption is not universally accepted. The multinuclear hydrolysis products, $M_n(OH)_m$, that are the precursors to the formation of a solid hydroxide phase (255) have been suggested to be the species that are actively adsorbed (249, 254). As multiple binding of solute $OH^-$ groups on a surface is possible, the preferential adsorption of these polymeric hydroxo complexes is facilitated (254). These larger molecular weight species can also be attracted to the surface as a result of van der Waals cohesive forces (252), and their adsorption may be responsible for charge reversal rather than only neutralizing the negative charge on cells and other surfaces.

The precipitation on the surface of a separate hydroxide phase rather than the specific adsorption of some particular aqueous species may be responsible for adsorption of the metals and their subsequent reversal of the charge of the adsorbent. Oxide adsorbents attain EPM values that are characteristic of the colloidal hydroxide of the adsorbate metal, supporting the concept of surface precipitation (244, 245, 253).

The adsorption of metals on surfaces of microbial and other cells shows similarities to the adsorption of metals on mineral surfaces, for example, reversal of charge at high pH values (e.g., Fig. 2.5). These similarities suggest that the mechanisms of adsorption that have been proposed for the adsorption of hydrolyzed metal ions on mineral surfaces may apply also to the adsorption of metal ions on cellular surfaces. The toxicity of most heavy metals varies with pH, and these variations in toxicity appear to be related, in part, to the different speciation forms of the metal that occur with changes in pH and to the relative ability of these speciation forms to bind to the cell surface and exert toxic effects (148, 149).

## 2.10  USE OF MICROBIAL CELLS IN THE LEACHING AND RECOVERY OF METALS

Microorganisms have been used in mineral exploration (8), the leaching of metals, for example, Cu and U, from ores and solid wastes, and to accumulate metals from solutions (256–258) (see Chapter 12). Bioprocessing of metals by microorganisms is an aspect of biotechnology that is being actively investigated (259, 260). In addition to the production of $H_2SO_4$, metabolic

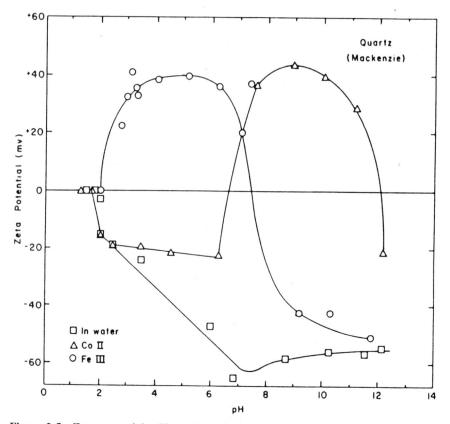

**Figure 2.5** Zeta potential–pH relationship for quartz in the presence of $4 \times 10^{-3}$ $M$ $Co(NO_3)_2$ and $6 \times 10^{-3}$ $M$ $FeCl_3$ (With the permission of the authors and Trans. A.I.M.E., Ref. 253).

products of microorganisms (e.g., methyl iodide that is produced by algae and fungi) can be used to solubilize various metals and metal sulfides (260–262). The use of mixed microbial cultures in metal recovery has been reviewed (263).

Microbial cells can also be used as biosorbents for heavy metals (86). For example, *S. cerevisiae* and *P. aeruginosa* accumulated U as $UO_2^{2+}$ and other hydrolysis products, such as $UO_2(OH)^+$, and the U could then be chemically removed from the cells. The chemical composition and structure of the cell walls of fungi were altered during growth in the presence of $Cu^{2+}$ and $Co^{2+}$, which enhanced the ability of the fungal cell walls to bind metals and suggests that chemically modified fungal cell walls could be used as biosorbents for the removal of heavy metal pollutants from the environment (99–101).

Waste products of coal and coke processing contain Ge (e.g., coal ash may contain 20–280 mg Ge kg$^{-1}$) (264), which can be recovered with microorganisms, as significant amounts of Ge were accumulated from the wastewaters by a mixed population of microorganisms from activated sludge (265). The biomass of *R. arrhizus* accumulated U, Th (266–268), and other cations (e.g., Cu, Zn, Cd) (105), and waste microbial biomass and *Penicillium chrysogenum* adsorbed $^{226}$Ra from solutions (269).

## 2.11  MICROORGANISMS AND CORROSION OF METALS

Numerous microorganisms (e.g., algae, fungi, aerobic and anaerobic bacteria) can cause corrosion of metals, but sulfate-reducing bacteria are the chief agents of anaerobic microbial corrosion (270–273). Sulfate-reducing bacteria settle on iron and steel pipes and accelerate their corrosion (274). *Arthrobacter siderocapsulatus*, a chemoorganotrophic bacterium, also settles on the surface of iron pipes and produces zones of differential oxygen tension that results in intensification of corrosion. This occurs as a result of a high rate of respiration and the presence of a mucus capsule (or sheath) on the bacterium (275).

## 2.12  CONCLUSIONS

Microorganisms interact with metals in various ways: many metals are essential to microorganisms, because they are electron acceptors or cofactors in enzymes, whereas other metals are toxic. Metals can be classified as hard and soft acids and bases (HSAB theory) or as Class A, Class B, and borderline metals. Essential metals are either hard acids or borderline metals, whereas nonessential metals are soft acids or Class B metals. Nonessential metals may inhibit growth and biochemical activities and cause morphological changes in microbes. The toxicity of heavy metals to microorganisms is affected by the physicochemical characteristics of the environment (e.g., pH, $E_h$, anionic and cationic composition, clay minerals, organic matter). Microorganisms have evolved several mechanisms of resistance (e.g., precipitation, volatilization) to the increasing levels of toxic metals that are increasingly being released into the environment. Heavy metals can also affect the electrokinetic properties of microorganisms (e.g., reversing the net negative charge on microorganisms to a net positive charge). Microbial cells exhibit colloidal characteristics similar to those of mineral oxides with respect to the adsorption of hydrolyzed metals. Hence theories that have been proposed for the mechanisms of adsorption of metals on inanimate oxide surfaces may also be applicable to the mechanism of adsorption of these metals on microbial cells. Microorganisms are being used increasingly in mining and metal recovery by utilizing microbial interactions with metals, such as indirect biotransformation of metals by extracellular microbial metabolites.

## ACKNOWLEDGMENTS

The preparation of this chapter and some of the studies discussed were made possible, in part, by grants R808329, R809067, CR812484, CR813431, and CR813650 from the U.S. Environmental Protection Agency, the latter three being cooperative agreements with the Corvallis Environmental Research Laboratory. The views expressed herein are not necessarily those of the agency.

## REFERENCES

1. H. Babich and G. Stotzky. Physicochemical factors that influence the toxicity of heavy metals and gaseous pollutants to microorganisms, CRC Crit. Rev. Microbiol., *8*, 99 (1980).

2. H. Babich and G. Stotzky. "Gaseous and heavy metal pollutants," in R. G. Burns and J. H. Slater, Eds., *Experimental Microbial Ecology*, Blackwell, Oxford, England, 1982, p. 631.

3. H. Babich and G. Stotzky. Developing standards for environmental toxicants: the need to consider abiotic environmental factors on microbe-mediated ecologic processes, Environ. Health Perspect., *49*, 247 (1983).

4. H. Babich and G. Stotzky. Heavy metal toxicity to microbe-mediated ecologic processes: a review and potential application to regulatory policies, Environ. Res., *36*, 111 (1985).

5. H. Babich and G. Stotzky. "Environmental factors affecting the utility of microbial assays for the toxicity and mutagenicity of chemical pollutants," in B. J. Dutka and G. Bitton, Eds., *Toxicity Testing Using Microorganisms*, CRC Press, Boca Raton, FL, 1986, p. 9.

6. G. Stotzky and H. Babich. "Mediation of the toxicity of pollutants to microbes by the physicochemical composition of the recipient environment," in D. Schlessinger, Ed., *Microbiology–1980*, American Society for Microbiology, Washington, DC, 1980, p. 352.

7. G. Stotzky and H. Babich. Physicochemical environmental factors influence the toxicity of heavy metals to microbes, Les Feuillets de l'U.E.R., Universite de Nancy, Nancy, France, *5*, 104 (1985).

8. G. Stotzky and H. Babich. "Physicochemical environment factors affect the response of microorganisms to heavy metals: implications for the application of microbiology to mineral exploration," in D. Carlisle, W. L. Berry, I. R. Kaplan, and J. Watterson, Eds., *Mineral Exploration: Biological Systems and Organic Matter*, Prentice-Hall, Englewood Cliffs, NJ, 1986, p. 238.

9. L. Friberg, T. Kjellstrom, G. Nordberg, and M. Piscator. "Cadmium," in L.

Friberg, G. F. Nordberg, and V. B. Vouk, Eds., *Handbook on the Toxicology of Metals*, Elsevier/North Holland Biomedical Press, New York, 1979, p. 355.

10. T. Norseth and M. Piscator. "Nickel," in L. Friberg, G. F. Nordberg, and V. B. Vouk, Eds., *Handbook on the Toxicology of Metals*, Elsevier/North-Holland Biomedical Press, New York, 1979, p. 541.

11. K. Tsuchiya. "Lead," in L. Friberg, G. F. Nordberg, and V. B. Vouk, Eds., *Handbook on the Toxicology of Metals*, Elsevier/North Holland Biomedical Press, New York, 1979, p. 451.

12. J. Berlin. "Mercury," in L. Friberg, G. F. Nordberg, and V. B. Vouk, Eds., *Handbook on the Toxicology of Metals*, Elsevier/North Holland Biomedical Press, New York, 1979, p. 503.

13. D. N. Lapedes. *Dictionary of Scientific and Technical Terms*. McGraw-Hill, New York, 1974, p. 674.

14. R. G. Pearson. Hard and soft acids and bases, J. Am. Chem. Soc., *85*, 3533 (1963).

15. R. G. Pearson. Hard and soft acids and bases, HSAB, Part 1, J. Chem. Educ., *45*, 581 (1968).

16. R. G. Pearson. Hard and soft acids and bases, Part II. Underlying theories, J. Chem. Educ., *45*, 643 (1968).

17. R. G. Pearson. Hard and soft acids and bases, Surv. Prog. Chem., *5*, 1 (1969).

18. R. G. Pearson. *Hard and Soft Acids and Bases*, Wiley, New York, 1973.

19. E. Nieboer and D. H. S. Richardson. The replacement of the nondescript term "heavy metals" by a biologically and chemically significant classification of metal ions, Environ. Pollut. (Ser. B), *1*, 3 (1980).

20. S. Ahrland, J. Chatt, and N. R. Davies. The relative affinities of ligand atoms for acceptor molecules and ions, Quart. Rev. Chem. Soc., *12*, 265 (1958).

21. A. Fiil and D. Branton. Changes in the plasma membrane of *Escherichia coli* during magnesium starvation, J. Bacteriol., *98*, 1320 (1969).

22. S. W. Rogers, H. E. Gilleland, Jr., and R. G. Eagon. Characterization of a protein–lipopolysaccharide complex released from cell walls of *Pseudomonas aeruginosa* by ethylenediaminetetraacetic acid, Can. J. Microbiol., *15*, 743 (1969).

23. H. E. Gilleland, Jr., J. D. Stinnett, and R. G. Eagon. Ultrastructural and chemical alteration of the cell envelope of *Pseudomonas aeruginosa*, associated with resistance to ethylenediaminetetraacetate resulting from growth in a $Mg^{2+}$-deficient medium, J. Bacteriol., *117*, 302 (1974).

24. R. T. Irvin, A. K. Chatterjee, K. E. Sanderson, and J. W. Costerton. Comparison of the cell envelope structure of a lipopolysaccharide-defective (heptose deficient) strain and a smooth strain of *Salmonella typhimurium*, J. Bacteriol., *124*, 930 (1975).

25. T. J. Beveridge and R. G. E. Murray. Superficial cell wall layers on *Spirillum* "Ordal" and their *in vitro* assembly, Can. J. Microbiol., *22*, 567 (1976).

26. T. J. Beveridge and R. G. E. Murray. Reassembly *in vitro* of the superficial cell wall components of *Spirillum putridiconchylium*, J. Ultrastruct. Res., *55*, 105 (1976).

27. F. L. A. Buckmire and R. G. E. Murray. The substructure and *in vitro* assembly of the outer, structured layer of *Spirillum serpens*, J. Bacteriol., *125*, 290 (1976).

28. R. Fontana, P. Canepari, and G. Satta. Alterations in peptidoglycan chemical composition associated with rod-to-sphere transition in a conditional mutant of *Klebsiella pneumoniae*, J. Bacteriol., *139*, 1028 (1979).

29. M. K. Rayman and R. A. MacLeod. Interaction of $Mg^{2+}$ with peptidoglycan and its relation to the prevention of lysis by a marine pseudomonad, J. Bacteriol., *122*, 650 (1975).

30. H. L. T. Mobley, A. L. Koch, R. J. Doyle, and U. N. Streips. Insertion and fate of the cell wall in *Bacillus subtilis*, J. Bacteriol., *158*, 169 (1984).

31. B. L. Vallee and D. D. Ulmer. Biochemical effects of mercury, cadmium and lead, Ann. Rev. Biochem., *41*, 91 (1972).

32. R. G. Pearson and R. J. Mawby. "The nature of metal-halogen bonds," in V. Gutman, Ed., *Halogen Chemistry*, Vol. 3, Academic, London, 1967, p. 55.

33. S. Ahrland. Thermodynamics of complex formation between hard and soft acceptors and donors, Struct. Bonding, *5*, 118 (1968).

34. M. W. Williams and J. E. Turner. Comments on softness parameters and metal ion toxicity, J. Inorg. Nucl. Chem., *43*, 1689 (1981).

35. M. W. Williams, J. D. Hoeschele, J. E. Turner, K. B. Jacobson, N. T. Christie, C. L. Paton, L. H. Smith, H. R. Witschi, and E. H. Lee. Chemical softness and acute metal toxicity in mice and *Drosophila*, Toxicol. Appl. Pharm., *63*, 461 (1982).

36. A. W. Hsie, R. L. Schenley, E.-L. Tan, S. W. Perdue, M. W. Williams, T. L. Hayden, and J. E. Turner. "The toxicity of sixteen metallic compounds in chinese hamster ovary cells: A comparison with mice and *Drosophila*," in A. M. Goldberg, Ed., *Acute Toxicity Testing*, Mary Ann Liebert Inc., New York, 1984, p. 117.

37. H. Babich, J. A. Puerner, and E. Borenfreund. *In vitro* cytotoxicity of metals to bluegill (BF-2) cells, Arch. Environ. Contam. Toxicol., *28*, 452 (1986).

38. M. M. Jones and W. K. Vaughn. HSAB theory and acute metal ion toxicity and detoxification processes, J. Inorg. Nucl. Chem., *40*, 2081 (1978).

39. F. W. Sunderman, Jr. "Metal carcinogenesis," in R. A. Goyer and M. A. Mehlman, Eds., *Advances in Modern Toxicology*, Vol. 1, Hemisphere Publishing Corp., Washington, DC, 1977, p. 257.

40. H. Babich, M. A. Devanas, and G. Stotzky. The mediation of mutagenicity and clastogenicity of heavy metals by physicochemical factors, Environ. Res., *37*, 253 (1985).

41. D. H. S. Richardson, E. Nieboer, P. Lavoie, and D. Padovan. The role of metal-ion binding in modifying the toxic effects of sulphur dioxide on the lichen *Umbilicaria muhlenbergii*. II. $^{14}$C-fixation studies, New Phytol., *82*, 633 (1979).

42. E. Nieboer, D. H. S. Richardson, P. Lavoie, and D. Padovan. The role of metal-ion binding in modifying the toxic effects of sulphur dioxide on the lichen *Umbilicaria muhlenbergii*. I. Potassium efflux studies, New Phytol., *82*, 621 (1979).

43. H. Irving and R. J. P. Williams. Order of stability of metal complexes, Nature, *162*, 746 (1948).

44. R. H. Crist, K. Oberholser, N. Shank, and M. Nguyen. Nature of bonding between metallic ions and algal cell walls, Environ. Sci. Technol., *15*, 1212 (1981).

45. H. Babich and G. Stotzky. Toxicity of nickel to microbes: environmental aspects, Adv. Appl. Microbiol., *29*, 195 (1983).

46. L. Kiremidjian-Schumacher and G. Stotzky. Influence of mono- and multivalent cations on the electrokinetic properties of normal human and Burkitt lymphoma cells, Experientia, *33*, 312 (1976).

47. J. Ashida. Adaptation of fungi to metal toxicants, Ann. Rev. Phytopath., *3*, 153 (1965).

48. H. Babich and G. Stotzky. Air pollution and microbial ecology, CRC Crit. Rev. Environ. Contr., *4*, 353 (1974).

49. H. Babich and G. Stotzky. Atmospheric sulfur compounds and microbes, Environ. Res., *15*, 405 (1978).

50. H. Babich and G. Stotzky. "Influence of chemical speciation on the toxicity of heavy metals to the microbiota," in J. O. Nriagu, Ed., *Aquatic Toxicology*, Wiley, New York, 1983, p. 1.

51. G. Stotzky and H. Babich. "Physicochemical factors that affect the toxicity of heavy metals to microbes in aquatic habitats," in R. R. Colwell and J. Foster, Eds., *Proceedings of the ASM Conference, Aquatic Microbial Ecology*, University of Maryland Sea Grant Publication, College Park, MD, 1980, p. 181.

52. A. Jernelov and A. L. Martin. Ecological implications of metal metabolism by microorganisms, Ann. Rev. Microbiol., *29*, 61 (1975).

53. H. L. Ehrlich. "How microbes cope with heavy metals, arsenic, and antimony in their environment," in D. J. Kushner, Ed., *Microbial Life in Extreme Environments*, Academic, London, 1978, p. 381.

54. M. Gadd and A. J. Griffiths. Microorganisms and heavy metal toxicity, Microb. Ecol., *4*, 303 (1978).

55. A. O. Summers and S. Silver. Microbial transformation of metals, Ann. Rev. Microbiol., *32*, 637 (1978).

56. J. T. Trevors, G. W. Stratton, and G. M. Gadd. Cadmium transport, resistance, and toxicity in bacteria, algae, and fungi, Can. J. Bacteriol., *32*, 447 (1986).

57. H. Babich and G. Stotzky. Toxicity of zinc to fungi, bacteria, and coliphages: influence of chloride ions, Appl. Environ. Microbiol., *36*, 904 (1978).

58. M. L. Failla. "Zinc: functions and transport in microorganisms," in E. D. Weinberg, Ed., *Microorganisms and Minerals*, Dekker, New York, 1977, p. 151.

59. T. Duxbury. "Ecological aspects of heavy metal responses in microorganisms," in K. C. Marshall, Ed., *Advances in Microbial Ecology*, Vol. 8, Plenum, New York, 1985, p. 185.

60. H. Babich, D. L. Davis, and J. Trauberman. Environmental quality criteria: some considerations, Environ. Management, *5*, 191 (1981).

61. H. Babich, R. J. F. Bewley, and G. Stotzky. Application of the "ecologic dose" concept to the impact of heavy metals on some microbe-mediated ecologic processes in soil. Arch. Environ. Contam. Toxicol., *12*, 421 (1983).

62. H. Babich and G. Stotzky. Nickel toxicity to fungi: Influence of environmental factors, Ecotoxicol. Environ. Safety, 6, 577 (1982).

63. H. Babich and G. Stotzky. "Physicochemical factors of natural reservoirs affect the transformation and exchange of heavy metals toxic to microbes," in R. O. Hallberg, Ed., *Environmental Biogeochemistry*, Proceedings of the Fifth International Symposium on Environmental Biogeochemistry, Ecol. Bull., Vol. 35, Ecological Bulletins Publishing House, Stockholm, 1983, p. 315.

64. S. Hepinstall, A. R. Archibald, and J. Baddiley. Teichoic acids and membrane function in bacteria. Selective destruction of teichoic acids reduces the ability of bacterial cell walls to bind $Mg^{2+}$ ions, Nature (London), 225, 519 (1970).

65. P. A. Lambert, I. C. Hancock, and J. Baddiley. The interaction of magnesium ions with teichoic acid, Biochem. J., 149, 519 (1975).

66. P. A. Lambert, I. C. Hancock, and J. Baddiley. Influence of alanyl ester residues on the binding of magnesium ions to teichoic acids, Biochem. J., 151, 671 (1975).

67. T. J. Beveridge and R. G. E. Murray. Uptake and retention of metals by cell walls of *Bacillus subtilis*, J. Bacteriol., 127, 1502 (1976).

68. T. J. Beveridge and R. G. E. Murray. Sites of metal deposition in the cell wall of *Bacillus subtilis*, J. Bacteriol., 141, 876 (1980).

69. R. E. Marquis, K. Mayzel, and E. L. Cartensen. Cation exchange in cell walls of gram-positive bacteria, Can. J. Microbiol., 22, 975 (1976).

70. T. J. Beveridge. The response of cell walls of *Bacillus subtilis* to metals and to electron microscopic stains, Can. J. Microbiol., 24, 89 (1978).

71. L.-T. Ou and R. E. Marquis. Coccal cell wall compactness and the swelling action of denaturants, Can. J. Microbiol., 18, 623 (1972).

72. C. W. Einolf, Jr. and E. L. Cartensen. Passive electrical properties of microorganisms V. Low-frequency dielectric dispersion of bacteria, Biophys. J., 13, 8 (1973).

73. T. M. McCalla. Physicochemical behavior of soil bacteria in relation to the soil colloid, J. Bacteriol., 40, 33 (1940).

74. T. J. Beveridge. Ultrastructure, chemistry and function of the bacterial wall, Int. Rev. Cytol., 72, 229 (1981).

75. B. D. Hoyle and T. J. Beveridge. Binding of metallic ions to the outer membrane of *Escherichia coli*, Appl. Environ. Microbiol., 46, 749 (1983).

76. L. Leive. Studies on the permeability change produced in coliform bacteria by ethylenediaminetetraacetate, J. Biol. Chem., 243, 2373 (1968).

77. H. E. Gilleland, Jr., J. D. Stinnett, and R. G. Eagon. Ultrastructural and chemical alteration of the cell envelope of *Pseudomonas aeruginosa*, associated with resistance to ethylenediaminetetraacetate resulting from growth in a $Mg^{2+}$-deficient medium, J. Bacteriol., 117, 302 (1974).

78. L. Leive. A non-specific increase in permeability in *Escherichia coli* produced by EDTA, Proc. Natl. Acad. Sci. U.S.A., 53, 745 (1965).

79. L. Leive. "Toward a study of supramolecular structure and function," in L. Leive, Ed., *Bacterial Membranes and Walls*, Dekker, New York, 1973, p. xi.

80. S. W. Rogers, H. E. Gilleland, Jr., and R. G. Eagon. Characterization of a

protein–lipopolysaccharide complex released from cell walls of *Pseudomonas aeruginosa* by ethylenediaminetetraacetic acid, Can. J. Microbiol., *15*, 743 (1969).

81. H. E. Gilleland, Jr., J. D. Stinnett, I. L. Roth, and R. G. Eagon. Freeze-etch study of *Pseudomonas aeruginosa*: localization within the cell wall of an ethylenediaminetetraacetate-extractable component, J. Bacteriol., *113*, 417 (1973).

82. T. M. McCalla. Cation adsorption by bacteria, J. Bacteriol., *40*, 23 (1940).

83. J. J. Doyle, R. T. Marshall, and W. H. Pfander. Effects of cadmium on the growth and uptake of cadmium by microorganisms, Appl. Microbiol., *29*, 562 (1975).

84. E. Kurek, J. Czaban, and J.-M. Bollag. Sorption of cadmium by microorganisms in competition with other soil constituents, Appl. Environ. Microbiol., *43*, 1011 (1982).

85. J.-M. Bollag and M. Duszota. Effect of the physiological state of microbial cells on cadmium sorption, Arch. Environ. Contam. Toxicol., *13*, 265 (1984).

86. G. W. Strandberg, S. E. Shumate, and J. R. Parrott, Jr. Microbial cells as biosorbents for heavy metals: Accumulation of uranium by *Saccharomyces cerevisiae* and *Pseudomonas aeruginosa*, Appl. Environ. Microbiol., *41*, 237 (1981).

87. G. N. Flatau, R. L. Clement, and M. J. Gauthier. Cadmium binding sites on a marine pseudomonad, Chemosphere, *14*, 1409 (1985).

88. C. L. Haber, T. G. Tornabene, and R. K. Skogerboe. Regulation of bacterial abstraction of lead by cell surface charge and chemical equilibria, Chemosphere, *9*, 21 (1980).

89. T. Horikoshi, A. Nakajima, and T. Sakaguchi. Studies on the accumulation of heavy metal elements in biological systems. XIX. Accumulation of uranium by microorganisms, Eur. J. Appl. Microbiol. Biotechnol., *12*, 90 (1981).

90. B. Klapcinska and J. Chmielowski. Binding of germanium to *Pseudomonas putida* cells, Appl. Environ. Microbiol., *51*, 1144 (1986).

91. J. Chmielowski and B. Klapcinska. Bioaccumulation of germanium by *Pseudomonas putida* in the presence of two selected substrates, Appl. Environ. Microbiol., *51*, 1099 (1986).

92. T. J. Beveridge, J. D. Meloche, W. S. Fyfe, and R. G. E. Murray. Diagenesis of metals chemically complexed to bacteria: Laboratory formation of metal phosphates, sulfides, and organic condensates in artificial sediments, Appl. Environ. Microbiol., *45*, 1094 (1983).

93. R. T. Coughlin, S. Tonsager, and E. J. McGroarty. Quantitation of metal cations bound to membranes and extracted lipopolysaccharide of *Escherichia coli*, Biochemistry, *22*, 2002 (1983).

94. F. G. Ferris and T. J. Beveridge. Binding of a paramagnetic metal cation to *Escherichia coli* K-12 outer membrane vesicles, FEMS Microbiol. Lett., *24*, 43 (1984).

95. E. M. Sonnenfeld, T. J. Beveridge, and R. J. Doyle. Asymmetric distribution of charge in the cell wall of *Bacillus subtilis*, Abstr. Ann. Mtng. ASM, 1985, p. 193.

96. E. M. Sonnenfeld, T. J. Beveridge, and R. J. Doyle. Discontinuity of charge on cell wall poles of *Bacillus subtilis*, Can. J. Microbiol., *31*, 875 (1985).

97. M. W. Mittelman and G. G. Geesey. Copper-binding characteristics of exopolymers from a freshwater-sediment bacterium, Appl. Environ. Microbiol., *49*, 846 (1984).

98. T. Rudd, R. M. Sterritt, and J. N. Lester. Formation and stability constants of complexes formed between heavy metals and bacterial extracellular polymers, Water Res., *18*, 379 (1984).

99. G. Venkateswerlu and G. Stotzky. Copper and cobalt alter the cell wall composition of *Cunninghamella blakesleeana*, Can. J. Microbiol., *32*, 654 (1986).

100. G. Venkateswerlu and G. Stotzky. Morphological, ultrastructural, and chemical changes induced in *Cunninghamella blakesleeana* by copper and cobalt (1988) (in preparation).

101. G. Venkateswerlu and G. Stotzky. Binding of metals by cell walls of *Cunninghamella blakesleeana* grown in the presence of copper or cobalt (1988) (in preparation).

102. A. Garcia-Toledo, H. Babich, and G. Stotzky. Training of *Rhizopus stolonifer* and *Cunninghamella blakesleeana* to copper: cotolerance to cadmium, cobalt, nickel, and lead, Can. J. Microbiol., *31*, 485 (1985).

103. M. Galun, P. Keller, D. Malki, H. Feldstein, E. Galun, S. M. Siegel, and B. Z. Siegel. Removal of uranium(VI) from solution by fungal biomass and fungal wall-related biopolymers, Science, *219*, 285 (1983).

104. M. Galun, E. Galun, B. Z. Siegel, P. Keller, H. Lehr, and S. M. Siegel. Removal of metal ions from aqueous solutions by *Penicillium* biomass: kinetic and uptake parameters, Water Air Soil Poll., *33*, 359 (1987).

105. J. M. Tobin, D. G. Cooper, and R. J. Neufeld. Uptake of metal ions by *Rhizopus arrhizus* biomass, Appl. Environ. Microbiol., *47*, 821 (1984).

106. S. Siegel, P. Keller, M. Galun, H. Lehr, B. Siegel, and E. Galun. Biosorption of lead and chromium by *Penicillium* preparations, Water Air Soil Poll., *27*, 69 (1986).

107. G. M. Gadd and C. White. Copper uptake by *Penicillium ochro-chloron*: Influence of pH on toxicity and demonstration of energy-dependent copper influx using protoplasts, J. Gen. Microbiol., *131*, 1875 (1985).

108. H. Brunnert and F. Zadrazil. The translocation of mercury and cadmium into the fruiting bodies of six higher fungi. A comparative study on species specificity in five lignocellulolytic fungi and the cultivated mushroom *Agaricus bisporus*, Eur. J. Appl. Microbiol. Biotechnol., *17*, 358 (1983).

109. E. Nieboer, P. Lavoie, R. L. P. Sasseville, K. J. Puckett, and D. H. S. Richardson. Cation-exchange equilibrium and mass balance in the lichen *Umbilicaria muhlenbergii*, Can. J. Bot., *54*, 720 (1975).

110. A. Rothstein. Cell membrane as a site of action of heavy metals, Fed. Proc., *18*, 1026 (1959).

111. M. Itoh, M. Yuasa, and T. Kobayashi. Adsorption of metal ions on yeast cells at varied cell concentrations, Plant Cell Physiol., *16*, 1167 (1975).

112. H. Passow and A. Rothstein. The binding of $Hg^{2+}$ by the yeast cell in relation to changes in permeability, J. Gen. Physiol., *43*, 621 (1960).

113. G. F. Fuhrmann and A. Rothstein. The transport of zinc, cobalt and nickel into yeast cells, Biochim. Biophys. Acta, *163*, 325 (1968).

114. M. L. Failla, C. D. Benedict, and E. D. Weinberg. Accumulation and storage of zinc by *Candida utilis*, J. Gen. Microbiol., *94*, 23 (1976).

115. P. R. Norris and D. P. Kelly. Accumulation of cadmium and cobalt by *Saccharomyces cerevisiae*, J. Gen. Microbiol., *99*, 317 (1977).

116. J. Stary and K. Kratzer. The cumulation of toxic metals on alga, J. Environ. Anal. Chem., *12*, 65 (1982).

117. T. Skowronski and M. Przytocka-Jusiak. Cadmium removal by green alga *Stichococcus bacillaris*, Chemosphere, *15*, 77 (1986).

118. A. Nakajima, T. Horikoshi, and T. Sakaguchi. Distribution and chemical state of heavy metal ions absorbed by *Chlorella* cells, Agric. Biol. Chem., *45*, 903 (1981).

119. B. A. Hart, P. E. Bertram, and B. D. Scaife. Cadmium transport by *Chlorella pyrenoidosa*, Environ. Res., *18*, 327 (1979).

120. K. Drbal, K. Veber, and J. Zahradnik. Toxicity and accumulation of copper and cadmium in the alga *Scenedesmus obliquus* LH., Bull. Environ. Contam. Toxicol., *34*, 904 (1985).

121. H. J. Geisweid and W. Urbach. Sorption of cadmium by the green microalgae *Chlorella vulgaris, Ankistrodesmus braunii*, and *Eremosphaera viridis*, Z. Pflanzenphysiol. Bd., *109*, S127 (1983).

122. P. Van Cutsem and C. Gillet. A thermodynamic study of $Cu^{++}$–$Zn^{++}$ ion exchange in the *Nitella flexilis* cell wall, Plant Soil, *62*, 367 (1981).

123. P. Van Cutsem and C. Gillet. Activity coefficients and selectivity values of $Cu^{++}$, $Zn^{++}$, and $Ca^{++}$ ions adsorbed in the *Nitella flexilis* L. cell wall during triangular ion exchanges, J. Exp. Bot., *33*, 847 (1982).

124. T. Sakaguchi, A. Nakajima, and T. Horikoshi. Studies on the accumulation of heavy metal elements in biological systems. XVIII. Accumulation of molybdenum by green microalgae, Eur. J. Appl. Microbiol. Biotechnol., *12*, 84 (1981).

125. A. Nakijima, T. Horikoshi, and T. Sakaguchi. Studies on the accumulation of heavy metal elements in biological systems. XVII. Selective accumulation of heavy metal ions by *Chlorella regularis*, Eur. J. Appl. Microbiol. Biotechnol., *12*, 76 (1981).

126. J. B. Neilands. "Microbial iron transport compounds (siderophores)," in W. F. Anderson and M. C. Hiller, Eds., *Development of Iron Chelators for Clinical Use*, National Institutes of Health, Bethesda, MD, 1973, p. 5.

127. J. B. Neilands. Microbial envelope proteins related to iron, Ann. Rev. Microbiol., *36*, 285 (1982).

128. T. J. Beveridge and S. F. Koval. Binding of metals to cell envelopes of *Escherichia coli* K-12, Appl. Environ. Microbiol., *42*, 325 (1981).

129. T. J. Beveridge, C. W. Forsberg, and R. J. Doyle. Major sites of metal binding in *Bacillus licheniformis* walls, J. Bacteriol., *150*, 1438 (1982).

130. F. G. Ferris and T. J. Beveridge. Functions of bacterial cell surface structures, BioScience, *35*, 172 (1985).

131. F. G. Ferris and T. J. Beveridge. Site specificity of metallic ion binding in *Escherichia coli* K-12 lipopolysaccharide, Can. J. Microbiol., *32*, 52 (1986).

132. G. Bitton and V. Freihofer. Influence of extracellular polysaccharides on the toxicity of copper and cadmium toward *Klebsiella aerogenes*, Microb. Ecol., *4*, 119 (1978).

133. T. R. Cassity and B. J. Kolodziej. Role of the capsule produced by *Bacillus megaterium* ATCC 19213 in the accumulation of metallic cations, Microbios, *41*, 117 (1984).

134. G. Stotzky. "Influence of soil mineral colloids on metabolic processes, growth, adhesion, and ecology of microbes and viruses," in P. M. Huang and M. Schnitzer, Eds., *Interaction of Soil Minerals with Natural Organics and Microbes*, Soil Science Society of America, Madison, WI, 1986, p. 305.

135. F. M. Patrick and M. W. Loutit. Passage of metals in effluents, through bacteria to higher organisms, Water Res., *10*, 699 (1976).

136. P. Doelman, G. Nieboer, J. Schrooten, and M. Visser. Antagonistic and synergistic toxic effects of Pb and Cd in a simple food chain: nematodes feeding on bacteria or fungi, Bull. Environ. Contam. Toxicol., *32*, 717 (1984).

137. A. Zirino and S. Yamamoto. A pH-dependent model for the chemical speciation of copper, zinc, cadmium, and lead in seawater, Limnol. Oceanogr., *17*, 661 (1972).

138. H. C. H. Hahne and W. Kroontje. The simultaneous effect of pH and chloride concentrations upon mercury (II) as a pollutant, Soil Sci. Am. Proc., *37*, 838 (1973).

139. H. C. H. Hahne and W. Kroontje. Significance of pH and chloride concentration on behavior of heavy metal pollutants: mercury (II), cadmium (II), zinc (II), and lead (II), J. Environ. Qual., *2*, 444 (1973).

140. H. Babich and G. Stotzky. Sensitivity of various bacteria, including actinomycetes, and fungi to cadmium and the influence of pH on sensitivity, Appl. Environ. Microbiol., *33*, 681 (1977).

141. H. Babich and G. Stotzky. Effects of cadmium on the biota: influence of environmental factors, Adv. Appl. Microbiol., *23*, 55 (1978).

142. H. Babich and G. Stotzky. Differential toxicities of mercury to bacteria and bacteriophages in sea and in lake water, Can. J. Microbiol., *25*, 1252 (1979).

143. J. O. Leckie. Conceptual model for metal–ligand surface interactions during adsorption, Environ. Sci. Tech., *15*, 1050 (1981).

144. H. Farrah and W. F. Pickering. The effect of pH and ligands on the sorption of heavy metal ions by cellulose, Aust. J. Chem., *31*, 1501 (1978).

145. H. Babich and G. Stotzky. Further studies on environmental factors that modify the toxicity of nickel to microbes, Regul. Toxicol. Pharmacol., *3*, 82 (1983).

146. H. Korkeala and T. J. Pekkanen. The effect of pH and potassium phosphate buffer on the toxicity of cadmium for bacteria, Acta Vet. Scand., *19*, 93 (1978).

147. J. F. Gipps and B. A. W. Coller. Effect of physical and culture conditions on uptake of cadmium by *Chlorella pyrenoidosa*, Aust. J. Mar. Freshwater Res., *31*, 747 (1980).

148. H. Babich and G. Stotzky. Nickel toxicity to microbes: effect of pH and implications for acid rain, Environ. Res., *29*, 335 (1982).

149. H. Babich and G. Stotzky. Temperature, pH, salinity, hardness, and particu-

lates mediate nickel toxicity to eubacteria, an actinomycete, and yeasts in lake, simulated estuarine, and sea waters, Aquat. Toxicol., *3*, 195 (1983).

150. H. Babich and G. Stotzky. Toxicity of nickel to microorganisms in soil: Influence of some physicochemical characteristics, Environ. Pollut., *29A*, 303 (1982).

151. R. O. Richter and T. L. Theis. "Nickel speciation in a soil/water system," in J. O. Nriagu, Ed., *Nickel in the Environment*, Wiley, New York, 1980, p. 189.

152. G. M. Gadd and A. J. Griffiths. Influence of pH on toxicity and uptake of copper in *Aureobasidium pullulans*, Trans. Br. Mycol. Soc., *75*, 91 (1980).

153. E. Steemann Nielsen and L. Kamp-Neilsen. Influence of deleterious concentrations of copper on the growth of *Chlorella pyrenoidosa*, Physiol. Plant., *23*, 828 (1970).

154. E. Steemann Nielsen, L. Kamp-Nielsen, and W. Wium-Anderson. The effect of deleterious concentrations of copper on the photosynthesis of *Chlorella pyrenoidosa*, Physiol. Plant., *22*, 1121 (1969).

155. J. G. Horsfall. *Principles of Fungicidal Action*, Chronica Botanica Co., Waltham, MA, 1956.

156. W. D. Schecher and C. T. Driscoll. Interactions of copper and lead with *Nostoc muscorum*, Water Air Soil Poll., *24*, 85 (1985).

157. J. W. Hargreaves and B. A. Whitton. Effect of pH on tolerance of *Hormidium rivulare* to zinc and copper, Oecologia, *26*, 235 (1977).

158. P. J. Say and B. A. Whitton. Influence of zinc on lotic plants. II. Environmental effects of zinc to *Hormidium rivulare*, Freshwater Biol., *7*, 377 (1977).

159. L. C. Rai, J. P. Gaur, and H. D. Kumar. Protective effects of certain environmental factors on the toxicity of zinc, mercury, and methylmercury to *Chlorella vulgaris*, Environ. Res., *25*, 250 (1981).

160. M. D. Baker, C. I. Mayfield, W. E. Inniss, and P. T. S. Wong. Toxicity of pH, heavy metals, and bisulfite to a freshwater green alga, Chemosphere, *12*, 35 (1983).

161. J. Stary, B. Havlik, K. Kratzer, J. Prasilova, and J. Hanusova. Cumulation of zinc, cadmium, and mercury on the alga *Scenedesmus obliquus*, Acta Hydrochim. Hydrobiol., *11*, 401 (1983).

162. T. Skowronski. Adsorption of cadmium on green microalga *Stichococcus bacillaris*, Chemosphere, *15*, 69 (1986).

163. H. Babich, M. Schiffenbauer, and G. Stotzky. Comparative toxicity of trivalent and hexavalent chromium to fungi, Bull. Environ. Contam. Toxicol., *28*, 452 (1982).

164. H. Babich and G. Stotzky. Influence of chloride ions on the toxicity of cadmium to fungi, Zbl. Bakt. Hyg., I. Abt. Orig., *C3*, 421 (1982).

165. K. H. Wong, K. Y. Chan, and S. L. Ng. Cadmium uptake by the unicellular green alga *Chlorella salina* Cu-I from culture media with high salinity, Chemosphere, *8*, 887 (1979).

166. M. J. Gauthier and G. N. Flatau. Etude de l'accumulation du cadmium par une bacterie marine en fonction des conditions de cultures, Chemosphere, *9*, 713 (1980).

167. H. Babich and G. Stotzky. Abiotic factors affecting the toxicity of lead to fungi, Appl. Environ. Microbiol., *38*, 506 (1979).

168. H. Babich and G. Stotzky. Components of water hardness that reduce the toxicity of nickel to fungi, Microbios Lett., *18*, 17 (1981).

169. B. C. Rana and H. D. Kumar. The toxicity of zinc to *Chlorella vulgaris* and *Plectonema boryanum* and its protection by phosphate, Phykos, *13*, 60 (1974).

170. F. H. A. Shehata and B. A. Whitton. Zinc tolerance in strains of the blue-green alga *Anacystis nidulans*, Br. Phycol. J., *17*, 5 (1982).

171. H. Schulze and J. J. Brand. Lead toxicity and phosphate deficiency in *Chlamydomonas*, Plant Physiol., *62*, 727 (1978).

172. H. Babich and G. Stotzky. Influence of pH on inhibition of bacteria, fungi, and coliphages by bisulfite and sulfite, Environ. Res., *15*, 513 (1978).

173. J. S. Kuwabara. Phosphorus–zinc interactive effects on growth by *Selenastrum capricornutum* (Chlorophyta), Environ. Sci. Technol., *19*, 417 (1985).

174. H. Babich and G. Stotzky. Nickel toxicity to estuarine/marine fungi and its amelioration by magnesium in sea water, Water Air Soil Poll., *19*, 193 (1983).

175. M. Webb. Interrelationships between the utilization of magnesium and the uptake of other bivalent cations by bacteria, Biochim. Biophys. Acta, *222*, 428 (1970).

176. M. Webb. The mechanism of acquired resistance to $Co^{2+}$ and $Ni^{2+}$ in Gram-positive and Gram-negative bacteria, Biochim. Biophys. Acta, *222*, 440 (1970).

177. P. H. Abelson and E. Aldous. Ion antagonisms in microorganisms: interference of normal magnesium metabolism by nickel, cobalt, cadmium, and manganese, J. Bacteriol., *60*, 401 (1950).

178. H. Babich, M. Schiffenbauer, and G. Stotzky. Sensitivity of coliphage T1 to nickel in fresh and salt waters, Curr. Microbiol., *8*, 101 (1983).

179. F. Laborey and J. Lavollay. Sur la nature des antagonismes responsables de l'interaction des ions $Mg^{++}$, $Cd^{++}$, et $Zn^{++}$ dans la croissance d'*Aspergillus niger*, C. R. Acad. Sci. (Paris), *276D*, 529 (1973).

180. M. A. Ainsworth, C. P. Tompsett, and A. C. R. Dean. Cobalt and nickel sensitivity and tolerance in *Klebsiella pneumoniae*, Microbios, *27*, 175 (1980).

181. F. Laborey and J. Lavollay. Sur l'antitoxicite du calcium et du magnesium a l'egard du cadmium dans la croissance d'*Aspergillus niger*, C. R. Acad. Sci. (Paris), *284D*, 639 (1977).

182. J. G. Reuter, K. T. O'Reilly, and R. R. Petersen. Indirect aluminum toxicity to the green alga *Scenedesmus* through increased cupric ion activity, Environ. Sci. Technol., *21*, 435 (1987).

183. Environmental Protection Agency. *Quality Criteria for Water*. Washington, DC, 1976.

184. H. Babich and G. Stotzky. Reductions in the toxicity of cadmium to microorganisms by clay minerals, Appl. Environ. Microbiol., *33*, 696 (1977).

185. H. Babich and G. Stotzky. Effect of cadmium on fungi and on interactions between fungi and bacteria in soil: influence of clay minerals and pH, Appl. Environ. Microbiol., *33*, 1059 (1977).

186. K. Debosz, H. Babich, and G. Stotzky. Toxicity of lead to soil respiration:

mediation by clay minerals, humic acids, and compost, Bull. Environ. Contam. Toxicol., *35*, 517 (1985).

187. R. J. F. Bewley and G. Stotzky. Effects of cadmium and zinc on microbial activity in soil: influence of clay minerals. Part I: Metals added individually, Sci. Total Environ., *31*, 41 (1983).

188. R. J. F. Bewley and G. Stotzky. Effects of cadmium and zinc on microbial activity in soil: influence of clay minerals. Part II: Metals added simultaneously, Sci. Total Environ., *31*, 57 (1983).

189. H. E. Allen, R. H. Hall, and T. D. Brisbin. Metal speciation: Effects on aquatic toxicity, Environ. Sci. Technol., *14*, 441 (1980).

190. G. S. Canterford and D. R. Canterford. Toxicity of heavy metals to the marine diatom *Ditylum brightwellii* (West) Grunow: correlation between toxicity and metal speciation, J. Mar. Biol. Assoc., U.K., *60*, 227 (1980).

191. J. M. Gentile, K. Hyde, and J. Schubert. Chromium genotoxity as influenced by complexation and rate effects, Toxicol. Lett., *7*, 439 (1981).

192. D. Hongve, O. K. Skogheim, A. Hindar, and H. Abrahamsen. Effects of heavy metals in combination with NTA, humic acid, and suspended sediment on natural phytoplankton photosynthesis, Bull. Environ. Contam. Toxicol., *25*, 594 (1980).

193. W. F. Jardim and H. W. Pearson. Copper toxicity to cyanobacteria and its dependence on extracellular ligand concentration and degradation, Microb. Ecol., *11*, 139 (1985).

194. C. M. G. Van den Berg, P. T. S. Wong, and Y. K. Chau. Measurement of complexing materials excreted from algae and their ability to ameliorate copper toxicity, J. Fish Res. Bd., Can. *36*, 901 (1979).

195. S. Ramamoorthy and D. J. Kushner. Binding of mercuric and other heavy metal ions by microbial growth media, Microb. Ecol., *2*, 162 (1975).

196. C. Szeto and D. Nyberg. The effect of temperature on copper tolerance of *Paramecium*, Bull. Environ. Contam. Toxicol., *21*, 131 (1979).

197. J. Huisman, H. J. G. Ten Hoopen, and A. Fuchs. The effect of temperature upon the toxicity of mercuric chloride in *Scenedesmus acutus*, Environ. Pollut., *22A*, 33 (1980).

198. J. S. Thayer and F. E. Brinckman. "The biological methylation of metals and metalloids," in F. G. A. Stone and R. West, Eds., *Advances in Organometallic Chemistry*, Vol. 20, Academic, New York, 1982, p. 313.

199. J. M. Wood and H-K. Wang. Microbial resistance to heavy metals, Environ. Sci. Technol., *17*, 582A (1983).

200. J. B. Robinson and O. H. Tuovinen. Mechanisms of microbial resistance and detoxification of mercury and organomercury compounds. Physiological, biochemical, and genetic analyses, Microbiol. Rev., *48*, 95 (1984).

201. G. J. Olson, W. P. Iverson, and F. E. Brinckman. Volatilization of mercury by *Thiobacillus ferrooxidans*, Curr. Microbiol., *5*, 115 (1981).

202. W. P. Iverson and F. E. Brinckman. "Microbial metabolism of metals," in R. Mitchell, Ed., *Water Pollution Microbiology*, Vol. 2, Wiley, New York, 1978, p. 201.

203. R. W. Olafson, K. Abel, and R. G. Sim. Procaryotic metallothionein: Prelim-

inary characterization of a blue-green alga heavy metal-binding protein, Biochem. Biophys. Res. Commun., *89*, 36 (1979).

204. W. N. Kuo. Partial purification and characterization of the cation-binding protein and megamodulin from *E. coli*, Microbios, *37*, 189 (1983).

205. W. R. Blair, J. A. Jackson, G. J. Olson, F. E. Brinckman, and W. P. Iverson. "Biotransformations of tin," in W. H. O. Ernst, Ed., *Proceedings International Conference Heavy Metals in the Environment, Amsterdam*, CEP Consultants, Edinburgh, 1981, p. 235.

206. M. Fukami, S. Yamazaki, and S. Toda. Distribution of copper in the cells of a heavy metal tolerant fungus, *Penicillium ochro-chloron*, cultured in concentrated copper medium, Agric. Biol. Chem., *47*, 1367 (1983).

207. Z. Tynecka, Z. Gos, and J. Zajac. Energy-dependent efflux of cadmium coded by a plasmid resistance determinant in *Staphylococcus aureus*, J. Bacteriol., *147*, 313 (1981).

208. Z. Tynecka, Z. Gos, and J. Zajac. Reduced cadmium transport determined by a resistance plasmid in *Staphylococcus aureus*, J. Bacteriol., *147*, 305 (1981).

209. R. A. Laddaga, R. Bessen, and S. Silver. Cadmium-resistant mutant of *Bacillus subtilis* 168 with reduced cadmium transport, J. Bacteriol., *162*, 1106 (1985).

210. B. E. Burke and R. M. Pfister. Cadmium transport by a $Cd^{2+}$-sensitive and a $Cd^{2+}$-resistant strain of *Bacillus subtilis*, Can. J. Microbiol., *32*, 539 (1986).

211. R. A. Laddaga and S. Silver. Cadmium uptake in *Escherichia coli* K-12, J. Bacteriol., *162*, 1100 (1985).

212. R. W. Olafson, S. Loya, and R. G. Sim. Physiological parameters of prokaryotic metallothionein induction, Biochem. Biophys. Res. Commun., *95*, 1495 (1980).

213. M. B. Khazaeli and R. S. Mitra. Cadmium-binding component in *Escherichia coli* during accommodation to low levels of this ion, Appl. Environ. Microbiol., *41*, 46 (1981).

214. I. Mahler, H. S. Levinson, Y. Wang, and H. O. Halvorson. Cadmium- and mercury resistance *Bacillus* strains from a salt marsh and from Boston Harbor, Appl. Environ. Microbiol., *52*, 1293 (1986).

215. T. Duxbury and B. Bicknell. Metal-tolerant bacterial populations from natural and metal-polluted soils, Soil Biol. Biochem., *15*, 243 (1983).

216. D. J. Shaw. *Electrophoresis*, Academic, New York, 1969.

217. D. V. Richmond and D. J. Fisher. The electrophoretic mobility of microorganisms, Adv. Microb. Physiol., *9*, 1 (1973).

218. A. M. James. Molecular aspects of biological surfaces, Chem. Soc. Rev., *8*, 389 (1979).

219. A. M. James. The electrical properties and topochemistry of bacterial cells, Adv. Colloid Interface Sci., *15*, 171 (1982).

220. T. Santoro and G. Stotzky. Sorption between microorganisms and clay minerals as determined by the electrical sensing zone particle analyzer, Can. J. Microbiol., *14*, 299 (1968).

221. K. C. Marshall. *Interfaces in Microbial Ecology*, Harvard University Press, Cambridge, MA, 1976.

222. G. Stotzky. Activity, ecology, and population dynamics of microorganisms in soil, CRC Crit. Rev. Microbiol., *2*, 59 (1972).

223. G. Stotzky, "Surface interactions between clay minerals and microbes, viruses, and soluble organics, and the probable importance of these interactions to the ecology of microbes in soil," in R. C. W. Berkeley, J. M. Lynch, J. Melling, P. R. Rutter, and B. Vincent, Eds., *Microbial Adhesion to Surfaces*, Ellis Harwood, Chichester, United Kingdom, 1980, p. 231.

224. G. Stotzky. "Surface interactions of microorganisms, viruses, and organics with clay minerals and the probable importance of these interactions in microbial ecology and in migration of clay–organic complexes," in *Migrations Organo-Minerales dans les Sols Temperes*, C.N.R.S., Paris, 1981, p. 173.

225. G. Stotzky. "Mechanisms of adhesion to clays, with reference to soil systems," in D. C. Savage and M. M. Fletcher, Eds., *Bacterial Adhesion: Mechanisms and Physiological Significance*, Plenum, New York, 1985, p. 195.

226. L. Kiremidjian and G. Stotzky. Effects of natural microbial preparations on the electrophoretic potential of bacterial cells and clay minerals, Appl. Microbiol., *25*, 964 (1973).

227. T. Santoro and G. Stotzky. Effect of electrolyte composition and pH and particle size distribution of microorganisms and clay minerals as determined by the electrical sensing zone method, Arch. Biochem. Biophys., *122*, 664 (1967).

228. Y. E. Collins. Effects of heavy metals on the electrokinetic properties of bacteria, yeasts, and clay minerals, Ph.D. thesis, New York University, New York, 1987.

229. Y. E. Collins and G. Stotzky. Influence of heavy metals on the electrokinetic properties of bacteria, Abstr. Ann. Mtg. Am. Soc. Microbiol., 1982, p. 229.

230. Y. E. Collins and G. Stotzky. Heavy metals alter the electrokinetic properties of bacteria, yeasts, and clay minerals, Abstr. Third Int. Symp. Microb. Ecol., 1983, p. 76.

231. T. Santoro and G. Stotzky. Effect of cations and pH on the electrophoretic mobility of microbial cells and clay minerals, Bacteriol. Proc., A15, (1967).

232. M. C. Fuerstenau, D. A. Elgillani, and J. D. Miller. Adsorption mechanisms in nonmetallic systems, Trans. A.I.M.E., *247*, 11 (1970).

233. E. A. Forbes, A. M. Posner, and J. P. Quirk. The specific adsorption of inorganic Hg(II) species and Co(II) complex ions on goethite, J. Colloid Interface Sci., *49*, 403 (1974).

234. J. Garcia-Miragaya and A. L. Page. Influence of ionic strength and inorganic complex formation on the sorption of trace amounts of Cd by montmorillonite, Soil Sci. Soc. Am. J. *40*, 659 (1976).

235. L. Kiremidjian and G. Stotzky. Influence of mono- and multivalent cations on the electrokinetic properties of *Rana pipiens* kidney cells, J. Cell Physiol., *85*, 125 (1975).

236. L. Kiremidjian-Schumacher, G. Stotzky, V. Likhite, J. Schwartz, and R. Dickstein. Influence of cadmium, lead, and zinc on the ability of sensitized guinea pig lymphocytes to interact with specific antigen and to produce lymphokine, Environ. Res., *24*, 96 (1981).

237. L. Kiremidjian-Schumacher, G. Stotzky, R. Dickstein, and J. Schwartz. Influence of cadmium, lead, and zinc on the ability of guinea pig macrophages to interact with macrophage migration inhibitory factor, Environ. Res., *24*, 106 (1981).

238. J. M. Diamond and E. M. Wright. Biological membranes: The physical basis of ion and nonelectrolyte selectivity, Ann. Rev. Physiol., *31*, 581 (1969).

239. H. Schott and C. Y. Young. Electrokinetic studies of bacteria. III: Effect of polyvalent metal ions on electrophoretic mobility and growth of *Streptococcus faecalis*, J. Pharm. Sci., *62*, 1797 (1973).

240. T. Matsuoka, M. Sugiyama, and Y. Shigenaka. Electrophoretic migration of the heliozoan, *Echinosphaerium akamae*, Cytobios, *40*, 107 (1984).

241. D. H. Taylor and H. B. Bosmann. The electrokinetic properties of Reovirus Type 3: Electrophoretic mobility and zeta potential in dilute electrolytes, J. Colloid Interface Sci., *83*, 153 (1981).

242. D. H. Taylor and H. B. Bosmann. Measurement of the electrokinetic properties of vaccinia and reovirus by laser-illuminated whole-particle microelectrophoresis, J. Virol. Meth., *2*, 251 (1981).

243. T. Santoro and G. Stotzky. Influence of cations on flocculation of clay minerals by microbial metabolites as determined by the electrical zone particle analyzer, Soil Sci. Amer. Proc., *31*, 761 (1967).

244. R. O. James and T. W. Healy. Adsorption of hydrolyzable metal ions at the oxide-water interface. I. Co(II) adsorption on $SiO_2$ and $TiO_2$ as model systems, J. Colloid Interface Sci., *40*, 42 (1972).

245. R. O. James and T. W. Healy. Adsorption of hydrolyzable metal ions at the oxide–water interface. III: A thermodynamic model of adsorption, J. Colloid Interface Sci., *40*, 65 (1972).

246. H. A. Elliott and C. P. Huang. The effect of complex formation on the adsorption characteristics of heavy metals, Environ. Int., *2*, 145 (1979).

247. J. N. Butler. *Ionic Equilibrium, A Mathematical Approach*, Addison-Wesley, Reading, MA, 1964.

248. W. Stumm and H. Bilinski. "Trace metals in natural waters: Difficulties of interpretation arising from our ignorance on their speciation," in Proc. Sixth Int. Conf. Wat. Poll. Res., Pergamon Press, New York, 1972, p. 39.

249. T. W. Healy, R. O. James, and R. Cooper. "The adsorption of aqueous Co(II) at the silica-water interface," in W. J. Weber Jr., and E. Matijevic, Eds., *Adsorption from Aqueous Solution*, Adv. Chem. Ser., Vol. 79, American Chemical Society, Washington, DC, 1968, p. 62.

250. E. Matijevic. "Charge reversal of lyophobic colloids," in S. D. Faust and I. V. Hunter, Eds., *Principles and Applications of Water Chemistry*, Wiley, New York, 1967, p. 328.

251. D. W. Newton, R. Ellis, Jr., and G. M. Paulsen. Effect of pH and complex formation on mercury (II) adsorption by bentonite, J. Environ. Qual., *5*, 251 (1976).

252. R. O. James, P. J. Stiglich, and T. W. Healy. Analysis of models of adsorption of metal ions at oxide/water interfaces, Disc. Farad. Soc., *59*, 142 (1973).

253. J. M. W. MacKenzie and R. T. O'Brien. Zeta potential of quartz in the presence of nickel(II) and cobalt(II), Trans. A.I.M.E., *244*, 168 (1969).

254. W. Stumm and C. R. O'Melia. Stoichiometry of coagulation, J. Am. Water Works Assoc., *60*, 514 (1968).

255. A. G. Langdon, K. W. Perrott, and A. T. Wilson. Iron(III) enhanced phosphate

and sulphate adsorption at the 001 face of mica, J. Colloid Interface Sci., *44*, 486 (1973).

256. A. Bruynesteyn. "Biological and chemical processing of low grade ores," in H. Grunewald, Ed., *Chemistry for the Future*, Pergamon, Oxford, 1983, p. 301.

257. D. G. Lundgren and M. Silver. Ore leaching by bacteria, Ann. Rev. Microbiol., *34*, 263 (1980).

258. F. E. Brinckman and G. J. Olson. "Chemical principles underlying bioleaching of metals from ores and solid wastes, and bioaccumulation of metals from solutions," Biotechnol. Bioengin. Symp., Vol. 16, Wiley, New York, 1986, p. 35.

259. G. J. Olson and F. E. Brinckman. Inorganic materials biotechnology: A new industrial measurement challenge, J. Res. NBS, *91*, 139 (1986).

260. J. S. Thayer, G. J. Olson, and F. E. Brinckman. A novel flow process for metal and ore solubilization by aqueous methyl iodide, J. Appl. Organometal. Chem., *1*, 1 (1987).

261. W. R. Manders, G. J. Olson, F. E. Brinckman, and J. M. Bellama. A novel synthesis of methyltin triiodide with environmental implications, J. Chem. Soc. Chem. Commun., *1984*, 538 (1984).

262. J. S. Thayer, G. J. Olson, and F. E. Brinckman. Iodomethane as a potential metal mobilizing agent in nature, Environ. Sci. Technol., *18*, 726 (1984).

263. P. R. Norris and D. P. Kelly. "The use of mixed microbial cultures in metal recovery," in A. T. Bull and J. H. Slater, Eds., *Microbial Interactions and Communities*, Academic, London, 1982, p. 443.

264. V. Vouk. "Germanium," in L. Friberg, G. F. Nordberg, and V. B. Vouk, Eds., *Handbook on the Toxicology of Metals*, Elsevier/North Holland Biomedical Press, New York, 1979, p. 421.

265. J. Chmielowski and C. Olczak. Abstr. Tenth FEBS Meeting, Paris, France, abstr. no. 1119, 1975.

266. M. Tsezos and B. Volesky. Biosorption of uranium and thorium, Biotechnol. Bioeng., *23*, 583 (1981).

267. M. Tsezos and B. Volesky. The mechanism of uranium biosorption by *Rhizopus arrhizus*, Biotechnol. Bioeng., *24*, 385 (1982).

268. M. Tsezos and B. Volesky. The mechanism of thorium biosorption by *Rhizopus arrhizus*, Biotechnol. Bioeng., *24*, 955 (1982).

269. M. Tsezos and D. M. Keller. Adsorption of radium-226 by biological origin absorbents, Biotechnol. Bioeng., *25*, 201 (1983).

270. W. A. Hamilton. Sulphate-reducing bacteria and anaerobic corrosion, Ann. Rev. Microbiol., *39*, 195 (1985).

271. A. K. Tiller. "Electrochemical aspects of microbial corrosion: an overview," in *Microbial Corrosion*, The Metals Society, London, 1983, p. 54.

272. A. K. Tiller. "Is stainless steel susceptible to microbial corrosion?," in *Microbial Corrosion*, The Metals Society, London, 1983, p. 104.

273. W. P. Iverson and G. J. Olson. "Anaerobic corrosion by sulfate-reducing bacteria due to highly reactive volatile phosphorus compound," in *Microbial Corrosion*, The Metals Society, London, 1983. p. 46.

274. I. V. Ulanovski, E. K. Rudenko, E. A. Suprun, and A. V. Ledenev. Electrokinetic properties of sulfate-reducing bacteria, Microbiology, *49*, 98 (1980).

275. E. A. Suprun, E. K. Rudenko, and I. B. Ulvanovskii. Electrokinetic properties of *Arthrobacter siderocapsulatus*, Microbiology, *49*, 276 (1980).

276. W. H. Smith. Influence of heavy metal leaf contaminants on the *in vitro* growth of urban-tree phylloplane fungi, Microb. Ecol., *3*, 231 (1977).

277. Z. A. Avakyan. Comparative toxicity of heavy metals for certain microorganisms, Microbiology, *36*, 366 (1967).

278. A. G. Cobet, C. Wirsen, and G. E. Jones. The effect of nickel on a marine bacterium, *Arthrobacter marinus* sp. nov., J. Gen. Microbiol., *62*, 159 (1970).

279. Z. Vaituzis, J. D. Nelson, Jr., L. W. Wan, and R. R. Colwell. Effects of mercuric chloride on growth and morphology of selected strains of mercury resistant bacteria, Appl. Microbiol., *29*, 275 (1975).

280. M. R. Blundell and D. G. Wild. Inhibition of bacterial growth by metal salts. A survey of the effects on the synthesis of ribonucleic acid and protein, Biochem. J., *115*, 207 (1969).

281. D. C. Sigee and R. H. Al-Rabaee. Nickel toxicity in *Pseudomonas tabaci*: single cell and bulk sample analysis of bacteria cultured at high cation levels, Protoplasma, *130*, 171 (1986).

282. J. W. Bhattacherjee. Effect of cadmium and zinc on microbial adhesion, growth, and metal uptake, Bull. Environ. Contam. Toxicol., *36*, 396 (1986).

283. L. F. Adams and W. C. Ghiorse. Influence of manganese on growth of a sheathless strain of *Leptothrix discophora*, Appl. Environ. Microbiol., *49*, 556 (1985).

284. D. S. Ross, R. E. Sjogren, and R. J. Bartlett. Behavior of chromium in soils: IV. Toxicity to microorganisms, J. Environ. Qual., *10*, 145 (1981).

285. T. Duxbury. Toxicity of heavy metals to soil bacteria, FEMS Microbiol. Lett., *11*, 217 (1981).

286. S. E. Williams and A. G. Wollum, II. Effect of cadmium on soil bacteria and actinomycetes, J. Environ. Qual., *10*, 142 (1981).

287. T. W. Jeffries and R. G. Butler. Growth inhibition of *Rhodopseudomonas capsulata* by methylmercury acetate, Appl. Microbiol., *30*, 156 (1975).

288. B. Mora and J. Fabregas. The effect of inorganic and organic mercury on growth kinetics of *Nitzschia acicularis* W. Sm. and *Tetraselmis suecica* Butch., Can. J. Microbiol., *26*, 930 (1980).

289. T. Kallqvist and B. S. Meadows. The toxic effect of copper on algae and rotifers from a soda lake (Lake Nakuru, East Africa), Water Res., *12*, 771 (1978).

290. M. E. Starodub, P. T. S. Wong, and C. I. Mayfield. Short-term and long-term studies on individual and combined toxicities of copper, zinc, and lead to *Scenedesmus quadricauda*, Sci. Tot. Environ., *63*, 101 (1987).

291. W. Barrow and T. G. Tornabene. Chemical and ultrastructural examination of lead-induced morphological convertants of *Bacillus subtilis*, Chem.-Biol. Interactions, *26*, 207 (1979).

292. W. Barrow, M. Himmel, P. G. Squire, and T. G. Tornabene. Evidence for alteration of the membrane-bound ribosomes in *Micrococcus luteus* cells exposed to lead, Chem.-Biol. Interactions, *23*, 387 (1978).

293. C. C. Lindegren and G. Lindegren. Mitochondrial modification and respiratory deficiency in the yeast cell caused by cadmium poisoning, Mut. Res., *21*, 315 (1973).

294. W. D. Rosenzweig and D. Pramer. Influence of cadmium, zinc, and lead on growth, trap formation, and collagenase activity of nematode-trapping fungi, Appl. Environ. Microbiol., *40*, 694 (1980).

295. J. W. Rachlin, T. E. Jensen, M. Baxter, and V. Jani. Utilization of morphometric analysis in evaluating response of *Plectonema boryanum* (Cyanophyceae) to exposure to eight heavy metals, Arch. Environ. Contam. Toxicol., *11*, 323 (1982).

296. G. W. Stratton and C. T. Corke. The effect of nickel on the growth, photosynthesis, and nitrogenase activity of *Anabaena inaequalis*, Can. J. Microbiol., *25*, 1094 (1979).

297. P. C. Adshead-Simonsen, G. E. Murray, and D. J. Kushner. Morphological changes in the diatom, *Tabellaria flocculosa*, induced by very low concentrations of cadmium, Bull. Environ. Contam. Toxicol., *26*, 745 (1981).

298. A. Massalski, V. M. Laube, and D. J. Kushner. Effects of cadmium and copper on the ultrastructure of *Ankistrodesmus braunii* and *Anabaena* 7120, Microb. Ecol., *7*, 183 (1981).

299. G. Roderer. Hemmung der Cytokinese und Bildung von Riesenzellen bei *Poterioochromonas malhamensis* durch organische Bleiverbindungen und andere Agenzien, Protoplasma, *99*, 39 (1979).

300. S. Duret, J. Bonaly, A. Bariaud, A. Vannereau, and J-C. Mestre. Cadmium induced ultrastructural changes in *Euglena* cells, Environ. Res., *39*, 96 (1986).

301. S. Rebhun and A. Ben-Amotz. The distribution of cadmium between the marine alga *Chlorella stigmatophora* and sea water medium, Water Res., *18*, 173 (1984).

302. C. W. Forsberg. Effects of heavy metals and other trace metals on the fermentative activity of the rumen microbiota and growth of functionally important rumen bacteria, Can. J. Microbiol., *24*, 298 (1978).

303. K. J. Puckett, E. Nieboer, M. J. Gorzynski, and D. H. S. Richardson. The uptake of metal ions by lichens: a modified ion-exchange process, New Phytol., *72*, 329 (1979).

304. C. Guha and A. Mookerjee. Effect of nickel on macromolecular synthesis in *Escherichia coli* K-12, Nucleus, *22*, 45 (1979).

305. M. Flavin and C. Slaughter. Microtubule assembly and function in *Chlamydomonas*: inhibition of growth and flagellar regeneration by antitubulins and other drugs and isolation of resistant mutants, J. Bacteriol., *118*, 59 (1974).

306. C. Andrivon. The stopping of ciliary movements by nickel salts in *Paramecium caudatum*: The antagonism of $K^+$ and $Ca^{2+}$ ions, Acta Protozool., *11*, 373 (1972).

307. V. Ya. Kostyaev. Effects of some heavy metals on cyanobacteria, Microbiology, *49*, 665 (1980).

308. G. W. Stratton and C. T. Corke. The effect of mercuric, cadmium, and nickel ion combinations on a blue-green alga, Chemosphere, *8*, 731 (1979).

309. J. L. Malanchuk and G. K. Greundling. Toxicity of lead nitrate to algae, Water Air Soil Poll., *2*, 181 (1973).

310. S. M. Saifullah. Inhibitory effects of copper on marine dinoflagellates, Mar. Biol., *44*, 299 (1978).

311. N. T. Christie and M. Costa. *In vitro* assessment of the toxicity of metal compounds. III. Effects of metals on DNA structure and function in intact cells, Biol. Trace Elem. Res., *5*, 55 (1983).

312. G. B. Diekert, E. G. Graf, and R. K. Thauer. Nickel requirement for carbon monoxide dehydrogenase formation in *Clostridium pasteurianum*, Arch. Microbiol., *122*, 117 (1979).

313. G. Diekert, H.-H. Gilles, R. Jaenchen, and R. K. Thauer. Incorporation of 8 succinate per mol nickel into factors $F_{430}$ by *Methanobacterium thermoautotrophicum*, Arch. Microbiol., *128*, 256 (1980).

314. G. Diekert, B. Klee, and R. K. Thauer. Nickel, a component of factor $F_{430}$ from *Methanobacterium thermoautotrophicum*, Arch. Microbiol., *124*, 103 (1980).

315. G. Diekert, U. Konheiser, K. Piechulla, and R. K. Thauer. Nickel requirement and factor $F_{430}$ content of methanogenic bacteria, J. Bacteriol., *148*, 459 (1981).

316. W. L. Ellefson, W. B. Whitman, and K. S. Wolfe. Nickel-containing factor $F_{430}$ chromophore of the methyl reductase of *Methanobacterium*, Proc. Natl. Acad. Sci., *79*, 3707 (1982).

317. R. K. Thauer. Nickel tetrapyrroles in methanogenic bacteria: structure, function, and biosynthesis, Zbl. Bakt. Hyg. I. Abt. Orig. *C3*, 265 (1982).

318. R. Tabillion, F. Weber, and H. Kaltwasser. Nickel requirement for chemolithotrophic growth in hydrogen-oxidizing bacteria, Arch. Microbiol., *124*, 131 (1980).

319. R. Bartha and E. J. Ordal. Nickel-dependent chemolithotrophic growth of two *Hydrogenomonas* strains, J. Bacteriol., *89*, 1015 (1965).

320. R. Tabillion and H. Kaltwasser. Energieabhangige $^{63}$Ni-Aufnahme bei *Alcaligenes eutrophus* Stamm H1 und H16, Arch. Microbiol., *113*, 145 (1977).

321. D. Bertrand and A. DeWolf. Le nickel, oligelement dynamique, pour les vegetaux superieurs, C. R. Acad. Sci. (Paris), *265*, 1053 (1967).

322. L. E. Hendriksson and E. J. DaSilva. Effects of some inorganic elements on nitrogen-fixation in blue-green algae and some ecological aspects of pollution, Zeitschr. Allg. Mikrobiol., *18*, 487 (1978).

323. C. Van Baalen and R. O'Donnell. Isolation of a nickel-dependent blue-green alga, J. Gen. Microbiol., *105*, 351 (1978).

324. W. Stumm. "Metal ions in aqueous solutions," in S. D. Faust and I. V. Hunter, Eds., *Principles and Applications of Water Chemistry*, Wiley, New York, 1967, p. 544.

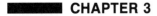 **CHAPTER 3**

# Inorganic Ion Gradients in Methanogenic Archaebacteria: A Comparative Analysis to Other Prokaryotes

G. DENNIS SPROTT

Division of Biological Sciences
National Research Council of Canada
Ottawa, Ontario, Canada

## Contents

NRCC Publication No. 29833. G. Dennis Sprott prepared this work as part of his official duties as a Canadian government employee. Therefore, copyright may not be claimed for this chapter.

**91**

## 3.1   INTRODUCTION

Living organisms have been classified into three major lineages (1): *Eukaryota, Eubacteria,* and *Archaebacteria.* Although the concept of the latter third major lineage was postulated from comparisons of base sequences of the ribosomal 16S RNA obtained from various microbes (2), other biochemical features have supported the separation of the prokaryotes into two separate groupings as well. These features have been reviewed a number of times (including Refs. 3 and 4) and are discussed here only with respect to the structural properties of the outer cell layers of the methanogenic bacteria. Despite these similarities, the archaebacteria are bacteria with widely differing features, from obligately anaerobic to aerobic and autotrophic to heterotrophic. The archaebacteria, then, consist of those prokaryotes that are not eubacteria, namely, the methanogens, the extremely halophilic archaebacteria (halobacteria), and the sulfur-dependent extreme thermophiles.

Methanogenic bacteria represent a diverse group of obligately anaerobic bacteria capable of growth through the conversion of simple $C_1$ or $C_2$ compounds to methane and cell biomass. The taxonomy of these bacteria and their growth substrates have been reviewed recently (4). Similarly, detailed reports are available of their unique assimilatory pathways (4–6) and energy-generating (methanogenesis) pathway (3, 4, 7).

For the convenience of those not working with methanogens the genera, all of which begin with the letter *M.*, are abbreviated as follows: *Msp., Methanospirillum; Mb., Methanobacterium; Mc., Methanococcus; Mbr., Methanobrevibacterium; Ms., Methanosarcina; Mtx., Methanothrix; Mg., Methanogenium; Mcp., Methanocorpusculum;* and *Mcc., Methanococcoides.*

It has long been recognized that prokaryotes maintain a closely controlled mix of inorganic cations and anions through the action of specific transport systems located in their cytoplasmic membranes. The translocation of inorganic ions in prokaryotes has been studied frequently in only a few eubacteria and in halobacteria. Perhaps the ions most studied include the cations $H^+$, $Na^+$, $K^+$, $NH_4^+$, $Fe^{3+}$, $Ca^{2+}$, $Mg^{2+}$, $Mn^{2+}$ and $Zn^{2+}$, and the anions $Cl^-$, $PO_4^{3-}$, $SO_4^{2-}$, $NO_3^-$, and arsenate (8–13).

Much has been done, in particular, on the cycles of $H^+$ and $Na^+$, because they are often intimately involved in the bioenergetics of the cell, and in pH regulation. Various bacteria have developed different strategies to expel these ions from their cytoplasm (Table 3.1). In the case of protons, primary pumps [the terminology of primary and secondary transport is described by West (14)] have been identified that use directly the energy of cytochrome-linked electron flow, ATP hydrolysis, or light energy. Other primary proton pumps, not shown in Table 3.1, exist as well. The excretion of metabolic end products (e.g., lactate) in symport with protons generates a proton motive force during the anaerobic growth of *Streptococcus cremoris* (15). An exciting mechanism suggested recently is the membrane coupling of a periplasmic, proton-generating system to proton consumption in the cytoplasm, perhaps typical in autotrophic bacteria. Evidence for such a scheme has been presented for the oxidation of small molecules such as $H_2$ in sulfate-reducing bacteria (16) and $NH_3$ in *Nitrosomonas europaea* (17). Speculations are that this mechanism may be extended to the oxidation of $NO_2^-$, reduced sulfur compounds, CO, $U^{4+}$, $Cu^+$, and $Mn^+$ (16, 17).

Primary sodium pumps identified in specific prokaryotes include a $Na^+$-dependent ATPase, and certain membrane-localized, $Na^+$-dependent decarboxylases shown in Table 3.1. Another mechanism found in certain moderate halophiles (*Vibrio* species) invokes a change in the respiratory chain from a $H^+$ to a $Na^+$ pump at alkaline pH (18). $Na^+$ efflux may occur also by coupling the activity of a $Na^+/H^+$ antiporter to the proton motive force in *Vibrio costicola* (19). The interconversion of the $H^+$ or $Na^+$ motive forces, and conversion to other ion motive forces, may be accomplished by the secondary antiporters shown.

In addition to protons and $Na^+$, other ions may be used as energy storage forms. For example, the $K^+$ gradient may be used in *E. coli* for the inward movement of ammonia by $NH_4^+/K^+$ antiport, and in *S. lactis* cytoplasmic phosphate may be exchanged for hexose 6-phosphates (Table 3.1).

With the exception of the halobacteria, no reviews have dealt specifically with ion movement in archaebacteria. Here this topic is addressed with comparative reference to the more extensive work done with eubacteria and halobacteria. Because little is known about ion gradients in the extreme thermophiles, the topic is further restricted to the methanogenic archaebacteria. Little reference is made here to ion movements in eukaryotic cells, but researchers might draw fruitfully from this body of knowledge, bearing in mind that certain biochemical features of the methanogens are more eukaryotic than prokaryotic (4).

## 3.2  METHANOGEN SURFACE FEATURES

### 3.2.1  Walls

A brief description of methanogen walls is warranted in recognition that they differ from those found in eubacteria, and that cations may be expected to

**TABLE 3.1  Some Mechanisms for Cation Movement Across Prokaryotic Cytoplasmic Membranes**

| Activity | Mechanism | Representative Bacteria* | Ref. |
|---|---|---|---|
| Primary proton pumps | Cytochrome-linked electron flow | *E. coli* | 20, 21 |
| | $F_0F_1$ ATPase | *E. coli* | 22 |
| | Light-driven, cyclic electron flow | Phototrophic bacteria | 23 |
| | Bacteriorhodopsin | Halobacteria | 24 |
| Primary sodium pumps | $Na^+$ ATPase | *Streptococcus faecalis* | 25 |
| | | *Mycoplasma mycoides* | 26 |
| | | *Acholeplasma laidlawii* | 27 |
| | Oxaloacetate CoA decarboxylase | *Klebsiella aerogenes* | 28 |
| | Glutaconyl CoA decarboxylase | *Acidiminococcus fermentens* | 29 |
| | Methylmalonyl CoA decarboxylase | *Micrococcus lactilyticus* | 30 |
| | Cytochrome-linked electron flow | *Vibrio alginolyticus* | 18 |
| Secondary cation/proton antiport | Sodium/proton | *E. coli* | 31–33 |
| | | *Vibrio costicola* | 34 |
| | Potassium/proton | *E. coli* | 35 |
| | Calcium/proton | *E. coli* | 32, 36 |
| | Calcium phosphate/proton | *E. coli* | 36 |
| Other antiporters | Sodium/potassium | *Mycoplasma mycoides* | 26 |
| | | *Streptococcus faecalis* | 37 |
| | Sodium/calcium | *Halobacterium halobium* | 12 |
| | Ammonium/potassium | *E. coli* | 38 |
| | Phosphate/hexose 6-phosphate | *Streptococcus lactis* | 39 |

* The bacteria listed are representative only, and not meant to be inclusive.

bind to bacterial walls (see Chapters 1, 9–11). Kandler and König determined that methanogens can be divided into four groups based on our present knowledge of wall structures (40). The first group consists of those species that have pseudomurein, resembling the murein of eubacteria but with substitutions of N-acetyltalosaminuronic acid for N-acetylmuramic acid and L- for D-amino acids. Second, the *Methanosarcina* spp. form a wall polymer similar in structure to the chondroitin sulfate of animal connective tissue (41). The polymer consists of N-acetyl-D-galactosamine and D-glucuronic acid with only small amounts of sulfate or phosphate. A third grouping of methanogens, typified by *Methanococcus* spp., possess only a regularly structured (RS) layer external to the cytoplasmic membrane (42, 43). Finally, *Methanospirillum* spp. and *Methanothrix* spp. consist of chains of cells within a tubular sheath. In an ultrastructural sense each of these organisms is unique to the prokaryotic world (40, 44), and each has a novel means of cell division (45, 46). The sheaths of *Methanospirillum hungatei* GP1 and JF1 and of *Methanothrix concilii* have been purified and analyzed. Major cross striations clearly represent hoops (rings) of varying widths (47), stacked to form the tube. Stacking of the hoops was most clearly shown in the case of *Msp. hungatei* GP1 by disassembly of the sheath using β-mercaptoethanol and heat, thus releasing the hoops sometimes as separate entities (Fig. 3.1). The hoops of all three methanogens consist of a backing, or matrix, upon which is crystallized a surface array of surprisingly small and identical subunit arrangement, with $p2$ symmetry ($a = 5.6$ nm, $b = 2.8$ nm, and $\gamma = 86°$) (49). A sieving role in controlling permeability is suggested by the compact nature of the surface array (47). Each sheath type contains a predominant amount of different divalent cations, $Ca^{2+}$, $Mg^{2+}$ for *Msp. hungatei* JF1, $Ca^{2+}$ for *Msp. hungatei* GP1, and $Zn^{2+}$ for *Mtx. concilii* (49). The resilience of these sheath structures to various chemical treatments is remarkable (50), and varies among the types (49). Presently the importance of divalent ions to the sheath structures is unknown. Cation contents of the other methanogen wall types have yet to be reported.

### 3.2.2  Cytoplasmic Membrane

A difficulty initially discouraging experimentation with membrane vesicles is the resistance of the methanogen wall types to lytic enzymes, including lysozyme (40, 50). Methods presently available to release osmotically fragile cell forms (protected from lysis by $Mg^{2+}$ or sucrose) include the formation of spheroplasts by dithiothreitol treatment of *Msp. hungatei* GP1 or JF1 (51) and *Mtx. concilii* (44); and spontaneous protoplast formation in *Mb. bryantii* during growth in a medium limiting in both $Ni^{2+}$ and $NH_4^+$ (52). Protoplast formation is now possible in certain pseudomurein-containing methanogens using a peptidase from autolysates of *Mb. wolfei* (53). Spheroplasts of *Msp. hungatei* (54) and protoplasts of *Mb. thermoautotrophicum* (55) retain about 50% of their methanogenic activity.

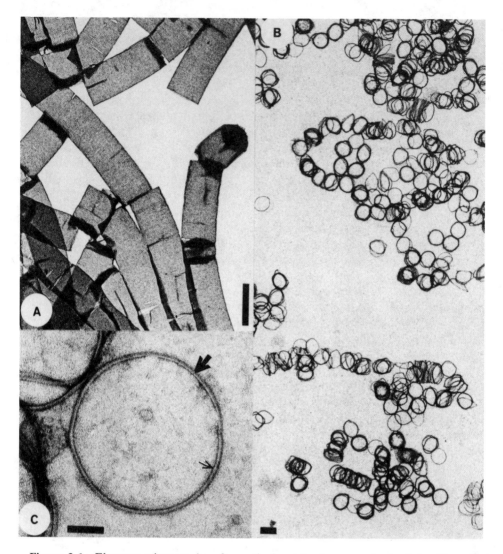

**Figure 3.1** Electron micrographs of negatively stained preparations of the *Msp. hungatei* GP1 sheath (*A*) before and (*B* and *C*) after treatment with 2% β-mercaptoethanol (90°C, 30 min). *A* and *B*, bar = 500 nm; *C*, bar = 100 nm. In *C* note the surface array (large arrow) and the matrix upon which the array is crystallized (small arrow). Reproduced with permission from Canadian Journal of Microbiology (48).

Cytoplasmic membrane isolated from *Msp. hungatei* (56) consists of protein (45–50%), lipid (35–37%), and carbohydrate (10–12%). The protein fraction separates into at least 22 polypeptides upon SDS-gel electrophoresis.

The diversity among methanogens is no more apparent than in the variety of structures found in their membrane lipids. As do other archaebacteria, the methanogens contain ether lipids in place of the ubiquitous, well-known ester-linked lipids of eubacteria (57). This polar fraction represents a large proportion, often about 90%, of the total cell lipids; the remaining neutral lipid fraction consists mainly of squalenes. Structures of several ether lipids have been completed for only a few methanogens, namely, *Msp. hungatei* GP1 (58, 59), *Mc. voltae* (60), *Mb. thermoautotrophicum* (61), *Mbr. arboriphilus* (62), and *Mtx. concilii* (62a). A striking feature evolving from these studies is that each genus contains predominant ether lipids that distinguish it from other genera.

The most extensive work on the polar lipids of a methanogen has been with *Msp. hungatei* GP1, as summarized in Figure 3.2. This methanogen contains only 4.2% of the cell dry weight as lipid, of which 92% is polar lipids. All of the polar lipids presently characterized are either glycerol diethers with $C_{20}C_{20}$ phytanyl chains in the *sn*-2 and *sn*-3 positions of glycerol, or the corresponding diglycerol tetraethers. The remaining *sn*-1 carbon of glycerol is typically linked glycosidically to sugar residues or via phosphodiester linkage to glycerol, to *N,N*-dimethylaminopentanetetrol, or to *N,N,N*-trimethylaminopentanetetrol. The relative amounts of these lipids is shown in the figure on a weight percent basis; seven very minor lipids are not included (59).

In *Mb. thermoautotrophicum* phosphoethanolamine has been identified in the *sn*-1[1] position of a glycerol tetraether lipid (61), and in *Mbr. arboriphilus* phosphatidylserine forms the polar group of a diether lipid (62). Diether analogs of phosphatidylinositol and α-D-mannopyranosyl-β(1→3)-D-galactopyranose in *Mtx. concilii* represent the first completed structures for methanogen lipids containing mannose or inositol (62a). Variations occur not only in the polar head groups, but in the core lipid structure as well. Some methanogens lack tetraether lipids (57) or make diether lipids with $C_{20}C_{25}$ chains, with cyclized $C_{20}$ to $C_{20}$, or even with tetritol in place of glycerol (4, 57, 59). In *Mtx. concilii* two major $C_{20}C_{20}$-diether core lipids are found; the standard 2,3-di-o-phytanyl-*sn*-glycerol, and a variation containing an hydroxyl group on C-3 of the *sn*-3 phytanyl chain (62b).

Unfortunately, little is known yet about the properties that these unusual archaebacterial lipids impart to the cytoplasmic membrane. It is expected that the $C_{40}$ phytanyl chains would span the membrane, raising the question of sidedness of the *sn*-1 and *sn*-1[1] polar head groups. Most of the physicochemical studies have been on the tetraether lipids of thermoacidophiles, rather than methanogens (63). We must be content here with the functional

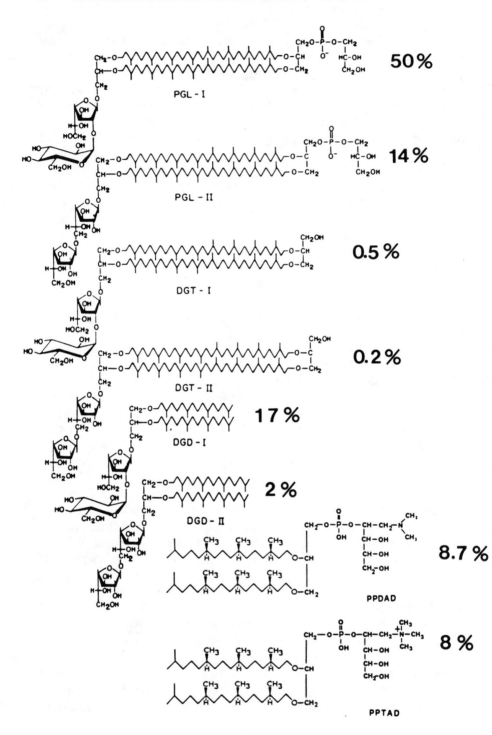

PGL - I  50%

PGL - II  14%

DGT - I  0.5%

DGT - II  0.2%

DGD - I  17%

DGD - II  2%

PPDAD  8.7%

PPTAD  8%

aspect of measuring ion pumping and ion gradients in whole methanogen cells.

## 3.3 ION REQUIREMENTS

Because the carbon substrates supporting growth are few (3, 4), it follows that their transport systems are limited primarily to inorganic ions. Certain strains requiring vitamins are probable exceptions, and an active transport system for coenzyme M occurs in *Mbr. ruminantium,* a strain auxotrophic for coenzyme M (64). Also exceptional is *Mc. voltae*, requiring leu and ile for growth (65) and actively transporting these and other amino acids (66, 67). Nutritional studies have identified a number of cations essential for growth (Table 3.2). Because cation requirements may vary depending on the growth substrate and the bacterial strain, these are specified in the table. The concentrations of cations shown to support maximum growth in batch cultures is valid, of course, only for the mixture of ingredients used in each respective growth medium. The occurrence of synergistic and antagonistic effects of ions is well known (82); for example, the $Na^+$ optimum for methane production in *Mb. thermoautotrophicum* increases as the $K^+$ content of the buffer increases (69). Reports suggesting that certain ions are not required for growth are absent from the table, because of uncertainty introduced by the technical difficulty in removing trace elements from growth media (65). Also note that the ion requirements shown for the moderate halophile *Mc. voltae* and for *Mg. tatii* isolated from a solfataric pool are often higher than for most of the methanogens studied. In many marine bacteria the effects of ions are, however, not very different from those on terrestrial types (83). Other trace elements usually present in methanogen media (84), for which no growth requirement has been demonstrated, include $Cu^{2+}$ and $Al^+$. Counter anions in methanogen media are primarily phosphate, $Cl^-$, and $SO_4^{2-}$.

Ammonium ion was included in the survey as the usual nitrogen source for growth, although in its absence several methanogens can fix diatomic nitrogen (4).

The scant information available on inorganic anion requirements relate

---

**Figure 3.2** Structures of ether lipids of *Msp. hungatei* GP1. PGL, phosphodiglycosyldibiphytanyldiglycerol tetraethers; DGT, diglycosyldibiphytanyldiglycerol tetraethers; DGD, diglycosyldiphytanylglycerol diethers; PPDAD, phosphopentanetetrol dimethylamino diether; PPTAD, phosphopentanetetrol trimethylamino diether. The percentage of the total lipid extract contributed by each component is shown in the figure. These data were taken from Kushwaha et al. (58) and Ferrante et al. (59).

**TABLE 3.2   Concentrations of Cations for Maximum Growth of Methanogenic Bacteria in Batch Culture**

| Ion | Concentration | Methanogen | Growth Substrate | Ref. |
|---|---|---|---|---|
| K | ~1 mM | *Mb. thermoautotrophicum* | $CO_2/H_2$ | 68 |
| Na | 400 mM | *Mc. voltae* | $CO_2/H_2$ | 65 |
| | 5 mM | *Mb. thermoautotrophicum* | $CO_2/H_2$ | 69 |
| | 170 mM | *Mg. tatii* | $CO_2/H_2$ | 70 |
| $NH_4$ | 5 mM | *Mc. voltae* | $CO_2/H_2$ | 65 |
| | >2 mM | *Ms. thermophila* TM1 | Methanol or acetate | 71 |
| | 6.8 mM | *Mtx. concilii* | Acetate | 72 |
| | 5 mM | *Mb. thermoautotrophicum* and TM1 | $CO_2/H_2$ | 73 |
| Mg | 84 mM | *Mc. voltae* | $CO_2/H_2$ | 65 |
| | 0.5 mM | *Mtx. concilii* | Acetate | 72 |
| Ca | 1 mM | *Mc. voltae* | $CO_2/H_2$ | 65 |
| | 13.6 μM | *Ms. thermophila* | Methanol | 71 |
| | 0.25 mM | *Mtx. concilii* | Acetate | 72 |
| Mn | 2.5 μM | *Mtx. concilii* | Acetate | 72 |
| Co | 1 μM | *Ms. barkeri* | Methanol | 74 |
| | ~0.04 μM | *Mb. thermoautotrophicum* | $CO_2/H_2$ | 75 |
| | 10 μM | *Mtx. concilii* | Acetate | 72 |
| | 0.1 μM | *Mcc. methylutens* | Trimethylamine | 76 |
| Fe | 10 μM | *Mc. voltae* | $CO_2/H_2$ | 65 |
| | ~20 μM | *Mb. thermoautotrophicum* | $CO_2/H_2$ | 75 |
| | 1–5 μM | *Mtx. concilii* | Acetate | 72 |
| | 0.3–0.9 mM | *Mb. bryantii; Msp. hungatei* | $CO_2/H_2$ | 77 |
| | 5 μM | *Mcc. methylutens* | Trimethylamine | 76 |
| Ni | 0.2 μM | *Mc. voltae* | $CO_2H_2$ | 65 |
| | 0.1 μM | *Mtx. concilii* | Acetate | 72 |
| | 1 μM | *Mb. thermoautotrophicum* | $CO_2/H_2$ | 75 |
| | 0.5 μM | *Ms. barkeri* | Methanol | 74 |
| | 0.25 μM | *Mcc. methylutens* | Trimethylamine | 76 |
| Zn | 5 μM | *Mtx. concilii* | Acetate | 72 |
| Se | 10 μM | *Mc. voltae* | $CO_2/H_2$ | 65 |
| | 1 μM | *Mc. thermolithotrophicus* | Formate | 78 |
| | 0.5 μM | *Ms. barkeri* | Methanol | 74 |
| | 1 μM | *Mc. vannielii* | Formate | 79 |
| Mo | ~0.04 μM | *Mb. thermoautotrophicum* | $CO_2/H_2$ | 75 |
| | 0.5 μM | *Ms. barkeri* | Methanol | 74 |
| W | 1 μM | *Mcp. parvum* | $CO_2/H_2$ | 80 |
| | 100 μM | *Mc. vannielli* | Formate | 79 |
| | 8 μM | *Mb. wolfei* | $CO_2/H_2$ | 81 |

to the sulfur source for growth (phosphate is described below). With $H_2$ as reductant, various methanogens can reduce $SO_4^{2-}$, $SO_3^{2-}$, $S^0$, and thiosulfate to sulfide (72, 85–87). All are capable of growth with sulfide as the sulfur source, whereas $SO_4^{2-}$ reduction, in particular, is less common. A requirement for about 0.3 m$M$ $SO_4^{2-}$, to achieve maximum growth in media reduced by cys–$Na_2S$, is found for *Mb. bryantii* (77). Cellular concentrations of these anions and their uptake have not been studied.

Efficient scavenging mechanisms for trace elements can be inferred not only from the low amounts required in the medium for growth, but also from their cellular contents. A thorough quantitative study of the elements present in 10 methanogens has been done by inductively coupled plasma emission spectroscopy of cell hydrolysates (88). Representatives were analyzed from three orders: I, Methanobacteriales; II, Methanococcales; and III, Methanomicrobiales. Orders II and III contained high $Ca^{2+}$ contents, which were approximately 10 times greater than that of Order I, probably reflecting binding by the acidic wall of *Methanosarcina* and by the RS layers characteristic of *Methanococcus* spp. $Mg^{2+}$ was present at high amounts in all methanogens. $Mo^{2+}$ values were generally low; $Zn^{2+}$ and $Cu^{2+}$ varied greatly from strain to strain. In a separate study, cells of *Ms. barkeri* were found to incorporate the heavy metals Pb and Cd, whereas cell-associated Zn and Cu levels were less (89).

The biochemical uses for trace elements can be obtained from other articles dealing with methanogens (references in Table 3.2; 3, 88–92). For example, the reader is referred to the well-known nickel–tetrapyrrole ($F_{430}$) prosthetic group of methylcoenzyme M reductase (90), the $F_{420}$-reducing hydrogenase containing (molar ratios) 33 atoms of Fe and 24 atoms of sulfur (91), and $F_{420}$-formate dehydrogenase containing 1 Mo, 2 Zn, 21–24 Fe, and 25–29 sulfur atoms (92). A Se-dependent formate dehydrogenase is found in *Mc. vannielii* (93) and Co in the corrinoid, Factor III (94). Metalloenzymes are described in another chapter.

## 3.4  PROTON MOTIVE FORCE

Methanogenesis is a respiratory, energy-yielding process from which methanogens must satisfy their energy requirements (3). In other prokaryotes respiratory processes, and/or the $F_0F_1$-ATPase (Table 3.1), may serve as primary pump to cause efflux of $H^+$ across the cytoplasmic membrane, thus generating an electrical potential (interior negative) and a chemical potential (interior alkaline). The resulting inward force on the protons is called the proton motive force (pmf) and is represented in millivolts as

$$\text{pmf} = \Delta\psi - Z\Delta\text{pH}$$

where $\Delta\psi$ is the membrane potential, $Z = 2.3\ RT/F$, $R$ is the gas constant,

$T$ the absolute temperature, and $F$ the Faraday constant (22, 95). Both components of the pmf have been measured in a variety of methanogens (3). Using a probe sensitive to the lipophilic cation tetraphenylphosphonium, in *Mb. thermoautotrophicum* a membrane potential of $-150$ to $-200$ mV was formed upon the initiation of methanogenesis (96). Similarly, addition of the methanogenic substrate methanol to *Ms. barkeri* resulted in formation of a protonophore-sensitive pmf coupled to the synthesis of ATP (97). Addition of $Na^+$ to *Mc. voltae* initiated methanogenesis establishing a $\Delta pH$, alkaline inside (66). Recently, several models for the formation of a pmf were reviewed (3). One possibility for growth on $CO_2/H_2$ is that the methanogenic enzymes are localized in the cytoplasm, linked via the membrane to periplasmic hydrogenase activity. There is presently no conclusive evidence for such a scheme, but it remains most attractive.

Localization is required of the several key electron transfer enzymes (3). These studies have been initiated using colloidal gold–antibody to localize the methylcoenzyme M reductase. In *Mc. voltae* the enzyme is in the vicinity of the cytoplasmic membrane, consistent with a role in pmf formation (98). This and other evidence (3, 7, 97) indicate that the energy conserved as a pmf from the exergonic methylcoenzyme M reductase reaction is used in the initial endergonic step of $CO_2$ reduction. As for the $F_{420}$-reducing hydrogenase, its release from *Msp. hungatei* occurred only upon lysis of spheroplasts, suggesting association with the spheroplast (99). The enzyme was very hydrophobic, as found for the $F_{420}$-reducing hydrogenase of *Mb. formicicum* (100). Indeed, in the case of *Mb.* strain G2R (101) and *Mb. formicicum* (100) the enzyme is associated with cytoplasmic membranes in cell lysates. In *Msp. hungatei* only about 10% of the hydrogenase co-migrated with the cytoplasmic membrane fraction (99), indicating a weak interaction. It is important to determine if any association of this large enzyme with cytoplasmic membranes favors the inner or outer face of the membrane and has relevance to the physiology of the intact cell.

During growth in media of pH near neutrality the pmf is composed of a membrane potential and no measurable $\Delta pH$ (Fig. 3.3). Over the external pH range of 6–7 where growth was optimal the cytoplasmic pH remained constant at about 6.8, indicating an adequate mechanism for pH homeostasis. If an analogy can be made with the eubacteria (95), this implies not only a mechanism for proton extrusion, but also proton/cation antiporters to return protons to the cytoplasm, when required. The current, scant evidence for antiporters in methanogens is discussed below.

Intracytoplasmic membranes (methanochondria) have been observed in thin sections of a number of methanogens, and suggested to have a role in energy coupling (103). However, these membranes serve no essential role for growth, because they are absent from certain strains and depend on growth conditions (104). Also, part of the evidence favoring the methanochondrion hypothesis, based on the presence of an ADP/ATP translocase atypical of bacteria, has now been discounted (105). Recently fast freezing

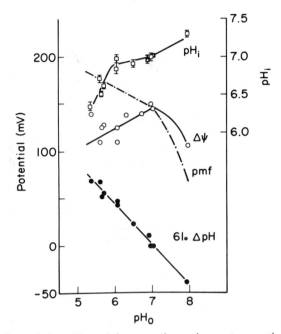

**Figure 3.3** Effect of the pH used for growth on the proton motive force and cytoplasmic pH of *Mb. bryantii*. Samples were removed from pH-controlled fermentors and the cells analyzed for (●) chemical potential; (○) membrane potential; (□) cytoplasmic pH; and ·—·—·—·) pmf. Reproduced with permission from Canadian Journal of Microbiology (102).

methods have shown the internal membranes to be artifacts of specimen preparation for electron microscopy (106). As a whole, these results might suggest that the frequency of membrane artifacts could depend on the specific ether lipids, and therefore unique membrane composition and properties, which vary among the methanogens (see Section 3.2.2).

Anabolic pathways in methanogens center on acetate synthesis (or uptake from the medium in aceticlastic methanogens) and its further metabolism to form cell constituents via a partial TCA pathway, also called the acetyl-coenzyme A pathway (5). Because glycolysis is absent in methanogens, ATP synthesis via substrate level phosphorylation was initially discounted. However, in the moderate halophile *Mc. voltae* there is evidence for substrate level phosphorylation coupled directly to a methanogenic reaction (107). This view is not widespread (97); in fact, acetylphosphate is a likely intermediate in methane formation from acetate in *Ms. barkeri* (7) indicating consumption, rather than formation, of ATP. It is conceivable that two mechanisms for ATP synthesis exist in this diverse grouping of bacteria. In the first the flow of energy is $CH_4 \rightarrow ATP \rightarrow pmf$, whereas in the second it is $CH_4 \rightarrow pmf \rightarrow ATP$. Either mechanism implies a proton-pumping ATPase (a $Na^+$-ATPase is a possible primary pump, also) in analogy to anaerobic streptococci that use glycolytic ATP to establish a pmf via the $F_0F_1$-ATPase (15), or other eubacteria that use the pmf formed by cytochrome-linked electron transport to reverse the ATPase reaction for ATP synthesis (22). Another complicating feature making it difficult to generalize among the methanogenic bacteria is that under certain growth conditions cytochromes of unknown function have been detected in a *Methanosarcina* spp. and a *Methanothrix* spp. (3).

Most, if not all, methanogens appear to contain an $F_0F_1$ ATPase typical of eubacteria. Dicyclohexylcarbodiimide-sensitive ATP synthesis has been observed in several genera (3, 97, 108, 109), and apparent insensitivity is uncertain unless the cell wall is removed to exclude binding (109). Inhibition of methanogenesis by dicyclohexylcarbodiimide, in protoplasts of a methanogen strain utilizing methanol + $H_2$, is relieved by a protonophore; this suggests coupling of methyl coenzyme M reduction to pmf formation and ATP synthesis (110). In *Mb. thermoautotrophicum* and *Ms. barkeri* the ATPase activity has been solubilized from membranes with EDTA or LiCl, and shown to require $Mg^{2+}$ (111, 112); $Ca^{2+}$ was ineffective for *Ms. barkeri* ATPase activity (112). Stalked particles similar to $F_0F_1$ ATPase are seen on cytoplasmic membranes of strain Göl, which cross-react with antibody prepared against the β subunit of *E. coli* $F_1$-ATPase (113).

## 3.5  SODIUM

### 3.5.1  Halobacteria

Of the archaebacteria studied, ion translocation is best known in *Halobacterium halobium* (23, 114). The extrusion of protons occurs by the primary light-driven pump bacteriorhodopsin or by cytochrome-linked respiration. The pmf, so formed, can be converted to a sodium motive force via an $Na^+/H^+$ antiporter (115). In turn, the $Na^+$ gradient ($[Na^+]_{in} < [Na^+_{out}]$) is used as energy for the transport of organic (e.g., amino acids) substrates by symport, or used to catalyze a $Ca^{2+}/Na^+$ antiporter (12). In addition, halobacteria can grow anaerobically in the dark if provided with arg for ATP synthesis by substrate phosphorylation (116).

### 3.5.2  Methanogens

The essential biochemical roles that $Na^+$ plays in methanogens are beginning to emerge. Not only is $Na^+$ required for methane synthesis in cell suspensions (117), but it also stimulates ATP synthesis driven by a $K^+$ diffusion potential in *Mb. thermoautotrophicum*. The effect was suggested to be either the result of ATP synthesis by $Na^+$ influx through a $Na^+$-ATPase similar to the $Na^+$-ATPases found in several eubacteria (Table 3.1), or to cytoplasmic pH regulation through $Na^+/H^+$ antiport activity (118). Neither $Na^+$-ATPase nor $Na^+/H^+$ antiporter activities were measured.

Now, two mechanisms for $Na^+$ translocation have been identified in methanogens. In *Mb. thermoautotrophicum* a $Na^+/H^+$ antiporter is implicated in pH homeostasis and used to explain why $Na^+$ is needed for methanogenesis (119). Certainly methanogenesis in *Msp. hungatei* exhibits a fairly narrow pH range in the cytoplasmic pH, and in $pH_0$ as well (120). An additional, but not fully understood, role for $Na^+$ in the oxidation of methanol to the level of formaldehyde occurs in *Ms. barkeri* growing on methanol (121). Also, an electrogenic $Na^+$-translocating ATPase appears to explain why $Na^+$ is required for ATP synthesis coupled to a valinomycin-induced $K^+$ diffusion potential in *Mc. voltae* (122). Physiologically, the $Na^+$-ATPase in *Mc. voltae* is expected to serve as a primary $Na^+$ pump using ATP, produced during methanogenesis, to move $Na^+$ out of the cell (122). The resulting electrochemical $Na^+$ gradient may be used in $Na^+$-dependent active transport systems for amino acids (66, 67). Other $Na^+$ pumps have not been reported in methanogens, including the $Na^+$-dependent decarboxylases (Table 3.1) or the mammalian $Na^+$, $K^+$-ATPase sensitive to ouabain.

## 3.6 POTASSIUM

### 3.6.1 K$^+$ Contents

Like the eubacteria and halobacteria (123), methanogens accumulate $K^+$ from their environments (124, 125). The amount accumulated varies widely among the methanogens, with highest capacity of about 1 $M$ in those strains most closely related phylogenetically to the extreme halophiles (Table 3.3). The reason for this wide variation is likely to relate to the different needs

**TABLE 3.3  Intracellular K$^+$ Concentration of Several Methanogenic Bacteria**

| Organism | Intracellular K$^+$ (mM) | Ref. |
|---|---|---|
| *Mbr. smithii* | 1065 ± 48 | 125 |
| *Mbr. arboriphilus* | 1225 ± 33 | 125 |
| *Mb. thermoautotrophicum* | 1103 ± 66 | 125 |
| *Mb. bryantii* | 861 ± 43 | 125 |
| *Mb.* strain G2R | 886 ± 10 | 125 |
| *Mc. voltae* | 725 ± 20 | 125 |
| *Ms. barkeri* | 183 ± 17 | 125 |
| *Msp. hungatei* GP1 | 218 ± 25 | 125 |
| *Msp. hungatei* JF1 | 172 ± 27 | 125 |
| *Mtx. concilii* | 55–160 | 126 |

of each strain to satisfy the same roles for $K^+$ as established for other pro-karyotes (i.e., *E. coli*), namely, for enzyme requirements, for osmoregula-tion, and for regulation of cytoplasmic pH (8, 127). Indeed, in *Msp. hungatei* $K^+$ and $H^+$ movements are linked, and the cytoplasmic content changes in response to the osmolarity of the medium (128). Another role for the $K^+$ gradient is to serve as a long-term storage of energy, especially in extreme halophiles where the cytoplasmic content can reach about 3 $M$ (123).

### 3.6.2   NH₃/K⁺ Exchange

Here, the term ammonia is used to describe either $NH_3$ or $NH_4^+$; whereas the protonation state is indicated by the chemical formulas $NH_3$ or $NH_4^+$.

A dramatic exchange between ammonia and cytoplasmic $K^+$ ($K_i^+$) oc-curs in several methanogens, and in the eubacteria *E. coli* and *Bacillus po-lymyxa*, whereas other methanogens suffer only a small decline in $K_i$ during incubation with ammonia (120). The exchange was studied in *Msp. hungatei* (120) which lost up to 98% of $K_i^+$ when exposed to ammonia at pH 8 in a $K^+$-free buffer. The exchange was immediate, occurring in cells poisoned by air or by metabolic inhibitors. The driving force for the exchange was the transmembrane $K^+$ gradient, and as expected, an external $K^+$ concen-tration sufficient to abolish the gradient ($K_i^+$ 0.2 $M$) largely prevented am-monia influx. The possibility of a novel $NH_4^+/K^+$ antiporter was discounted because the exchange occurred best at alkaline $pH_o$ (external pH), suggesting that $NH_3$, rather than $NH_4^+$, was the active species crossing the membrane. Furthermore, the ratio of $K_{efflux}$/ammonia$_{influx}$ varied depending on the $pH_o$ and concentration of ammonia. This exchange dissipated the transmembrane $\Delta pH$, but had little effect on the membrane potential (negative inside) until concentrations of ammonia were used above that needed to abolish the $K^+$ gradient. A model to explain these effects (Fig. 3.4) shows ammonia entering the cell as the $NH_3$ species at alkaline $pH_o$, combining with a $H^+$ in the cytoplasm to dissipate the $\Delta pH$ (acidic inside) and form $NH_4^+$, which ac-

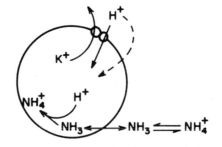

**Figure 3.4**   Model hypothesized to illustrate ammonia/$K^+$ exchange in *Msp. hun-gatei*. The dashed line indicates the possibility of passive entry of protons.

cumulates. Because of an hypothesized $K^+/H^+$ antiporter, ammonia influx may continue, depending on the concentration of $NH_3$ in the medium. At high $pH_0$ and high ammonia concentrations a passive influx of protons (dashed line) and continued influx of $NH_3$ would result in the observed quenching of the membrane potential. For *Msp. hungatei,* we suggested that ammonia/$K^+$ exchange serves to help prevent the loss of membrane potential coupled to ammonia uptake (126).

Methanogens exhibiting the dramatic exchange reaction include *Msp. hungatei* strains GP1 and JF1, *Ms. barkeri,* and *Mtx. concilii* (120, 126, 128). Because cytoplasmic membranes are generally freely permeable to the $NH_3$ species of ammonia (129), it is suggested that $K^+/H^+$ antiporter activity may be absent in those methanogens lacking dramatic ammonia/$K^+$ exchange.

### 3.6.3 Ammonia Uptake/Toxicity

Ammonia/$K^+$ exchange appears to be a method of accumulating $NH_4^+$ using the $K^+$ gradient as driving force. The mechanism is electroneutral and, because a transmembrane $\Delta pH$ is absent in many methanogens at growth pH (6.6–7.0), the pmf is conserved. The $NH_4^+$ gradient achieved would depend, in part, on the concentration of ammonia in the medium and the $pH_0$ (i.e., the $NH_3$ concentration), and on the rate of $K^+/H^+$ exchange (see Fig. 3.4).

The first case of an $NH_4^+/K^+$ antiporter driven by the electrochemical $K^+$ gradient has been found recently in *E. coli* (130). Cell suspensions of *Msp. hungatei, Ms. barkeri,* and *Mtx. concilii,* and several other methanogens to a lesser degree, lost $K_i^+$ when suspended in an $NH_4Cl$ buffer (pH 7.0) (126). At this $pH_0$ the $NH_3$ species represents only about 1% of the total ammonia, suggesting that a $NH_4^+/K^+$ antiporter, or some other means of transporting the $NH_4^+$ species, should be looked for. An active transport of $NH_4^+$ occurs in a number of eubacteria (129).

In growth studies, methanogens could be separated into those relatively resistant to $NH_4Cl$ and those that are sensitive (126). These effects were attributed to $NH_4^+$, not to $Cl^-$. In general, the sensitive strains are those exhibiting either ammonia/$K^+$ exchange or inhibition of methanogenesis by ammonia. The latter effect was studied in *Msp. hungatei,* where ammonia appears to exchange with essential $Mg^{2+}$ (or $Ca^{2+}$) at an unidentified site on the outer surface of the cytoplasmic membrane, thereby abolishing methanogenesis (128). The growth studies were complicated by the effect of competing ions, which could counter the effect of ammonia in causing either the loss of $K_i^+$ or inhibition of methane synthesis, depending on the methanogen being tested (126). It is difficult also to distinguish whether toxicity is caused by the high internal ammonia content or by the lowering of $K_i^+$ content. *Msp. hungatei* grew normally in a medium containing sufficient ammonia to decrease $K_i^+$ to 30 m$M$, at which point the cytoplasmic ammonia had reached about 170 m$M$ (126).

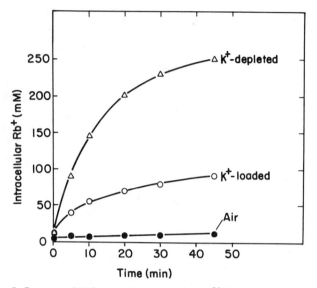

**Figure 3.5**  Influence of $K^+$ depletion and air on $^{86}Rb^+$ uptake in *Msp. hungatei*. Reproduced with permission from Journal of Biological Chemistry (128).

### 3.6.4  Rb⁺ Uptake

The ammonia/$K^+$ exchange reaction provided a convenient method to prepare $K^+$-depleted cells of *Msp. hungatei* for $K^+$ transport studies (128). Following treatment of the cell suspension with ammonia to remove $K_i^+$, it was necessary, however, to restore methanogenesis from $CO_2/H_2$ by adding $Mg^{2+}$ ($Ca^{2+}$ or $Mn^{2+}$). Because $K^+$-depleted cells retain their cytoplasmic $Mg^{2+}$ content, the necessity for $Mg^{2+}$ addition appears to indicate activation at a site exposed to the medium.

The stable isotope $^{86}Rb^+$ can be used as an $K^+$ analog in *Msp. hungatei*. Competition studies indicated no preference by the $K^+$ transport system for either ion. The effect of $K^+$-depletion on $Rb^+$ transport (Fig. 3.5) indicates a feedback regulation by cytoplasmic $K^+$, typical of eubacteria (131). Transport exhibited Michaelis–Menten kinetics. At steady state the concentration gradient (in/out) was 300-fold, and the cytoplasmic $Rb^+$ content approached the initial $K^+$ content before depletion. The $Rb^+$ transport system had a $K_m$ of 0.42 m$M$ and $V_{max}$ of 29 nmol min$^{-1}$ mg$^{-1}$. Transport was energy dependent, requiring both $CO_2$ and $H_2$, and inhibited by air, valinomycin, or nigericin. Protonophores caused a partial decline in ATP content and dramatically collapsed $Rb^+$ transport. Considering that the $Rb^+$ gradient was too large to be in equilibrium with the pmf alone, and from other inhibitor effects, a role is suggested for both ATP and the pmf in $Rb^+$ transport. In these respects, the transport system in *Msp. hungatei* resembles the low-affinity $K^+$ transport system of the eubacteria *E. coli* (132) and *Strepto-*

*coccus faecalis* (131). Also, $K^+$ uptake in *Msp. hungatei* is electrogenic and associated with $H^+$ efflux. A sodium requirement could not be demonstrated. $K^+$ uptake is linked to the efflux of $H^+$ or $Na^+$ in several eubacteria (10), and to $Na^+$ in *Halobacterium halobium* (123). No evidence was found for a $Na^+$, $K^+$-ATPase, typical of higher organisms and found in a eubacterium, *Mycoplasma mycoides* (133).

## 3.7 CALCIUM/MAGNESIUM

Prokaryotes actively excrete $Ca^{2+}$ from their cytoplasm, but concentrate $Mg^{2+}$ (12, 13). Work on transmembrane $Ca^{2+}$ movements in methanogens has not been done, but in eubacteria both a primary $Ca^{2+}$ pump and secondary antiporters ($Ca^{2+}/H^+$, $Ca^{2+}/Na^+$, and $CaHPO_4/H^+$) have been identified (12). Also, the primary $Ca^{2+}$ pumping ATPase of eukaryotic cells (134) is well known. In the case of $Mg^{2+}$, comparisons of extraction with $HClO_4$ and *n*-butanol suggested that approximately half of the $Mg^{2+}$ content of *Msp. hungatei,* and most of the $Mg^{2+}$ content of *Mb. thermoautotrophicum,* was in a bound state (124). $Mg^{2+}$ released by *n*-butanol from *Msp. hungatei* was about 100 nmol $mg^{-1}$ dry weight (128).

## 3.8 TRACE ELEMENTS

### 3.8.1 $Ni^{2+}$ Uptake

Detailed analyses of transport systems for trace elements are complicated by the presence of the element as a contaminant of laboratory reagents, their low $K_m$ for transport, and the difficulty of separating often high amounts of cell-surface binding from active transmembrane flux. Systems for $Ni^{2+}$ transport in microorganisms have not been extensively studied. In eubacteria, uptake occurs either via the $Mg^{2+}$-transport system or by a $Ni^{2+}$-specific transport system. In most cases energy is thought to be required (see Ref. 135 for review).

The first report on $Ni^{2+}$ transport in a methanogen was for the pseudomurein-containing bacterium *Mb. bryantii* (136). The initial fast step of uptake, likely representing binding to the cell surface, was subtracted by measuring rates of uptake between 1 and 10 min from the point of $^{63}Ni^{2+}$ addition to the cells. Nickel was transported against a gradient by a high affinity system ($K_m$ 3.1 $\mu M$) dependent on methanogenesis. Transport was resistant to inhibitors of either ATP synthesis or the membrane potential, but appeared to be linked to a $H^+$ circuit. Not only was transport best at acidic $pH_0$, where an appreciable transmembrane $\Delta pH$ occurred, but also protonophore-sensitive uptake was driven by injections of HCl to generate an artificial $\Delta pH$. Upon dissipation of the artificial $\Delta pH$, $^{63}Ni^{2+}$ efflux occurred from

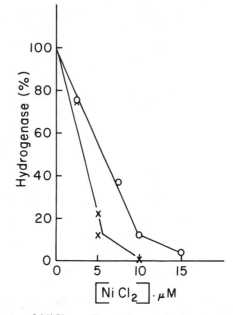

**Figure 3.6**   Influence of NiCl$_2$ on F$_{420}$-reducing hydrogenase activity. Crude cell extracts of *Msp. hungatei* GP1 ($\times$) and *Mb. bryantii* M.o.H. (○) were prepared by French pressure cell lysis. Reduction of F$_{420}$ by H$_2$ was measured spectrophotometrically at 420 nm under anaerobic conditions, as described in Ref. 99. Additions of an anaerobic solution of NiCl$_2$ were made to the assay systems, and the assay begun by injecting aliquots of the crude enzyme.

the cells. Magnesium did not compete with $^{63}$Ni$^{2+}$ for transport, although Co$^{2+}$ did. The possibility should be tested that Co$^{2+}$, needed for corrinoid biosynthesis, is transported solely by the Ni$^{2+}$ transport system.

During growth *Mtx. concilii* incorporated $^{63}$Ni$^{2+}$ into the CO dehydrogenase and the F$_{430}$ prosthetic group of the methylcoenzyme M reductase (136a). In cell suspensions, Ni$^{2+}$ was taken up by a system that was saturated, was time dependent, and was independent of methanogenesis. The K$_m$ (91μ$M$) and V$_{max}$ (23 nmol min$^{-1}$/mg$^{-1}$) for Ni$^{2+}$ uptake by the cells could be reproduced in isolated, empty sheath tubes, showing that adsorption to the sheath accounted for uptake. Any active transport that may be present in active cell preparations would be masked by the large amount of surface adsorption.

Crude extracts of *Msp. hungatei* and *Mb. bryantii* contained F$_{420}$-reducing hydrogenase activity, which was sensitive to NiCl$_2$ concentrations exceeding 5 μ$M$ (Fig. 3.6). The implications of these results is that, during growth, these methanogens contain only low concentrations of free nickel.

### 3.8.2 Other Trace Elements

As reported in Section 3.3, a number of trace elements have been implicated in the nutrition of the methanogens. Even less is known regarding the scavenging mechanisms for these elements than is known for $Ni^{2+}$. Recently, it was shown that many methanogens take up $^{185}W$ during growth (80), although the mechanism for its uptake is unknown.

## 3.9 ANION TRANSPORT

### 3.9.1 Phosphate

A new phosphorus-containing compound designated cyclic 2,3-diphosphoglycerate (cDPG) is present in *Mb. thermoautotrophicum* with concentrations varying from 2 to 200 m$M$, depending on growth conditions (3, 137, 138). Both phosphoryl groups of cDPG turn over during growth, indicating an important role in phosphorus metabolism (137). Cells grown in continuous, phosphate-limited conditions take up phosphate by a single, high-affinity transport system. The $K_m$ was 25 n$M$ and $V_{max}$ 58 mmol phosphate $min^{-1}$ $g^{-1}$ (dry weight). For growth the Monod constant was only 5 n$M$, perhaps explained by the high rates of uptake (high $V_{max}$). Accumulation against large concentration gradients occurred, and was abolished by interruption of the $H_2$ (energy) supply. The incoming phosphate may be stored as cDPG, rather than as polyphosphate common in most microorganisms.

### 3.9.2 Other Anions

The identity of counterions, balancing the charge of the often high $K_i^+$ content in the cytoplasm, has yet to be determined. At $K_i^+$ concentrations above about 300 m$M$ a correlation is seen between cDPG and the $K_i^+$ concentration of *Mb. thermoautotrophicum*, suggesting that $K^+$ may balance the three negative charges of cDPG, or vice versa (138). This did not explain $K^+$ accumulation in phosphate-limited cultures where cDPG was low, or in methanogens (other than the methanobacteria) in which cDPG was not detected (139). The anionic content of methanogens has not been examined, although the anions of sulfur reduced by some species (Section 3.3) and $Cl^-$ are possibilities. Sulfate, selenate, and selenite are actively transported by the same carrier in *E. coli* (140). In *Halobacterium halobium*, halorhodopsin is a light-driven pump moving $Cl^-$ into the cytoplasm (141), but this mechanism appears unique to the extreme halophiles.

The possibility should be considered, for the bulk of methanogens capable of utilizing $CO_2$, that $CO_2$ may be actively transported, rather than penetrating by simple diffusion. A $CO_2$-concentrating mechanism has been found in cyanobacteria, green algae, and green plants involving transport of $CO_2$

or $HCO_3^-$, and most recently uptake of $CO_2$ in *Thiobacillus neapolitanus* was shown to require a pmf and electron transfer (142). Also of possible relevance to future studies with methanogens is the occurrence of electrogenic $Na^+/HCO_3^-$ co-transport in basolateral membranes isolated from rabbit renal cortex (143). Such a mechanism may explain, in part, why $Na^+$ is needed for methanogenesis from $CO_2/H_2$.

As a final example of eubacterial anion transport, the plasmid-encoded arsenical pump of *E. coli* (8) may be cited. Whether this mechanism for extrusion of toxic anions is present in methanogens is unknown.

## 3.10  SUMMARY

The cell walls and cytoplasmic membranes of methanogens differ chemically from eubacteria, which may effect the accumulation and uptake of ions. Transmembrane ion translocating systems are implied from nutritional studies (Table 3.2) showing requirements for those ions typically required by eubacteria, and for those elements present in only trace amounts in normal growth media (i.e., Ni, Fe, Mo, Zn, Se, W). The primary proton pump may differ mechanistically in methanogens, in which the novel methylcoenzyme M reductase reaction appears to be linked to the formation of a pmf. Iontranslocating systems of methanogens have seldom been sufficiently studied to allow a detailed comparison; however, the systems known are not atypical of certain of the eubacteria. These include $K^+$ transport, $Na^+/H^+$ antiport, and $Na^+$-ATPase activity. Only a few methanogen species have been tested in these studies, and considering the diversity expected among methanogens (3, 4), it is dangerous to draw analogies among species. Obviously, a great deal remains unknown; for example, whether iron transport occurs using the same types of natural chelators discovered in eubacteria remains to be established. The possibility exists for novel chelation mechanisms for certain other trace elements as well. The next few years should prove most exciting.

## REFERENCES

1. N. G. Mehta. An alternative view of the origin of life, Nature (London), *324*, 415 (1986).
2. C. R. Woese, L. J. Magrum, and G. E. Fox. Archaebacteria, J. Mol. Evolution, *11*, 245 (1978).
3. L. Daniels, R. Sparling, and G. D. Sprott. The bioenergetics of methanogenesis, Biochim. Biophys. Acta, *768*, 113 (1984).
4. W. J. Jones, D. P. Nagle, Jr., and W. B. Whitman. Methanogens and the diversity of archaebacteria, Microbiol. Rev., *51*, 135 (1987).
5. G. Fuchs. $CO_2$ fixation in acetogenic bacteria: variations on a theme, FEMS Microbiol. Rev., *39*, 181 (1986).

6. I. Ekiel, G. D. Sprott, and G. B. Patel. Acetate and $CO_2$ assimilation by *Methanothrix concilii*, J. Bacteriol., *162*, 905 (1985).

7. K. Laufer, B. Eikmanns, U. Frimmer, and R. K. Thauer. Methanogenesis from acetate by *Methanosarcina barkeri:* catalysis of acetate formation from methyl iodide, $CO_2$, and $H_2$ by the enzyme system involved, Z. Naturforsch., *42c*, 360 (1987).

8. B. P. Rosen. Recent advances in bacterial ion transport, Ann. Rev. Microbiol. *40*, 263 (1986).

9. S. Silver and R. D. Perry. "Bacterial inorganic cation and anion transport systems," in A. N. Martonosi, Ed., *Membranes and Transport,* Vol. 2, Plenum Press, New York, 1982, pp. 115–128.

10. F. M. Harold and K. Altendorf. Cation transport in bacteria; $K^+$, $Na^+$, and $H^+$, Current Topics in membranes and Transport, *5*, 1 (1974).

11. A. Rothstein. "Ion transport in microorganisms," in L. E. Hokin, Ed., *Metabolic Transport,* Vol. 6, Academic, New York and London, 1972, pp. 17–39.

12. B. P. Rosen. Bacterial calcium transport, Biochim. Biophys. Acta, *906*, 101 (1987).

13. B. P. Rosen and S. Silver, Eds. *Ion Transport in Prokaryotes,* Academic, New York, 1987.

14. I. C. P. West. Energy coupling in secondary active transport, Biochim. Biophys. Acta, *604*, 91 (1980).

15. W. N. Konings and R. Otto. Energy transduction and solute transport in streptococci, Antonie van Leeuwenhoek, *49*, 247 (1983).

16. J. M. Odom and H. D. Peck, Jr. Hydrogenase, electron-transfer proteins, and energy coupling in the sulfate-reducing bacteria *Desulfovibrio*, Ann. Rev. Microbiol., *38*, 551 (1984).

17. A. B. Hooper, A. A. DiSpirito, T. C. Olson, K. K. Andersson, W. Cunningham, and L. R. Taaffe. "Generation of a proton gradient by a periplasmic dehydrogenase," in R. L. Crawford and R. S. Hanson, Eds., *Microbial Growth on $C_1$ Compounds,* American Society for Microbiology, Washington, DC, 1984, pp. 53–58.

18. H. Tokuda and T. Unemoto. Characterization of the respiration-dependent $Na^+$ pump in the marine bacterium *Vibrio alginolyticus*, J. Biol. Chem., *257*, 10,007 (1982).

19. F. Hamaide, D. J. Kushner, and G. D. Sprott. Proton circulation in *Vibrio costicola*, J. Bacteriol., *161*, 681 (1985).

20. P. Mitchell. Chemiosmotic coupling in oxidative and photosynthetic phosphorylation, Biol. Rev., *41*, 445 (1966).

21. B. A. Haddock and C. W. Jones. Bacterial respiration, Bacteriol. Rev., *41*, 47 (1977).

22. P. Mitchell. A chemiosmotic molecular mechanism for proton-translocating adenosine triphosphatases, FEBS Lett., *43*, 189 (1974).

23. D. B. Knaff. Active transport in phototrophic bacteria, Photosynthesis Res., *10*, 507 (1986).

24. W. Stoeckenius and R. A. Bogomolni. Bacteriorhodopsin and related pigments of halobacteria, Ann. Rev. Biochem., *52*, 587 (1982).

25. D. L. Heefner and F. M. Harold. ATP-driven sodium pump in *Streptococcus faecalis*, Proc. Natl. Acad. Sci. U.S., *79*, 2798 (1982).

26. M. Benyoucef, J.-L. Rigaud, and G. Leblanc. Cation transport mechanisms in *Mycoplasma mycoides* var. Capri cells, Biochem. J., *208*, 539 (1982).

27. D. C. Jinks, J. R. Silvius, and R. N. McElhaney. Physiological role and membrane lipid modulation of the membrane-bound ($Mg^{2+}$, $Na^+$)-adenosine triphosphatase activity in *Acholeplasma laidlawii*, J. Bacteriol., *136*, 1027 (1978).

28. P. Dimroth. The generation of an electrochemical gradient of sodium ions upon decarboxylation of oxaloacetate by the membrane-bound and $Na^+$-activated oxaloacetate decarboxylase from *Klebsiella aerogenes*, Eur. J. Biochem., *121*, 443 (1982).

29. W. Buckel and R. Semmler. A biotin-dependent sodium pump: glutaconyl-CoA decarboxylase from *Acidaminococcus fermentans*, FEBS Lett., *148*, 35 (1982).

30. W. Hilpert and P. Dimroth. Conversion of the chemical energy of methylmalonyl-CoA decarboxylation into a $Na^+$ gradient, Nature (London), *296*, 584 (1982).

31. T. A. Krulwich. $Na^+/H^+$ antiporters, Biochim. Biophys. Acta, *726*, 245 (1983).

32. T. Nakamura, C. Hsu, and B. P. Rosen. Cation/proton antiport systems in *Escherichia coli*, J. Biol. Chem., *261*, 678 (1986).

33. I. C. West and P. Mitchell. Proton/sodium ion antiport in *Escherichia coli*, Biochem. J., *144*, 87 (1974).

34. F. Hamaide, D. J. Kushner, and G. D. Sprott. Proton motive force and $Na^+/H^+$ antiport in a moderate halophile, J. Bacteriol., *156*, 537 (1983).

35. R. N. Brey, B. P. Rosen, and E. N. Sorensen. Cation/proton antiport systems in *Escherichia coli*, J. Biol. Chem., *255*, 39 (1980).

36. S. V. Ambudkar, G. W. Zlotnick, and B. P. Rosen. Calcium efflux from *Escherichia coli*, J. Biol. Chem., *259*, 6142 (1984).

37. Y. Kabinuma and F. M. Harold. ATP-driven exchange of $Na^+$ and $K^+$ ions by *Streptococcus faecalis*, J. Biol. Chem., *260*, 2086 (1985).

38. A. Jayakumar, W. Epstein, and E. M. Barnes, Jr. Characterization of ammonium (methylammonium)/potassium antiport in *Escherichia coli*, J. Biol. Chem., *260*, 7528 (1985).

39. P. C. Maloney, S. V. Ambudkar, J. Thomas, and L. Schiller. Phosphate/hexose 6-phosphate antiport in *Streptococcus lactis*, J. Bacteriol., *158*, 238 (1984).

40. O. Kandler and H. König. "Cell envelopes of archaebacteria," in C. R. Woese and R. S. Wolfe, Eds., *The Bacteria*, Vol. 8, Academic, New York, 1985, pp. 413–457.

41. P. Kreisl and O. Kandler. Chemical structure of the cell wall polymer of *Methanosarcina*, System. Appl. Microbiol., *7*, 293 (1986).

42. H. König and K. O. Stetter. Studies on archaebacterial S-layers, System. Appl. Microbiol., *7*, 300 (1986).

43. U. B. Sleytr, P. Messner, M. Sára, and D. Pum. Crystalline envelope layers of archaebacteria, System. Appl. Microbiol., *7*, 310 (1986).

44. T. J. Beveridge, G. B. Patel, B. J. Harris, and G. D. Sprott. The ultrastructure of *Methanothrix concilii*, a mesophilic aceticlastic methanogen, Can. J. Microbiol., *32*, 703 (1986).

45. T. J. Beveridge, B. J. Harris, and G. D. Sprott. Septation and filament splitting in *Methanospirillum hungatei,* Can. J. Microbiol., *33,* 725 (1987).

46. T. J. Beveridge, B. J. Harris, G. B. Patel, and G. D. Sprott. Cell division and filament splitting in *Methanothrix concilii,* Can. J. Microbiol., *32,* 779 (1986).

47. M. Stewart, T. J. Beveridge, and G. D. Sprott. Crystalline order to high resolution in the sheath of *Methanospirillum hungatei:* a cross-beta structure, J. Mol. Biol., *183,* 509 (1985).

48. G. D. Sprott, T. J. Beveridge, G. B. Patel, and G. Ferrante. Sheath disassembly in *Methanospirillum hungatei* strain GP1, Can. J. Microbiol., *32,* 847 (1986).

49. G. B. Patel, G. D. Sprott, R. W. Humphrey, and T. J. Beveridge. Comparative analysis of the sheath structures of *Methanothrix concilii* GP6 and *Methanospirillum hungatei* strains GP1 and JF1, Can. J. Microbiol., *32,* 623 (1986).

50. T. J. Beveridge, M. Stewart, R. J. Doyle, and G. D. Sprott. Unusual stability of the *Methanospirillum hungatei* sheath, J. Bacteriol., *162,* 728 (1985).

51. G. D. Sprott, J. R. Colvin, and R. C. McKellar. Spheroplasts of *Methanospirillum hungatei* formed upon treatment with dithiothreitol, Can. J. Microbiol., *25,* 730 (1979).

52. K. F. Jarrell, J. R. Colvin, and G. D. Sprott. Spontaneous protoplast formation in *Methanobacterium bryantii,* J. Bacteriol., *149,* 346 (1982).

53. H. König, R. Semmler, C. Lerp, and J. Winter. Evidence for the occurrence of autolytic enzymes in *Methanobacterium wolfei,* Arch. Microbiol., *141,* 177 (1985).

54. G. D. Sprott and K. F. Jarrell. "Electrochemical potential and membrane properties of methanogenic bacteria," in W. R. Strohl and O. H. Tuovinen, Eds., *Microbial Chemoautotrophy,* The Ohio State University Press, Columbus, 1984, pp. 255–273.

55. D. O. Mountfort, E. Mörschel, D. B. Beimborn, and P. Schönheit. Methanogenesis and ATP synthesis in a protoplast system of *Methanobacterium thermoautotrophicum,* J. Bacteriol., *168,* 892 (1986).

56. G. D. Sprott, K. M. Shaw, and K. F. Jarrell. Isolation and chemical composition of the cytoplasmic membrane of the archaebacterium *Methanospirillum hungatei,* J. Biol. Chem., *258,* 4026 (1983).

57. T. A. Langworthy and J. L. Pond. Archaebacterial ether lipids and chemotaxonomy, System. Appl. Microbiol., *7,* 253 (1986).

58. S. C. Kushwaha, M. Kates, G. D. Sprott, and I. C. P. Smith. Novel polar lipids from the methanogen *Methanospirillum hungatei* GP1, Biochim. Biophys. Acta, *664,* 156 (1981).

59. G. Ferrante, I. Ekiel, and G. D. Sprott. Structures of diether lipids of *Methanospirillum hungatei* containing novel head groups N,N-dimethylamino- and N,N,N-trimethylamino pentanetetrol, Biochim. Biophys. Acta, *921,* 281 (1987).

60. G. Ferrante, I. Ekiel, and G. D. Sprott. Structural characterization of the lipids of *Methanococcus voltae,* including a novel N-acetylglucosamine 1-phosphate diether, J. Biol. Chem., *261,* 17062 (1986).

61. M. Nishihara, H. Morii, and Y. Koga. Structure determination of a quartet of novel tetraether lipids from *Methanobacterium thermoautotrophicum,* J. Biochem., *101,* 1007 (1987).

62. H. Morii, M. Nishihara, M. Ohga, and Y. Koga. A diphytanyl ether analog of phosphatidylserine from a methanogenic bacterium, *Methanobrevibacter arboriphilus*, J. Lipid Res., *27*, 724 (1986).

62a. G. Ferrante, I. Ekiel, G. B. Patel, and G. D. Sprott. Structure of the major polar lipids isolated from the aceticlastic methanogen, *Methanothrix concilii*, GP6 Biochim. Biophys. Acta, *963*, 162–172 (1988).

62b. G. Ferrante, I. Ekiel, G. B. Patel, and G. D. Sprott. A novel core lipid isolated from the aceticlastic methanogen, *Methanothrix concilii* GP6, Biochim. Biophys. Acta, *963*, 173–182 (1988).

63. M. De Rosa, A. Gambacorta, and A. Gliozzi. Structure, biosynthesis, and physicochemical properties of archaebacterial lipids, Microbiol. Rev., *50*, 70 (1986).

64. W. E. Balch and R. S. Wolfe. Transport of coenzyme M (2-mercaptoethanesulfonic acid) in *Methanobacterium ruminantium*, J. Bacteriol., *137*, 264 (1979).

65. W. B. Whitman, E. Ankwanda, and R. S. Wolfe. Nutrition and carbon metabolism of *Methanococcus voltae*, J. Bacteriol., *149*, 852 (1982).

66. K. F. Jarrell and G. D. Sprott. Importance of sodium to the bioenergetic properties of *Methanococcus voltae*, Can. J. Microbiol., *31*, 851 (1985).

67. I. Ekiel, K. F. Jarrell, and G. D. Sprott. Amino acid biosynthesis and sodium-dependent transport in *Methanococcus voltae*, as revealed by $^{13}C$ NMR, Eur. J. Biochem., *149*, 437 (1985).

68. P. Schönheit, D. B. Beimborn, and H.-J. Perski. Potassium accumulation in growing *Methanobacterium thermoautotrophicum* and its relation to the electrochemical proton gradient, Arch. Microbiol., *140*, 247 (1984).

69. H. J. Perski, J. Moll, and R. K. Thauer. Sodium dependence of growth and methane formation in *Methanobacterium thermoautotrophicum*, Arch. Microbiol., *130*, 319 (1981).

70. H. P. Zabel, H. König, and J. Winter. Isolation and characterization of a new coccoid methanogen, *Methanogenium tatii* spec. nov. from a solfataric field on Mount Tatio, Arch. Microbiol., *137*, 308 (1984).

71. P. A. Murray and S. H. Zinder. Nutritional requirements of *Methanosarcina* sp. strain TM1, Appl. Env. Microbiol., *50*, 49 (1985).

72. G. B. Patel, C. Baudet, and B. J. Agnew. Nutritional requirements for growth of *Methanothrix concilii*, Can. J. Microbiol., *34*, 73 (1987).

73. P. H. Rönnow and L. A. H. Gunnarsson. Response of growth and methane production to limiting amounts of sulfide and ammonia in two thermophilic methanogenic bacteria. FEMS Microbiol. Lett., *14*, 311 (1982).

74. P. Scherer and H. Sahm. Effect of trace elements and vitamins on the growth of *Methanosarcina barkeri*, Acta Biotechnologia I, *1*, 57 (1981).

75. P. Schönheit, J. Moll, and R. K. Thauer. Nickel, cobalt, and molybdenum requirement for growth of *Methanobacterium thermoautotrophicum*, Arch. Microbiol., *123*, 105 (1979).

76. K. R. Sowers and J. G. Ferry. Trace metal and vitamin requirements of *Methanococcoides methylutens* grown with trimethylamine, Arch. Microbiol., *142*, 148 (1985).

77. G. B. Patel, A. W. Khan, and L. A. Roth. Optimum levels of sulphate and iron

for the cultivation of pure cultures of methanogens in synthetic media, J. Appl. Bacteriol., *45*, 347 (1978).

78. N. Belay, R. Sparling, and L. Daniels. Relationship of formate to growth and methanogenesis by *Methanococcus thermolithotrophicus,* Appl. Env. Microbiol., *52*, 1080 (1986).

79. J. B. Jones and T. C. Stadtman. *Methanococcus vannielii:* culture and effects of selenium and tungsten on growth, J. Bacteriol., *130*, 1404 (1977).

80. G. Zellner and J. Winter. Growth promoting effect of tungsten on methanogens and incorporation of tungsten-185 into cells, FEMS Microbiol. Lett., *40*, 81 (1987).

81. J. Winter, C. Lerp, H.-P. Zabel, F. X. Wildenauer, H. König, and F. Schindler. *Methanobacterium wolfei,* sp. nov., a new tungsten-requiring, thermophilic autotrophic methanogen, System. Appl. Microbiol., *5*, 466 (1984).

82. I. J. Kugelman and K. K. Chin. "Toxicity, synergism, and antagonism in anaerobic waste treatment processes," in R. F. Gould, Ed., *Anaerobic Biological Waste Treatment Processes,* Advances in Chemistry Series 105, American Chemical Society, Washington, DC, 1971, pp. 55–90.

83. R. A. MacLeod. Marine microbiology far from the sea, Ann. Rev. Microbiol., *39*, 1 (1985).

84. E. A. Wolin, M. J. Wolin, and R. S. Wolfe. Formation of methane by bacterial extracts, J. Biol. Chem., *238*, 2882 (1963).

85. L. Daniels, N. Belay, and B. S. Rajagopal. Assimilatory reduction of sulfate and sulfite by methanogenic bacteria, Appl. Env. Microbiol., *51*, 703 (1986).

86. T. K. Mazumder, N. Nishio, S. Fukuzaki, and S. Nagai. Effect of sulfur-containing compounds on growth of *Methanosarcina barkeri* in defined medium, Appl. Env. Microbiol., *52*, 617 (1986).

87. B. S. Rajagopal and L. Daniels. Investigation of mercaptans, organic sulfides, and inorganic sulfur compounds as sulfur sources for the growth of methanogenic bacteria, Curr. Microbiol., *14*, 137 (1986).

88. P. Scherer, H. Lippert, and G. Wolff. Composition of the major elements and trace elements of 10 methanogenic bacteria determined by inductively coupled plasma emission spectrometry, Biological Trace Element Research, *5*, 149 (1983).

89. P. A. Scherer and H.-P. Bochem. Energy-dispersive X-ray microanalysis of the methanogen *Methanosarcina barkeri* 'Fusaro' grown on methanol and in the presence of heavy metals, Curr. Microbiol., *9*, 187 (1983).

90. P. L. Hartzell and R. S. Wolfe. Requirement of the nickel tetrapyrrole $F_{430}$ for *in vitro* methanogenesis: Reconstitution of methylreductase component C from its dissociated subunits, Proc. Natl. Acad. Sci. USA, *83*, 6726 (1986).

91. F. S. Jacobson, L. Daniels, J. A. Fox, C. T. Walsh, and W. H. Orme-Johnson. Purification and properties of an 8-hydroxy-5-deazaflavin-reducing hydrogenase from *Methanobacterium thermoautotrophicum,* J. Biol. Chem., *257*, 3385 (1982).

92. N. L. Schauer and J. G. Ferry. Composition of the coenzyme $F_{420}$-dependent formate dehydrogenase from *Methanobacterium formicicum,* J. Bacteriol., *165*, 405 (1986).

93. J. B. Jones and T. C. Stadtman. Selenium-dependent and selenium-independent formate dehydrogenases of *Methanococcus vannielii*, J. Biol. Chem., *256*, 656 (1981).

94. V. Höllriegl, P. Scherer, and P. Renz. Isolation and characterization of the Co-methyl and Co-aquo derivative of 5-hydroxybenzimidazolylcobamide (factor III) from *Methanosarcina barkeri* grown on methanol, FEBS Lett., *151*, 156 (1983).

95. E. Padan, Z. Zilberstein, and S. Schuldiner. pH homeostasis in bacteria, Biochim. Biophys. Acta. *650*, 151 (1981).

96. B. M. Butsch and R. Bachofen. The membrane potential in whole cells of *Methanobacterium thermoautotrophicum*, Arch. Microbiol., *138*, 293 (1984).

97. M. Blaut and G. Gottschalk. Coupling of ATP synthesis and methane formation from methanol and molecular hydrogen in *Methanosarcina barkeri*, Eur. J. Biochem., *141*, 217 (1984).

98. R. Ossmer, T. Mund, P. L. Hartzell, U. Konheiser, G. W. Kohring, A. Klein, R. S. Wolfe, G. Gottschalk, and F. Mayer. Immunochemical localization of component C of the methylreductase system in *Methanococcus voltae* and *Methanobacterium thermoautotrophicum*, Proc. Natl. Acad. Sci. USA, *83*, 5789 (1986).

99. G. D. Sprott, K. M. Shaw, and T. J. Beveridge. Properties of the particulate enzyme $F_{420}$-hydrogenase isolated from *Methanospirillum hungatei*, Can. J. Microbiol., *33*, 896 (1987).

100. S. F. Baron, D. P. Brown, and J. G. Ferry. Locations of the hydrogenases of *Methanobacterium formicicum* after subcellular fractionation of cell extract, J. Bacteriol., *169*, 3823 (1987).

101. R. C. McKellar and G. D. Sprott. Solubilization and properties of a particulate hydrogenase from *Methanobacterium* strain G2R, J. Bacteriol., *139*, 231 (1979).

102. G. D. Sprott, S. E. Bird, and I. J. McDonald. Proton motive force as a function of the pH at which *Methanobacterium bryantii* is grown, Can. J. Microbiol., *31*, 1031 (1985).

103. D. B. Kell, H. J. Doddema, J. G. Morris, and G. D. Vogels. "Energy coupling in methanogens," in H. Dalton, Ed., *Microbial Growth on $C_1$ Compounds*, Heyden, London, 1981, pp. 159–170.

104. G. D. Sprott, L. C. Sowden, J. R. Colvin, and K. F. Jarrell. Methanogenesis in the absence of intracytoplasmic membranes, Can. J. Microbiol., *30*, 594 (1984).

105. R. Krämer and P. Schönheit. Testing the "methanochondrion concept": are nucleotides transported across internal membranes in *Methanobacterium thermoautotrophicum?* Arch. Microbiol., *146*, 370 (1987).

106. H. C. Aldrich, D. B. Beimborn, and P. Schönheit. Creation of artifactual internal membranes during fixation of *Methanobacterium thermoautotrophicum*, Can. J. Microbiol., *33*, 844 (1987).

107. B. P. Crider, S. W. Carper, and J. R. Lancaster, Jr. Electron transfer-driven ATP synthesis in *Methanococcus voltae* is not dependent on a proton electrochemical gradient, Proc. Natl. Acad. Sci. USA, *82*, 6793 (1985).

108. D. O. Mountfort. Evidence for ATP synthesis driven by a proton gradient in *Methanosarcina barkeri*, Biochem. Biophys. Res. Commun., *85*, 1346 (1978).

109. G. D. Sprott and K. F. Jarrell. Sensitivity of methanogenic bacteria to dicyclohexylcarbodiimide, Can. J. Microbiol., *28*, 982 (1982).

110. A. Jussofie, F. Mayer, and G. Gottschalk. Methane formation from methanol and molecular hydrogen by protoplasts of new methanogenic isolates and inhibition by dicyclohexylcarbodiimide, Arch. Microbiol., *146*, 245 (1986).

111. R. Roth, R. Duft, A. Binder, and R. Bachofen. Isolation and characterization of a soluble ATPase from *Methanobacterium thermoautotrophicum*, System. Appl. Microbiol., *7*, 346 (1986).

112. K.-I. Inatomi. Characterization and purification of the membrane-bound ATPase of the archaebacterium *Methanosarcina barkeri*, J. Bacteriol., *167*, 837 (1986).

113. F. Mayer, A. Jussofie, M. Salzmann, M. Lübben, M. Rohde, and G. Gottschalk. Immunoelectron microscopic demonstration of ATPase on the cytoplasmic membrane of the methanogenic bacterium strain Göl, J. Bacteriol., *169*, 2307 (1987).

114. J. K. Lanyi. The role of $Na^+$ in transport processes of bacterial membranes, Biochim. Biophys. Acta, *559*, 377 (1979).

115. B. F. Luisi, J. K. Lanyi, and H. J. Weber. $Na^+$ transport via $Na^+/H^+$ antiport in *Halobacterium halobium* envelope vesicles. FEBS Lett., *117*, 354 (1980).

116. R. Hartmann, H.-D. Sickinger, and D. Oesterhelt. Anaerobic growth of halobacteria, Proc. Natl. Acad. Sci. USA, *77*, 3821 (1980).

117. H. J. Perski, P. Schönheit, and R. K. Thauer. Sodium dependence of methane formation in methanogenic bacteria, FEBS Lett., *143*, 323 (1982).

118. P. Schönheit and H. J. Perski. ATP synthesis driven by a potassium diffusion potential in *Methanobacterium thermoautotrophicum* is stimulated by sodium, FEMS Microbiol. Lett., *20*, 263 (1983).

119. P. Schönheit and D. B. Beimborn. Presence of a $Na^+/H^+$ antiporter in *Methanobacterium thermoautotrophicum* and its role in $Na^+$ dependent methanogenesis, Arch. Microbiol., *142*, 354 (1985).

120. G. D. Sprott, K. M. Shaw, and K. F. Jarrell. Ammonia/potassium exchange in methanogenic bacteria, J. Biol. Chem., *259*, 12602 (1984).

121. M. Blaut, V. Müller, and G. Gottschalk. Mechanism of ATP synthesis and role of sodium ions in *Methanosarcina barkeri* growing on methanol, System. Appl. Microbiol., *7*, 354 (1986).

122. S. W. Carper and J. R. Lancaster, Jr. An electrogenic sodium-translocating ATPase in *Methanococcus voltae*, FEBS Lett., *200*, 177 (1986).

123. G. Wagner, R. Hartmann, and D. Oesterhelt. Potassium uniport and ATP synthesis in *Halobacterium halobium*, Eur. J. Biochem., *89*, 169 (1978).

124. G. D. Sprott and K. F. Jarrell. $K^+$, $Na^+$, and $Mg^{2+}$ content and permeability of *Methanospirillum hungatei* and *Methanobacterium thermoautotrophicum*, Can. J. Microbiol., *27*, 444 (1981).

125. K. F. Jarrell, G. D. Sprott, and A. T. Matheson. Intracellular potassium concentration and relative acidity of the ribosomal proteins of methanogenic bacteria, Can. J. Microbiol., *30*, 663 (1984).

126. G. D. Sprott and G. B. Patel. Ammonia toxicity in pure cultures of methanogenic bacteria, System. Appl. Microbiol., *7*, 358 (1986).

127. W. Epstein and L. Laimins. Potassium transport in *Escherichia coli:* diverse systems with common control by osmotic forces, Trends Biochem. Sci., *5*, 21 (1980).

128. G. D. Sprott, K. M. Shaw, and K. F. Jarrell. Methanogenesis and the K$^+$ transport system are activated by divalent cations in ammonia-treated cells of *Methanospirillum hungatei*, J. Biol. Chem., *260*, 9244 (1985).

129. D. Kleiner. The transport of $NH_3$ and $NH_4^+$ across biological membranes, Biochim. Biophys. Acta, *639*, 41 (1981).

130. A. Jayakumar. W. Epstein, and E. M. Barnes, Jr. Characterization of ammonium (methylammonium)/potassium antiport in *Escherichia coli*, J. Biol. Chem., *260*, 7528 (1985).

131. E. P. Bakker and F. M. Harold. Energy coupling to potassium transport in *Streptococcus faecalis*, J. Biol. Chem., *255*, 433 (1980).

132. D. B. Rhoads and W. Epstein. Energy coupling to net K$^+$ transport in *Escherichia coli* K12, J. Biol. Chem., *252*, 1394 (1977).

133. M. Benyoucef, J.-L. Rigaud, and G. Leblanc. Cation transport mechanisms in *Mycoplasma mycoides* var. Capri cells, Na$^+$-dependent K$^+$ accumulation, Biochem. J., *208*, 529 (1982).

134. M. Michalak, K. Famulski, and E. Carafoli. The Ca$^{2+}$-pumping ATPase in skeletal muscle sarcolemma, J. Biol. Chem., *259*, 15540 (1984).

135. R. P. Hausinger. Nickel utilization by microorganisms, Microbiol. Rev., *51*, 22 (1987).

136. K. F. Jarrell and G. D. Sprott. Nickel transport in *Methanobacterium bryantii*, J. Bacteriol., *151*, 1195 (1982).

136a.C. Baudet, G. D. Sprott, and G. B. Patel. Adsorption and uptake of nickel in *Methanothrix concilii*, Arch. Microbiol., *150*, 338–342 (1988).

137. R. D. Krueger, J. W. Campbell, and D. E. Fahrney. Turnover of cyclic 2,3-diphosphoglycerate in *Methanobacterium thermoautotrophicum*, J. Biol. Chem., *261*, 11945 (1986).

138. R. D. Krueger, R. J. Seeley, and D. E. Fahrney. Intracellular K$^+$ and cyclic diphosphoglycerate pools and transients in *Methanobacterium thermoautotrophicum*, System. Appl. Microbiol., *7*, 388 (1986).

139. C. J. Tolman, S. Kanodia, M. F. Roberts, and L. Daniels. $^{31}$P-NMR spectra of methanogens: 2,3-cyclopyrophosphoglycerate is detectable only in methanobacteria strains, Biochim. Biophys. Acta, *886*, 345 (1986).

140. C. Lindblow-Kull, F. J. Kull, and A. Shrift. Single transporter for sulfate, selenate, and selenite in *Escherichia coli* k-12, J. Bacteriol., *163*, 1267 (1985).

141. B. Schobert and J. K. Lanyi. Halorhodopsin is a light-driven chloride pump, J. Biol. Chem., *257*, 10306 (1982).

142. Y. A. Holthuijzen, F. F. M. van Dissel-Emiliani, J. G. Kuenen, and W. N. Konings. Energetic aspects of $CO_2$ uptake in *Thiobacillus neapolitanus*, Arch. Microbiol., *147*, 285 (1987).

143. S. M. Grassl and P. S. Aronson. Na$^+$/HCO$_3^-$ co-transport in basolateral membrane vesicles isolated from rabbit renal cortex, J. Biol. Chem., *261*, 8778 (1986).

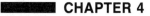 

# CHAPTER 4

# Bacterial Resistance to Toxic Heavy Metals

SIMON SILVER and TAPAN K. MISRA

Department of Microbiology and Immunology
University of Illinois College of Medicine
Chicago, Illinois

RICHARD A. LADDAGA

Department of Biological Sciences
Bowling Green State University
Bowling Green, Ohio

## Contents

## 4.1  INTRODUCTION

Bacterial cells have coexisted with toxic heavy metals since the origin of life, perhaps 3 or 4 $\times$ $10^9$ years ago. In the early stages of the evolution of life, when volcanic activity and other sources of toxic heavy metals were

This manuscript is an altered version of one which will appear in R. K. Poole and G. M. Gadd (Eds.) *Metal-Microbe Interactions*, IRL Press, Oxford, in press, which is the report from a 1988 Society of General Microbiology meeting in Warwick, U.K.

ubiquitous, it was essential to invent mechanisms to cope with—to be resistant to—the toxic heavy metals that were abundant in the environment (Chapter 1). Perhaps later in prokaryotic evolution, the genes for resistances to toxic heavy metals were less essential, and it became important to minimize the genetic burden of carrying these sometimes essential, sometimes burdensome genes. Then, as best as we can reconstruct, the genes for toxic heavy metal resistances, quite similarly to the genes for antibiotic resistances and other ancillary functions, were "packaged" into bacterial plasmids and transposons. These small circular pieces of DNA and linear "hopping genes," respectively, could be lost from particular lines of bacterial cells easily without endangering the rest of the cellular genetic heritage, and even more importantly could move from place to place, from cell to cell, in a facile fashion by mechanisms of intercellular gene transfer; such transfer facilitated the spread of a resistance among a population of bacteria including more than a single strain or species, when stress from toxic heavy metal pollution made this resistance an asset for cellular survival. With this view of how bacterial toxic heavy metal resistances came about, we can recognize that they should be quite ancient, and we can expect the genetic and biochemical mechanisms involved to share properties with those for essential cellular roles, such as growth, metabolism of energy and carbon sources, and biosynthesis of essential nutrients.

In common with resistances to antibiotics, bacterial resistances to toxic heavy metals appear to have only a small number of basic mechanisms:

1. There are enzymes, oxidases and reductases, to convert metal ions from more toxic into less toxic. There are alkylating enzymes and dealkylating lyases that add and remove covalently attached components of organometal compounds. Reduction and dealkylation are the major mechanisms of resistance to inorganic and organic mercury compounds. Arsenite oxidation and chromate reduction can be mechanisms of resistance for those toxic metal ions, but they have not been demonstrated (as yet) to be plasmid resistance mechanisms.

2. There is the possibility of sequestration and binding of toxic heavy metals either in the cell wall (preventing them from reaching the intracellular cytoplasm) (Chapters 9–11) or intracellularly in highly specific binding components, such as metallothionein (Chapter 6). Again, there is no clear-cut example in which this has been demonstrated to be a plasmid gene-determined resistance mechanism.

3. There is the possibility of blocking cellular uptake by altering the uptake pathway available in sensitive cells. Although this is the mechanism of chromosomally determined resistance to arsenate, cadmium, chromate, and perhaps other heavy metal ions, there is no known example of this mechanism for plasmid-governed resistance.

4. Once the toxic heavy metal ion has reached the intracellular cytoplasm,

it can be pumped out again rapidly by a highly specific efflux system, which might derive its energy either from the membrane potential or more directly from ATP. Efflux pumps seem to be the mechanism of tetracycline (an antibiotic) resistance in bacteria and for resistance to arsenic, cadmium, and chromate, at least in some cases. In the last few years, DNA sequencing analysis has clarified the nature of an arsenic ATPase and a cadmium ATPase efflux system, both of which are highly specific.

5. There is the possibility of altering intracellular targets for the toxic action of heavy metals, but in the case of metal ions, rather than antibiotics, the mechanisms of toxicity are generally so broad and nonspecific that this might be impossible. It might be necessary to change all of the thiol-containing enzymes that are sensitive to cadmium or arsenite in order to obtain resistance to these toxic ions. In terms of genetically determined biochemical functions, that is not feasible.

This brief overview emphasizes recent findings from DNA sequence analysis that has provided detailed understanding for cadmium, arsenic, and mercury resistance governed by bacterial plasmids. A more detailed coverage of bacterial heavy metal resistance appeared recently (1).

## 4.2  CADMIUM RESISTANCE

There are perhaps six known mechanisms of cadmium resistance (1), and only one of these has been studied and understood at a reasonable level from DNA sequencing analysis. This is the *cadA* determinant from *Staphylococcus aureus* plasmids (2). Weiss et al. (3) showed that cadmium accumulation occurs via the chromosomally determined manganese transport system in sensitive cells and that less net cadmium accumulation occurs in resistant cells. Rather than a direct block on $Cd^{2+}$ uptake, Tynecka et al. (4) demonstrated that an energy-dependent efflux system functions in resistant cells but is missing in sensitive cells. Based on studies of inhibition of cadmium efflux by membrane-perturbing antibiotics, Tynecka et al. (4) concluded that the fundamental mechanism was a $Cd^{2+}/2H^+$ exchange (Fig. 4.1). It remained to be seen whether the efflux system was powered by the pH gradient across the cellular membrane or directly coupled to ATP energy. Recent DNA sequence analysis of the *cadA* determinant has clarified the mode of energy coupling (5, 6). The cadmium resistance determinant contains only a single, but very long, open reading frame. The *cadA* gene potentially encodes a polypeptide of 727 amino acids. It is surprising that a protein whose function is to confer cadmium resistance is so unusually low in cysteine content, with only 4 out of 727 being cysteine residues. However, these residues are strategically positioned so that for both pairs specific functional roles can be postulated. Mutagenesis studies will test these hypotheses.

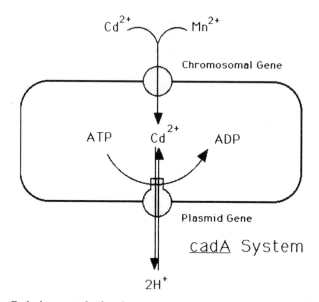

**Figure 4.1** Cadmium uptake by the manganese transport system and efflux by the *cadA* $Cd^{2+}$ efflux ATPase (modified from Ref. 1).

The comparison of the *cadA* amino acid sequence with other polypeptide sequences in DNA-derived polypeptide sequence libraries showed that the $Cd^{2+}$ resistance protein was a member of a growing family of cation-translocating El,E2 ATPases, which includes the previously determined $K^+$ uptake ATPases of both Gram-positive (7) and Gram-negative (8) bacteria, the $H^+$ efflux ATPases of yeast and *Neurospora*, and even the $Ca^{2+}$ ATPase of mammalian muscle and the $Na^+/K^+$ ATPases of animal cell membranes (5, 6, 8). The basic properties of these enzymes, deduced from 25 years of direct biochemistry on the $Ca^{2+}$ and $Na^+/K^+$ ATPases plus the close sequence analogies with the other El,E2 ATPases are diagrammed in Figure 4.2 (6). This model can be considered no more than a cartoon at the moment. Although the basic properties of this yet-to-be directly measured protein seem clear, the model should be taken cautiously. The CadA polypeptide starts with an amino-terminal substrate recognition sequence. The first two cysteines at positions 23 and 26 are closely homologous in sequence to $Hg^{2+}$ binding regions hypothesized in the mercuric reductase and mercury-binding protein that are components of the mercury resistance system (see below). A recurring pattern seems to be developing with a "soft" metal dithiol binding motif, now in two of these resistance systems. Following a pair of transmembrane segments (perhaps from residues 106–126 and 130–150), there is an approximately 186-residue domain on the cytoplasmic side of the membrane that constitutes a cation "funnel" accepting the $Cd^{2+}$ cation from the cysteine pair and guiding it to the transmembrane channel. In the case of

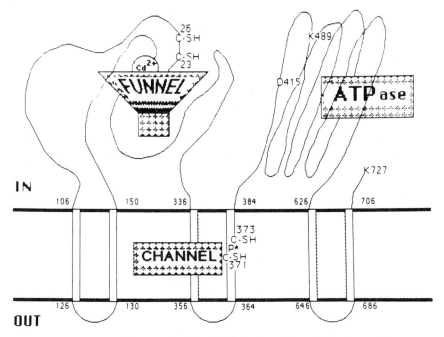

**Figure 4.2**  Hypothetical model of the $Cd^{2+}$ ATPase from the amino acid sequence and homology with E1,E2 ATPases (see text) (modified from Ref. 6).

the $Ca^{2+}$ ATPase, there are direct data for this (summarized in Ref. 9). For the new $Cd^{2+}$ ATPase, this is entirely hypothetical and is derived from DNA sequence analysis. The second pair of transmembrane, potentially $\alpha$-helical segments at approximately 336–356 and 364–384 are positioned in a comparable setting to the transmembrane components thought to constitute the "channel" itself in the other E1,E2 ATPases. The second cysteine pair occurs here at positions 371 and 373, bounding a proline residue (Fig. 4.2) that occurs in a comparable position in all these enzymes (6). Then follows a ATPase domain approximately 250 amino acids long, including an aspartate residue at position 415, which starts a seven amino acid sequence that is unaltered in all of these proteins (6). Lysine$_{489}$ is a candidate for binding ATP (by analogy to the $Ca^{2+}$ and $Na^+/K^+$ enzymes) prior to donating the phosphate to aspartate$_{415}$. The end of the ATPase domain and the next potential membrane-spanning segment are the most conserved sequences in all of this family of proteins (6, 9). Following a third pair of membrane-spanning potentially $\alpha$-helical segments, the protein ends on the cytoplasmic side with lysine$_{727}$ (Fig. 4.2). This general pattern of (a) substrate recognition domain, followed by (b) a pair of closely positioned membrane spanning segments, (c) a substrate sequestering funnel on the cytoplasmic side, (4) another pair of transmembrane peptides, potentially lining the cation-specific transmembrane channel, (e) a large highly conserved ATPase domain, followed by (f) a third pair of membrane-spanning segments is common to all of these proteins. The model in Figure 4.2 is similar to those for better studied $Ca^{2+}$ and $Na^+/K^+$ ATPases in that the bulk of the amino acid residues (perhaps 75%) are cytoplasmic, with perhaps 20% of the residues being in the membrane of this integral membrane protein; only a very small portion of the polypeptide is extracellular. This pattern should be subject to limited proteolysis, as has been done with the $Ca^{2+}$ and $Na^+/K^+$ ATPases. The reader should be warned that the model in Figure 4.2 (although detailed in its structural and functional specifics) is based entirely on the DNA sequence analysis, without direct biochemical data at the moment. For a system for which the DNA sequence has not as yet been published, the supporting experimental efforts have not been undertaken.

## 4.3 ARSENIC RESISTANCE

The arsenic resistance ATPase of Gram-negative bacteria has been more thoroughly studied at the biochemical level (1, 10, 11), following earlier physiological studies (12) and then DNA sequence analysis (10). A plasmid-determined resistance system for As(III), As(V), and Sb(III) is found on plasmids of both Gram-negative and Gram-positive bacteria. Silver et al. (12) showed that arsenate enters the bacterial cells via the chromosomally determined phosphate transport systems (Fig. 4.3), of which for *Escherichia coli* (and perhaps for many other bacteria) there are two. As summarized in Figure 4.3, the Pit (*Pi transport*) system has low specificity, with a $K_m$ of 25 $\mu M$ phosphate and an equivalent $K_i$ of 25 $\mu M$ arsenate. The Pst (*phosphate specific transport*) system has 100 times higher affinity for phosphate than for arsenate. Arsenate, however, enters both systems with kinetic constants apparently unchanged by the plasmid resistance system (12). With whole-cell experiments (13, 14), it was demonstrated that efflux of accumulated arsenate was an energy-dependent process with characteristics indicative of an ATPase mechanism. The DNA sequence analysis indicated the existence of four genes. The first (*arsR*) determines a regulatory protein that binds to the DNA, switching on the arsenic resistance system when induced (12). The DNA sequence of the *arsR* gene is complete (B. P. Rosen, personal communication). The DNA sequence analysis (10) of the other three genes (*arsA*, *arsB*, and *arsC*) has shed significant light upon the mechanism of arsenic efflux, but has not allowed the detailed understanding (by homology to other systems) that was true for the cadmium ATPase. This is because the arsenic ATPase has little similarity to other known ATPases.

The ArsA protein is a loosely membrane-associated protein that has been purified to homogeneity and shown to function in vitro as an arsenic-stimulated ATPase (11). From the amino acid sequence, this polypeptide has two potential ATP-binding regions, homologous to those found in other

Chromosomal Genes

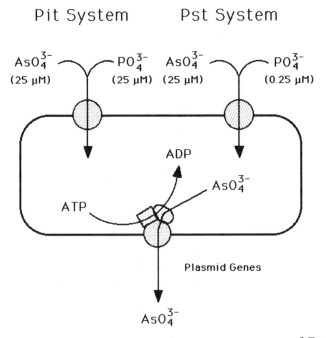

**Figure 4.3** Arsenate uptake by the phosphate transport systems of *E. coli* and arsenate efflux by the plasmid-determined arsenic ATPase (modified from Ref. 1).

ATPases of both bacterial and eukaryotic origin (10). The homologies of these ATP binding sequences have recently been discussed in more detail (6). The ArsB protein potentially encodes a very highly hydrophobic, probably integral membrane protein. From its sequence and computer modeling, ArsB is thought to go back and forth across the membrane as many as 12 times (1, 6, 10). The ArsB protein potentially contains the arsenic and antimony transmembrane channel, but these residues have not yet been identified. ArsA and ArsB are essential for the working of the arsenic/antimony efflux pump. Both are large polypeptides, approximately 500 amino acids long. In comparison, the ArsC polypeptide is smaller, only 141 amino acids long, and it appears to determine the substrate specificity of the efflux ATPase rather being essential for its functioning. When the *arsC* gene was removed by deletion from the end, the system still functioned and afforded arsenite resistance, but arsenate resistance was lost (10).

Comparison of the amino acid sequences of the ArsA and ArsC polypeptides (from the DNA sequences) with those of other recently published polypeptide sequences led B. P. Rosen (personal communication) to a tentative hypothesis as to the origin of the *ars* operon. The ArsA and ArsC polypeptides are related to components of the bacterial nitrogenase system, a complex system of at least 17 gene products involved in atmospheric nitrogen fixation and a system that is rather conserved among otherwise dissimilar nitrogen-fixing bacteria. The ArsA polypeptide has two recognizable ATP-binding regions that are homologous with the *nifH*-determined iron-containing nitrogenase structural component (of which there are 12 from different bacteria in our currently available polypeptide sequence library). This ArsA/NifH homology is closer for the amino-half ATP-binding sequence of ArsA than for the carboxyl-half ATP-binding sequence of ArsA (Refs. 6 and 10 show the actual matches) but NifH is the best match in the library of ATP-binding sites for both halves of ArsA. B. P. Rosen (personal communication) thinks it significant that ArsA is a double fusion polypeptide with similar N- and C-half sequences (undoubtedly arising from DNA duplication and fusion), whereas NifH is found functionally as a homo-dimeric protein.

Nitrogenase requires oxyanions such as vanadate and molybdate for function, but whether this has any ancestral relationship to the oxyanion (arsenite, arsenate, and antimonate) recognition sites of ArsA (1, 11, 12) is not known. The ArsB membrane polypeptide has no recognizable homology to other known amino acid sequences to date. However, the small soluble ArsC sequence is significantly related (25% identities over 96 amino acid aligned segments) with a new *nif* open reading frame (ORF3) from *Azotobacter vinelandii* (15). Although it is clearly in a cluster of *nif* genes, this open reading frame is not homologous to any previously known *nif* genes and its function is still unknown (15).

## 4.4 MERCURY RESISTANCE

The mercury resistance systems from a wide variety of bacterial sources, both Gram positive and Gram negative, have been studied in considerable detail (1, 16, 17). At the level of DNA sequencing, six have been sequenced to date, whereas there is only a single published sequence for the arsenic resistance system, and the first cadmium resistance sequence is in preparation. Thus DNA sequence analysis has provided the greatest impact to date on understanding the mercury resistance system. From studies of mutants using cloning as well as DNA sequence analysis, the model shown in Figure 4.4 has been deduced for mercury systems of Gram-negative bacteria. There is a large (more than 3000 bp) segment of DNA given over to the determination of perhaps half a dozen proteins, which are involved in mercury resistance. Not all the proteins occur in all of the systems studied. Starting from the left in Figure 4.4, the first gene, *merR*, produces a trans-acting regulatory protein. This is followed by an operator/promotor (OP) site for the association of the MerR protein to the DNA and for RNA polymerase attachment, initiating mRNA transcription. Then follows a series of struc-

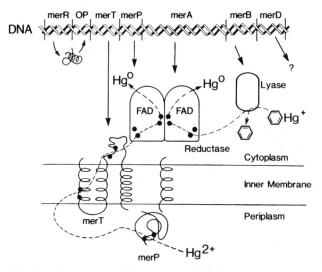

**Figure 4.4** Model of the genetic determination of the system for detoxifying inorganic $Hg^{2+}$ (from Ref. 1 and earlier reports). Top line shows order of the genes on the DNA (see text). The remainder of the figure shows the protein products of the genes and their known or postulated locations and functions.

tural genes, determining components of the resistance system. For the three systems from Gram-negative bacteria studied to date (18–22), these genes are *merT*, *merP*, *merC* [present only in R100 (18) and not in the two other systems], *merA* (the determinant of the mercuric reductase enzyme), *merB* [the determinant of the organomercurial lyase, present only in the pDU1358 system (20) of the three Gram-negative systems sequenced to date], and *merD*. From the DNA sequence analysis, followed by direct studies on the proteins and their functions (in some cases), a very sophisticated understanding is emerging. The MerR protein of Gram-negative mercuric resistant systems is a small (144 amino acids long) dimeric (23) protein that is transcribed from a gene in the opposite (right to left) orientation (24) from the remainder of the genes shown in Figure 4.4 (transcribed left to right). The MerR protein binds to the operator promoter region (23), repressing transcription of *merR* itself and the synthesis of mRNA for the remaining genes (24, 25). In the absence of the protein, MerR is synthesized, and a low level of structural gene products as well (24–26). When MerR is bound to the DNA and $Hg^{2+}$ is added, transcription of the structural genes occurs at a high rate (25), and the proteins are synthesized (27).

The MerR protein appears to have at least four determinants encoded in its small structure: (1) There is a DNA-binding region, which appears to be a member of the "helix-turn-helix" motif common to many DNA-binding regulatory proteins (28). (2) There are amino acid residues, probably including four cysteines per dimer (25) that bind $Hg^{2+}$ turning the system on.

(3) There is an organomercurial-binding region apparently at the carboxyl end of the pDU1358 version of this protein (which responds to phenylmercury as well as inorganic mercury) that can be eliminated leaving the inorganic mercury response intact (21). And then (4) There must be amino acids determining the specific interactions between the monomers forming the dimeric structure.

In all three versions of the Gram-negative mercuric resistance system, the first structural gene is *merT*, which determines a 116-amino acid membrane-transport protein (18, 21). The protein (from its amino acid sequence) may pass across the cell membrane three times, as diagrammed in Figure 4.4. The MerT protein contains two cysteine pairs, the first of which may be in the first membrane "pass" as shown. The second cysteine pair appears to be located on the inner surface of the membrane between the second and third transmembrane segment. Deletion analysis (29) shows that this segment of the system determines a mercury uptake system, which in the absence of the detoxifying enzyme results in hyperaccumulation and hypersensitivity to $Hg^{2+}$ (30).

The next gene, *merP*, determines a small periplasmic mercury binding protein that contains only 91 amino acids. As shown in Figure 4.4, this protein appears to be processed, leaving a 19-amino acid "leader sequence" and resulting in a 72-amino acid periplasmic binding protein (16), which contains a single pair of cysteine residues. This mercury binding protein shows close sequence homology to the N-terminal end of the *cadA* ATPase (above) and to the N-terminal domain found in most versions of the *merA*-determined mercuric reductase enzyme.

The mercuric reductase protein is determined by the next gene *merA*. This protein is highly conserved (80–90% amino acid identities) in the three Gram-negative versions sequenced (Table 4.1) and also quite conserved (about 40% identities) when comparing the Gram-negative with the Gram-positive versions (Table 4.1). Although the Gram-negative and Gram-positive versions of the enzyme share only 40% of their acid residues, when those residues known to play functional roles (the active site residues, and those involved in binding of FAD and NADPH) are considered, the conservation of amino acids increases to more than 90% (32).

The locations of the FAD and NADPH binding regions of mercuric reductase are known from the close sequence and functional homologies between mercuric reductase and the enzymes of central cellular metabolism glutathione reductase and lipoamide dehydrogenase (33, 34). For human glutathione reductase, a high resolution X-ray diffraction structure has been determined (35), so the location of the amino acid residues is well established. Mercuric reductase (in most versions of the enzyme available) starts with an 80-amino acid N-terminal segment that is closely homologous in sequence to the mercury binding protein (1). There then follow a series of domains that can be identified by homology with glutathione reductase. Firstly comes the 15-amino acid active site region, which is the most con-

**TABLE 4.1  Mercuric Reductase Sequence Homologies (Percent Identical Amino Acids) of Aligned Polypeptide Sequences Translated for Three Glutathione Reductases, Lipoamide Dehydrogenease, and Mercuric Reductase[a]**

| Enzyme | Percent Identities | | | | | | | | Length (Amino Acids) |
|---|---|---|---|---|---|---|---|---|---|
| Glutathione reductase (*Pseudomonas*) | 100 | 44.7 | 44.2 | 28.9 | 30.7 | 31.0 | 32.7 | 31.8 | 451 |
| Glutathione reductase (*E. coli*) | | 100 | 54.8 | 27.7 | 31.5 | 30.0 | 31.5 | 31.5 | 450 |
| Glutathione reductase (man) | | | 100 | 28.8 | 28.5 | 28.0 | 29.4 | 28.4 | 478 |
| Lipoamide dehydrogenase (*E. coli*) | | | | 100 | 29.6 | 27.4 | 28.9 | 30.2 | 473 |
| Mercuric reductase (*Pseudomonas*) | | | | | 100 | 85.0 | 41.5 | 41.2 | 561 |
| Mercuric reductase (*Shigella*) | | | | | | 100 | 40.1 | 39.6 | 564 |
| Mercuric reductase (*S. aureus*) | | | | | | | 100 | 67.2 | 547 |
| Mercuric reductase (*Bacillus* sp.) | | | | | | | | 100 | 631 |

[a] See text and Ref. 1 for details. Boxes surround glutathione reductase comparisons, mercuric reductase comparisons, and comparisons of glutathione reductase with mercuric reductase. Alignments in Tables 4.1 through 4.4 were made with the Feng and Doolittle (31) multiple alignment program.

served part of this family of enzymes of all (1). The NADPH and FAD binding regions and even the interface region between the two subunits are significantly conserved. The C-terminal end of the enzyme is highly conserved, but differs from that of glutathione reductase and lipoamide dehydrogenase (1, 32), indicating that this may be the site for mercury binding and coordinating its entrance into the active site domain. This intricate model of how mercuric reductase functions is now being derived from direct enzymological studies and specific site-directed mutagenesis (34). Table 4.1 summarizes the overall amino acid homologies among this family of enzymes, showing that glutathione reductases are more closely related one to another (44–55% identities) than they are related to mercuric reductases (about 30%). Similarly, the mercuric reductases are more closely related one to the other than they are to glutathione reductase.

The next gene in the pDU1358 sequence is *merB* (20), the determinant of the organomercurial lyase enzyme. This polypeptide, for which there are now four sequenced versions [two published (20, 32) and two in preparation (Ref. 36 and J. Altenbuchner, personal communication] is smaller (212–218 amino acids long) and monomeric (37). The basic enzymatic mechanism of reaction (hydrolysis) of organomercurials has been clarified (38). The *merB* gene is found only in the pDU1358 version of the three sequenced Gram-negative *mer* operons, but it occurs in all three currently sequenced Gram-positive *mer* operons. After *merB*, all three Gram-negative versions of the mercuric resistance determinant end with still another gene, *merD*, which appears to play a role in regulation of the mercury resistance system (22). MerD shows significant sequence homology with MerR (22) (Table 4.2), but the actual function of MerD is yet to be determined.

The three Gram-positive versions of the mercuric resistance system known today are each quite different, one from the other. The first version sequenced (32) was from *Staphylococcus aureus* plasmid pI258 and consists of a series of six or seven genes, starting with a gene for a MerR protein (which shows significant homology with that from the Gram-negative systems) followed by a series of genes that (from deletion analysis; M. Horwitz and T. K. Misra, unpublished) determine a mercuric transport function, analogous to that from the Gram-negative systems. However, the amino acid sequences of the Gram-positive transport region are rather dissimilar from those of the Gram-negative *merT–merP* transport system.

After this series of perhaps four genes, the pI258 DNA sequence has a well-defined *merA* and a well-defined *merB* gene. As described above, the sequence identities between the Gram-positive and the Gram-negative versions of these two proteins are about 40%. For the *merA* gene product, the amino acid homologies are stronger in all the known functional regions of that protein. For the MerB protein, where the functional domains have not been determined, the amino acid homology is stronger in the middle part of the polypeptide and much weaker at the amino and carboxyl ends (20, 32). The next Gram-positive *mer* sequence determined came from a soil *Bacillus*

**TABLE 4.2** Amino Acid Sequence Homologies (Percent Identical Amino Acids) Between the Regulatory Polypeptides (MerR) of the Gram-positive and Gram-negative *mer* Systems and the *merD* Gene Products

| Sequence | Percent Identities | | | | | | | Length (Amino Acids) |
|---|---|---|---|---|---|---|---|---|
| S. aureus ORF2 | 100 | 59.0 | 36.1 | 35.3 | 33.8 | 19.2 | 18.5 19.2 | 135 |
| Bacillus ORF1 | | 100 | 36.2 | 36.9 | 36.2 | 22.5 | 19.3 21.7 | 132 |
| Tn501 merR | | | 100 | 93.8 | 87.5 | 25.6 | 26.7 25.6 | 144 |
| R100 merR | | | | 100 | 87.5 | 26.5 | 26.7 26.5 | 144 |
| pDU1358 merR | | | | | 100 | 25.6 | 25.0 25.6 | 144 |
| Tn501 merD | | | | | | 100 | 80.0 90.9 | 121 |
| R100 merD | | | | | | | 100 79.2 | 120 |
| pDU1358 merD | | | | | | | 100 | 121 |

strain, and it occurs on the bacterial chromosome, rather than on a plasmid or transposon. We do not know the origin of these genes and how they incorporated into the chromosome. Wang et al. (36) have recently sequenced the *Bacillus mer* determinant, and it is considerably different in structure from that of pI258. Both Gram-positive systems start with recognizably similar (about 59% amino acid identities) *merR* genes, followed by operator/promoter DNA-binding regions. The *Bacillus* and *S. aureus* MerR proteins are also significantly homologous with the three sequenced versions of the Gram-negative *merR* gene product (34–37% amino acid identities) and *merD* gene product (19–23% amino acid identities) (Table 4.2).

There then follows a series of three genes that are not closely related in the two systems and that in both cases may determine a mercury transport system. When optimally aligned, the *S. aureus* ORF5 amino acid sequence (possibly functionally equivalent to the Gram-negative MerT polypeptide) shows significant homologies (18–28% amino acid identities) with the *Bacillus* ORF2 product, with the ORF2 product of a new *Streptomyces* sequence (see next), and with the Gram-negative *merT*-gene product (Table 4.3).

Then in both cases, there is the long *merA* gene that determines the mer-

**TABLE 4.3** Amino Acid Sequence Homologies (Percent Identical Amino Acids) Between Aligned Sequences of Presumed $Hg^{2+}$ Transport Proteins

| Sequence | Percent Identities | | | | Length (Amino Acids) |
|---|---|---|---|---|---|
| R100 merT | 100 | 18.5 | 28.1 | 19.6 | 116 |
| S. aureus ORF5 | | 100 | 20.4 | 22.5 | 128 |
| Bacillus ORF2 | | | 100 | 18.2 | 98 |
| Streptomyces ORF2 | | | | 100 | 100 |

curic reductase subunit. Surprisingly, the *Bacillus* version of this gene has a duplication and therefore the protein has two copies head to tail of the initial mercury binding domain. The remainders of the two mercuric reductase sequences seem basically quite similar. Whereas the pI258 *merA* gene is followed immediately by *merB* gene (32), there is a 2.5-kb gap between *merA* and *merB* in the *Bacillus* sequence (36). What genetic determinants lie in this gap are unknown, and how this "broken operon" is regulated is still to be determined.

The newest of the mercuric resistance operons sequenced comes from a *Streptomyces lividans* strain (J. Altenbuchner, personal communication). It differs from all of the previously described systems, in that all of the genes other than *merA* and *merB* are transcribed separately and in the opposite direction from the *merA* and *merB* genes. *merA* and *merB* are continuous in this system (J. Altenbuchner, personal communication). When aligned with the three previously sequenced *merB* gene products, the *Streptomyces* organomercurial lyase is somewhat (but not strikingly) more similar to those from low-G+C Gram-positive organisms than it is to the Gram-negative organomercurial lyase from plasmid pDU1358 (Table 4.4). All four organomercurial lyase sequences are more closely similar in the middle than at the N- and C-termini; all four sequences have conserved residues for 4 Phe, 1 Trp, 1 Tyr, 4 Pro, 2 His, and 3 Cys residues (including a conserved Trp-Cys-Ala-Leu-Asp-Thr-Leu heptapeptide) (data not shown). These conserved residues from DNA sequence analysis are candidates for essential functional residues that can be studied by mutagenesis analysis.

Continuing with surprises from the DNA sequence analysis, the *Streptomyces* version of mercuric reductase lacks the N-terminal mercury binding domain. Thus we have three Gram-negative versions of this enzyme with closely related 80-amino acid binding domains, one of the three Gram-positive versions of the enzyme with a similar domain, another with two, and a third with none!

From this description of the six mercuric resistance determinants that have been sequenced, it may be clear that similarities and differences shed light on functional roles and detailed biochemical mechanisms. We hope that

**TABLE 4.4  Amino Acid Sequence Homologies (Percent Identical Amino Acids) Between Aligned Organomercurial Lyase Sequences**

| Sequence Source | Percent Identities | | | | Length (Amino Acids) |
|---|---|---|---|---|---|
| *Streptomyces* | 100 | 53.5 | 54.9 | 41.8 | 215 |
| *Bacillus* | | 100 | 73.2 | 40.7 | 218 |
| *S. aureus* | | | 100 | 41.4 | 216 |
| pDU1358 | | | | 100 | 212 |

additional sequences of arsenic, cadmium, and other heavy metal resistance determinants will shed equal light on the biological function of these systems.

## 4.5  OTHER HEAVY METAL RESISTANCE SYSTEMS

There are two other heavy metal resistance systems for which DNA sequences have been determined. These are the tellurium resistance determinant from one plasmid (39) and the copper resistance determinant from another (40). An outline of the DNA sequence results of these systems is shown in Figure 4.5. However, the sequence analysis in these two cases has not led immediately to biochemical or molecular understanding, so these are presented here as examples of the limitations of DNA analysis.

The tellurium resistance determinant consists of five ORFs (open reading frames) which appear to govern five proteins, running from 13,700 to 38,200 Da in size. Whereas the first two of these gene products appear to be involved in regulation (39), how this might work is yet unknown. The last three gene products may be involved in the resistance mechanism itself (39).

For the copper resistance determinant (40), the DNA sequence of a 4.5-kb segment contains four ORFs (Fig. 4.5), identified as probable genes. Deletions of or mutations in ORFA and ORFB lead to copper sensitivity. ORFC and ORFD are required for full, but not for partial resistance (40). A tandemly repeated octapeptide [Asp-His-Ser-Gln(or Lys)-Met-Gln-Gly-Met] occurs five times toward the beginning of ORFB and related octapeptides occur four times in the middle region of ORFA. The methionine sulfurs and histidine imidazole nitrogens were considered candidates for copper-binding residues (40). The first three gene products appear (from the se-

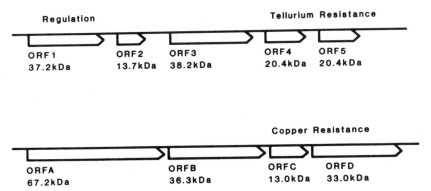

**Figure 4.5**  Diagram of the open reading frames from the DNA sequence analysis of the tellurium resistance determinant (*top*) (ref. 39) and of the copper resistance determinant (*bottom*) (ref. 40).

quences) to be soluble polypeptides, although they contain hydrophobic N-terminal segments characteristic of membrane signal sequences. Sequence homology with known regulatory proteins led to the hypothesis that the ORFC product may be a positively acting regulatory protein (40). The ORFD product has several potential membrane-spanning hydrophobic stretches, making the ORFD product a candidate for a copper transport protein (40). These hypothesized roles for the four copper resistance ORFs from sequence analysis are less convincing than those described above for the cadmium, arsenic, and mercury resistance systems.

With the cloning and analysis of a second resistance determinant (41), the potential for better understanding of copper resistance mechanisms from DNA sequencing grows. The four genes of this second copper resistance determinant are not, however, similar in apparent size and location (41) to those of the first system. It appears in this case as if the second gene is the regulatory gene and the fourth (smaller) gene is involved in copper binding (41). Once the sequence analysis of this second copper resistance determinant is reported then we shall be able to judge whether two quite separate systems are being studied or not.

In summary, the DNA sequence analysis of the first plasmid resistance systems for cadmium and for arsenic and of six distinct genetic determinants of mercury resistance has provided sophisticated understanding of the physiological and biochemical mechanisms of these resistances. This is very similar to the impact of DNA sequence analysis in other areas of molecular biology. For many additional heavy metal resistance determinants, DNA sequence analysis has yet to be effective. [Two more sequencing projects are currently underway in our laboratory: one for the determinant of cadmium, zinc, and cobalt resistance in *Alcaligenes* (42, 43) and the other for the chromate resistance system in *Pseudomonas* (44).] The application of such modern tools as recombinant DNA analysis will continue radically to advance our understanding of bioinorganic chemistry.

## ACKNOWLEDGMENTS

The research in this report has been supported in part by grants from the National Institutes of Health and the National Science Foundation.

## REFERENCES

1. S. Silver and T. K. Misra. Plasmid-mediated heavy metal resistances. Ann. Rev. Microbiol., *42*, 717 (1988).

2. R. P. Novick, E. Murphy, T. J. Gryczan, E. Baron, and I. Edelman. Penicillinase plasmids of *Staphylococcus aureus*: restriction-deletion maps. Plasmid, *2*, 109 (1979).

3. A. A. Weiss, S. Silver, and T. G. Kinscherf. Cation transport alteration associated with plasmid-determined resistance to cadmium in *Staphylococcus aureus*. Antimicrob. Agents Chemother., *14*, 856 (1978).

4. Z. Tynecka, Z. Gos, and J. Zajac. Energy-dependent efflux of cadmium coded by a plasmid resistance determinant in *Staphylococcus aureus*. J. Bacteriol., *147*, 313 (1981).

5. G. Nucifora, L. Chu, T. K. Misra, and S. Silver. Cadmium resistance from *Staphylococcus aureus* plasmid pI258 *cadA* results from a cadmium efflux ATPase. Proc. Natl. Acad. Sci. USA., 1989 (in press).

6. S. Silver, G. Nucifora, L. Chu, and T. K. Misra. Bacterial resistance ATPases: primary pumps for exporting toxic cations and anions. Trends Biochem. Sci., *14*, 76 (1989).

7. M. Solioz, S. Mathews, and P. Furst. Cloning of the $K^+$-ATPase of *Streptococcus faecalis*. J. Biol. Chem., *262*, 7358 (1987).

8. M. O. Walderhaug, D. C. Dosch, and W. Epstein. "Potassium transport in bacteria," in B. P. Rosen and S. Silver. Eds., *Ion Transport in Prokaryotes*. Academic, New York, 1987. p. 85.

9. C. J. Brandl, N. M. Green, B. Korczak, and D. H. MacLennan. Two $Ca^{2+}$ ATPase genes: homologies and mechanistic implications of deduced amino acid sequences. Cell, *44*, 597 (1986).

10. C. M. Chen, T. K. Misra, S. Silver, and B. P. Rosen. Nucleotide sequence of the structural genes for an anion pump. The plasmid encoded arsenical resistance operon. J. Biol. Chem., *261*, 15030 (1986).

11. B. P. Rosen, U. Weigel, C. Karkaria, and P. Gangola. Molecular characterization of an anion pump. J. Biol. Chem., *263*, 3067 (1988).

12. S. Silver, K. Budd, K. M. Leahy, W. V. Shaw, D. Hammond, R. P. Novick, G. R. Willsky, M. H. Malamy, and H. Rosenberg. Inducible plasmid-determined resistance to arsenate, arsenite, and antimony (III) in *Escherichia coli* and *Staphylococcus aureus*. J. Bacteriol., *146*, 983 (1981).

13. S. Silver and D. Keach. Energy-dependent arsenate efflux: the mechanism of plasmid-mediated resistance. Proc. Natl. Acad. Sci. USA., *79*, 6114 (1982).

14. H. L. T. Mobley and B. P. Rosen. Energetics of plasmid-mediated arsenate resistance in *Escherichia coli*. Proc. Natl. Acad. Sci. USA., *79*, 6119 (1982).

15. R. D. Joerger and P. E. Bishop. Nucleotide sequence and genetic analysis of the *nifB-nifQ* region from *Azotobacter vinelandii*. J. Bacteriol., *170*, 1475 (1988).

16. A. O. Summers. Organization, expression, and evolution of genes for mercury resistance. Ann. Rev. Microbiol., *40*, 607 (1986).

17. T. J. Foster. The genetics and biochemistry of mercury resistance. CRC Crit. Rev. Microbiol., *15*, 117 (1987).

18. T. K. Misra, N. L. Brown, D. C. Fritzinger, R. D. Pridmore, W. M. Barnes, L. Haberstroh, and S. Silver. Mercuric ion-resistance operons of plasmid R100 and transposon Tn*501*: the beginning of the operon including the regulatory region and the first two structural genes. Proc. Natl. Acad. Sci. USA., *81*, 5975 (1984).

19. T. K. Misra, N. L. Brown, L. Haberstroh, A. Schmidt, D. Goddette, and S.

Silver. Mercuric reductase structural genes from plasmid R100 and transposon Tn*501*: functional domains of the enzyme. Gene, *34*, 253 (1985).

20. H. G. Griffin, T. J. Foster, S. Silver, and T. K. Misra. Cloning and DNA sequence of the mercuric- and organomercurial-resistance determinants of plasmid pDU1358. Proc. Natl. Acad. Sci. USA., *84*, 3112 (1987).

21. G. Nucifora, L. Chu, S. Silver, and T. K. Misra. Mercury operon regulation by the *merR* gene of the organomercurial resistance system of plasmid pDU1358. J. Bacteriol., 1989 (submitted).

22. N. L. Brown, T. K. Misra, J. N. Winnie, A. Schmidt, M. Seiff, and S. Silver. The nucleotide sequence of the mercuric resistance operons of plasmid R100 and transposon Tn*501*: further evidence for *mer* genes which enhance the activity of the mercuric ion detoxification system. Mol. Gen. Genet., *202*, 143 (1986).

23. T. O'Halloran and C. Walsh. Metalloregulatory DNA-binding protein encoded by the *merR* gene: isolation and characterization. Science, *235*, 211 (1987).

24. T. J. Foster and N. L. Brown. Identification of the *merR* gene of R100 by using *mer-lac* gene and operon fusions. J. Bacteriol., *163*, 1153 (1985).

25. T. O'Halloran. "Metalloregulatory proteins: Metal-responsive molecular switches governing gene expression," in H. Sigel, Ed., *Metal Ions in Biological Systems*, Vol. 25, Dekker, New York, 1988 (in press).

26. N. Ni'Bhriain, S. Silver, and T. J. Foster. Tn*5* insertion mutations in the mercuric ion resistance genes derived from plasmid R100. J. Bacteriol., *155*, 690 (1983).

27. J. Jackson and A. O. Summers. Biochemical characterization of HgCl$_2$-inducible polypeptides encoded by the *mer* operon of plasmid R100. J. Bacteriol., *151*, 962 (1982).

28. C. O. Pabo and R. T. Sauer. Protein-DNA recognition. Ann. Rev. Biochem., *53*, 293 (1984).

29. P. A. Lund and N. L. Brown. Role of the *merT* and *merP* gene products of transposon Tn*501* in the induction and expression of resistance to mercuric ions. Gene, *52*, 207 (1987).

30. H. Nakahara, S. Silver, T. Miki, and R. H. Rownd. Hypersensitivity to Hg$^{2+}$ and hyperbinding activity associated with cloned fragments of the mercurial resistance operon of plasmid NR1. J. Bacteriol., *140*, 161 (1979).

31. D.-F. Feng and R. F. Doolittle. Progressive sequence alignment as a prerequisite to correct phylogenetic trees. J. Mol. Evol., *25*, 351 (1987).

32. R. A. Laddaga, L. Chu, T. K. Misra, and S. Silver. Nucleotide sequence and expression of the mercurial-resistance operon from *Staphylococcus aureus* plasmid pI258. Proc. Natl. Acad. Sci. USA., *84*, 5106 (1987).

33. C. T. Walsh, M. D. Distefano, M. J. Moore, L. M. Shewchuk, and G. L. Verdine. Molecular basis of bacterial resistance to organomercurial and inorganic mercuric salts. FASEB J., *2*, 124 (1988).

34. M. D. Distefano, K. G. Au, and C. T. Walsh. Mutagenesis of the redox-active disulfide in mercuric ion reductase: catalysis by mutant enzymes restricted to flavin redox chemistry. Biochemistry, in press (1989).

35. R. Thieme, E. F. Pai, R. H. Schirmer, and G. E. Schulz. Three-dimensional structure of glutathione reductase at 2 A resolution. J. Mol. Biol., *152*, 763 (1981).

36. Y. Wang, M. Moore, H. S. Levinson, S. Silver, C. Walsh, and I. Mahler. Nu-

cleotide sequence of a chromosomal mercury resistance determinant from a *Bacillus* sp. with broad-spectrum mercury-resistance. J. Bacteriol., *171*, 83 (1989).

37. T. P. Begley, A. E. Walts, and C. T. Walsh. Bacterial organomercurial lyase: overproduction, isolation, and characterization. Biochemistry, *25*, 7186 (1986).

38. T. P. Begley, A. E. Walts, and C. T. Walsh. Mechanistic studies of a protonlytic organomercurial cleaving enzyme: bacterial organomercurial lyase. Biochemistry, *25*, 7192 (1986).

39. M. G. Jobling and D. A. Ritchie. The nucleotide sequence of a plasmid determinant for resistance to tellurium anions. Gene, *66*, 245 (1988).

40. M. A. Mellano and D. A. Cooksey. Nucleotide sequence and organization of copper resistance genes from *Pseudomonas syringeae* pv. *tomato*. J. Bacteriol., *170*, 2879 (1988).

41. D. Rouch, B. T. O. Lee, and J. Camakaris. "Genetic and molecular basis of copper resistance in *Escherichia coli*," in D. Winge and D. Hamer, Eds., *Metal Ion Homeostasis: Molecular Biology and Chemistry*. Liss, New York, 1989 (in press).

42. D. Nies, M. Mergeay, B. Friedrich, and H. G. Schlegel. Cloning of plasmid genes enoding resistance to cadmium, zinc, and cobalt in *Alcaligenes eutrophus* CH34. J. Bacteriol., *169*, 4865 (1987).

43. D. H. Nies and S. Silver. Plasmid-determined inducible efflux is responsible for resistance to cadmium, zinc and cobalt in *Alcaligenes eutrophus*. J. Bacteriol., *171*, 896 (1989).

44. H. Ohtake, C. Cervantes, and S. Silver. Decreased chromate uptake in *Pseudomonas fluorescens* carrying a chromate resistance plasmid. J. Bacteriol., *169*, 3853 (1987).

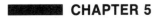 **CHAPTER 5**

# Siderophore Systems of Bacteria and Fungi

J. B. NEILANDS

Department of Biochemistry
University of California, Berkeley
Berkeley, California

## Contents

## 5.1   OVERVIEW

### 5.1.1   Introduction

Siderophores (Greek, "iron carriers") are relatively low-molecular-weight, virtually ferric-specific coordination compounds excreted under low iron stress by aerobic and facultative anaerobic bacteria and by fungi for the purpose of securing iron from the environment. Siderophores were early shown to have the attributes expected of a transport form of iron: a general preponderance of oxygen atoms in the coordination sphere, a relatively weak affinity for Fe(II), substantial water solubility, and enhanced synthesis at low iron growth. Organisms producing siderophores could be shown to use efficiently the ferrated form of the molecule as a source of iron. A few natural auxotrophes were found to respond to siderophores, certain other biologically derived chelates, and synthetic metal-binding agents that had in common only the capacity to complex Fe(III). To this impressive body of data must be added the conclusive genetic evidence obtained with mutant strains of enteric bacteria. Thus mutants of *Escherichia coli* blocked in the biosynthesis of enterobactin fail to grow in media where the available iron has been complexed by a coordination agent such as deferriferrichrome A, a fungal siderophore almost univerally not used by bacteria (1). Similar mutants of *Salmonella typhimurium* will not grow in the presence of citrate because, although *E. coli* has an inducible system for uptake of ferric citrate, this transport system is absent from *S. typhimurium* and consequently growth can proceed only when sufficient iron has been added to titrate out the tricarboxylic acid ligand. These are some of the reasons that all workers in the field agree that siderophores, of which about 100 individual compounds have by now been described from different microbial species, are fabricated for the solubilization and transport of iron. Some typical siderophores and the source organisms are listed in Table 5.1.

Gram-negative bacteria transport amino acids, monosaccharides, and other small molecules via water-filled pores in the outer membrane of the cell envelope. These pores, lined with special proteins (porins) apparently cannot accommodate siderophores, which typically have molecular weights in the range of 500–1000 Da. The evolutionary response to this difficulty has been the synthesis of specific receptor proteins designed first to recognize the Fe(III) complex form of the molecule and then, with the aid of other transport components, to guide the coordinated iron to the cytoplasmic membrane or to the cytoplasm. Later in evolutionary time certain lethal agents such as bacteriophages, bacteriocins, and antibiotics have discovered how to adapt themselves to siderophore receptors as a means of penetration of the bacterial envelope. Thus a commonly observed ancillary biological activity of siderophores is antagonism of one or more of the lethal agents just described. The first example of this type of competition with a siderophore acting against a well-known receptor was observed with ferrichrome

**TABLE 5.1  Some Well-Characterized Siderophores from Bacterial and Fungal Species**

| Microorganism | Siderophore |
|---|---|
| **Bacteria** | |
| *Escherichia coli, Salmonella typhimurium* | Enterobactin, aerobactin |
| *Agrobacterium tumefaciens* | Agrobactin |
| *Rhizobium meliloti* DM4 | Rhizobactin |
| *Pseudomonas* sp. | Pyochelin, pseudobactins, pyoverdines |
| *Anabaena* sp., *Bacillus megaterium* | Schizokinen |
| *Arthrobacter* sp. | Arthrobactin |
| *Azotobacter* sp. | Azotobactin |
| *Vibrio* sp. | Vibriobactin, anguibactin |
| *Actinomyces* sp. | Ferrioxamines |
| *Mycobacteria* | Mycobactins |
| **Fungi** | |
| *Penicillia, Aspergilli, Neurospora, Ustilago* | Ferrichromes, coprogen |
| *Fusaria* | Fusarinines |
| *Rhodotorula* sp. | Rhodotorulic acid |

negating the lethal group comprised of bacteriophages T1, T5, Φ80, colicin M, and albomycin (2). Since the initial observation of this phenomenon with ferrichrome and enterobactin in *E. coli*, many additional examples of this type of biochemical ecology have been described.

Thus far Fe is the only essential element observed to require a specific organic ligand for its dissolution and subsequent transport. There are probably several reasons why this is so. The solubility product constant of ferric hydroxide, $< 10^{-38}$, means that at biological pH the maximum concentration of free $Fe^{3+}$ that can exist in solution is of the order of $10^{-18}$ $M$, a value too low to support microbial growth. Among the first-row transition elements Fe is generally involved in more metabolic events and hence is required in larger amounts than Mn, Co, or Cu. The hydroxides of these elements have substantially greater solubility than the hydroxide of ferric iron. The level of Zn in cells is appreciable, but there appears to be no problem with its solubility. All the divalent ions just listed have reasonable binding affinities for amino acids and tend to find their way into the side chains of apoproteins to become an integral component of specific metalloenzymes. The intracellular pathway of Fe is further complicated by the fact that the metal must, in addition, be diverted to heme and to regulation of the synthesis of the siderophore biosynthesis and transport pathways.

This chapter focuses on the regulation of siderophore-mediated iron absorption, because other aspects of the subject have been reviewed extensively in recent years. The most comprehensive reference on the general aspects of siderophores and their relation to animal and plant metabolism of iron is the recently published tome *Iron Transport in Microbes, Plants and Animals* (3). After a brief overview of the field we turn to a discussion of regulation of siderophore-mediated iron assimilation in *E. coli*, for it is here that it has been possible to propose the first molecular mechanism for control of absorption of a nutritious mineral element in any living species.

### 5.1.2  Determination. CAS: The "Swiss Army Knife" of Siderophore Technology

Basically there are two general procedures for the detection and determination of siderophores, namely, chemical and microbiological (1). The chemical methods have the advantage of convenience, but have traditionally suffered from lack of sensitivity and specificity. Because most siderophores contain either the hydroxamic acid or the catechol functional groups, probes can be directed at these moieties. The blue color of the 1:1 ferric complex of a monohydroxamic acid, which exists at a pH of about 2, has an extinction of about 1000 $M^{-1}$ cm$^{-1}$. Although this is too feeble for analytical purposes, the reaction has important diagnostic application because on adjustment of the pH to 7, Fe is thrown out and the color assumes a golden hue. With the addition of two more hydroxamate rings around the Fe the extinction, which now peaks at about 430 nm, advances to about 3000 $M^{-1}$ cm$^{-1}$. A much more sensitive probe for the hydroxamic acid group is the so-called Csaky test, which is based on I oxidation of hydroxylamines to nitrite (4). Depending on the conditions, the extinction of the pink azo dye at 530–540 nm may exceed 30,000 $M^{-1}$ cm$^{-1}$. However, all hydroxamate siderophores contain bound (*N*-substituted) hydroxylamine and must be hydrolyzed prior to analysis.

Because of the presence of a substituent on the N, oxidation of hydroxamate siderophores with periodate leads to formation of a *cis*-nitroso dimer (5). These molecules have a very sharp absorption band at 240 nm in the ultraviolet and exhibit an extinction of 10,000 $M^{-1}$ cm$^{-1}$. However, because two moles of hydroxamic acid are required to form 1 mol of dimer, the effective extinction is 5000 $M^{-1}$ cm$^{-1}$.

Catechols are routinely measured with the Arnow reaction, which is based on nitrosation of the ring and its subsequent conversion to the molybdate complex, which is yellow in acid and red in alkaline media (6). The extinction at 515 nm is about 9000 $M^{-1}$ cm$^{-1}$. This is close to the same value, 9600 $M^{-1}$ cm$^{-1}$, obtained by measuring the band intensity of a tricatechol, such as enterobactin, at its peak in the near ultraviolet at 315–320 nm. The charge transfer band of the ferric catechols, like those of the ferric hydroxamates, are of the order of a few thousand $M^{-1}$ cm$^{-1}$.

Bioassays on solid or in liquid media are orders of magnitude more sensitive than the usual chemical test, but are plagued by their own drawbacks.

Not only must viable stocks of the appropriate test organisms be maintained, but there is no such thing as a universal microbial response to siderophores. *Arthrobacter flavescens* JG-9ATCC 29091 is stimulated by the hydroxamic acid line of siderophores, but the catechol type is unable to support its growth. The best situation is to possess a biosynthesis mutant of the producing organism. Failing this, one can devise a bioassay based on reversal of inhibition of growth inhibition invoked by the presence of a chelating agent, such as ethylenediamine-$N,N'$-bis(2-hydroxyphenylacetic acid) (EDDA), which is generally not utilized by bacteria.

Finally, there is a growing collection of siderophores that have neither the hydroxamic acid nor the catechol functionalities. Thus structures of the genre of rhizobactin (7) and rhizobactin 1021 (8) are certain to be encountered as the search for siderophores is extended to diverse types of microbial species.

It was a consideration of some of the problems just enumerated that stimulated a search for a universal chemical method for detection and determination of siderophores. The result was the development of the method based on deferration of the ferric complex of chrome azurol S (CAS), a procedure somewhat immodestly described as "universal" (9). The extremely high extinction coefficient of ferric chrome azurol S, a value in excess of 100,000 $M^{-1}$ cm$^{-1}$, means that the complex is at least 10 times as potent in absorption as compared to the charge transfer bands of the ferric siderophores. The affinity of CAS for Fe(III) seems to be just less than that of the siderophores and hence the metal ion is quantitatively released to the competing ligand.

The CAS test can be applied to column effluents either quantitatively by measuring an aliquot of solution or qualitatively by use of the spot plate. The molar concentration of the siderophore ligand can be determined because, particularly with added shuttle, the deep blue color of the standard potion is instantly converted to the equally pigmented but now orange-colored free form of CAS. Without the shuttle the rate of leaching of the ferric ion from the CAS complex gives important clues regarding the nature of the siderophore, hydroxamates being relatively slow compared to catechols.

The CAS reagent can be applied as a spray to thin layer or paper chromatograms. On paper electrophoresis inorganic phosphate serves as a fast moving marker.

A particularly attractive feature of the CAS method is the fact that the dye can be implanted in agar media and, at least with several Gram-negative species, it will identify siderophore-excreting clones through the orange halos that surround the colonies. Wild-type colonies of *E. coli* K-12 exhibit discrete orange halos whereas mutants defective in enterobactin synthesis form no halo. Both transport and regulatory mutants exhibit large halos. These mutants can be distinguished on the basis of their response to a competing ligand not utilized by the cells. The transport mutants survive on their low-affinity iron uptake pathway and are nonviable if this is blocked out by deferriferrichrome A or EDDA. These chelators are without effect on growth of the regulatory mutants because in this case the high affinity, siderophore-mediated pathway is still operative. Additionally, very high levels of iron will selectively reduce the halo size of transport mutants.

There are some limitations of the CAS method, the most serious being the apparent toxicity of the cetyltrimethylammonium bromide that must be present to disperse the triphenylmethane reagent. As a replacement for this cationic detergent we have employed the zwitterionic 3-(dimethyldodecy-lammonium)propane sulfonate. This additive, which gives a green complex in the ferric chelate and a yellow color to the free dye, has been used successfully in this laboratory by Jason Cheung for detection of mutants of the basiomycetous fungus, *Rhodotorula pilimanae*, which is defective in synthesis of the siderophore rhodotorulic acid. The interference by phosphate can be serious, which is why we "lean down" the standard M9 medium in this constituent. Other difficulties arise with media that are excessively complex or when the pH is too low or too high.

### 5.1.3  Production of Siderophores

To test for production of siderophores the organism must first be demonstrated to be iron deficient. The most desirable situation is when the microbe will grow in synthetic media, because these are normally of the order of $0.1$–$1.0$ $\mu M$ in total iron. A carbon source such as succinate or Tris has been found to impose a higher demand for iron. If the organism has complex nutritional requirements, all is not lost because the medium can be extracted with 8-hydroxyquinoline in chloroform, or supplemented with an iron-complexing agent such as EDDA, bipyridyl, or ovotransferrin. Much will depend on the idiosyncrasies of the particular species; for example, we have already seen that citrate will serve as deferration agent with *S. typhimurium* whereas in *E. coli* this organic acid would induce a special transport system for its ferric complex. Before it can be concluded that the organism does not elaborate a siderophore, the culture must be shown to exhibit a faster growth rate after addition to the medium of a trace of ferric or ferrous salt.

Once some development work has been done on a siderophore, the routine production of the compound is greatly facilitated by the growth of mutants. Both transport and regulatory mutants can be expected to overproduce siderophores. The transport mutants are chronically iron starved and will sometimes pump out very high levels of the siderophores. The regulatory mutants can be grown in rich, high iron media and these will, at least in *E. coli*, elaborate high levels of siderophores.

### 5.1.4  Isolation of Siderophores

After the cultural conditions for maximum production of siderophore are established, the next problem is the isolation of the compound(s) from the supernatant medium. No universal recipe can be given here because the route to be adopted depends on the properties of the individual siderophore. The initial decision must be whether or not to ferrate. Addition of an excess of ferrous sulfate with agitation will afford the ferric complex, which is often colored, and its purification can then be monitored on this basis. However, several of the most useful characterization steps can be performed only on the metal-free ligand and eventual removal of the iron should be possible.

An initial extraction into an organic solvent is highly recommended because this will separate the siderophore from the salts and the major polar ingredients of the medium. Benzyl alcohol and chloroform:phenol (1:1) are the two solvents most commonly employed for removal of siderophores from culture supernatants after addition of a high level of a soluble salt such as ammonium sulfate to the aqueous phase. Dilution of the organic layer with several volumes of diethyl ether will generally drive the compound back into the aqueous phase. Very aromatic siderophores such as enterobactin and other members of the catechol series can be extracted directly into ethyl acetate which, unlike benzyl alcohol or chloroform–phenol, can be easily removed by evaporation. Highly water-soluble siderophores bearing charged groups should be isolated with the aid of ion exchange resins because such adsorbents have high capacity. The polymeric resin XAD has found favor for adsorption of very water-soluble, uncharged siderophores such as ferrichrome. Exceptionally polar siderophores are difficult to isolate and some attention should be paid to development of general methods for the preparation of such compounds.

### 5.1.5  Characterization of Siderophores

The superior method for characterization in the siderophore series is crystallography, preferably of the Fe(III) complex. Unfortunately, only half or less of the well-known siderophores have been crystallized and thus fully described in such important details as the stereochemistry, whether lambda or delta, around the centrally coordinated iron. In the absence of crystals resort can be made to the various modes ($^1$H, $^{13}$C) of nuclear magnetic resonance and mass spectroscopy. It must be stressed that the paramagnetic $Fe^{3+}$ will eliminate resonance lines in NMR analysis. However, the $Fe^{3+}$ can be substituted by either $Al^{3+}$ or $Ga^{3+}$, both of which are diamagnetic and which appear to afford complexes that are isostructural with that derived from $Fe^{3+}$. Much useful information on the nature of hydroxamate siderophores can be obtained by measuring the electronic absorption spectrum at various pH levels because, as already noted, mono-, di-, and trihydroxamates exhibit predictable shifts. In addition, in the iron-free form these siderophores are readily cleaved by periodate without an attack on ester or amide bonds elsewhere in the molecule (5). Hydrolysis in 6 $N$ HCl enables recovery of the amino acids and polyamines bearing the iron-chelating moieties, but again this must be done with the metal-free species because the presence of the iron leads to extensive degradation by redox reactions.

Only one siderophore is commercially available at the moment of writing. This is deferriferrioxamine B, a product of *Streptomyces pilosus* and the Ciba-Geigy Company. Although the compound has been synthesized, it is more economically prepared by low iron microbial fermentation. The main use of this siderophore is for deferration therapy in patients suffering from the excessive iron loading resulting from the transfusion regime for thalassemia and aplastic anemia. Because the drug, which is offered as the mesylate salt under the trade name Desferal, must be injected there is an urgent need for an orally effective nostrum for such therapeutic applications.

### 5.1.6   Iron in Infection and Bio-control

The classical work of Schade and Caroline (10) identified transferrin as a principal antibacterial agent in blood. They proved that the inhibitory effect could be assigned to the iron-binding activity of the newly discovered protein. In subsequent years many reports have appeared that link iron to infection in man and animals, and there has recently been published a monograph on the subject (11). It seems that the iron-binding proteins, transferrin, ovotransferrin, and lactoferrin, serve in the first line of defense against infection. For their part, microbes have evolved powerful, siderophore-mediated mechanisms for acquiring iron that are specifically induced to overproduction under the low-iron conditions that prevail in tissues.

The fish pathogen *Vibrio anguillarum* carries a plasmid-coded siderophore synthesis and transport system that is connected to the virulence of the organism (12). The particular siderophore has been isolated and named anguibactin; its characterization is in progress. The best established correlation with siderophores and virulence is found in the hospital isolates of *E. coli*, which are capable of causing disseminating infections in various organs and tissues. In this case the siderophore responsible has been identified as aerobactin (13).

A catechol-type siderophore, apparently different from any described thus far, appears to be involved in the virulence of *Erwinia chrysanthemi*, an organism infecting stored vegetables (14).

It has been observed that frequent cropping reduces potato yields and that sterilization of the soil eliminates the effect (15). The crops suffered from no obvious pathogenic infestation, although the frequently cropped plants could be seen to have smaller root systems. Treatment with cultures of fluorescent *Pseudomonas* species restored root vigor. Apparently the *Pseudomonas* act by inhibiting deleterious organisms in the rhizosphere.

The fluorescent *Pseudomonads* are known to excrete, under iron stress, a line of siderophores variously known as pseudobactins, pyoverdines, or azotobactins. These compounds are linear and cyclic peptides containing six to nine residues of D or L amino acid residues. Deployed along the chain for effective binding of Fe(III) are found a quinoline moiety, which imparts fluorescence, as well as α-hydroxyl acid and ornithine hydroxamate functional groups. Some progress has been made in cloning the gene complexes coding these siderophores (16). Like the enterobactin gene cluster in *E. coli* the system is comprised of regulatory, biosynthetic, and transport determinants and is organized into several transcriptional units. As yet no regulatory mutants have been described, so it is not possible to compare this system with the control circuits observed in *E. coli* K-12. Typically some species of *Pseudomonas* can use a variety of different siderophores, whereas others are more fastidious regarding the particular chelate that will be accepted. From a study of enantio-enterobactin and linear catechols related to enterobactin, it was concluded that a major element of this specificity is vested in the outer membrane receptor protein (17). In the case of the pseudobactins this has been taken a step further by genetically switching receptor proteins, a substitution that was found to alter specificity.

## 5.2  REGULATION OF IRON ABSORPTION

### 5.2.1  Iron Potentiates Oxygen Toxicity

The need to regulate absorption of iron is readily appreciated when the potential enhancing effect of the metal on oxygen stress is considered (18). Although cytochrome *c* oxidase quite effectively guides four electrons to the oxygen molecule to generate 2 moles of water, this reaction is not 100% efficient and results in the simultaneous formation of partially reduced oxygen species such as superoxide anion and hydrogen peroxide. Although these intermediates have a certain level of cytotoxicity, their real damage is probably a consequence of conversion to hydroxyl radical, which can oxidize any organic molecule. Redox active metal ions, particularly iron and copper, catalytically yield hydroxyl radical from superoxide and hydrogen peroxide. Traces of ferric iron are reduced by superoxide and the resulting ferrous iron then reoxidized by peroxide to afford the hydroxyl radical with regeneration of a ferric ion ready for a new turn of the cycle. Iron is needed by aerobic organisms for efficient generation of ATP, for electron transport generally, for reduction of ribotides to deoxyribotides, and for many other essential metabolic reactions. Hence the regulation of assimilation of iron is the key step in determination of the biological efficacy of the mineral.

### 5.2.2  All Species Regulate Assimilation of Iron

Irrespective of species, in a gross sense and without regard to detailed mechanism, uptake of iron appears to be negatively regulated. This was first established in experimental animals where it was shown that individuals replete with respect to iron stores did not remove more of the metal from the diet. The upper region of the small intestine is the site of iron absorption and also the locus of the control mechanism, regarding which little has been elucidated a half century after the initial work on the subject. The human contains 3–5 g of iron, of which the bulk is in hemoglobin, most of the remainder in ferritin, and a few milligrams in the various enzymes. Iron is carried into all proliferating cells as a complex with the 80-kDa glycoprotein transferrin. There are two ferric iron-binding centers in transferrin, and normally the protein is only about 30% saturated with iron. The iron-laden transferrins interact with a surface receptor complex that is subsequently incorporated by endocytosis. By some means, not yet entirely clear, the iron is released and the receptor returned to the cell membrane. Synthesis of the receptor is regulated by iron, possibly at the transcriptional level (19). Few details are yet available regarding regulation of synthesis of transferrin itself although, because sequence data are available for all of these proteins, such information will soon be forthcoming.

Plants are as dependent as animals on a supply of iron. Two general strategies, which may not encompass all of the possibilities, are currently recognized (20). Strategy I, characteristic of dicotyledenous and non-grass monocotyledenous species, involves extrusion of $H^+$ and reducing agents and enhanced uptake rates for $Fe^{2+}$. Strategy II, typical of the grasses, involves excretion of a line of Fe(III) complexing agents generically called phytosiderophores. Mugineic acid is the single member of the series best studied so far. Although it has not yet been possible to carry out a genetic analysis of the mugineic acid pathway, the mechanism whereby the system is turned on at low iron is of great interest. This is because the grains constitute the most important food crops in the world. Iron deficiency in plants results in inability to synthesize chlorophyll and consequent poor crop yields. The condition is most severe in the calcareous soils of the intermountain region of the United States and wide areas of almost all countries around the globe.

### 5.2.3 Regulation of Siderophore Synthesis

The mechanism of regulation of siderophore-mediated iron assimilation, which we now purport to understand at the molecular level, is a continuing investigation in this laboratory that dates to the isolation of ferrichrome from the smut fungus *Ustilago sphaerogena* in 1952 (21). This fungus has the quirk of overproducing cytochrome *c*. When the hemoprotein had been isolated by precipitation from saturated ammonium sulfate solution, a substantial amount of colored material remained in the salt solution. The color was extracted into benzyl alcohol and the compound responsible crystallized from methanol. Considering the source, a fungus rich in cytochrome, and the fact that it bound only the higher oxidation state of iron, ferrichrome was suspected to be a transport form of iron. This suspicion was substantiated when efforts to increase the yield by varying the trace element composition of the medium disclosed iron to be the key ingredient regulating the synthesis of the deferriferrichrome molecule. Whereas ferrichrome had been isolated by extraction from the cell paste, growth at low iron led to excretion of relatively massive quantities of the ligands of the ferrichromes. This afforded abundant quantities of crystalline ferrichrome A with which pilot characterization experiments could be run while hoarding the supply of ferrichrome, which was only available in much smaller quantities.

Armed with the technique of iron starvation as a tool, a search was made through other fungal and bacterial species to see if this growth regime would induce microorganisms generally to elaborate ferric specific ligands. *Aspergillus niger, Bacillus megaterium,* and *Baccillus subtilis* behaved as did *U. sphaerogena,* and it was concluded that the effect was quite general and likely a common device employed to combat iron deficiency in the microbial world (22). Interestingly, *Escherichia coli* did not appear to form a siderophore and it was surmised incorrectly that in this facultative anaerobe the iron requirement may have been too low to enable observation of the effect.

Meanwhile the catechol from *B. subtilis* was characterized as the 2,3-dihydroxybenzoyl conjugate of glycine and the structure of ferrichrome and ferrichrome A were worked out. In succeeding years a catalogue of siderophores was compiled, all of them either hydroxamates or catechols. We were not to come back to the enteric bacteria until B. N. Ames of this Department isolated some "iron mutants" of *S typhimurium*. These mutants were grouped into two classes depending on the presence or absence of 2,3-dihydroxybenzoic acid in the growth medium (23). This pointed to a defect in the biosynthesis of a siderophore derived from this catechol compound. The product was eventually isolated from *S. typhimurium* and *E. coli* and named enterobactin and enterochelin, respectively. Mutants of enteric bacteria unable to synthesize the siderophore grow well on most minimal media and the discovery of enterobactin came about only because of our habit of supplying carbon as citrate. This tricarboxylic acid ties up the iron in a form that is unavailable to *S. typhimurium,* whereas in *E. coli* ferric citrate induces a special transport system (see above).

Mutants of *S. typhimurium* defective in enterobactin synthesis were found capable of growth on ferrichrome as an alternative source of iron. Albomycin, a structural analogue of ferrichrome, was used to collect a library of resistant mutants, most of which mapped at *panC*. Because albomycin was similarly toxic to *E. coli,* attention was directed to the linkage map of the latter organism in the region of *panC*. The most obvious marker at this site was the *tonA* gene imparting resistance to bacteriophages T1 and an array of other lethal agents (2). Following the identification of the ferrichrome receptor as the target for the lethal agents, it has become routine to suspect the receptors of such agents to have a beneficial biochemical function such as the transport of a nutritious substance, of which iron is a prime example.

### 5.2.4   The Escherichia coli K-12 (pColV-K30) Model

***5.2.4.1   Cloning the Aerobactin Operon.***   The enterobactin siderophore system of *E. coli* is a *priori* the obvious choice for studies aimed at understanding the molecular genetics of the system. The siderophore itself is the cyclic trimer of 2,3-dihydroxybenzoylserine, which is not an excessively complicated molecule. Expression of the siderophore is coordinately coupled to synthesis of the outer membrane receptor protein, which serves also as receptor for colicin B. However, preliminary cloning experiments proved the enterobactin system to be surprisingly complex. The determinants were found to be spread over more than 20 kb of DNA and to be organized into several transcriptional units (24, 25).

It was about this time that reports began to appear in the literature on a novel iron uptake system in clinical, pColV-bearing isolates of *E. coli*. The new system was shown to be hydroxamate in nature and to be independent of colicin V. The latter bacteriocin may account for some selective advantage for host species in the gut but could not explain the invasive character of the hospital isolates, which was attributed to the novel hydroxamate siderophore. Although common in fungi, the hydroxamate-type siderophores had only rarely been encountered in bacterial species and with the exception of mycobactin from mycobacteria were confined to the citrate-hydroxamate type of compound, namely, aerobactin, schizokinen, and arthrobactin (Terregens factor). Because aerobactin had previously been identified from the enteric species *Aerobacter aerogenes* 62-I, the novel siderophore was suspected to be aerobactin and this was proven by isolation and characterization of the compound (13).

Because aerobactin is a relatively simple compound of citrate, $N^6$-hydroxylysine, and acetate, a minimum of three enzymes could be required for its synthesis. An outer membrane receptor was shown to serve as the common binding site for ferric aerobactin and cloacin, a bacteriocin from *Enterobacter cloacae*. This happy coincidence provided a most effective means of cloning the receptor because recombinant plasmids carrying the receptor gene should be susceptible to cloacin. This facilitated the design of a successive positive and negative selection screen and resulted in insolation of a 16-kb fragment carrying the receptor gene (26). By chance, the fragment also coded for biosynthetic genes for the siderophore. This immediately suggested an operon structure comprised of not many more genes than the absolute minimum. Thus, unlike the enterobactin gene complex, the aerobactin system appeared much more amenable to genetic dissection.

***5.2.4.2   Organization of the Aerobactin Gene Complex.***   A systematic study of the aerobactin system of pColV-K30 showed it to be composed of only five genes, four for biosynthesis and one for transport of the siderophore (27). The genes were designated *iucA, B, C,* and *D*, where *iuc* refers to "iron uptake chelate," and *iutA,* where *iut* designated "iron uptake transport."

The genes occur in an array consisting of *iucA, B, C, D, iutA* and are transcribed in this sequence. The gene products were shown to have $M_r$ values on SDS-PAGE gels of 63, 33, 62, 53 and 74 kDa, respectively. As regards function, the only immediately obvious assignment was that of the 74 kDa component, which had previously been recognized as the outer membrane receptor for cloacin–ferric aerobactin. A key finding was the observation that a deletion in the *iucC* gene eliminated synthesis of aerobactin and resulted in the accumulation in the growth medium of the aerobactin side chain, $N^6$-acetyl-$N^6$-hydroxylysine, and an anionic compound. The latter was identified by isolation and characterization as citric acid bearing a single aerobactin side chain. A similar type of deletion analysis coupled with examination of metabolic products showed gene *iucD* to be an oxygenase that carried out the initial oxygenation of lysine on the $N^6$ nitrogen. The next step, catalyzed by the product of *iucB*, is the acetylation of the hydroxylamino group of the oxidized lysine. There then follows the synthesis of aerobactin in two steps, the first catalyzed by the product of *iucA* and resulting in formation of the anionic hydroxamate, and the second, promoted by the *iucC* product, affording aerobactin. The biosynthetic sequence for aerobactin is shown in Figure 5.1.

Some progress has been achieved in delineation of the properties of the enzymes of the aerobactin operon. The 63-kDa protein, subunit A of the synthetase, has been isolated in an apparently homogeneous form. The next translational product, the acetylase, has been isolated and the kinetic and specificity parameters of the protein have been charted (28). The product of gene *iucC*, a subunit of the synthetase, has yet to be prepared in pure form. The most interesting enzyme in the series is the oxygenase, the product of gene *iucD*, for a nontoxic specific inhibitor of this step in assembly of aerobactin could have therapeutic application. The enzyme has been sequenced and shown to contain 426 amino acid residues (29). The protein is intimately associated with the cytoplasmic membrane. A study of *iucD'–'lacZ* and *iucD'–'phoA* fusions, constructed in vitro and in vivo, respectively, suggest that protein IucD extends across the cytoplasmic membrane with domains contacting both cytosol and periplasmic space. A sequence resembling that of signal peptides was detected in the first 25 amino acid region of the protein.

### 5.2.4.3 *The Aerobactin Promoter.*

Once the operon nature of the aerobactin complex had been established, it became immediately possible to identify the single promoter driving the transcription unit (30). This was achieved by the standard technique of mapping with S1 nuclease, following which the message was sequenced. Two start sites were found in vitro. The first, major initiation site was detected just downstream from the -10 box. The second, minor, start site was located some 50 bp further upstream. Only the major start site could be detected in vivo. The sequence of the promoter indicated it could be classed as a typical "strong" *E. coli* promoter in which

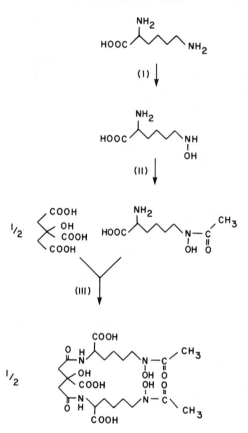

**Figure 5.1** Biosynthetic pathway of aerobactin from L-lysine, acetic acid, and citric acid. The sequence requires an oxygenase (1), an acetylase (11), and two subunits of a synthetase (111), which are coded by genes *iucD*, *iucB*, and *iucAB*, respectively (see Refs. 27, 29).

the -10 and -35 sites are separated by the optimal 17 bp and deviate only slightly from the accepted consensus sequence (Fig. 5.2).

The strength of the aerobactin promoter enabled the setting up of a novel quantitative S1 protection assay to pinpoint the site of action of iron as regulator of expression of the operon. Determination of the degree of protection at low, intermediate, and high iron enabled the conclusion that regulation occurs directly at the transcriptional level (30). This was further confirmed by construction of both operon and protein fusions with *lacZ* minus its promoter. This left no doubt that the iron acts directly on the operator region of the aerobactin promoter to negatively regulate downstream transcription. This is the first iron-regulated promoter of a gene or operon to be characterized by direct methods.

```
        -35        HinfI              -10              +1

TTGATAATGAGAATCATTATTGACATAATTGTTATTATTTTA

       T             C       G      GA A    C     A C
```

**Figure 5.2** Comparison of the sequence of the main (P1) aerobactin promoter of pColV-K30 with a consensus sequence derived from other iron-regulated genes and operons in *Escherichia coli*. The sequence at the P1 promoter of the aerobactin operon is shown in the first row of bases. The −10 and −35 RNA polymerase binding sites, the unique *Hinf*I site, and the +1 site for initiation of the transcript are shown lined above the sequence. The primary and secondary Fur binding sites are indicated by single and double underlining, respectively. The second row of bases records the substitutions in the aerobactin sequence that must be made in order to achieve a consensus sequence derived from promoters of the following iron-regulated genes and operons in *Escherichia coli*: *iuc*, *fhu*, *fepA*, *slt*, and *fur* (see Ref. 37).

### 5.2.4.4 The Product of the fur Gene Identified as a trans-Acting Repressor Protein.

The naked ions of ferrous or ferric iron are not sufficiently "semantic" to interact directly with DNA without the mediation of one or more adapter molecules. Indeed, in 1978 a mutation, designated *fur* (*f*erric *u*ptake *r*egulation), was described in *S. typhimurium* (31). The lesion was found to result in constitutive expression of enterobactin and the outer membrane proteins known to be under iron regulation. Subsequently, similar mutations were generated in *E. coli* and tentatively mapped near *lac* (32). The operon fusions that were prepared for the purpose of identifying the site of regulation by iron enabled us to search for additional *fur* type, constitutive mutations. One such Tn5 mutant was found and mapped at 15.7 min, well separated from *lac* (33). However, the original mapping had been in error and it was concluded that the mutant isolated in our laboratory was identical to that previously described from *E. coli*. The *fur* gene was cloned, sequenced, and shown to code for a 17-kDa protein rich in histidine (34).

Because we were interested in the mechanism of action of the Fur protein, its gene was recloned in our laboratory (35). The kanamycin resistance of the *fur* mutant was first cloned and the wild-type gene then recovered by homologous recombination. The *fur* gene was transferred to an inducible expression vector and the 17-kDa protein isolated by affinity chromatography over zinc-iminodiacetate agarose. These steps made the Fur protein available in the amounts needed for in vitro experiments designed to illuminate its mechanism of action.

An obvious role for the Fur protein is that of a repressor that uses iron, or some derivative of iron, as co-repressor. The properties of iron render a demonstration of such a role in vitro experimentally difficult. Fe(III) is quantitatively insoluble at biological pH, and Fe(II) in an aerobic atmosphere is very rapidly oxidized to the higher valence state. If Fur should be an iron-binding protein it should be rather highly dissociated and hence, like other metal-activated proteins, not entirely specific for iron. We hence performed some preliminary experiments to see if iron could be substituted by some other metal, or metals, less subject to oxidation and precipitation.

Cells harboring the *lacZ* operon fusion were cultured in the presence of varying levels of Mn, Fe, and Co, all added to the growth medium as divalent ions, and the effect of the metals on the level of $\beta$-galactosidase was measured in cell extracts (36). All three metals severely depressed expression of the indicator enzyme and it was concluded that Mn(II), because it is relatively resistant to oxidation, would be a suitable substitute for iron in subsequent in vitro experiments. In vitro transcription–translation from the fusion was found to be strongly repressed by Mn(II), but not by Fe(II), when the experiments were performed aerobically. When care was taken to remove all traces of oxygen, however, iron added as Fe(II) was found to be as effective as Mn(II). This suggested immediately that Fur is a ferrous iron-binding protein. Measurement of the effect of Fur concentration on repressor activity further indicated that the protein acts at the level of a dimer.

Inspection of the promoter sequence of the aerobactin operon revealed the presence of a *Hin*fI site strategically located between the -10 and -35 boxes (Fig. 5.2). This enabled a simple experimental test of the capacity of Fur to protect this site. A plasmid was constructed to contain the aerobactin promoter in a vector carrying a total of seven *Hin*fI sites. Fur was shown to protect only the one provided by the aerobactin promoter (Fig. 5.3) (36). This test system is much cleaner than the in vitro transcription–translation assay and consists of only plasmid DNA, the two proteins, and the activating metal ion. Regarding the latter, it was now possible to survey a range of metal ions. Panel A of Figure 5.3 shows that the Fur protein in the absence of any added metal has some protective effect on the *Hin*fI site. Because this is eliminated by addition of EDTA, it may be safely concluded that the effect is due to contaminating metal ions at a trace level. The data also show that Mn(II) serves as an efficient co-repressor. Passing to panel B of Figure 5.3, we see that even freshly prepared solutions of ferrous sulfate are active, as are also salts of cobalt and cadmium. Panel C indicates that in this test system it is possible to obtain a zero blank without added metal ion, depending on the adventitious contamination of the particular preparations used, and that aluminum, a trivalent ion, is without activity.

### 5.2.4.5  *Definition of the "Iron Box" Operator Consensus Sequence.*
The use of the Fur protein to protect the *Hin*fI site in the aerobactin promoter brought us close to the operator site, but did not allow a designation of the particular bases that make up the repressor binding site. To achieve this level of resolution we turned to the use of the footprinting technique, in which the DNA-binding protein is used to ward off digestion by DNAase I (37). By this methodology Fur was found to bind at a primary site located just upstream of the -10 box, and then at a secondary site almost adjacent to this site but displaced by two bases toward the operon. The particular bases involved are shown in Figure 5.2. Although the aerobactin promoter was the only thoroughly characterized 5′ region of any iron-regulated gene at the time this study was made, sequences were available for a number of relevant genes from *E. coli,* including that of the Fur protein itself. Other published sequences were for the promoters of the *fhu* operon and for *fepA*, the latter the gene for the outer membrane receptor for ferric enterobactin. From these limited data, it was possible to propose a palindromic "iron box" consensus sequence, 5′GATAATGATAATCATTATC, as the preferred locus of Fur binding to the operator. Figure 5.2 gives the substitutions that must be made in the primary and secondary binding sites to reach the suggested consensus sequence. As may be seen, only two changes are necessary at the primary binding site, whereas several are required at the secondary site. Undoubtedly this accounts for the superior binding at the former position in the aerobactin promoter.

Since this study was published a second iron-sensing promoter in *E. coli* has been investigated in depth and the start site defined by primer extension

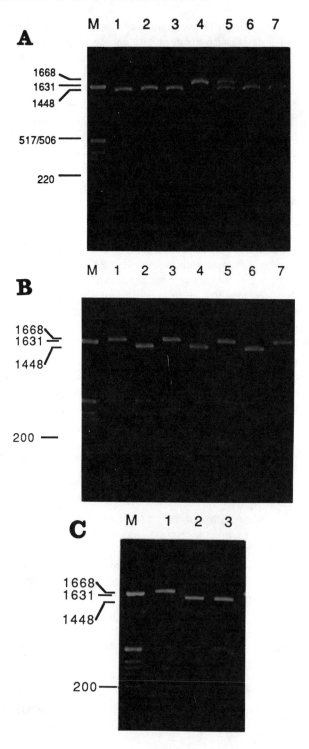

(38). This is the Shiga-like toxin (SLT), which is encoded by a family of bacteriophages associated with enteropathogenic isolates of *E. coli* and which is closely related to toxins produced by *Shigella dysenteriae*. Like the diphtheria toxin, the toxins from the enteric bacteria are produced at low iron concentration. In recent years at least two laboratories have performed a molecular-genetic analysis of a particular bacteriophage coding an SLT, namely, H-19B (38, 39). The two-cistron SLT operon of H-19B has a much longer leader than occurs in other iron-regulated promoters in *E. coli*. Comparison of the 21-pb dyad around the -10 region with the aerobactin promoter and the putative promoters of *fhu* and *fur* gave the same consensus sequence previously deduced from comparison of the aerobactin promoter with a somewhat larger number of 5' regions of iron-regulated genes. Although it is virtually certain that this is the site of binding of the Fur protein, this needs to be confirmed by footprinting experiments. Thus in at least certain strains of *E. coli* the Fur protein may behave as an exceptionally versatile regulator in that it can control bacteriophage (H-19B) and plasmid (ColV-K30) as well as chromosomal genes, which are all regulated by iron.

## 5.3 SUMMARY

An impressive body of knowledge concerning the chemistry and biology of siderophores has accumulated in the three and a half decades since the first report on the isolation of ferrichrome. However, much remains to be accomplished before we can fully understand the mechanism of high-affinity iron assimilation in microorganisms and the regulation of this process.

The molecular genetics of the aerobactin system borne on the ColV K-30 plasmid is currently the best understood in terms of its organization and regulation. The most outstanding problem regarding the operon is the isolation of protein IucD (oxygenase) and identification of its cofactor(s). Pro-

---

**Figure 5.3** Restriction site protection assay for demonstration of the approximate site of action of the Fur repressor and detection of metal ions acting as co-repressor. (A) Lane 1, Fur + $MnSO_4$ + pre-digested plasmid; Lane 2, $MnSO_4$; Lane 3, 100 $\mu M$ EDTA; Lane 4, Fur + $MnSO_4$; Lane 5, Fur; Lane 6, Fur + 50 $\mu M$ EDTA; Lane 7, Fur + 100 $\mu M$ EDTA. (B) Lane 1, Fur + $FeSO_4$; Lane 2, $FeSO_4$; Lane 3, Fur + $CoCl_2$; Lane 4, $CoCl_2$; Lane 5, Fur + $CdCl_2$; Lane 6, $CdCl_2$; Lane 7, Fur + $MnSO_4$. (C) Lane 1, Fur + $MnSO_4$; Lane 2, Fur; Lane 3, Fur + $AlCl_3$. Reprinted with permission from Anne Bagg and J. B. Neilands, Ferric Uptake Regulation Protein Acts as a Repressor, Employing Iron (II) as a Cofactor To Bind the Operator of an Iron Transport Operon in *Escherichia coli*. *Biochemistry*, *26*, 5471–5477. Copyright (1987) American Chemical Society. Note: The particular *Hin*fI site protected by the Fur repressor is shown in Figure 5.2. Protection at this site results in fusion of a 1448- and a 220-bp fragment to give a new 1668-bp fragment.

tein IucC, a subunit of the synthetase, should be isolated and the mechanism of formation of the nonpeptide amide bonds of aerobactin established. Because the aerobactin determinants occur frequently on the chromosome of *E. coli* and in both plasmids and on the chromosome of other Gram-negative bacteria, the possible role of the IS1 elements located fore and aft of the gene cluster in pColV-K30 should be suspected as contributing to the mobility of the operon (40).

At present we do not know if the model devised for regulation of the 30-odd genes in *E. coli* K-12 by the Fur repressor and its co-repressor ferrous iron can be applied to other strains of *E. coli*, let alone to other bacterial and to fungal species. It has so far been impossible to demonstrate hybridization of the *fur* gene to DNA from any bacterial species other than the source organism. We already know that siderophore transport systems are sometimes highly specific, and this may apply as well to the regulatory proteins. The CAS method should facilitate the search for constitutive mutants provided that such mutations are not lethal and single lesions are sufficient to disconnect the regulation circuit. Some methods need to be developed to monitor the fluctuations in levels of Fur and Fe(II) inside the bacterial cell.

Growth of *E. coli* in an iron-restricted environment results in failure of methylthiolation at the 2 position of the hypermodified adenosine residue adjacent to the anticodon loop of tRNAs for phenylalanine, tyrosine, tryptophan, and serine (41). This lack of modification causes lower translational efficiency, relaxation of transcriptional termination at the attenuator, and enhanced expression of genes in the aromatic biosynthesis pathway. This would favor formation of enterobactin, a siderophore that arises from chorismic acid via a series of intermediates, including 2,3-dihydroxybenzoic acid. In addition, methylthiolation of tRNA stimulates, by some unknown mechanism, uptake of aromatic amino acids from the medium. There is as yet no completely satisfying explanation for this phenomenon, which was first noted in 1968. However, the *fur* gene is regarded as the main regulator of high-affinity iron uptake in *E. coli* (41).

At this point nothing is known about the molecular genetics of siderophore systems in fungi. Unfortunately, *Saccharomyces cerevisiae* definitely does not elaborate a siderophore, at least as investigated by the CAS test. This is much to be regretted because cloning technology into yeast is essentially as advanced as in *E. coli*. On the other hand, *S. cerevisiae* could serve as a possible siderophore-less recipient into which fungal siderophore genes might be cloned.

What kind of model can be suggested for iron regulation of siderophore synthesis in fungi? If the metal acts negatively as a co-repressor and in the divalent form, as in *E. coli*, about the only locus where this would be possible would be in the interior of the mitochondrion, which is the most anaerobic site in the eukaryotic cell. In extending the *E. coli* work to fungi, the first objective should be to locate the cellular source of the siderophore genes.

Thus far the pColV-K30 aerobactin operon is the only virulence related system where the chemical structure of the particular siderophore is known, and it happened to be a product already characterized over a decade earlier from *A. aerogenes* 62-I. Anguibactin, the virulence-specifying siderophore from the fish pathogen *Vibrio anguillarum*, belongs to the catechol line of siderophores but the structure has not yet been completely elucidated. The same comment applies to the siderophore of *Erwinia chrysanthemi*, the causative agent of soft rot of vegetables.

Some classical biochemistry remains to be performed with the Fur protein. From the data recorded in Figure 5.3, it is obvious that it is a divalent heavy metal ion-binding protein, but the number, affinity constants, and sites of metal attachment have still to be determined. Probably ferrous iron is the only divalent heavy metal ion available intracellularly in sufficient quantity to activate the repressor. This requires a highly anaerobic cytoplasm in *E. coli*, a condition that fits with the fact that the cell contains a substantial level of glutathione. It is possible that Fur has some other function in view of the fact that our *fur* mutant fails to utilize certain carbon sources. All of this indicates that additional *fur* type mutations should be isolated from Gram-negative bacteria and their properties compared with the primary standard, *E. coli* K-12. This should be feasible through application of the CAS assay.

## REFERENCES

1. J. B. Neilands, Methodology of siderophores, *Structure & Bonding, 58*, 1–24 (1984).
2. R. Wayne and J. B. Neilands, Evidence for a common binding site for ferrichrome compounds and bacteriophage Φ80 in the cell envelope of *Escherichia coli, J. Bacteriol., 121*, 497–501 (1975).
3. G. Winkelmann, D. van der Helm, and J. B. Neilands, Eds., in *Iron Transport in Microbes, Plants and Animals,* VCH Publishers, Weinheim, 1987.
4. A. H. Gillam, A. G. Lewis, and R. J. Andersen, Quantitative determination of hydroxamic acids, *Anal. Chem., 53*, 841–844 (1981).
5. T. F. Emery and J. B. Neilands, Further observations concerning the periodic acid oxidation of hydroxylamine derivatives, *J. Org. Chem., 27*, 1075–1076 (1962).
6. L. E. Arnow, Colorimetric determination of the components of 3,4-dihydroxyphenylalanine–tyrosine mixtures, *J. Biol. Chem., 118*, 531–537 (1937).
7. M. J. Smith, J. N. Shoolery, B. Schwyn, I. Holden, and J. B. Neilands, Rhizobactin, a structurally novel siderophore from *Rhizobium meliloti, J. Am. Chem. Soc., 107*, 1739–1743 (1985).
8. B. Schwyn and J. B. Neilands, Siderophores from agronomically important species of the *Rhizobiacae, Comments Agric. Food Chem., 2*, 1–19 (1987).
9. B. Schwyn and J. B. Neilands, Universal chemical assay for the detection and determination of siderophores, *Anal. Biochem., 160*, 47–56 (1987).

10. A. L. Schade and L. Caroline, An iron binding component in human blood plasma, *Science, 104,* 340–341 (1946).

11. J. J. Bullen and E. Griffiths, Eds., *Iron and Infection,* Wiley, New York, 1987.

12. L. A. Actis, W. Fish, J. H. Crosa, K. Kellerman, S. R. Ellenberger, F. M. Hauser, and J. Sanders-Loehr, Characterization of anguibactin, a novel siderophore from *Vibrio anguillarum* 775(pJM1), *J. Bacteriol., 167,* 57–65 (1986).

13. P. J. Warner, P. H. Williams, A. Bindereif, and J. B. Neilands, ColV plasmid specified aerobactin synthesis by invasive strains of *Escherichia coli, Infect. Immun., 33,* 540–545 (1981).

14. D. Expert and A. Toussaint, Bacteriocin-resistant mutants of *Erwinia chrysanthemi*: Possible involvement of iron acquisition in phytopathogenicity, *J. Bacteriol., 163,* 221–227 (1985).

15. L. A. de Weger, B. Schippers, and B. Lugtenberg, in G. Winkelmann, D. van der Helm, and J. B. Neilands, Eds., *Iron Transport in Microbes, Plants, and Animals,* VCH Publishers, Weinheim, 1987, p.385.

16. J. Leong, Siderophores: Their biochemistry and possible role in the bio-control of plant pathogens, *Ann. Rev. Phytopathol., 24,* 187–209 (1986).

17. J. B. Neilands, T. Peterson, and S. A. Leong, "High Affinity Iron Transport in Microorganisms," in A. E. Martell, Ed., *Inorganic Chemistry in Biology and Medicine,* American Chemical Society, Washington, DC, 1980, p. 263.

18. W. Flitter, D. A. Rowley, and B. Halliwell, Superoxide-dependent formation of hydroxyl radicals in the presence of iron salts, *FEBS Lett., 158,* 310–312 (1983).

19. K. Rao, J. B. Harford, T. Rouault, A. McClelland, R. H. Ruddle, and R. D. Klausner, Transcriptional regulation by iron of the gene for the transferrin receptor, *Mol. Cell Biol., 6,* 236–240 (1986).

20. V. Romheld, in G. Winkelmann, D. van der Helm, and J. B. Neilands, Eds., *Iron Transport in Microbes, Plants, and Animals,* VCH Publishers, Weinheim, 1987, p. 351.

21. J. B. Neilands, A crystalline organo-iron pigment from a smut fungus, *Ustilago sphaerogena, J. Am. Chem. Soc., 74,* 4846–4847 (1952).

22. J. A. Garibaldi and J. B. Neilands, Formation of iron binding compounds by microorganisms, *Nature, 177,* 526–527 (1956).

23. J. R. Pollack, B. N. Ames, and J. B. Neilands, Iron transport in *Salmonella typhimurium, J. Bacteriol., 104,* 635–639 (1970).

24. A. J. Laird, D. W. Ribbons, G. C. Woodrow, and I. G. Young, Bacteriophage µ mediated gene transposition and *in vitro* cloning of the enterochelin gene cluster of *Escherichia coli, Gene, 11,* 347–357 (1980).

25. A. J. Laird and I. G. Young, Tn5 mutagenesis of the enterochelin gene cluster of *Escherichia coli, Gene, 11,* 359–366 (1980).

26. A. Bindereif and J. B. Neilands, Cloning of the aerobactin mediated iron assimilation system of plasmid ColV, *J. Bacteriol., 153,* 1111–1113 (1983).

27. V. de Lorenzo and J. B. Neilands, Characterization of *iucA* and iucC genes of the aerobactin system of plasmid ColV K-30 in *Escherichia coli, J. Bacteriol., 167,* 350–355 (1986).

28. M. Coy, B. H. Paw, A. Bindereif, and J. B. Neilands, Isolation and properties

of $N^\epsilon$-hydroxylysine:acetyl coenzyme A $N^\epsilon$-transacetylase from *Escherichia coli* (pABN11), *Biochemistry, 25*, 2485–2489 (1986).

29. M. Herrero, V. de Lorenzo, and J. B. Neilands, Nucleotide sequence of *iucD* gene of the aerobactin operon of pCol-K30 and topology of its product studied with *phoA* and *lacZ* gene fusions, *J. Bacteriol., 170*, 56–74 (1988).

30. A. Bindereif and J. B. Neilands, Promoter mapping and transcriptional regulation of the iron assimilation system of plasmid ColV-K30 in *Escherichia coli* K-12. *J. Bacteriol., 162*, 1039–1046 (1985).

31. J. F. Ernst, R. L. Bennett, and L. I. Rothfield, Constitutive expression of the iron enterochelin and ferrichrome uptake systems in a mutant strain of *Salmonella typhimurium, J. Bacteriol., 135*, 928–934 (1978).

32. K. Hantke, Regulation of ferric iron transport in *Escherichia coli*. Isolation of a constitutive mutant, *Mol. Gen. Genet., 182*, 288–292 (1981).

33. A. Bagg and J. B. Neilands, Mapping of a mutation affecting regulation of iron uptake systems in *Escherichia coli* K-12, *J. Bacteriol., 161*, 450–453 (1985).

34. S. Schaffer, K. Hantke, and V. Braun, Nucleotide sequence of the iron regulatory gene *fur, Mol. Gen. Genet., 201*, 204–212 (1985).

35. A. Bagg and J. B. Neilands, Molecular mechanism of regulation of siderophore mediated iron assimilation, *Microbiol Rev., 51*, 509–518 (1987).

36. A. Bagg and J. B. Neilands, Ferric uptake regulation protein acts as a repressor, employing iron (II) as a cofactor to bind the operator of an iron transport operon in *Escherichia coli, Biochemistry, 26*, 5471–5477 (1987).

37. V. de Lorenzo, S. Wee, M. Herrero, and J. B. Neilands, Operator sequences of the aerobactin operon of plasmid ColV-K30 binding the ferric uptake regulation (*fur*) repressor, *J. Bacteriol., 169*, 2624–2630 (1987).

38. S. De Grandis, J. Ginsberg, M. Toone, S. Climie, J. Friesen, and J. Brunton, Nucleotide sequence and promoter mapping of the *Escherichia coli* Shiga-like toxin operon of bacteriophage H-19B, *J. Bacteriol., 169*, 4313–4319 (1987).

39. S. B. Calderwood and J. J. Mekalanos, Iron regulation of Shiga-like toxin expression in *Escherichia coli* is mediated by the *fur* locus, *J. Bacteriol., 170*, 1015–1017 (1988).

40. S. McDougal and J. B. Neilands, Plasmid- and chromosomal-coded aerobactin synthesis in enteric bacteria, *J. Bacteriol., 169*, 300–305 (1984).

41. E. Griffiths, in J. J. Bullen and E. Griffiths, Eds., *Iron and Infection*, Wiley, New York, 1987, p. 69.

**CHAPTER 6**

# Transition Metal Enzymes in Bacterial Metabolism

LAWRENCE P. WACKETT

Department of Biochemistry
Gray Freshwater Biological Institute
University of Minnesota
Navarre, Minnesota

WILLIAM H. ORME-JOHNSON and CHRISTOPHER T. WALSH*

Department of Chemistry
Massachusetts Institute of Technology
Cambridge, Massachusetts

## Contents

* *Current affiliation*: Department of Biological Chemistry and Molecular Pharmacology, Harvard Medical School, Boston, Massachusetts

## 6.1 OVERALL PROPERTIES AND SIGNIFICANCE OF BACTERIAL METALLOENZYMES

### 6.1.1 Introduction

Elemental analysis of dehydrated *E. coli* reveals that carbon, oxygen, nitrogen, hydrogen, and phosphorus make up 95% of the cell mass (1). In this context, one can think of the structural framework of a bacterial cell to be composed largely of organic molecules. Interspersed in this organic milieu are the metallic elements that serve as osmotic regulators, as structural glue, and as catalytic centers for hundreds of cellular reactions. The significance of metals in biological catalysis is underscored by the fact that greater than one-third of all characterized enzymes are metalloenzymes (2). Thus metals serve important functions in all facets of bacterial metabolism.

### 6.1.2 Metalloenzymes in Elemental Cycles in Nature

Bacterial metalloenzymes exert a major catalytic force on the biosphere by mediating a large number of important reactions in elemental cycles where biological systems play important roles (Fig. 6.1). Because microorganisms are the key players in recycling carbon, hydrogen, nitrogen, oxygen, and sulfur on the Earth's surface, bacterial enzymes that contain iron, molybdenum, manganese, nickel, and copper are, by transference, the agents responsible for the cycling of these elements. Although the elemental cycles of Figure 6.1 are shown as independent units for clarity of presentation, they operate in nature as a complex, interactive web. In anaerobic environments occupied by methanogens and sulfate reducers, hydrogen oxidation is obligately coupled to carbon dioxide reduction and sulfate reduction, respectively (3). Methane formed by methanogenic bacteria is utilized by methanotrophic bacteria as a source of carbon and energy through the action of the iron-containing enzyme methane monooxygenase (4). In this reaction one atom of molecular oxygen is inserted into the C–H bond of methane to form methanol. Methanotropic and methylotrophic bacteria further oxidize methanol and assimilate $C_1$ units into cellular constituents. Oxygen that is fixed into organic material can be released as water that in turn is recycled to the atmosphere as oxygen through the action of the photosynthetic cyanobacteria, eukaryotic algae, and plants (5). This reaction contains an array of light-harvesting molecules, iron-containing electron transfer proteins, and a reaction center that utilizes manganese to form molecular oxygen and produce electrons for cellular metabolism.

In biological systems, the nitrogen and sulfur cycles act mutually with carbon metabolism. As shown in Figure 6.1, nitrogen is reduced to ammonia by nitrogen-fixing bacteria and sulfate can be reduced to sulfide by a variety of bacteria. At these oxidation states, nitrogen and sulfur are readily incorporated into biomolecules and so become important elements in intermediary

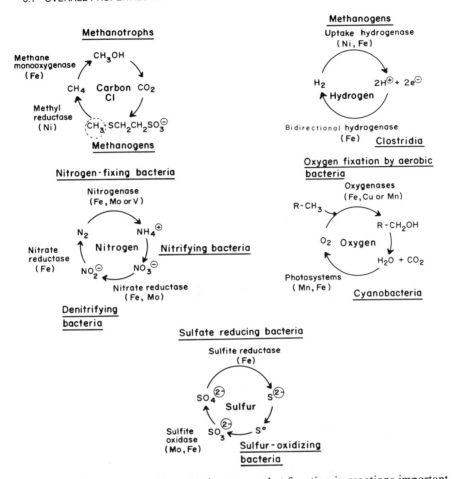

**Figure 6.1** Bacterial transition metal enzymes that function in reactions important in elemental cycling in the biosphere. Representative groups of bacteria that catalyze a given reaction(s) are shown underlined.

metabolism. Following cell death, biomolecules are degraded, carbon–heteroatom bond cleavage is accomplished by a large array of catabolic enzymes, and the elements again enter the inorganic cycles depicted in Figure 6.1. Bacterial metalloenzymes representing each of these elemental cycles are discussed in greater detail in Section 6.3.

### 6.1.3  Properties of Metalloenzymes and the Scope of the Review

Given the formidable array of bacterial enzymes that require a metal to conduct catalysis, we will focus our attention on enzymes containing a transition metal that is redox active in biological reactions (Fig. 6.2). This is

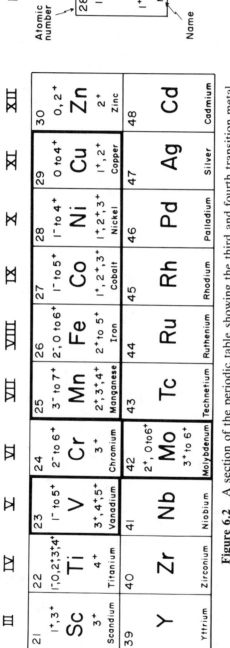

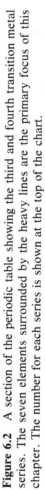

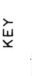

**Figure 6.2** A section of the periodic table showing the third and fourth transition metal series. The seven elements surrounded by the heavy lines are the primary focus of this chapter. The number for each series is shown at the top of the chart.

generally not the case for enzymes utilizing group I and II metals or zinc-containing enzymes. Bacteria have largely called on Mg(II), Ca(II), Mn(II), Ni(II), and first and foremost Zn(II) to act in enzymes that catalyze Lewis acid chemistry (6), but we do not discuss this group here.

Even though we are restricting ourselves to redox-active transition metals there is still a vast array of enzymes, so the list of enzymes covered here is by no means complete. Those covered, especially in depth, necessarily reflect our biases. In general, we discuss protein catalysts that bind a specific transition metal firmly such that extreme conditions are required to remove it. In quantitative terms, a somewhat arbitrary definition of tight binding of metals is those proteins with dissociation constants below $10^{-7}-10^{-8}$ $M$ for their respective metal. Almost invariably, the enzyme in question functions exclusively with a specific transition metal(s), although metal replacement studies coupled with biophysical methodologies can prove valuable in developing insight into ligand and protein structure.

It is worth pointing out some key properties of the transition metals that come to have a bearing on both their biological roles in enzymes and on the repertoire of physicochemical methodologies that has been focused on metalloenzymes. The transition metals, excluding the lanthanides and actinides, can be loosely defined as those elements that possess a partially filled set of $d$ orbitals. Thus, in contrast to the $s$- and $p$-block metals, which form ions in one or, at most, two oxidation states, the transition metals can exist in a variety of oxidation states (Fig. 6.2). This versatility comes into play in enzyme catalysis as well as the ability to tune oxidation states by changing ligands of biological significance, generally nitrogen-, oxygen-, or sulfur-containing donor groups.

Nature has devised two general methods for coordinating metals to enzymes (Fig. 6.3). In the first, the metal is coordinated directly by amino acid side chains. Histidine, glutamic acid, aspartic acid, cysteine, lysine, arginine, serine, threonine, and tryptophan can serve in this capacity (Fig. 6.3a–c). Alternatively, the metal is held by a prosthetic group such as heme Fe, the corrin ring of coenzyme $B_{12}$ (Co), or the tetrahydrocorphinoid cofactor $F_{430}$ (Ni) (Fig. 6.3d–g). In turn, the prosthetic group is tightly bound by the enzyme, largely through ionic interactions between charged groups on the ligand periphery and complementary charges of amino acid side chains. In general, it has been pointed out (14) that the interplay between enzyme evolution, which modifies amino acid–ligand composition and geometries, and the physicochemical properties of transition metals has given rise to a variety of highly efficient biological catalysts that are, in a sense, optimized for conducting a given chemical reaction.

### 6.1.4 Physical Methods of Studying Metalloenzymes

An appreciation of the properties of transition metals has furnished biochemists with a window for examining metal environments in proteins. Even

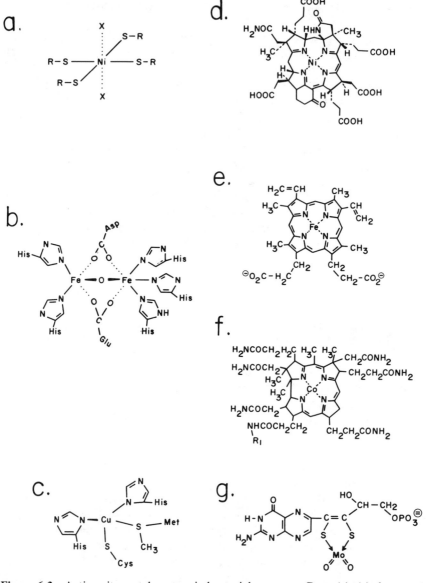

**Figure 6.3** Active-site metal centers in bacterial enzymes. Parts (a)–(c) show metal ligated directly to enzyme: (*a*) the nickel center in $F_{420}$-reducing hydrogenase from *Methanobacterium thermoautotrophicum* (7); (*b*) the binuclear iron center found in methemerythrin (8) and a similar one in *E. coli* ribonucleotide reductase; (*c*) the copper site in *Pseudomonas* azurin (9). Parts (d)–(g) show metal bound in a prosthetic group: (*d*) the nickel chromophore, $F_{430}$, that serves as a cofactor for methanogen methyl reductase (10); (*e*) protoporphyrin IV, which acts as an electron carrier in various cytochromes and catalytic proteins (11); (*f*) coenzyme $B_{12}$, which is found in various enzymes (12) including ribonucleotide reductase from *Lactobacillus leichmanii*; and (*g*) molybdopterin (13), the form of molybdenum in enzymes other than nitrogenase. In some enzymatic examples, molybdopterin may contain one or two sulfur atoms in place of oxygen as ligands for the molybdenum atom.

**TABLE 6.1  Physical Methods Used for Studying Metalloenzymes**

| Method Studied | Metal Species Studied | Information Derived | Ref. |
|---|---|---|---|
| Optical absorption | Fe, Co, Ni, Cu, Mo | Type of transition gives insight into ligands | 90 |
| EPR | Mn(II), Fe(III), Co(II), Mo(V), Cu(II) | Ligand structure | 91 |
| Mössbauer | Fe | Oxidation state; symmetry of electric field | 92 |
| NMR | Mn, $^{57}$Co | Bonding nature and structure | 93 |
| EXAFS | Fe, Co, Ni, Cu, Mo | Coordination number and ligand–metal distances | 94 |

though the metal may constitute a small fraction of the total mass of the enzyme, the metal and its immediate environment can often be examined selectively. Some of the useful physicochemical techniques are listed in Table 6.1 along with the types of information that they can impart. For more detailed information, excellent reviews of these techniques applied to proteins are available (15). In this chapter, more specific uses of these methodologies are discussed in the context of their utility in deriving mechanistic insights into metalloenzyme catalysis.

## 6.2  A WALK THROUGH THE TRANSITION METAL SERIES WITH A FOCUS ON BACTERIAL ENZYMES

Although their electronic configurations formally place scandium and titanium at the front of the first transition series, they exist largely in $+3$ and $+4$ oxidation states, respectively. As a result, their ions have no $d$ electrons and a closed-shell configuration which precludes biologically relevant redox chemistry. It should be noted, however, that the dinoflagellate *Gymnodinum brevis* concentrates titanium intracellularly by a factor of $8 \times 10^4$ against seawater, but no role for this metal has been shown (16). Vanadium was identified as a biologically important element over 60 years ago with its demonstration in *Ascidia* deep-sea worms. Only in 1986, however, has vanadium been shown to have a distinct function in microbial enzymes. In two well documented investigations, a bromoperoxidase (17) and a unique nitrogenase activity (18) have been shown to require vanadium specifically to catalyze their respective reactions (Table 6.2).

In moving to group VI in the periodic table (Fig. 6.2), the $4d$, $4f$, and $5d$ rows are represented by chromium, molybdenum, and tungsten, respec-

**TABLE 6.2  Transition Metal Enzymes in Bacteria**

| Element/Enzyme | E.C. # | Organism | Reaction/Role | Other Data | Ref. |
|---|---|---|---|---|---|
| **Vanadium** | | | | | |
| Nitrogenase | | *Azotobacter chroococcum* strain MCD1155 | $N_2 + 6H^+ + 6e^- \rightarrow 2NH_3$ | Distinct from Mo nitrogenase | 18 |
| Bromoperoxidase | | *Ascophyllum nodosum* | $R-H + H_2O_2 + Br^- + H^+ \rightarrow R-Br + 2H_2O$ | | 17 |
| **Molybdenum** | | | | | |
| Nitrogenase | 1.19.2.1 | *Klebsiella pneumoniae*, other bacteria | $N_2 + 6H^+ + 6e^- \rightarrow 2NH_3$ | Also contains Fe | 58 |
| Xanthine oxidase | 1.2.3.2 | *Arthrobacter* S-2 | $\text{Xanthine} + H_2O + O_2 \rightarrow \text{urate} + H_2O_2$ | Also contains Fe and FAD | 95 |
| Sulfite oxidase | 1.8.3.1 | *Thiobacillus thioparus*, and other bacteria | $SO^{2-} + H_2O \rightarrow SO_4^{3-} + 2H^+ + 2e^-$ | Also contains heme iron | 96 |
| Nitrate reductase | 1.7.99.4 | *Micrococcus denitrificans* | $NO_3^- + 2H^+ + 2e^- \rightarrow NO_2 + H_2O$ | Also contains nonheme iron and acid-labile sulfur | 97 |
| Formate dehydrogenase | | *Methanobacterium formicicum* | $HCOOH \rightarrow CO_2 + 2e^- + 2H^+$ | Also contains nonheme iron, acid-labile sulfur, zinc, and FAD | 98 |
| CO dehydrogenase | | *Pseudomonas carboxydovorans*, *Clostridium thermoaceticum*, and other bacteria | $CO + H_2O \rightarrow CO_2 + 2e^- + 2H^+$ | Also contains nonheme iron, acid-labile sulfur, and FAD | 65 |
| Dimethylsulfoxide dehydrogenase | | | $2e^- + 2H^+ + CH_3S(O)CH_3 \rightarrow CH_3SCH_3 + H_2O$ | | |
| Trimethylamine *N*-oxide reductase | | | $(CH_3)_3N(O) + 2e^- + 2H^+ \rightarrow (CH_3)_3N + H_2O$ | | 99 |

**Manganese**

| Enzyme | EC number | Source | Reaction | Properties | Ref |
|---|---|---|---|---|---|
| Pseudocatalase | | *Lactobacillus plantarum* | $H_2O_2 \rightarrow H_2O + \frac{1}{2}O_2$ | Pentamer; 2 Mn per subunit | 100 |
| 3,4-Dihydroxyphenyl-acetate 2,3-dioxygenase | | *Bacillus brevis* | 3,4-Dihydroxyphenyl-acetate $+ O_2 \rightarrow$ 5-carboxymethyl-2-hydroxy-*cis,cis*-muconic semialdehyde | 2 Mn per enzyme | 101 |
| Superoxide dismutase | | *E. coli* | $2O_2^{-} + 2H^{+} \rightarrow O_2 + H_2O_2$ | | 102 |
| Guanidinoacetate aminohydrolase | 3.4.3.2 | *Pseudomonas* sp. ATCC 14676 | Guanidinoacetate $+ H_2O \rightarrow$ glycine $+$ urea | | 103 |
| Allantoate amidino-hydrolase | 3.4.3.4 | *Pseudomonas aeruginosa* | Allantoate $+ H_2O \rightarrow$ (-)-ureidoglycollate $+$ urea | | 104 |
| α-Isopropylmalate synthetase | 4.1.3.12 | *Alcaligenes eutrophus* | 3-Hydroxy-4-methyl-3-carboxyvalerate $+$ CoA $\rightarrow$ Acetyl-CoA $+$ 2-oxo-3-methylbutyrate $+ H_2O$ | | 105 |
| D-Phosphoglycerate 2,3-phosphomutase | 5.4.2.1 | *Bacillus subtilis* or *Bacillus megaterium* | 2-phospho-D-glycerate $\rightarrow$ 3-phospho-D-glycerate | | 106 |

**Iron**

A. *Heme proteins*

| Enzyme | EC number | Source | Reaction | Properties | Ref |
|---|---|---|---|---|---|
| 1. Electron-transfer cytochromes | | Many bacteria | Electron transfer | | 11 |
| 2. Catalase/peroxidase | 1.11.1.6 | Many bacteria | $H_2O_2 \rightarrow H_2O + \frac{1}{2}O_2$ | | 107 |

**TABLE 6.2** *(continued)*

| Element/Enzyme | E.C. # | Organism | Reaction/Role | Other Data | Ref. |
|---|---|---|---|---|---|
| **3. Oxygenases** | | | | | |
| Cytochrome P450 | 1.14.15.1 | *Pseudomonas putida* | Camphor + $O_2$ + NADH → 5-*exo*-hydroxycamphor | Requires accessory flavoprotein and ferredoxin | 108 |
| L-Tryptophan 2,3-dioxygenase | 1.13.1.12 | *Pseudomonas fluorescens* | L-Tryptophan + $O_2$ → L-formylkynurenine | | 109 |
| **4. Other heme enzymes** | | | | | |
| Hydroxylamine oxidoreductase (nitrite reductase) | | *Nitrosomonas europeae* | $NO_3^- + 4e^- + 5H^+ \rightarrow NH_2OH + H_2O$ | Contains 21 c-type hemes and 3 unusual hemes | 110 |
| Sulfite reductase | 1.8.1.2 | *E. coli* | $SO_3^{2-} + 6e^- + 6H^+ \rightarrow S^{2-} + 3H_2O$ | Also contains $Fe_4S_4$ and FAD | 27 |
| p-Cresol hydroxylase | | *Pseudomonas putida* | p-Cresol + $NAD^+$ + $H_2O$ → p-hydroxybenzyl alcohol + NADH | Contains covalently bound FAD | 111 |
| ***B. Iron–sulfur proteins*** | | | | | |
| 1. Electron transfer only | | | | | |
| Rubredoxin (Fe) | | *Pseudomonas oleovorans* | Electron transfer to non-heme iron oxygenase | Contains 1 Fe coordinated by 4 cysteine sulfurs | 112 |
| Ferredoxin$_{CAM}$ ($Fe_2S_2$) | | *Pseudomonas putida* | Electron transfer to heme iron oxygenase | Contains 1 $Fe_2S_2$ | 108 |
| $Fe_3S_4$ ferredoxin | | *Azotobacter vinelandii* | Electron transfer | Also contains 1 $Fe_4S_4$ cluster | 113 |

| Enzyme | EC number | Source | Reaction | Properties | Ref. |
|---|---|---|---|---|---|
| Fe$_4$S$_4$ ferredoxin | | Clostridium acidi-urici | Electron transfer | | 26 |
| Reiske-type Fe$_2$S$_2$ | | Pseudomonas putida or Thermus thermophilus | Electron transfer to non-heme iron dixoygenases in Pseudomonas | Fe$_2$S$_2$ liganded by 2 cysteines and 2 non-cysteine amino acids | 114 |
| 2. Hydrogenase | 1.18.3.1 | Clostridium pasteurianum | $H_2 \rightleftarrows 2e^- + 2H^+$ | All hydrogenases contain FeS; some contain other redox groups as well | 115 |
| 3. Dehydratases: Aconitase | 4.2.1.3 | All organisms with citric acid cycle | Citrate $\rightarrow$ cis-aconitate + $H_2O$ | Contains Fe$_4$S$_4$, but one Fe readily lost | 107 |
| 4. Oxygenases containing iron in addition to FeS | | | | | |
| 4-Methoxybenzoate monooxygenase | | Pseudomonas putida | 4-Methoxybenzoate + $H^+$ + $O_2$ + NAD(P)H $\rightarrow$ HCHO + 4-hydroxybenzoate + $H_2O$ | 2-Component enzyme system | 116 |
| Toluene dioxygenase | | Pseudomonas putida | NADH + toluene + $O_2$ + $H^+ \rightarrow NAD^+$ + cis-toluene dihydrodiol | 3-Component enzyme system | 42 |
| Methane monooxygenase | | Methylococcus capsulatus | NADH + $H^+$ + $O_2$ + $CH_4 \rightarrow CH_3OH + H_2O$ | | 117 |
| C. *Nonheme iron (no acid-labile sulfur)* | | | | | |
| Catechol 1,2-dioxygenase | | Pseudomonas arvilla c-1 (ATCC 23974) | Catechol + $O_2 \rightarrow$ cis, cis-muconic acid | | 118 |

**TABLE 6.2** *(continued)*

| Element/Enzyme | E.C. # | Organism | Reaction/Role | Other Data | Ref. |
|---|---|---|---|---|---|
| p-Hydroxyphenyl-pyruvate hydroxyl-ase | | *Pseudomonas* sp. P.J. 874 | p-Hydroxyphenylpyruvate + $O_2 \rightarrow$ homogentisate + $CO_2$ | | 119 |
| Ribonucleotide reductase | | *E. coli* | Nucleoside diphosphate + $2e^- + 2H^+ \rightarrow$ deoxyribonucleoside diphosphate | | 49 |
| Superoxide dismutase | | *Photobacterium leiognathi* | $SO_2^- + 2H^+ \rightarrow O_2 + H_2O_2$ | | 120 |
| **Cobalt** | | | | | |
| **A. *$B_{12}$-containing enzymes*** | | | | | |
| 1. Reductases | | | | | |
| Ribonucleotide reductase | 1.17.4.2 | *Lactobacillus leichmanii* | Ribonucleotide triphos-phate + reduced thio-redoxin → deoxyribo-nucleotide triphosphate + thioredoxin disulfide | | 121 |
| 2. Internal redox reactions | | | | | |
| Propanediol dehy-drase | 4.2.1.28 | *Klebsiella pneumoniae* | 1,2-Propanediol → proionaldehyde | | 122 |
| Glycerol dehydrase | 4.2.1.30 | *Klebsiella pneumoniae* | Glycerol → β-hydroxy-propionaldehyde | | 123 |
| Ethanolamine deaminase (ethanol-amine ammonia lyase) | 4.3.1.7 | *E. coli* | Ethanolamine → acetalde-hyde + ammonia | | 124 |

## 3. Carbon skeletal rearrangements

| Enzyme | EC number | Organism | Reaction | Comments | Ref |
|---|---|---|---|---|---|
| Glutamate mutase (methylaspartate ammonia lyase) | 4.3.1.2 | *Clostridium tetanomorphum* | L-Glutamate → *threo*-β-methyl-L-aspartate | | 125 |
| Methylmalonyl-CoA mutase | 5.4.99.2 | *Propionobacterium shermanii* | R-Methylmalonyl-CoA → succinyl-CoA | | 126 |
| 2-Methyleneglutarate mutase | 5.4.99.4 | *Clostridium barkeri* | 2-Methyleneglutarate → 2-methylene-3-methyl-succinate | | 127 |

## 4. Amino group migrations

| Enzyme | EC number | Organism | Reaction | Comments | Ref |
|---|---|---|---|---|---|
| β-Lysine aminomutase | 5.4.3.3 | *Clostridium* sp. | L-3,6-Diamino-hexanoate → 3,5-diaminohexanoate | Also requires bound divalent cation and pyridoxal-5'-phosphate | 128 |
| D-α-Lysine aminomutase | 5.4.3.4 | *Clostridium* sp. | D-Lysine → 2,5-diaminohexanoate | Copurifies with β-lysine aminomutase but distinct active site | 128 |
| D-Ornithine 4,5-aminomutase | 5.4.3.5 | *Clostridium stricklandii* | D-Ornithine → D-*threo*-2,4-diaminopentanoate | | 129 |

## B. Non-B$_{12}$ Co Enzymes

| Enzyme | EC number | Organism | Reaction | Comments | Ref |
|---|---|---|---|---|---|
| Transcarboxylase | | *Propionobacterium shermanii* | S-Methylmalonyl-CoA + pyruvate → propionyl-CoA + oxaloacetate | Also contains Zn and biotin | 130 |
| Amidino aspartase (*N*-amidino-L-aspartate amidinohydrolase) | 3.5.3.14 | *Pseudomonas chlororaphis* | *N*-Amidino-L-aspartate + H$_2$O → L-aspartate + urea | | 131 |

**TABLE 6.2** (continued)

| Element/Enzyme | E.C. # | Organism | Reaction/Role | Other Data | Ref. |
|---|---|---|---|---|---|
| **Nickel** | | | | | |
| Hydrogenases | | *Methanobacterium thermoautotrophicum* ΔH | $H_2 \rightarrow 2e^- + 2H^+$ | Two in this organism. One reduces deaza-flavin cofactor $F_{420}$ | 132 |
| Hydrogenase | | Many other bacteria | | | 36 |
| Methyl-S-coenzyme M reductase | | *Methanobacterium thermoautotrophicum* ΔH | $CH_3SCH_2CH_2SO_3^- + 2e^- + 2H \rightarrow CH_4 + HSCH_2CH_2SO_3$ | Contains nickel cofactor, $F_{430}$ | 133 |
| CO dehydrogenase (involved in acetate biosynthesis) | | *Costridium thermoaceticum* | $H_2O + CO \rightleftarrows CO_2 + 2H + 2e$ | Also contains FeS and zinc | 67 |
| Urease | | *Selenomonas ruminantium* | Urea + $H_2O \rightarrow$ carbon dioxide + 2 ammonia | | 134 |
| **Copper** | | | | | |
| *A. Small "blue" copper proteins* | | | | | |
| Rusticyanin | | *Thiobacillus* ferrooxidans | $Fe^{2+} \rightarrow Fe^{3+} + 1e^-$ active at pH 2 | | 135 |
| Azurin | | *Pseudomonas aeruginosa* | Electron transfer | | 136 |
| Amicyanin | | *Pseudomonas* AM1 | Electron transfer | Electron acceptor from methylamine dehydrogenase | 137 |
| Plastocyanin | | *Anabaena variabilis* | Electron transfer | In photosynthetic electron transport | 138 |

**B. Oxygenases and oxidases**

| Enzyme | EC number | Organism | Reaction | Notes | Ref. |
|---|---|---|---|---|---|
| Methylamine oxidase | 1.4.3.6 | *Arthrobacter* P1 | $CH_3NH_2 + H_2O + O_2 \rightarrow HCHO + H_2O_2 + NH_3$ | Also contains pyrroloquinoline quinone | 139 |
| Cytochrome *c* oxidase | 1.9.3.1 | Many bacteria | 4 cytochrome *c* (Fe$^{2+}$) + $O_2 \rightarrow$ 4 cytochrome *c* (Fe$^{3+}$) + $2H_2O$ | Also contains heme iron | 39 |
| Phenylalanine hydroxylase | 1.14.16.1 | *Chromobacterium violaceum* | L-Phenylalanine + $2e^-$ + H + $O_2 \rightarrow$ L-tyrosine + $H_2O$ | | 140 |
| Tyrosinase | | *Streptomyces nigrifaciens* | $2H^+ + 2e^- + O_2 +$ p-coumarate $\rightarrow$ caffeate | | 141 |

**C. Other copper proteins**

| Enzyme | EC number | Organism | Reaction | Notes | Ref. |
|---|---|---|---|---|---|
| Superoxide dismutase | | *Pseudomonas diminuta* | $2H^+\ 2O_2^- \rightarrow O_2 + H_2O_2$ | Also contains zinc | 142 |
| Nitric oxide oxidoreductase | 1.7.99.3 | *Pseudomonas* sp. | Nitric oxide + $2H_2O$ + acceptor $\rightarrow$ 2 nitrite + reduced acceptor | | 143 |

tively. Although chromium is thought to play some role in the regulation of glucose and cholesterol metabolism in mammals (16), bacterial enzymes have apparently bypassed chromium as a catalytic cofactor. This is likely to be based on the substitution inertness of this element and its monovalency ($+3$) in the common biological redox range ($-0.4$ to $+0.8$ $V$). In contrast, molybdenum and tungsten can exist in multiple oxidation states ($+3$ to $+6$) in the biological milieu. Tungsten has been found in bacterial enzymes, for example, in formate dehydrogenase from *Clostridium thermoaceticum* (19), but a direct catalytic function for this element remains to be established. Thus the presence of group VI elements in bacterial enzymes is represented largely by molybdenum. In fact, molybdenum remains the only 4d element to have a documented role at the active site of bacterial enzymes.

Enzyme-bound molybdenum has been demonstrated to exist in only two environments, both of them as distinct cofactors that can be removed from their respective enzymes (20). One form is the MoFe cofactor of nitrogenase; the other is the molybdopterin cofactor of other molybdenum-containing enzymes (Fig. 6.3 and Table 6.2). Nitrogenase, the key enzyme in bacterial nitrogen fixation, is discussed in greater detail in Section 6.3. The other molybdenum enzymes of Table 6.2 contain the universal molybdenum cofactor. This insight has stemmed from the work of Nason et al. (21, 22), who developed an assay whereby the extracted molybdopterin cofactor can complement the *nit-1* mutant of *Neurospora crassa*. The present understanding of the structure of molybdopterin (Fig. 6.2) is derived from a series of investigations by Rajagopalan and others (13).

In general, the biochemistry of molybdenum, as shown in Table 6.2, involves multielectron transfers; six for nitrogen and two each for the molybdopterin-containing enzymes. The oxygen-transfer reactions catalyzed by sulfite and nitrate reductases are important reactions in global sulfur and nitrogen cycles (Fig. 6.1).

Manganese can exist in 11 oxidation states ($+7$ to $-3$), more than any other element (16). However, the aqueous chemistry of this element is largely restricted to $Mn^{2+}$ complexes; in enzymes $Mn^{2+}$ and $Mn^{3+}$ states are described. The ionic radius of 0.9Å places $Mn^{2+}$ midway between that of $Mg^{2+}$ and $Ca^{2+}$ so it is not surprising that there is overlap in function with this group in providing structural charge stabilization of enzymes and, in some cases, substrates such as Mn·ATP. In this regard, manganese has been useful in substitutions for $Mg^{2+}$ and $Ca^{2+}$ as a handle for NMR and EPR spectroscopic probes of active site architecture and catalysis (23). Manganese also acts as a superacid catalyst in several hydrolytic enzyme-catalyzed reactions, some of which are shown in Table 6.2.

In general, the relevant redox functions of manganese in enzymes comes into play largely with oxygen as the substrate or product. Because interactions with dioxygen in biological systems are largely carried out with iron enzymes and iron is very prevalent in the biosphere, the list of manganese-containing redox-active proteins is necessarily a small set overlapping with iron (see Table 6.2). Two manganese enzymes that protect bacterial cells from active oxygen species, superoxide dismutase and pseudocatalase, have been described. Furthermore, *Bacillus brevis* has been shown to utilize a unique manganese-containing aromatic ring cleavage dioxygenase. All other described examples of this latter enzyme contain iron.

Iron occupies a central region in the first row of transition-metal elements in the periodic table and, likewise, is central to many metabolic processes in bacteria. This prevalence of iron-containing proteins derives from the availability of iron in nature, where it exists in concentrations of $5 \times 10^5$ ppm in primary igneous rocks (16). Thus biological systems are constantly exposed to iron and evolutionary processes have capitalized on this metal's abundance in devising enzymes that catalyze a wide variety of reactions. In addition to its availability, iron also possesses chemical properties that allow it to conform to a diverse set of metabolic functions. Although inorganic complexes of $Fe^{1+}$ and $Fe^{4+}$ are known, biologically relevant free iron typically exists in $Fe^{2+}$ and $Fe^{3+}$ forms. Both $Fe^{2+}$ and $Fe^{3+}$ exist in low- and high-spin configurations and the facility of interconversion between the low- and high-spin forms has important biochemical implications, as discussed in detail by Spiro and Saltman (24). The energy difference between low- and high-spin forms for a given oxidation state can be very small. Thus the modulation of spin state by ligand charges and differences in geometry can be important in catalytic mechanisms. For example, the heme iron of cytochrome $P450_{CAM}$ from *Pseudomonas putida* undergoes a transition from low spin to a mixture of low- and high-spin forms when the protein binds the substrate camphor. This results in an increase of the redox potential of the iron, making the next step, electron input, easier (25).

Nature has also called upon the versatility of iron to use similar structures to operate at a wide range of redox potentials in biological systems. A dramatic illustration of this point is the observed difference in redox potentials between 4Fe4S proteins isolated from *Clostridium pasteurianum* ($-0.4$ V) and *Chromatium vinosum* ($+0.35$ V) (26). It is now understood that 4Fe4S clusters (Fig. 6.4) can accept and deliver two electrons and that the low potential form undergoes a $-2$ to $-3$ charge transition whereas the high potential form utilizes a $-1$ to $-2$ couple. The enormous variety of iron-containing enzymes found in nature precludes a treatment of any more than a small fraction of the total here. This diversity of evolution in putting iron to enzymatic usage necessitates an approach whereby iron enzymes are segmented into classes of different iron environments (Table 6.3). Proteins in both major divisions, the heme and nonheme iron proteins, catalyze a diverse set of reactions including electron transfer, oxygen dismutation and activation, and the oxidation or reduction of inorganic and organic substrates.

In the former group, heme iron reactivities are modulated by the structure of the porphyrin ligand and the nature of axial ligation. For example, *E. coli* sulfite reductase, which catalyzes the six-electron reduction of sulfite to

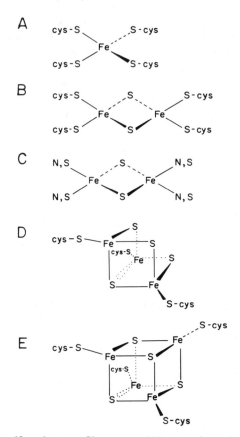

**Figure 6.4** Iron–sulfur clusters. Shown are (A) a one-iron cluster as found in rubredoxin from *Pseudomonas oleovorans*; (B) a spinach-type 2Fe2S cluster containing four cysteine sulfur ligands; (C) a Reiske-type 2Fe2S cluster that contains two nitrogen ligands, perhaps histidine, and two cysteine ligands; (D) a 3Fe4S cluster; and (E) a 4Fe4S cluster.

sulfide, contains the tetrahydroporphinoid heme cofactor, denoted siroheme, and is thought magnetically to couple heme iron and 4Fe4S cluster iron through a bridging sulfur ligand (27). This novel combination may be important in the multielectron reduction catalyzed by this protein. Heme proteins also play important roles in bacterial electron transport where cytochromes pass electrons for the ultimate reduction of dioxygen (most aerobes), nitrate (denitrifiers), and sulfate (sulfate reducers) (28). In addition, methanogenic bacteria that grow on methylamines as their sole source of carbon and energy produce cytochromes (29) but the function of these heme proteins in the physiology of these bacteria has yet to be determined.

Bacterial iron–sulfur proteins also function in electron transport and, as documented more recently, may play a direct catalytic role in important

**TABLE 6.3   Classes and Examples of Iron-Containing Enzymes**

A.  Heme
   1.  Siroheme
      a.  Sulfite reductase
      b.  Nitrite reductase
   2.  Heme b (protoporphyrin IX)
      a.  Elecron-transfer cytochromes
      b.  Catalytic proteins
         1.  Catalase
         2.  Oxygenases
            a.  Monooxygenase: e.g. cytochrome P450
            b.  Dioxygenases
         3.  Other reactions: Hydroxylamine oxidoreductase
   3.  Heme A: Cytochrome $c$ oxidase
   4.  Heme c: (covalently attached, but otherwise like b)
B.  Nonheme iron
   1.  Iron–sulfur
      a.  $Fe_1$-Rubredoxin
      b.  $Fe_2$-Ferredoxin
         1.  Spinach-type
         2.  Reiske-type
      c.  $Fe_3S_4$ centers
      d.  $Fe_4S_4$ centers
   2.  Mononuclear: Oxygenases
   3.  Binuclear: Mu-oxo bridged e.g., ribonucleotide reductase
   4.  Complex: Nitrogenase

hydration and dehydration reactions. For example, the enzyme aconitase, which contains a 4Fe4S cluster in its active form, catalyzes the reversible interconversion of citrate and isocitrate via the enzyme-bound intermediate *cis*-aconitate. The work of Beinert and associates has demonstrated coordination of substrate carboxylate oxygens to an iron atom of the iron–sulfur cluster in aconitase (30). Many oxygenase systems also contain iron–sulfur centers and one example of this group, toluene dioxygenase, is treated in greater detail in the following section. Both mononuclear and binuclear iron centers, which are characterized by direct coordination of iron to amino acid ligands, are found in a variety of proteins, as shown in Table 6.3.

Known cobalt compounds are largely composed of cobalt in oxidation states of I, II, and III (31). These are also biologically relevant oxidation states of cobalt. For example, Co(I)-$B_{12}$ is an important low-potential two-electron reduced form of this important cofactor found in bacterial enzymes. Cobalt is typically found in association with nickel in nature and it is in low abundance with respect to iron. Still, cobalt is an essential element in bacteria and is generally required in higher concentrations for anaerobic, as opposed to aerobic, bacteria.

The largest group of enzymes that require cobalt are the $B_{12}$ enzymes (12). In addition, cobalt sometimes has a role as an enzymatic superacid and, in this regard, has proven useful as an experimental substitute for zinc as a probe of the metal coordination environment (32). However, in these roles, the cobalt is nonredox active and so our focus is on those enzymes that contain the tetrapyrole cofactor $B_{12}$ (Fig. 6.3). The corrin ring system depicted in Figure 6.3 has a center Co(III) atom equatorially bound by the four pyrrole nitrogens and axial ligands that are not shown in the figure. The bottom ligand is often the free nitrogen of benzimidazole and the top ligand may be the 5'-methylene carbon of a 5'-deoxyadenosyl moiety. This stable cobalt–carbon bond is the only known covalent carbon–metal bond in biological systems. The low bond strength of 26 kcal mol$^{-1}$ and the propensity of the carbon–cobalt bond to undergo homolytic scission are important properties that underlie many of the biochemical functions of this coenzyme.

Three major types of enzymatic reactions that require coenzyme $B_{12}$ are (1) intramolecular 1,2 shifts, (2) methyl transfer in methionine and in acetate biosynthesis, and (3) reduction of a ribonucleotide to a deoxyribonucleotide. Most of the cobalt enzymes shown in Table 6.2 catalyze the first class of reactions, that of intramolecular rearrangements. The role of coenzyme $B_{12}$ in acetate synthesis and in DNA biosynthesis (ribonucleotide reductase) is discussed in more detail in the next section.

Nickel, which has a very rich organometallic chemistry, is often found in compounds as Ni(II). This element composes only 0.008% of the Earth's crust (33) and thus, like cobalt, it is less available to biological systems than iron.

The role of nickel in biological systems has become appreciated only since 1975, when urease was shown to be a nickel enzyme (34). Although the source of the urease in that study was jack bean, recent work has demonstrated that bacterial urease also contains nickel (35). Since 1975, three more nickel-containing enzymes have been discovered: hydrogenase, methyl-S-coenzyme M reductase, and carbon monoxide dehydrogenase, which functions in acetate biosynthesis (36). All three of these nickel enzymes are found in significant quantities in methanogenic bacteria. Methyl-S-coenzyme M reductase is unique to methanogens, whereas acetate-synthesizing CO dehydrogenase is also found in acetogenic bacteria such as *Clostridium thermoaceticum* and nickel-containing hydrogenases are found in many bacteria.

Copper trails only iron and zinc as the most abundant metallic element in biological systems (37). The organometallic and bioinorganic chemistry of copper is dominated by Cu(I) and Cu(II) oxidation states between these states. In enzymology, copper is somewhat similar to iron in that it functions in a series of oxidases, oxygenases, and low-molecular-weight electron transfer proteins that are reminiscent of ferredoxins (see Table 6.2). Furthermore, although one class of superoxide dismutases is known that contains iron, another class contains copper and zinc in which the copper undergoes redox change during catalysis (38).

Iron and copper sometimes act cooperatively in bacterial enzymes. Perhaps the most outstanding and widespread example is found in the terminal oxidase of bacterial respiratory chains, cytochrome $c$ oxidase (39). This integral membrane protein functions in aerobic bacteria to catalyze the four-electron reduction of molecular oxygen to water as the product. Cytochrome $c$ oxidase contains two types of $a$ cytochromes ($a$ and $a_3$) and two copper atoms. Although many mechanistic details remain to be elucidated, it appears that one heme center (cyt $a_3$) and one copper center are antiferromagnetically coupled, perhaps through a bridging imidazole. Initial electron input is through the other cytochrome $a$, which gets transferred rapidly to the other copper center. Dioxygen binds to the antiferromagnetically linked pair of cytochrome $a_3$ and Cu(I) center, which transfers two electrons to oxygen to give a peroxide equivalent. Subsequent two-electron transfer results in reduction of peroxide to water:

$$O_2 \xrightarrow[2e^-,2H^+]{Fe,Cu} \text{``}H_2O_2\text{''} \xrightarrow[2e^-,2H^+]{Fe,Cu} 2H_2O \tag{1}$$

Iron and copper interact in a different way with the blue copper protein rusticyanin (40). This periplasmic protein from *Thiobacillus ferrooxidans* serves at pH 2 to oxidize environmental $Fe^{2+}$ to $Fe^{3+}$. Reduced rusticyanin, in turn, passes electrons to a membrane respiratory chain, which allows the organism to derive energy from the oxidation of ferrous iron. The reduction potential of rusticyanin, at 680 mV, is much higher than in other small blue copper proteins but more closely matches the potential of the $Fe^{3+}$ to $Fe^{2+}$ half-reaction, which is 771 mV.

## 6.3  MECHANISTIC STUDIES OF SELECTED BACTERIAL METALLOENZYMES

### 6.3.1  Iron Enzymes

***6.3.1.1  Toluene Dioxygenase.*** Dioxygenases catalyze the incorporation of both atoms of molecular oxygen into a substrate molecule (41). These enzymes from bacteria may contain, in rare cases, manganese (2,3-dihydroxyphenylacetate dioxygenase) but largely have iron as an essential catalytic metal. Both heme iron and nonheme iron enzymes catalyze dioxygenation reactions. An interesting class of nonheme iron dioxygenases have been purified from bacteria that utilize aromatic compounds as growth substrates. Toluene dioxygenase (42) from *Pseudomonas putida* F1 is characteristic of this group that also includes benzoate dioxygenase (43), benzene dioxygenase (44), and naphthalene dioxygenase (45). All of these enzyme systems are multicomponent and utilize a mini-electron transport chain to oxidize reduced pyridine nucleotide and, ultimately, to pass electrons to oxygen for activation, which precedes substrate dioxygenation (Fig. 6.5).

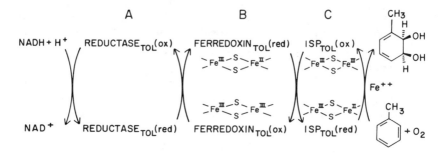

**Figure 6.5** Toluene dioxygenase. The three components of this enzyme form an electron-transport chain, passing electrons from NADH to ($A$) reductase$_{TOL}$, a flavoprotein, to ($B$) ferredoxin$_{TOL}$, a Reiske-type iron–sulfur protein, to ($C$) ISP$_{TOL}$, which contains both iron–sulfur centers and nonheme iron.

The three-component enzyme system of toluene dioxygenase is composed of a flavoprotein, ferredoxin$_{TOL}$ reductase, which passes electrons to a small 2Fe2S protein, ferredoxin$_{TOL}$, which, in turn, transfers electrons to the terminal oxygenase component, ISP$_{TOL}$. The ISP$_{TOL}$ component has an $\alpha_2\beta_2$ subunit structure and contains four to six iron atoms and four acid-labile sulfide. Spectroscopic studies indicate that four of the iron atoms are organized into two 2Fe2S clusters. The environment of the additional iron atoms, which may constitute the oxygen binding site, has not yet been determined for this enzyme nor has it been elucidated for other dioxygenases of this class.

All of the dioxygenases of this group, as well as the cytochrome P450$_{CAM}$ monooxygenase system, interpose one or more iron–sulfur centers between the flavoprotein components and the oxygen-activating iron proteins. This organization for electron flow results in the two-electron acceptor group, FAD, discharging one electron at a time to the obligate single-electron acceptor 2Fe2S group of ferredoxin$_{TOL}$ (46). The details of electron transfer between ferredoxin$_{TOL}$ and ISP$_{TOL}$ and between ISP$_{TOL}$ redox-active groups have not been clearly defined. It is worth noting here that the spectroscopic properties of ferredoxin$_{TOL}$ (47) and ISP$_{TOL}$ indicate that their 2Fe2S clusters are of the Reiske type, which contain two cysteine and two non-cysteine ligands, likely to be nitrogen (see Fig. 6.4 and Table 6.2). One additional property that emanates from the less electron-donating nitrogen ligands is a higher redox potential; this characteristic was also observed for ferredoxin$_{TOL}$ ($E_{1/2} = -109$ mV). A more detailed study of the interactions between the redox-active groups and between the enzyme, organic substrate, and dioxygen should prove instructive in understanding the mechanism of aromatic ring *cis*-dihydroxylation.

### 6.3.1.2 *Ribonucleotide Reductase.*

Ribonucleotide reductases catalyze the reduction of ribonucleotides or ribonucleotide triphosphates to the cor-

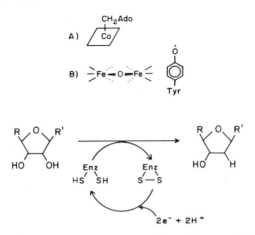

**Figure 6.6**   Two forms of bacterial ribonucleotide reductase. (*A*) The enzyme from *Lactobacillus leichmanii* contains adenosylcobalamin whereas (*B*) the enzyme from *Escherichia coli* is characterized by a binuclear iron center and a stable tyrosinate radical. Both forms of ribonucleotide reductase catalyze similar reactions and accept electrons from the oxidation of two protein cysteines, which form a disulfide.

responding 2′-deoxyribose forms (Fig. 6.6), a key reaction in de novo DNA biosynthesis (48). There are two distinct classes of ribonucleotide reductase. One type of enzyme, found in *E. coli*, contains a binuclear iron center in conjunction with a stable enzyme tyrosinate radical. The other group contains coenzyme $B_{12}$ and is found in *Lactobacillus leichmanii* and *Clostridium sp.* (Fig. 6.6). Thus nature has apparently drawn on two distinct metalloenzyme centers to perform similar chemistry. Both types of enzymes receive electrons from the oxidation of two protein thiols to a disulfide that supplies electrons for ribonucleotide reduction. The binuclear iron center is similar to that of methemerythrins, shown in figure 6.3. This resemblance has been observed by large Mössbauer quadrupole splittings (49) and Raman vibrations (50) that are a signature for an Fe–O–Fe site. Subtle differences were discerned in EXAFS studies that indicated 0.07 Å shorter ligand distances to the iron atoms in ribonucleotide reductase compared to those of methemerythrins (51). This suggested that two nitrogens may be replaced by oxygen ligands (see Fig. 6.3) in the former enzyme.

Mechanistic studies have been conducted with both the *E. coli* iron tyrosinate enzyme and the *Lactobacillus* coenzyme $B_{12}$ form of ribonucleotide reductase. A series of investigations by Stubbe and co-workers has utilized halogenated and radiolabeled substrates to delineate reaction pathways for both enzymes. It was demonstrated that 2′-chloro-2′-deoxynucleotides are processed to an intermediate that irreversibly inactivates the enzymes (52). More detailed studies on the mechanism of formation of the enzyme–nucleophile trap, 2-methylene-3(2*H*)-furanone, indicated mechanistic similarities between the iron and cobalt enzymes (53). Thus a generalized reaction

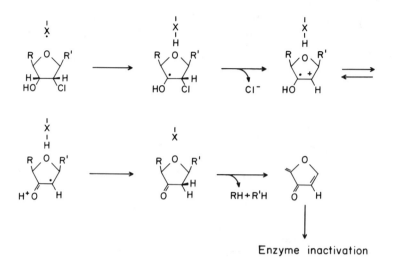

**Figure 6.7**  Proposed route of catalytic processing of a chlorinated ribonucleotide analog that leads to enzyme inactivation. Derived from Ref. 53.

scheme, derived from one proposed by Harris et al. (53), shows an enzyme radical that initiates catalytic events by abstracting a hydrogen from C-3 (Fig. 6.7). This radical could be either the iron tyrosinate or a methyl radical derived following homolytic cleavage of the Co–C bond of 5'-adenosylcobalamin.

## 6.3.2  Molybdenum Enzymes

***6.3.2.1  Nitrogenase.***  As far as is known, only bacteria can reduce dinitrogen to ammonia. This ability to manufacture an assimilatible form of nitrogen from freely available atmospheric nitrogen is found in both free-living and symbiotic bacteria and has recently been demonstrated in methanogens (54, 55). The genetics of nitrogen fixation has been most well-studied in *Klebsiella pneumoniae* and the biochemistry of the process has proceeded largely with this organism as well as *Azotobacter vinelandii* and *Clostridium pasteurianum* (56). Until recently, molybdenum was thought to be an obligate component of all enzyme systems that catalyze the nitrogenase reaction:

$$N_2 + 6e^- + 6H^+ \rightarrow 2NH_3 \qquad (2)$$

In 1986, convincing evidence was presented that a vanadium-dependent nitrogenase that lacks molybdenum could also catalyze the six-electron reduction of dinitrogen to ammonia (57). However, the molybdenum system has been investigated in much greater detail and is the subject of this discussion.

Both molybdenum and iron are integral components of two proteins that have been purified and shown to catalyze the six-electron reduction shown above with concomitant hydrolysis of ATP to ADP plus Pi (58). The first protein contains iron and is known as the Fe protein or, alternatively, component II or dinitrogenase reductase. The second requisite protein contains molybdenum and iron and is known as the MoFe protein. It is sometimes referred to as component I or dinitrogenase.

The Fe protein accepts electrons from either a flavodoxin or a ferredoxin in vivo whereas sodium dithionite is often used as a reductant in vitro. Electrons can be transferred in an ATP-dependent manner to the MoFe protein, which can reduce dinitrogen or other nonphysiological substrates. The Fe protein is a dimer of identical subunits and it contains four iron and four acid-labile sulfides. Most data support the idea that the iron atoms are arranged in a 4Fe4S cluster. Unusual spectroscopic features of the apparent 4Fe4S cluster could be explained by the proposal that a population of Fe protein contains clusters with a mixture of two spin states (for a discussion of this point, see Ref. 58). The symmetry of the protein and the chemical modification data of Hausinger and Howard (59) support the contention that the iron–sulfur cluster is located at the subunit–subunit interface with two cysteine ligands provided by each subunit. Electron transfer out to the MoFe protein requires MgATP where the stoichiometry of nucleotide hydrolysis to electron transfer appears to be minimally two to one.

As purified from a variety of sources the MoFe protein has been shown to be a tetramer of $\alpha_2\beta_2$ subunit structure containing four $Fe_4S_4$ clusters (P-centers), two $MoFe_6$ clusters (M-centers), and one or more S-centers of unknown composition (56). It is possible to remove the FeMo cofactor from dinitrogenase and, with it, to complement a cofactorless MoFe protein obtained from a mutant strain of *Azotobacter vinelandii* known as UW45 (60). The best estimate of the composition of the cofactor has been confounded by the cofactor's instability and its extreme lability in the presence of traces of oxygen. A number of model complexes have been synthesized with the intent of providing a basis of comparison to the dinitrogenase FeMo cofactor in spectroscopic and catalytic experiments (see Fig. 6.8).

Evidence for the participation of molybdenum in substrate reduction is at present indirect (56). Firstly, the bacteria require molybdenum to fix nitrogen. Secondly, the EPR signal assigned to the FeMo cluster disappears during reduction of the enzyme under turnover conditions. Thirdly, the isolated FeMo cofactor will reduce acetylene to ethylene, a reaction that is also catalyzed by the holoenzyme.

Furthermore, molybdenum dinitrogen complexes have been synthesized (61–63). The properties of their reduction have been examined in an effort to develop insight into possible mechanistic pathways that the enzyme might follow. A mechanism showing the six-electron reduction of dinitrogen at a

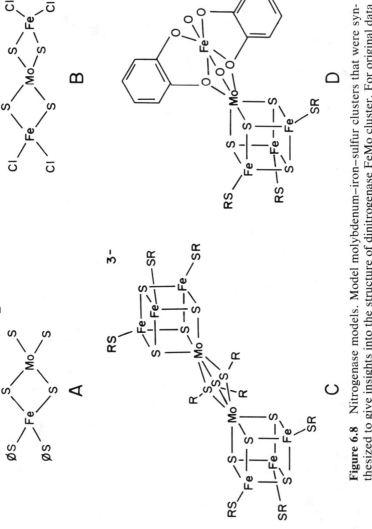

**Figure 6.8** Nitrogenase models. Model molybdenum–iron–sulfur clusters that were synthesized to give insights into the structure of dinitrogenase FeMo cluster. For original data see (*A*) Ref. 61, (*B*) Ref. 62, (*C*) Ref. 63, (*D*) Ref. 63a. In D, the aromatic ring from one set of catechol ligands is omitted for clarity.

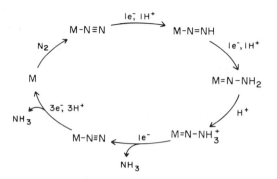

**Figure 6.9** Mechanistic model for nitrogenase. The scheme shows electron input and potential metal-bound intermediates for the six-electron reduction of nitrogen to ammonia. The pathway is derived from Ref. 64.

single site has been proposed by Chatt (Fig. 6.9; 64). Further progress on the mechanism of dinitrogenase, an enzyme of extreme importance in agriculture, will depend on understanding the nature of the catalytic center, the details of electron transfer, and the elucidation of enzyme-bound intermediates along the reaction pathway.

### 6.3.3 Nickel Enzymes

#### 6.3.3.1 Carbon Monoxide Dehydrogenase. Bacteria found in both aerobic and anaerobic environments catalyze the reversible interconversion of carbon monoxide and carbon dioxide:

$$CO + H_2O \rightleftharpoons CO_2 + 2e^- + 2H^+ \qquad (3)$$

In both aerobic and anaerobic bacteria, the enzyme that catalyzes the redox equilibration shown above is called carbon monoxide dehydrogenase. However, there is a large difference between the enzymes found in aerobes such as *Pseudomonas* and those found in acetogenic bacteria (*Clostridium thermoaceticum* and *Acetobacterium woodii*) and methanogens (65). In the former group, CO dehydrogenase is induced by CO and supports growth on CO as a sole carbon and energy source. In contrast, acetogens and methanogens produce CO dehydrogenase constitutively during chemolithoautotrophic growth on $CO_2$ and $H_2$. The carbon monoxide produced from $CO_2$ reduction is condensed with a methyl group to form acetate in a reaction requiring CO dehydrogenase. Thus CO dehydrogenase of acetogens and methanogens could be more appropriately called acetate (acetyl-CoA) synthase (Fig. 6.10).

The striking difference in function between aerobic and anaerobic CO dehydrogenases is reflected by the differences in the composition of redox

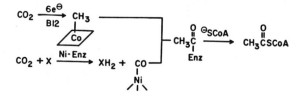

**Figure 6.10**  Acetate biosynthesis in acetogenic bacteria. CO dehydrogenase, designated Ni–Enz in this figure, brings together "$CH_3$," "CO," and HS–coenzyme A moieties to produce acetyl-S-CoA.

active groups of the respective enzymes. Whereas the pseudomonad enzymes contain molybdopterin, 2Fe2S clusters, FAD, and in some cases, copper and zinc (66), the anaerobe enzymes that have been characterized contain nickel, 4Fe4S clusters, and zinc (67, 68). The focus here will be on the nickel-containing enzymes and the intriguing process of acetate biosynthesis from $C_1$ precursors. In this context, CO dehydrogenase from *Clostridium thermoaceticum* has been most well-studied and will serve as a model for this class of enzyme. CO dehydrogenase from *Clostridium thermoaceticum* has an $\alpha_3\beta_3$ subunit structure (67). It contains 2 Ni, 1 or 2 Zn, 12 Fe, and 14 acid-labile sulfides per $\alpha\beta$ dimer. In the presence of carbon monoxide, methyltetrahydrofolate, coenzyme A, a $B_{12}$ enzyme, methyltetrahydrofolate $B_{12}$ methyltransferase, and disulfide reductase, the CO dehydrogenase will synthesize acetyl-CoA (69) (Fig. 6.10).

What events are occurring to form a net C–C bond and what role does CO dehydrogenase play in this process? These questions can best be answered by understanding the nature and interactions of redox active groups in CO dehydrogenase and by studying partial reactions that give insight into the central steps in acetate synthesis. Both EPR (70) and EXAFS (71) experiments indicate that at least some of the iron atoms are arranged into 4Fe4S clusters. Furthermore, EXAFS experiments with enzyme in the absence of CO show, as a best fit, nickel liganded by four sulfur atoms at a distance of 2.16Å. The nickel site has been examined in the presence of substrates by EPR spectrosocpy (72). Evidence for CO binding to nickel was obtained by the observation of [13]CO hyperfine broadening of the [61]Ni EPR signal. Furthermore, the EPR spectrum of the CO dehydrogenase–CO complex is changed by the addition of coenzyme A whereas other thiols have no effect. These observations are consistent with nickel being the site of carbon–carbon bond formation in acetyl–CoA biosynthesis.

Additional observations support the idea that CO dehydrogenase is the site of acetate biosynthesis (73). In addition to the redox equilibration of CO and $CO_2$ shown in Eq. 3, the enzyme catalyzes two exchange reactions: (1) *CoA $\rightleftharpoons$ acetyl–*CoA and (2) *Co $\rightleftharpoons$ *acetyl-CoA. In the first reaction, radiolabeled coenzyme A exchanges into acetyl–CoA and in the second, the labeled carbonyl carbon of the acetyl group of acetyl CoA exchanges with

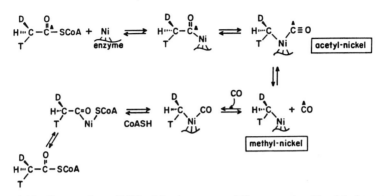

**Figure 6.11** Interaction of CO dehydrogenase (Ni-enzyme) with chiral acetyl-S-coenzyme A that is labeled at the carbonyl carbon. Shown is the cleavage of the carbon–carbon bond leading to exchange of the carbonyl carbon with carbon monoxide that is present in the reaction gas phase. During this overall process the chirality of the methyl group is retained.

unlabeled CO in the gas phase (Fig. 6.11). These reactions, which occur with freshly purified, homogeneous CO dehydrogenase, are suggestive of the enzyme being able to break acetyl–CoA into methyl, CO, and CoA fragments and recombine them. It is possible that the nickel is the site of this fragmentation and recombination because there is precedence for carbonylation of metal–methyl bonds in organotransition metal chemistry. If this were the case then it would be anticipated that the exchange reaction would occur with retention of configuration at the methyl group of acetyl–CoA (Fig. 6.11). This was tested experimentally and shown to be the case (73).

Studies on CO dehydrogenase are hampered by the loss of exchange activity on storage of the enzyme, suggesting that changes in active site structure may be occurring. Insight into the nature of these changes and further studies of potential changes in ligation to nickel during catalysis may unravel further mysteries surrounding this versatile enzyme.

### 6.3.3.2 *Methyl-S-coenzyme M Reductase.*

Methyl-S-coenzyme M reductase catalyzes the last two-electron reduction step in the methane-yielding metabolic pathway of methanogenic bacteria. Methanogens produce methane from the eight-electron reduction of carbon dioxide, from the acetoclastic reaction, or from metabolism of methylamines (28) (Fig. 6.12). As far as it is known, all the bacteria that catalyze these reactions contain methyl-S-coenzyme reductase which catalyzes methane formation by the following reaction:

$$CH_3\text{-}SCH_2CH_2SO_3^- + 2e^- + 2H^+ \rightarrow CH_4 \uparrow + HSCH_2CH_2SO_3^- \quad (4)$$

The bacteria that carry out this methane-forming reaction are widespread.

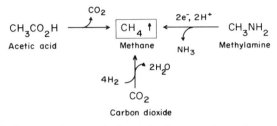

**Figure 6.12**   Various methanogenic bacteria form methane from carbon dioxide, acetic acid, or methylamine.

Hence the magnitude of global methane formation by this enzyme is estimated to be $10^{15}$g year$^{-1}$ (74). Further interest in methyl reductase stems from its content of two equivalents of a novel nickel-containing tetrapyrrole cofactor that has been denoted $F_{430}$. The structure of the tetrahydrocorphinoid cofactor, $F_{430}$, was elucidated in a landmark investigation by Pfaltz et al. (10) and is shown in Figure 6.3. At one time, multiple forms of $F_{430}$ were thought to exist in *Methanobacterium thermoautotrophicum*, but more recent studies demonstrated that only one form of the cofactor is present in vivo and the additional forms were artifacts arising during the purification protocol (75–77).

Attention was drawn to the $F_{430}$ nickel as a possible participant in thioether reductive cleavage as desulfurization reactions catalyzed by Raney nickel are well known. By this perception, methyl reductase may be a regioselective desulfurization catalyst (only one of two C–S bonds are cleaved) in which a potential nickel–sulfur intermediate is further processed to leave a free nickel center that can carry out another catalytic cycle. However, efforts to examine the potential role of the $F_{430}$–Ni have been hampered by (1) the oxygen lability of the proteins, (2) the complexity in reconstruction of activity in vitro (see Table 6.4a), and (3) the low observed in vitro activities that are 0.3% of the in vivo methanogenic rates (78). However, improvements have been made. For example, oxygen damage to components has been minimized by implementing better methods for maintaining anaerobiosis. In addition, a simplified assay system has been developed that replaces a minimum of three protein components with dithiothreitol and coenzyme $B_{12}$, which are thought to serve as alternative reductants (79). The problem of low in vitro rates still plagues investigators but potential causes that have been implicated are requirements for protein:protein (80) and/or protein:membrane interactions (81) and the possibility that components are missing as evidenced by the observation that the operon for the three subunit enzyme ($\alpha_2\beta_2\gamma_2$) contains five open reading frames (82).

In spite of the difficulties, progress has been made in understanding the potential role(s) of the nickel in catalysis. It would be predicted that participation of $F_{430}$ Ni in the desulfurization reaction would require that the nickel be axially reactive. Indeed, the nickel atom in both free $F_{430}$ and in the

**TABLE 6.4   Required Components for Reconstitution of
Methyl-S-Coenzyme M Reductase Activity in Vitro, by Assay**

**Hydrogen-Dependent Assay (Ref. 144)**

    $A_1$ (hydrogenase)

    $A_2$

    $A_3$

    Component B (7-mercaptoheptanoylthreonine phosphate)

    Component C (methyl reductase)

**DTT/$B_{12}$ Dependent Assay (Ref. 79)**

    Dithiothreitol

    Coenzyme $B_{12}$

    Component B (7-mercaptoheptanoylthreonine phosphate)

    Methyl reductase

enzyme-bound cofactor was shown by EXAFS to be hexacoordinate with oxygen and/or nitrogen axial ligands (83). This result directs one to consider three potential enzyme intermediates that could be generated by an axially reactive $F_{430}$ Ni. In Figure 6.13, the axial ligand in the resting enzyme, which might be water, is shown to be replaced by (*a*) the substrate methyl group, (*b*) the substrate thioester sulfur, or (*c*) a hydride equivalent. Alkylation of the nickel, as shown in Figure 6.13*a*, has precedence in $B_{12}$ chemistry. For example, methionine synthetase forms a methyl-$B_{12}$ intermediate for transfer to the thiol group of homocysteine (84). In methyl reductase, transfer of a methyl group from a methylthioether to the nickel could occur following homolytic or heterolytic C–S bond cleavage. Evidence for a Ni(I)–$F_{430}$ species has been reported for the pentamethylester form of $F_{430}$ by Jaun et al.

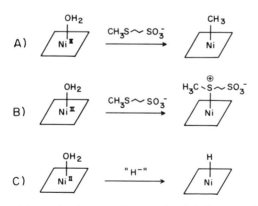

**Figure 6.13**   Potential reaction intermediates at the nickel center of methyl reductase leading to the reductive cleavage of methyl-S-coenzyme M to yield methane.

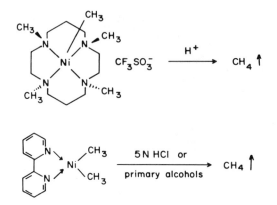

**Figure 6.14** Protonolysis of methyltetraazanickel and diazanickel species to yield methane.

(85) and, potentially, in the enzyme by Albracht et al. using EPR (86). Ni(I)–$F_{430}$ is a possible candidate for participation in C–S bond cleavage with subsequent methylation of the nickel. There is ample precedent for methyl–tetrazanickel complexes undergoing facile protonation to yield methane (87, 88) making this a plausible intermediate in the enzymatic reaction pathway (Fig. 6.14).

The reaction intermediate shown in Figure 6.13b could precede an enzyme nickel–methyl species or it could serve to labilize the C–S bond for attack by an incoming hydride equivalent. In either case, it would be predicted that changing the strength of nickel–heteroatom interaction could show up in altering substrate $K_m$, if $K_m$ is reflective of substrate binding. This proposition was tested by preparing methyl-S-coenzyme M substrate analogs with an altered thioether heteroatom (O or Se) or with decreasing electron density on the heteroatom by replacing hydrogen with electron-withdrawing fluorine on the methyl group (89). As shown in Table 6.5, methyl-Se-coenzyme M is a good substrate for methyl reductase whereas two fluorines on the methyl

**TABLE 6.5   Kinetic Parameters of Substrate Analogues Designed to Examine Potential Nickel–Heteroatom Interaction**

| Substrate or Inhibitor | $K_m$ (m$M$) | $K_{cat}$ (min$^{-1}$) | $K_i$ or $I_{50}$ (m$M$) |
|---|---|---|---|
| $CH_3SCH_2CH_2SO_3H$ | 0.1 | 11 | — |
| $CH_3SeCH_2CH_2SO_3H$ | 0.3 | 35 | — |
| $CF_2HSCH_2CH_2SO_3H$ | 2.5 | 20 | — |
| $CH_3OCH_2CH_2SO_3H$ | — | — | 8.3 |
| $CF_3SCH_2CH_2SO_3H$ | — | — | 7.0 |
| $CF_3SeCH_2CH_2SO_3H$ | — | — | 3.4 |

group substantially raises $K_m$. The placement of three fluorines on the methyl group or replacement of sulfur with oxygen results in analogs that are not substrates and observed inhibitor constants are substantially higher than the $K_m$ for the physiological substrate. These data are consistent with, but not proof of, nickel–thioether heteroatom recognition being important in substrate binding that would place the substrate at the nickel center.

A deeper understanding of the mechanism of methyl-S-coenzyme M reductase will require the further use of spectroscopic tools to examine changes in nickel redox state and axial ligation during catalysis. To this end, obtaining enzyme preparations with high in vitro activities is an important goal for future research. The simplified assay protocol of Ankel-Fuchs and Thauer (79) has provided an important method for testing potential means of increasing in vitro rates.

## 6.4  CONCLUSION

The importance of metalloenzymes in biological systems is underscored by the sheer numbers in this class as well as the elaborate biosynthetic pathways that have evolved to fashion metal-containing cofactors. Progress in understanding transition metal enzymes has traditionally come from examining the purified catalysts by various spectroscopic methods, by X-ray crystallography, and by kinetic and substrate-analog probes. It has been particularly useful to compare the properties of a metalloenzyme to relevant organometallic model compounds. Most recently, molecular biological techniques such as site-specific mutagenesis are allowing the selective modification of enzymes that contain metal centers, which can be instructive in making structure/function correlations.

## REFERENCES

1. J. L. Ingraham, O. Maaløe, and F. C. Neidhardt. *Growth of the Bacterial Cell*, Sinauer Associates, Sunderland, MA, 1983.
2. E. Ochiai. *Bioinorganic Chemistry*, Allyn and Bacon, Boston, 1977, p. 12.
3. L. Y. Young. "Anaerobic degradation of aromatic compounds," in D. T. Gibson, Ed., *Microbial Degradation of Organic Compounds*, Dekker, New York, 1982, p. 487.
4. C. Anthony. *The Biochemistry of Methylotrophs*, Academic, New York, 1982.
5. R. Y. Stanier, E. A. Adelberg, and J. Ingraham. *The Microbial World*, 4th ed., Prentice-Hall, Englewood Cliffs, NJ, 1976.
6. R. W. Hay. *Bio-inorganic Chemistry*, Ellis Horwood, Chichester, United Kingdom, 1984.
7. P. A. Lindahl, N. Kojima, R. P. Hausinger, J. A. Fox, B. K. Teo, C. T. Walsh, and W. H. Orme-Johnson. Nickel and iron EXAFS of F420-reducing hydro-

genase from *Methanobacterium thermoautotrophicum*, J. Am. Chem. Soc., *106*, 3062 (1984).

8. R. E. Stenkamp, L. C. Sieker, and L. H. Jensen. Binuclear iron complexes in methemerythrin and azidomethemerythrin. J. Am. Chem. Soc., *106*, 618 (1984).

9. A. E. G. Cass and H. A. O. Hill. "Copper proteins and copper enzymes," in *Biological Roles of Copper* (Ciba Foundation Symposium 79), Excerpta Medica, Amsterdam, 1980, p. 71.

10. A. Pfaltz, B. Jaun, A. Fassler, A. Eschenmoser, R. Jaenchen, H. H. Gilles, G. Diekert, and R. K. Thauer. Zur kenntnis des faktors F430 aus methanogenen bakterien: struktur des porphinoiden ligandsystems, Helv. Chim. Acta, *68*, 1338 (1982).

11. A. L. Lehninger. *Biochemistry*, 2nd ed., Worth, New York, 1975.

12. D. Dolphins. $B_{12}$, Vol. 1, Wiley, New York, 1982.

13. K. V. Rajagopalan. Chemistry and biology of the molybdenum cofactor, Biochem. Soc. Trans., *13*, 401 (1985).

14. R. J. P. Williams. Natural selection of the chemical elements, Proc. R. Soc. Lond. B, *213*, 361 (1981).

15. D. W. Darnall and R. G. Wilkins. *Methods for Determining Metal Ion Environments in Proteins* (*Advances in Inorganic Biochemistry*, Vol. 2), Elsevier, New York, 1980.

16. D. A. Phipps. *Metals and Metabolism*, Clarendon, Oxford, 1976.

17. E. de Boer, Y. van Kooyk, M. G. M. Tromp, H. Plat, and R. Wever. Bromoperoxidase from *Ascophyllum nodosum*: A novel class of enzymes containing vanadium as a prosthetic group? Biochim. Biophys. Acta, *869*, 48 (1986).

18. R. L. Robson, R. R. Eady, T. H. Richardson, R. W. Miller, M. Hawkins, and J. R. Postgate. The alternative nitrogenase of *Azotobacter chromooccum* is a vanadium enzyme, Nature, *322*, 388 (1986).

19. I. Yamamoto, T. Saiki, S. Liu, and L. G. Ljungdahl. Purification and properties of NADP-dependent formate dehydrogenase from *Clostridium thermaceticum*, a tungsten-selenium-iron protein, J. Biol. Chem., *258*, 1826 (1983).

20. E. I. Stiefel. "Structures and spectra of molybdenum active-sites," in M. Coughlan, Ed., *Molybdenum and Molybdenum-Containing Enzymes*, Pergamon, Oxford, 1980, p. 43.

21. A. Nason, A. D. Antoine, P. A. Ketchum, W. A. Frazier, and D. K. Lee. Formation of assimilatory nitrate reductase by *in vitro* inter-cistronic complementation in *Neurospora crassa*, Proc. Natl. Acad. Sci. USA, *65*, 137 (1970).

22. A. Nason, K.-Y. Lee, S.-S. Pan, P. A. Ketchum, A. Lamberti, and J. DeVries. *In vitro* formation of assimilatory reduced nicotinamide adenine dinucleotide phosphate: nitrate reductase from a *Neurospora* mutant and a component of molybdenum-enzymes, Proc. Natl. Acad. Sci. USA, *68*, 3242 (1971).

23. A. S. Mildvan and D. C. Fry. "NMR Studies of the mechanism of enzyme action," in A. Meister, Ed., *Advances in Enzymology*, Vol. 59, Wiley-Interscience, New York, 1987, p. 241.

24. T. Spiro and P. Saltman. In A. Jacobs and M. Worwood, Eds., *Iron in Biochemistry and Medicine*, Academic, New York, 1974, p. 1.

25. S. G. Sligar and I. C. Gunsalus. A thermodynamic model of regulation: modulation of redox equilibria in camphor monooxygenase. Proc. Natl. Acad. Sci. USA, *73*, 1078 (1976).

26. W. H. Orme-Johnson. "Iron-sulfur proteins: structure and function," in E. E. Snell, P. D. Boyer, A. Meister, and C. C. Richardson, Eds., *Annual Review of Biochemistry*, Vol. 51, Annual Reviews, Inc., Palo Alto, CA 1973, p. 159.

27. D. E. McRee, D. C. Richardson, J. S. Richardson, and L. M. Siegel. The heme and $Fe_4S_4$ cluster in the crystallographic structure of *Escherichia coli* sulfite reductase, J. Biol. Chem., *261*, 10277 (1986).

28. G. Gottschalk. *Bacterial Metabolism*, 2nd ed., Springer, New York, 1985.

29. W. Kühn and G. Gottschalk. Characterization of the cytochromes occurring in *Methanosarcina* species, Eur. J. Biochem., *135*, 89 F(1983).

30. J. Telser, M. H. Emptage, H. Merkle, M. C. Kennedy, H. Beinert, and B. M. Hoffman. $^{17}O$ Electron nuclear double resonance characterization of substrate binding to the $[4Fe-4S]^{1+}$ cluster of reduced active aconitase, J. Biol. Chem., *261*, 4840 (1986).

31. F. A. Cotton and G. Wilkinson. *Advanced Inorganic Chemistry*, 4th ed., Wiley-Interscience, New York, 1980, p. 766.

32. B. L. Vallee, A. Galdes, D. S. Auld, and J. F. Riordan. "Carboxypeptidase A," in T. Spiro, Ed., *Zinc Enzymes*, Wiley-Interscience, New York, 1983, p. 25.

33. National Research Council. Nickel, National Academy of Science, Washington, DC, 1975.

34. N. E. Dixon, C. Gazzola, R. L. Blakeley, and B. Zerner. Jack bean urease (EC 3.5.1.5). A metalloenzyme. A simple biological role for nickel? J. Am. Chem. Soc., *97*, 4131 (1975).

35. M. J. Todd and R. P. Hausinger. Purification and characterization of the nickel-containing multicomponent urease from *Klebsiella aerogenes*, J. Biol. Chem., *262*, 5963 (1987).

36. R. P. Hausinger. Nickel utilization by microorganisms, Microbiol Rev., *51*, 22 (1987).

37. F. A. Cotton and G. Wilkinson. *Advanced Inorganic Chemistry*, 4th ed., Wiley-Interscience, New York, 1980, p. 1334.

38. J. A. Fee. "The copper/zinc superoxide dismutase," in H. Sigel, Ed., *Copper Proteins (Metal Ions in Biological Systems*, Vol. 13), Dekker, New York, 1981, p. 259.

39. M. Brunori, E. Antonini, and M. T. Wilson. "Cytochrome c oxidase: an overview of recent work," in H. Sigel Ed., *Copper Proteins (Metal Ions in Biological Systems*, Vol. 13), Dekker, New York, 1981, p. 187.

40. J. G. Cobley and B. A. Haddock. Reversible uncoupling of the copper and cobalt spin systems in cobalt bovine superoxide dismutase at low pH, FEBS Lett., *60*, 29 (1975).

41. O. Hayaishi. "My life and oxygen," in M. Nozaki, S. Yamamoto, Y. Ishimura, M. J. Coon, L. Ernster, and R. W. Estabrook, Eds., *Oxygenases and Oxygen Metabolism*, Academic, New York, 1982, p. 1.

42. D. T. Gibson, W. K, Yeh, T. N. Liu, and V. Subramanian. "Toluene dioxy-

genase: a multi-component enzyme system from *Pseudomonas putida*," in M. Nozaki, S. Yamamoto, Y. Ishimura, M. J. Coon, L. Ernster, and R. W. Estabrook, Eds., *Oxygenases and Oxygen Metabolism*, Academic, New York, 1982, p. 51.

43. M. Yamaguchi and H. Fujisawa. Subunit structure of oxygenase component in benzoate-1,2-dioxygenase system from *Pseudomonas arvilla* C-1, J. Biol. Chem., *257*, 12497 (1982).

44. S. E. Crutcher and P. J. Geary. Properties of the iron-sulfur proteins of the benzene dioxygenase systems from *Pseudomonas putida*, Biochem. J., *177*, 393 (1979).

45. B. D. Ensley and D. T. Gibson. Naphthalene dioxygenase: purification and properties of a terminal oxygenase component, J. Bacteriol., *155*, 505 (1983).

46. V. Subramanian, T-N. Liu, W-K. Yeh, M. Narro, and D. T. Gibson. Purification and properties of NADH-ferredoxin$_{TOL}$ reductase: a component of toluene dioxygenase from *Pseudomonas putida*, J. Biol. Chem., *256*, 2723 (1981).

47. V. Subramanian, T-N. Liu, W-K. Yeh, C. Serdan, L. P. Wackett, and D. T. Gibson. Purification and properties of ferredoxin$_{TOL}$: a component of toluene dioxygenase from *Pseudomonas putida* F1, J. Biol. Chem., *260*, 2355 (1985).

48. L. Thelander and P. Reichard. "Reduction of ribonucleotides," in E. E. Snell, P. D. Boyer, A. Meister, C. C. Richardson, Eds., *Annual Review of Biochemistry*, Vol. 48, Annual Reviews, Inc., Palo Alto, CA 1979, p. 133.

49. C. L. Atkin, L. Thelander, P. Reichard, and G. Lang. Iron and free radical in ribonucleotide reductase, J. Biol. Chem., *248*, 7464 (1973).

50. B-M. Sjöberg, T. M. Loehr, and J. Sanders-Loehr. Raman spectral evidence for a μ-oxo bridge in the binuclear iron center of ribonucleotide reductase, Biochemistry, *21*, 96 (1982).

51. R. C. Scarrow, M. J. Maroney, S. M. Palmer, L. Que, S. P. Salowe, and J. Stubbe. EXAFS studies of the $\beta_2$ subunit of the ribonucleotide reductase from *E. coli*, J. Am. Chem. Soc., *108*, 6832 (1986).

52. G. Harris, M. Ator, and J. Stubbe. Mechanism of inactivation of *Escherichia coli* and *Lactobacillus leichmannii* ribonucleotide reductases by 2'-chloro-2'-deoxynucleotides: evidence for generation of 2-methylene-3(2H)-furanone, Biochemistry, *23*, 5214 (1984).

53. G. Harris, G. W. Ashley, M. J. Robins, R. L. Tolman, and J. Stubbe. 2'-Deoxy-2'-halonucleotides as alternate substrates and mechanism based inactivators of *Lactobacillus leichmannii* ribonucleotide reductase, Biochemistry, *26*, 1895 (1987).

54. P. A. Murray and S. H. Zinder. Nitrogen fixation by a methanogenic archaebacterium, Nature, *312*, 284 (1984).

55. N. Belay, R. Sparling, and L. Daniels. Dinitrogen fixation by a thermophilic methanogenic bacterium, Nature, *312*, 286 (1984).

56. M. J. Nelson, P. A. Lindahl, and W. H. Orme-Johnson. "Bioinorganic chemistry of nitrogenase," in G. L. Eichorn and L. G. Marzilli, Eds., *Advances in Inorganic Biochemistry*, Vol. 4, Elsevier, New York, 1982, p. 1.

57. R. L. Robson, R. R. Eady, T. H. Richardson, R. W. Miller, M. Hawkins, and J. R. Postgate. The alternative nitrogenase of *Azotobacter chroococcum* is a vanadium enzyme, Nature, *322*, 388 (1986).

58. W. H. Orme-Johnson. Molecular basis of biological nitrogen fixation, Ann. Rev. Biophys. Biophys. Chem., *14*, 419 (1985).

59. R. P. Hausinger and J. B. Howard. Thiol reactivity of the nitrogenase Fe-protein from *Azotobacter vinelandii*, J. Biol. Chem., *258*, 13486 (1983).

60. S-S. Yang, W-H. Pan, G. D. Friesen, B. K. Burgess, J. L. Corbin, E. I. Stiefel, and W. E. Newton. Iron-molybdenum cofactor from nitrogenase: modified extraction methods as probes for composition, J. Biol. Chem., *257*, 8042 (1982).

61. D. Coucouvanis, N. C. Baenziger, E. D. Simhon, P. Stremple, D. Swenson, A. Kostikas, A. Simopoulos, V. Petrouleas, and V. Papaefthymiou. Heterodinuclear di-μ-sulfidio bridged dimers containing iron and molybdenum or tungsten. Structures of $(Ph_4P)_2$ $FeMS_9$ complexes (M = Mo,W), J. Am. Chem. Soc., *102*, 1730 (1980).

62. D. Coucouvanis, N. C. Baenziger, E. D. Simhon, P. Stremple, D. Swenson, A. Kostikas, A. Simopoulos, V. Petrouleas, and V. Papafthymiou. Synthesis and structural characterization of the $(Ph_4P)_2$ $[Cl_2FeS_2MS_2FeCl_2]$ complexes (M = Mo,W). First example of a doubly bridging $MoS_4$ unit and its possible relevance as a structural feature in the nitrogenase active site, J. Am. Chem. Soc., *102*, 1732 (1980).

63. T. E. Wolf, J. M. Berg, K. O. Hodgson, R. B. Frankel, and R. H. Holm. Synthetic approaches to the molybdenum site in nitrogenase. Preparation and structural properties of the molybdenum-iron-sulfur "double-cubane" cluster complexes $[Mo_2Fe_6S_8(SC_2H_3)_9]^{3-}$ and $[Mo_2Fe_6S_9(SC_2H_5)_8]^{3-}$, J. Am. Chem. Soc., *101*, 4140 (1979).

63a. T. E. Wolff, J. M. Berg, and R. H. Holm. Synthesis, structure and properties of the cluster complex $[MoFe_4S_4(SC_2H_5)_3(C_6H_4O_2)_3]^{3-}$, containing a single cubane-type $MoFe_3S_4$ core, Inorg. Chem., *20*, 174 (1981).

64. J. Chatt, J. R. Dilworth, and R. L. Richards. Recent advances in the chemistry of nitrogen fixation, Chem. Rev., *78*, 589 (1978).

65. O. Meyer and K. Fiebig. "Enzymes oxidizing carbon monoxide," in H. Degn, R. P. Cox, and H. Toftlund, Eds., *Gas Enzymology*, D. Reidel, Dordrecht, 1985, p. 147.

66. O. Meyer and K. V. Rajagopalan. Molybdopterin in carbon monoxide oxidase from carboxydotrophic bacteria, J. Bacteriol., *157*, 643 (1984).

67. S. W. Ragsdale, J. E. Clark, L. G. Ljungdahl, L. L. Lundie, and H. L. Drake. Properties of purified carbon monoxide dehydrogenase from *Clostridium thermoaceticum*, a nickel, iron-sulfur protein, J. Biol. Chem., *258*, 2364 (1983).

68. S. W. Ragsdale, L. G. Ljungdahl, and D. V. Der Vartanian. Isolation of carbon monoxide dehydrogenase from *Acetobacterium woodii* and comparison of its properties with those of the *Clostridium thermoaceticum* enzyme, J. Bacteriol., *155*, 1224 (1983).

69. H. G. Wood, S. W. Ragsdale, and E. Pezacka. A new pathway of autotrophic growth utilizing carbon monoxide or carbon dioxide and hydrogen, Biochem. Int., *12*, 421 (1986).

70. S. W. Ragsdale, L. G. Ljungdahl, and D. V. Der Vartanian. EPR evidence for nickel-substrate interaction in carbon monoxide dehydrogenase from *Clostridium thermoaceticum*, Biochem. Biophys. Res. Commun., *108*, 658 (1982).

71. N. R. Bastian, G. Diekert, E. C. Niederhoffer, B-K. Teo, C. T. Walsh, and W. H. Orme-Johnson. Nickel and iron EXAFS of carbon monoxide dehydrogenase from *Clostridium thermoaceticum* strain DSM, J. Am. Chem. Soc., *110*, 5581 (1988).

72. S. W. Ragsdale, H. G. Wood, and W. E. Antholine. Evidence that an iron-nickel-carbon complex is formed by reaction of CO with the CO dehydrogenase from *Clostridium thermoaceticum*, Proc. Natl. Acad. Sci. USA, *82*, 6811 (1985).

73. S. A. Raybuck, N. R. Bastian, L. D. Zydowsky, K. Kobayashi, H. G. Floss, W. H. Orme-Johnson, and C. T. Walsh. Nickel-containing CO dehydrogenase catalyzes reversible decarbonylation of acetyl CoA with retention of stereochemistry at the methyl group, J. Am. Chem. Soc., *109*, 3171 (1987).

74. D. H. Enhalt. The atmospheric cycle of methane, Tellus, *26*, 58 (1974).

75. R. P. Hausinger, W. H. Orme-Johnson, and C. T. Walsh. Nickel tetrapyrole cofactor F430: a comparison of forms bound to methyl coenzyme M reductase and protein free in cells of *Methanobacterium thermoautotrophicum* ΔH, Biochemistry, *232*, 801 (1984).

76. D. A. Livingston, A. Pfaltz, J. Schreiber, A. Eschenmoser, D. Ankel-Fuchs, J. Moll, R. Jaenchen, and R. K. Thauer. Zur kenntnis des faktors F430 aus methanogenen bakterien: struktur des proteinfreien faktors, Helv. Chim. Acta, *67*, 334 (1984).

77. R. Hüster, H.-H. Gilles, and R. K Thauer. Is coenzyme M bound to factor F430 in methanogenic bacteria? Eur. J. Biochem., *148*, 107 (1985).

78. L. Daniels, R. Sparling, and D. Sprott. The bioenergetics of methanogenesis, Biochim. Biophys. Acta, *768*, 113 (1984).

79. D. Ankel-Fuchs and R. K. Thauer. Methane formation from methyl-coenzyme M in a system containing methyl-coenzyme M reductase, component B, and reduced cobalamin, Eur. J. Biochem., *156*, 171 (1986).

80. L. P. Wackett, E. A. Hartwieg, J. A. King, W. H. Orme-Johnson, and C. T. Walsh. Electron microscopy of nickel-containing methanogenic enzymes: methyl reductase and F420-reducing hydrogenase, J. Bacteriol., *169*, 718 (1987).

81. R. Ossmer, T. Mund, P. L. Hartzell, U. Konheiser, G. W. Kohring, A. Klein, R. S. Wolfe, G. Gottschalk, and F. Mayer. Immunocytochemical localization of component C of the methyl reductase system in *Methanococcus voltae* and *Methanobacterium thermoautotrophicum*, Proc. Natl. Acad. Sci. USA, *83*, 5789 (1986).

82. D. S. Cram, B. S. Sherf, R. T. Libby, R. J. Mattaliano, K. L. Ramachandran, and J. N. Reeve. Structure and expression of the genes, *mcrBDCGA*, which encode the subunits of component C of methyl coenzyme M reductase in *Methanococcus vannielii*, Proc. Natl. Acad. Sci. USA, *84*, 3992 (1987).

83. M. K. Eidsness, R. V. Sullivan, J. R. Schwartz, P. L. Hartzell, R. S. Wolfe, A. Flank, S. P. Cramer, and R. A. Scott. Structural diversity of F430 from *Methanobacterium thermoautotrophicum*. A nickel X-ray absorption spectroscopic study. J. Am. Chem. Soc., *108*, 3120 (1986).

84. R. T. Taylor and H. Weissbach. "N⁵-methyltetrahydrofolate-homocysteine methyltransferases," in P. D. Boyer, Ed., *Enzymes*, 3rd E., Vol. 9, Academic, New York, 1972, p. 121.

85. B. Jaun and A. Pfaltz. Coenzyme F430 from methanogenic bacteria: reversible one-electron reduction of F430 pentamethyl ester to the nickel (I) form, J. Chem. Soc. Chem. Commun., *1986*, 1327.

86. S. P. J. Albracht, D. Ankel-Fuchs, J. W. Vander Zwaan, R. D. Fontijn, and R. K. Thauer. A new EPR signal of nickel in *Methanobacterium thermoautotrophicum*, Biochim. Biophys. Acta, *870*, 50 (1986).

87. M. J. D'Aniello and E. K. Barefield. A paramagnetic square-pyramidal nickel (II) alkyl complex, J. Am. Chem. Soc., *98*, 1610 (1976).

88. G. Wilke and G. Herrman. Angew Chem. Int. Ed., *5*, 580 (1966).

89. L. P. Wackett, J. F. Honek, T. P. Begley, V. Wallace, W. H. Orme-Johnson, and C. T. Walsh. Substrate analogues as mechanistic probes of methyl-S-coenzyme M reductase, Biochemistry, *26*, 6012 (1987).

90. H. B. Gray. "Electronic absorption spectroscopy," in D. W. Darnall and R. G. Wilkins, Eds., *Methods for Determining Metal Ion Environments in Proteins* (*Advances in Inorganic Biochemistry*, Vol. 3), Elsevier, New York, 1980, p. 1.

91. A. Abragam and B. Bleaney. *EPR of Transition Ions*, Clarendon Press, Oxford, 1970.

92. J. G. Stevens and G. K. Shenoy. *Mössbauer Spectroscopy and its Chemical Applications*, American Chemical Society, Washington, DC, 1981.

93. O. Jardetsky and G. C. K. Roberts. *NMR in Molecular Biology*, Academic, New York, 1981.

94. B. K. Teo. *EXAFS: Basic Principles and Data Analysis*, Springer, Berlin, 1986.

95. M. P. Coughlan, "Aldehyde oxidase, xanthine oxidase, and xanthine dehydrogenase: hydroxylases containing molybdenum, iron-sulfur and flavin," in M. P. Coughlan, Ed., *Molybdenum and Molybdenum-Containing Enzymes*, Pergamon, Oxford, 1980, p. 119.

96. K. V. Rajagopalan. "Sulfite oxidase (sulfite: ferricytochrome C oxidoreductase)," in M. Coughlan, Ed., *Molybdenum and Molybdenum-Containing Enzymes*, Pergamon, Oxford, 1980, p. 243.

97. E. J. Hewitt and B. A. Notton. "Nitrate reductase systems in eukaryotic and prokaryotic organisms," in M. Coughlan, Ed., *Molybdenum and Molybdenum-Containing Enzymes*, Pergamon, Oxford, 1980, p. 275.

98. N. L. Shauer and J. G. Ferry. Composition of the coenzyme F420-dependent formate dehydrogenase from *Methanobacterium formicicum*, J. Bacteriol., *165*, 405 (1986).

99. I. Yamamoto, N. Okubo, and M. Ishimoto. Further characterization of trimethylamine N-oxide reductase from *Escherichia coli*, a molybdopterin, J. Biochem., *99*, 1773 (1986).

100. W. F. Beyer and I. Fridovich. Pseudocatalase from *Lactobacillus plantarum*: evidence for a homopentameric structure containing two atoms of manganese per subunit, Biochemistry, *24*, 6460 (1985).

101. L. Que, J. Widom, and R. L. Crawford. 3,4-Dihydroxyphenylacetate 2,3-dioxygenase: a manganese (II) dioxygenase from *Bacillus brevis*. J. Biol. Chem., *256*, 10941 (1981).

102. A. E. G. Cass. *Superoxide Dismutase*, Part 1 (*Topics in Molecular and Structural Biology*, Vol. 7) Verlag Chemie, Weinheim, 1985, p. 121.

103. H. Tamai, H. Usami, and T. Yorifuji. Role of thiol groups in $Mn^{2+}$ dependent guanidinoacetate aminohydrolase, Agric. Biol. Chem., *42*, 1295 (1978).

104. C. van der Drift and G. D. Vogels. Effect of metal and hydrogen ions on the activity and stability of allantoicase, Biochim. Biophys. Acta, *198*, 339 (1970).

105. J. Wiegel. $Mn^{++}$-specific reactivation of EDTA inactivated α-isopropylmalate synthase from *Alcaligenes eutrophus*, Biochem. Biophys. Res. Commun., *82*, 907 (1978).

106. Y. K. Oh and E. Freese. Manganese requirement of phosphoglycerate phosphomutase and its consequences for growth and sporulation of *Bacillus subtilis*, J. Bacteriol., *127*, 739 (1976).

107. C. T. Walsh. *Enzymatic Reaction Mechanisms*, W. H. Freeman, San Francisco, 1979.

108. I. C. Gunsalus and G. C. Wagner. Bacterial P-450$_{CAM}$ methylene monooxygenase components cytochrome M, putidaredoxin, and putidaredoxin reductase, in S. P. Colowick and N. O. Kaplan, Eds., *Methods in Enzymology*, Vol. 52, Academic, New York, 1978, p. 166.

109. Y. Ishimura, R. Makino, R. Ueno, K. Sakaguchi, F. O. Brady, P. Feigelson, P. Aisen, and O. Hayaishi. Copper is not essential for the catalytic activity of L-tryptophan 2,3-dioxygenase, J. Biol. Chem., *255*, 3835 (1980).

110. K. K. Andersson, T. A. Kent, J. D. Lipscomb, A. B. Hooper, and E. Münck. Mössbauer, EPR, and optical studies of the P-460 center of hydroxylamine oxidoreductase from *Nitrosomonas*, J. Biol. Chem., *259*, 6833 (1984).

111. W. McIntire, D. E. Edmondson, T. P. Singer, and D. J. Hopper. 8α-0-Tyrosyl-FAD: a new form of covalently bound flavin from *p*-cresol methylhydroxylase, J. Biol. Chem., *255*, 6553 (1980).

112. J. A. Peterson and M. J. Coon. Enzymatic ω-oxidation III. Purification and properties of rubredoxin, a component of the ω-hydroxylation system of *Pseudomonas oleovorans*, J. Biol. Chem., *243*, 329 (1968).

113. M. K. Johnson, D. E. Bennett, J. A. Fee, and W. V. Sweeney. Spectroscopic studies of the seven-iron-containing ferredoxins from *Azotobacter vinelandii* and *Thermus thermophilus*, Biochim. Biophys. Acta, *911*, 81 (1987).

114. J. A. Fee, K. L. Findling, T. Yoshida, R. Hille, G. E. Tarr, D. O. Hearshen, W. R. Dunham, E. P. Day, T. A. Kent, and E. Münck. Purification and characterization of the Rieske iron-sulfur protein from *Thermus thermophilus*, J. Biol. Chem., *259*, 124 (1984).

115. G. Nakos and L. E. Mortenson. Structural properties of hydrogenase from *Clostridium pasteurianum* W5, Biochemistry, *10*, 2442 (1971).

116. F. H. Bernhardt, N. Erdin, H. Staudinger, and V. Ullrich. Interactions of substrates with a purified 4-methoxybenzoate monooxygenase system (O-demethylating) from *Pseudomonas putida*, Eur. J. Biochem., *35*, 126 (1973).

117. M. P. Woodland and H. Dalton. Purification and characterization of component A of the methane monooxygenase from *Methylococcus capsulatus* (Bath), J. Biol. Chem., *259*, 53 (1984).

118. L. Que, Jr. The catechol dioxygenases, Adv. Inorg. Biochem., *5*, 167 (1983).

119. R. A. Pascal, M. A. Oliver, and Y.-C. Jack Chen. Alternate substrates and inhibitors of bacterial 4-hydroxyphenylpyruvate dioxygenase, Biochemistry, *24*, 3158 (1985).

120. D. Barra, M. E. Schinina, W. H. Bannister, J. V. Bannister, and F. Bossa. The primary structure of iron-superoxide dismutase from *Photobacterium leiognathi*, J. Biol. Chem., *262*, 1001 (1987).

121. H. Follman and H. Hogenkamp. Ribonucleotide reductase. Studies with $^{18}$O-labelled substrates, Biochemistry, *8*, 4372 (1969).

122. W. W. Bachovchin, R. G. Eager, K. W. Moore, and J. H. Richards. Mechanism of action of adenosylcobalamin; glycerol and other substrate analogues as substrates and inactivators for propanediol dehydrate—kinetics, stereospecificity, and mechanism, Biochemistry, *16*, 1082 (1977).

123. Z. Sneider, E. G. Larsen, G. Jacobson, B. C. Johnson, and J. Pawelkiewicz. Purification and properties of glycerol dehydrase, J. Biol. Chem., *245*, 3388 (1970).

124. C. M. Blackwell and J. M. Turner. Microbial metabolism of amino alcohols. Purification and properties of coenzyme $B_{12}$-dependent ethanolamine ammonia-lyase of *Escherichia coli*, Biochem. J., *175*, 555 (1978).

125. F. Suzuki and H. A. Barker. Purification and properties of component E of glutamate mutase, J. Biol. Chem., *241*, 878 (1966).

126. R. W. Kellermeyer, S. H. G. Allen, R. Stjernholm, and H. G. Wood. Methylmalonyl isomerase. IV. Purification and properties of the enzyme from propionibacteria, J. Biol. Chem., *239*, 2563 (1964).

127. H.-F. Kung, S. Cederbaum, L. Tsai, and T. C. Stadtman. Nicotinic acid metabolism, V. A cobamide coenzyme-dependent conversion of $\alpha$-methyleneglutaric acid to dimethylmaleic acid, Proc. Natl. Acad. Sci. USA, *65*, 978 (1970).

128. T. C. Stadtman. "Lysine metabolism by clostridia," in A. Meister, Ed., *Advances in Enzymology*, Vol. 38, Wiley-Interscience, New York, 1973, p. 413.

129. R. Somack and R. N. Costilow. Purification and properties of a pyridoxal phosphate and coenzyme $B_{12}$ dependent D-$\alpha$-ornithine 5,4-aminomutase, Biochemistry, *12*, 2597 (1973).

130. H. G. Wood and G. K. Zwolinski. Transcarboxylase: role of biotin, metals, and subunits in the reaction and its quarternary structure, Crit. Rev. Biochem., *4*, 47 (1976).

131. S. Milstein and P. Goldman. Metabolism of guanidinosuccinic acid. I. Characterization of a specific amidino hydrolase from *Pseudomonas chlororaphis*, J. Biol. Chem., *247*, 6280 (1972).

132. F. S. Jacobson, L. Daniels, J. A. Fox, C. T. Walsh, and W. H. Orme-Johnson. Purification and properties of an 8-hydroxy-5-deazaflavin-reducing hydrogenase from *Methanobacterium thermoautotrophicum*, J. Biol. Chem., *257*, 3385 (1982).

133. L. P. Wackett, J. F. Honek, T. P. Begley, S. L. Shames, E. C. Niederhoffer, R. P. Hausinger, W. H. Orme-Johnson, and C. T. Walsh. "Methyl-S-coenzyme M reductase: a nickel-dependent enzyme catalyzing the terminal redox step in methane biogenesis," in J. Lancaster Ed., *Bioinorganic Chemistry of Nickel*, VCH, Florida, 1988, pp. 249–274.

134. R. P. Hausinger. Purification of a nickel-containing urease from the rumen anaerobe *Selenomonas ruminantium*, J. Biol. Chem., *261*, 7866 (1986).

135. A. G. Lappin. "Properties of copper blue proteins," in H. Sigel, Ed., *Copper Proteins (Metal Ions in Biological Systems*, Vol. 13), Dekker, New York, 1981, p. 15.

136. T. D. Tullius, P. Frank, and K. O. Hodgson. Characterization of the blue copper site in oxidized azurin by extended X-ray absorption fine structure: determination of a short Cu-S distance, Proc. Natl. Acad. Sci. USA, *75*, 4069 (1978).

137. Y. Fukumari and T. Yamanaka. The methylamine oxidizing system of *Pseudomonas* AM1 reconstituted with purified components, J. Biochem., *101*, 441 (1987).

138. D. Boulter, B. G. Haslett, D. Peacock, J. A. M. Ramshaw, and M. D. Scawen. Chemistry, function and evolution of plastocyanin, Int. Rev. Biochem., *13*, 1 (1977).

139. J. van Iersel, R. A. van der Meer, and J. A. Dune. Methylamine oxidase from *Arthrobacter* P1, Eur. J. Biochem., *161*, 415 (1986).

140. S. Benkovic, D. Wallick, L. Bloom, B. J. Gaffney, P. Domanico, T. Dix, and S. Pember. On the mechanism of action of phenylalanine hydroxylase, Biochem. Soc. Trans., *13*, 436 (1985).

141. A. M. D. Nambudiri and J. V. Bhat. Conversion of *p*-coumarate into caffeate by *Streptomyces nigrifaciens*: Purification and properties of the hydroxylating enzyme, Biochem. J., *130*, 425 (1972).

142. H. M. Steinman. Bacteriocuprein superoxide dismutases in pseudomonads, J. Bacteriol., *162*, 1255 (1985).

143. H. Iwasaki and J. Matsubara. A nitrite reductase from *Achromobacter cycloclastes*, J. Biochem., *71*, 645 (1972).

144. D. P. Nagle and R. S. Wolfe. Component A of the methyl coenzyme M methylreductase system of *Methanobacterium*: resolution into four components. Proc. Natl. Acad. Sci. USA, *80*, 2151 (1983).

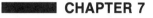 CHAPTER 7

# Importance of Iron in Bacterial Virulence

CHARLES D. COX

Department of Microbiology
University of Iowa
Iowa City, Iowa

## Contents

## 7.1   INTRODUCTION

We should be celebrating the 100th anniversary of a period that some medical historians have referred to as the "golden age of bacteriology." During the period 1880–1900 numerous reports were made of successful isolations and cultivations of bacteria from human and animal diseases. Although few present-day investigators read those early reports, we still use many of the same culture media. We have spent the past 100 years studying how bacteria lose pathogenicity on these media and how they regain that characteristic during experimental infections in animals and probably during infections in humans. The precise selective pressures governing the appearance of virulence during repeated animal infections are most important to a human understanding of pathogenicity. Perhaps it is time to understand the importance of selective pressures of inorganic nutrition on bacteria during growth in vivo and in vitro. This discussion focuses on the iron component of the field of inorganic nutrition and its relative importance to bacterial growth during infections of vertebrates.

Iron nutrition in the vertebrate must carry or transfer iron absorbed through the intestinal wall to tissues needing iron for biosynthesis or maintenance. According to numerous, recent reviews concerning this system (1–6), its iron-binding capacity and tenacity constitute such an imposing framework of innate defense against bacterial growth that it has been used as an example of nutritional immunity (7). Although the term nutritional immunity implies that normal vertebrate hosts and the sera from those hosts appear to deny bacteria many nutrients (hypothetically, carbon and nitrogen sources as well) necessary for growth, only iron-related nutrition and iron-related immunity have been studied in detail. This form of immunity is observed mainly through bacteriostatic activity.

If the theory of nutritional immunity is correct, then bacteria that are obligate parasites should have obvious characteristics that make them appear to have been under intense selective pressure to obtain iron. From the bacteriologist's perspective, the nutritional immunity theory implies that only those bacteria that succeed in obtaining iron from the vertebrate will succeed in being pathogenic, and those that cannot must remain saprophytic. Although this field has been reviewed numerous times in great detail, the theory of nutritional immunity has not been proven and may not even be presented or understood in its complete form for proper analysis. This chapter attempts to review some of the conflicting information behind the theory. The perspective is that of a bacteriologist studying pathogens, searching for possible evolutionary adaptations that bacteria might be interpreted to have undergone so as to occupy the ecological niche of mammalian tissue.

For this analysis, some terms must be defined. The word virulence is used here as it was intended by Miles (8). Although many scientists use the term synonymously with pathogenicity, this discussion has to deal with the applicability of the term ''virulence factor'' to describe bacterial mechanisms that promote iron acquisition during infection. Therefore, virulence is defined as the relative degree of pathogenicity demonstrated by a particular strain of bacteria, and a ''virulence factor'' is defined as any bacterial component or product contributing to the disease process. For example, during a consideration of the innate pathogenicity of *Salmonella typhimurium*, the task is to search among the strains of that species for expressions of higher virulence that are empowered by aggressive mechanisms for iron acquisition. Therefore, although there may be an indication that iron has effects on bacterial virulence, it must be stressed that virulence and the relationship between host and bacterium are extremely complex. The iron sequestering mechanism possessed by a particular bacterium is only a part of the bacterial phenotype. Once bacterial growth is initiated in the host, perhaps through or assisted by iron acquisition, then the bacteria can elicit numerous other factors that bring about direct harm to the host. These bacterial factors that bring about direct harm are the components that have traditionally been referred to as ''virulence factors.''

## 7.2  NUTRITIONAL IMMUNITY

Using simple colorimetric assays, investigators have been able to correlate both hyperferremic and hypoferremic states with the increased incidence of disease (9). The biochemistry of the control of iron concentration has been revealed largely through the protein chemistry of the serum glycoprotein transferrin (10). The antibacterial properties of this iron-binding protein have also resulted in its being named siderophilin (11). The antibacterial activity was further suggested by the discovery that those patients who survived prolonged agammaglobulinemia did so only because they had elevated serum concentrations of transferrin (12). In addition to transferrin, there is a very similar protein, lactoferrin (2, 13), that demonstrates some of the same antibacterial activity in secretions such as milk and inside phagocytic cells.

This section is intended to be a brief introduction to the study of bacterial interactions with the major components of the nutritional immune system. Transferrin and lactoferrin are mentioned, along with conalbumin (ovotransferrin), a similar glycoprotein from avian eggs. Although there are differences between the three iron chelators, the general structure consists of approximately 80,000-Da, single-polypeptide proteins having two separate domains, each of which binds one iron atom (two atoms per molecule). The overall binding coefficient for iron that would be found for transferrin in human serum appears to be between 1 and $6 \times 10^{22} \ M^{-1}$ (14). The site of the C-terminus, the end of the molecule containing the carbohydrate, binds iron with about five-fold more tenacity than the site at the N-terminus. However, when iron and transferrin are mixed, the N-terminus site is selectively occupied.

Invading bacteria must take advantage of any potential weaknesses in the structural or chemical features of iron binding by transferrin. The molecule is thought to possess two structural lobes, each containing one site. When iron is bound, the effective radius of the molecule becomes appreciably smaller. The ferric complexes of transferrin are more stable to denaturation and enzymatic digestion than the iron-free form. Excess bicarbonate (human serum contains approximately 20 m$M$ bicarbonate) promotes efficient binding. It is possible that this anion functions as a bridging ligand. Water and bicarbonate, along with either tyrosyl or histidyl ligands, have been thought to be important for iron binding. Relatively gentle mechanisms of iron release have been envisioned through an interference with the water or bicarbonate ligands. The addition of alternative anions, such as phosphate or pyrophosphate, leads to markedly reduced affinities for iron. Alternatively, reduction of the Fe(III) to Fe(II) is an effective means of iron release. Although acidification of the environment below pH 6.7 facilitates iron release (15) from transferrin, an extremely low pH (4.0) is necessary for facilitated release from lactoferrin. The evolutionary design of the nutritional immune system appears from the human viewpoint to be a bacteriostatic mechanism to slow down or stop bacterial growth until specific, acquired immune mechanisms can be formed for killing and clearing the bacteria.

If we examine the phenomenon of nutritional immunity from the microbial perspective, we see that it is important for most bacteria, except for those gaining entrance by bites, to colonize a mucosal surface before causing infection (16, 17). Once they are attached to the mucosal surface, growth must occur in the presence of lactoferrin (13). The iron binding at acid pH is so firm that this protein is capable of controlling intestinal colonization in the neonate following the ingestion of colostrum and milk (18–21), and of controlling iron concentration in the phagolysosome of the white cell (22).

Although the antibacterial activity of lactoferrin is believed to be exerted through iron deprivation, other investigators have found bactericidal effects, especially against *Legionella* and *Streptococci* (23–25). Therefore a bacterium attempting to colonize and grow on an epithelial surface may face the bacteriostatic and bactericidal effects of lactoferrin. Lactoferrin may also promote other ancillary antibacterial mechanisms, such as the promotion of polymorphonuclear leukocyte margination, which may be effective in the host (26) and will be important in the next stage of infection.

Following an expansion of the bacterial population and resultant inflammatory response, the colonizing bacteria may also confront lactoferrin-mediated antibacterial activities carried within polymorphonuclear leukocytes (27) called into the area. The lactoferrin, carried in specific granules of the leukocytes (22), acts not only by iron deprivation but also in the oxidative killing of the ingested bacteria (28). Both the extracellular (29) and intracellular (24, 30) activities of lactoferrin have been reported to be abrogated by the addition of iron. Therefore it is vital to the longevity of the human to maintain the mucosal epithelium free from compromising conditions. However, the various species of bacteria to be discussed can be arranged in a rank order of degrees of pathogenicity. Certain bacteria can resist being killed, will obtain iron to multiply, and will then invade the host without requiring significant compromise of defense mechanisms in the host. Alternatively, there are opportunistic bacteria that are eliminated by normal individuals, but are capable of causing invasive infections in humans with compromised immune mechanisms.

Some bacteria may invade the tissue and bloodstream directly. The invading bacteria initially confront a new iron-binding protein in the serum and site of inflammation, transferrin (7). This protein is found in serum at concentrations of 2–4 mg ml$^{-1}$ serum and is approximately 20–25% saturated with iron. Therefore, there are a considerable number of free sites that scrub the area of any released iron. The degree of inflammation controls the pH (31), which in turn determines the stability of the polymorphonuclear leukocytes in the area. As the pH drops to 6.5, the polymorphonuclear leukocytes begin dying and releasing their contents, including lactoferrin, into the exudate (32, 33). Under neutral conditions, a bacterium is in contact with only $10^{-18}$ $M$ ionic iron (1). Because the availability of iron appears to be so limited, infecting bacteria are left with few options. There is no possibility of growth determined by the exchange rate between transferrin and the solvent; this process is simply too slow.

The nutritional immune system also responds to infection in a manner further to deprive invading bacteria of iron. The hypoferremic state during infection can also be observed following injections of Gram-negative endotoxin (34, 35) and *Mycobacterium* (BCG strain) cell wall extracts (36). The fever resulting from infection or endotoxin administration also causes hypoferremia (37). Some mechanisms of hypoferremia have been discovered during recent experiments measuring the serum and organ levels of [$^{125}$I]transferrin and $^{59}$Fe during and after *Neisseria meningitidis* infections (38). It had been thought that transferrin concentration was regulated during infection. In opposition to this theory, investigators have found that the serum level of transferrin did not change during infection (38). The iron bound to the transferrin was rapidly deposited in the bone marrow, and the serum iron level decreased. The serum level decreased because the normal supply route to serum transferrin from the ferritin supply in the liver stopped functioning. Ceruloplasmin, enzymatically functioning as ferroxidase (39), appeared to control this process. Mice deficient in ceruloplasmin had increased resistance to *N. meningitidis* infection owing to low serum iron levels (28). When ceruloplasmin was administered to the mice, the iron saturation of transferrin increased. Conversely, during convalescence from infection, normal mice had high serum ceruloplasmin levels and increased serum iron. It was suggested that ceruloplasmin, which is under the control of copper concentration, oxidizes Fe(II) at the membranes of hepatocytes to Fe(III) for extracellular binding by transferrin. During infection, the ceruloplasmin concentration drops so that iron remains largely in the liver. During convalescence, when the host needs increased iron for repair, ferroxidase levels and activity increase to meet this need (28). Another study has also suggested that there may be changes in lactoferrin concentration at the mucosal surface. During infections with *Haemophilus*, an increase in lactoferrin concentration (40) has been implicated in increased bacteriostatic and bactericidal activity at the site of initial colonization.

## 7.3  IRON EFFECTS ON HOST AND PARASITE

### 7.3.1  Bacterial Responses to Iron Overload in Experimental Animals and in Serum

The nutritional immune system should cause formidable bacteriostatic effects. However, some bacteria have evolved over millions of years in close, obligate contact with the proteins of the nutritional immune system. There are also the different ecological niches of the extracellular and intracellular environments which would seem to place specific demands for evolutionary adaptations on pathogenic bacteria. The selective pressure on obligate parasites must be different from that experienced by opportunistic pathogens which have historically met the selective pressures of human tissue for only short periods. There should be examples of bacterial pathogenesis that would portray bacteria starving for iron in mammalian ecosystems and responding positively to iron supplied during infection.

There are several reports of comparisons of the pathogenicity of bacteria

**TABLE 7.1 Organization of Pathogens According to Growth in Embryonated Eggs Treated with Iron-binding Proteins or Iron Overload**

| Class I | Class III |
|---|---|
| N. meningitidis | N. gonorrhoeae |
| N. gonorrhoeae invasive strains | Avirulent N. meningitidis |
| S. typhimurium | V. cholerae strains |
| E. coli K1 | E. coli |
| P. aeruginosa | S. flexneri |
| H. influenzae | |
| **Class II** | **Class IV** |
| S. flexneri | Commensal Neiserria |
| S. dysenteriae | Avirulent Y. pestis |
| V. cholerae | E. coli |
| N. gonorrhoeae urogenital strains | S. flexneri–E. coli hybrid |

for different animal models that should aid in determination of different bacterial abilities to acquire and to use iron during infection. Payne and Finkelstein (41) were able to classify a number of bacteria into four groups (Table 7.1) on the basis of their responses to iron following injection into embryonated eggs. Bacteria in the first class (Class I), grew in the eggs regardless of the presence of added iron. Class II was composed of strains which were inhibited by conalbumin containing especially low iron saturation. Class III pathogens were strongly inhibited by serum transferrin or conalbumin in eggs and had to have exogenous iron administered before growth could occur. Congo Red is a stain which binds to certain bacterial strains according to their virulence and will be discussed later. Class IV strains were those that showed no growth even when iron was added (41).

The assay revealed some innate similarities among the bacteria in their responses to iron deprivation caused by conalbumin. There are problems relating this information to other investigations, such as the original findings by Shade et al. (42, 43) that demonstrated that conalbumin had dramatic inhibitory effects against *P. aeruginosa* and *S. dysenteriae*, both Class I pathogens (41). Although there are obvious problems with these assays, these important comparisons must be used to give some historical perspective to recent information that is being generated about these pathogens. It is also this information that will ultimately allow us to decide whether the theories of nutritional immunity and bacterial virulence based on iron acquisition have merit and to determine the kinds of experiments that must be constructed to test the theories.

In another review of various bacterial species, Miles et al. (45) measured diameters of skin lesions in guinea pigs to determine the infectivity of bacteria and the effects of iron, injected both systemically and locally, on 120 strains of bacteria from 17 different genera. Systemic iron stimulated 23%

of 115 strains and local iron stimulated 49% of 71 strains. Some of the strains stimulated the most were the vaccine strain (BCG) of *Mycobacterium tuberculosis*, *Listeria monocytogenes*, *Clostridium* sp., *Proteus*, *Aeromonas hydrophilla*, and some strains of *Klebsiella*. Quite contrary to the theory of iron starvation, some examples showed depressed infectivity with iron injection. Systemic iron depressed lesion diameters produced by strains of *Staphylococcus*, *Pseudomonas*, *Haemophilus* sp., and some strains of *Proteus*. The authors concluded that a depression of zone diameter was due to a lack of stimulation of bacterial growth and an inhibition of the inflammatory response (44). Maskell and Miles (45) used the guinea pig skin assay again to reveal additional variations in bacterial responses to the injection of iron-containing compounds. Eleven of 55 strains were enhanced by iron, but 27 of the 55 strains were stimulated by injection of the heme-iron protein hemoglobin. Although no strains of *P. aeruginosa* responded to iron, two of six strains tested were enhanced in skin pathogenicity assays by injected hemoglobin (45).

One of the most common animal models used to detect iron effects on pathogenicity is the lethality assay in rats and mice. One might expect that bacteria normally causing diseases in these rodents would have high virulence and therefore would be the bacteria of choice for experiments determining responses to iron injections. However, only a few investigators have reported iron-induced lethality by *Salmonella typhimurium* (46, 47). Other animal pathogens, *Pasteurella multocida* (48) and *P. hemolytica* (49), were also stimulated in lethality by injected iron. Interestingly, the opportunistic bacterium *E. coli* was dramatically more lethal when injected along with ferric ammonium citrate, hemoglobin, or hematin into guinea pigs (50%). Therefore, it appears that iron and iron-containing compounds shifted the equilibrium away from the inhibitory effect of transferrin toward the rapid growth of some species of infecting bacteria.

However, one Class I (41) pathogen, *P. aeruginosa* (an opportunistic pathogen), proved to be depressed or largely incapable of using iron in guinea pig skin. This bacterium has been extensively studied because it possesses low pathogenicity for mice, but demonstrates invasive characteristics when given opportunities in compromised hosts. Forseberg and Bullen (51) revealed a drop in the 50% lethal doses (LD$_{50}$ values) for mice from $1.2 \times 10^7$ without iron to $4.74 \times 10^5$ with added iron. They also found that *P. aeruginosa* gained additional lethality following repeated passage through animals, probably because of selection by host immune mechanisms. A strain passed through 16 serial infections in mice demonstrated an LD$_{50}$ of $4.09 \times 10^4$ but responded with an LD$_{50}$ of less than 10 when injected with iron. However, other investigators have found different results. For example, Martin and Finland (44) showed that iron injection only marginally affected the lethality of *P. aeruginosa*. In the same study they found that *Klebsiella pneumoniae* was markedly enhanced by iron. The site of iron injection was also found to be vital for the enhancement, because intraperitoneally injected iron stimulated *K. pneumoniae* but not the obligate aerobe *P. aeruginosa.* Another study, which took into account the aerobic properties of *P. aeruginosa*, compared the differences between bacteria passed through infections in the peritoneal cavity and bacteria passed through infections in the thoracic cavity (52) of compromised mice. Surprisingly, those bacteria passed through the intraperitoneal cavity had more virulence and responded with increased lethality to iron injections. Normal mice would not allow sufficient bacterial growth or survival for selection or adaptation to take place. Instead, the mice had to be compromised by injections of methotrexate and iron chloride to allow bacteria a chance to demonstrate changes in virulence with serial passage; eight passages were necessary to demonstrate significantly increased virulence (52). Earlier studies on the infectivity of this opportunist may have used avirulent strains (44, 45).

Although these examples indicated that iron and iron-containing compounds affected bacterial lethality, these injected compounds could be acting at sites other than transferrin. Attempts to answer this objection involved injecting both conalbumin (41) and transferrin into embryonated eggs and mice, respectively. These injections of iron-binding proteins inhibited the bacterial lethality that had been stimulated by injected iron. Although these experiments indicate that the damage done to the host by the injected iron was reversible through the nutritional immune system, the specific effects of the iron on bacterial lethality remain unknown.

Most of the studies on iron effects have utilized injections of bacteria into animals to compare the outcome of systemic infections. It would be valuable to find examples of iron effects on the lethality and infectivity of bacteria living on mucosal surfaces. Theoretically, bacteria at a mucosal surface must obtain iron from lactoferrin in order to colonize and grow. One report (53) indicated that mucin increased the survival of the cholera vaccine strain during colonization of the intestine. The growth-promoting effects of mucin have been attributed to iron because mucin is known to be a carrier of iron (54, 55), but the exact explanation has not been determined.

### 7.3.2  Effects of Previous Bacterial Exposure to Iron on the Outcome of Subsequent Infections and Growth Studies with Transferrin

The effects of iron supply have been observed in different kinds of experiments. Bacteria surviving passage through animal infections appeared to be the result of selective pressure for the most efficient iron-acquiring cells. Therefore it is reasonable that passage of bacteria through serial cultures in animal serum might also have yielded the same results. However, serum-passed *E. coli* and *S. typhimurium* appeared to be less capable of growing in serum (56). The authors concluded from this demonstration of complex antibacterial effects that serum forced bacteria to utilize their stored iron. Bacteria which were subject to growth inhibition could not utilize their reserves and remained relatively rich in iron. Virulent cells used their intracellular stores and (possibly with more metabolic time to adapt) eventually gained access to extracellular protein-bound iron. Therefore, investigators must be acutely aware of iron supplied to bacteria previous to injection for lethality studies. This iron may poise the bacterial physiology, either by pacifying the aggressive mechanisms for iron acquisition or by inducing those mechanisms. Not only the amount of stored iron, but also the readiness of the cells to obtain iron, must be appreciated in these assays.

For example, *Corynebacterium renale* had to be grown in the presence of high iron concentrations in order to be pathogenic in rats (57). In contrast, iron supplied to *P. aeruginosa*, strain PAO1, caused it to be avirulent when injected into rabbit corneas (58). However, the pathogenicity of the bacteria may not have depended on the insertion of iron, but controlled by iron supply. Toxin A production by *P. aeruginosa* is under control of iron concentration. Cells from iron-replete medium were unprepared to produce toxin when inoculated into the animal. Without toxin A production, the bacteria were rapidly cleared. Conversely, cells grown under iron starvation have the immediate capability to produce the toxin when injected into animals and were found to colonize the corneas and produce infection (58). Similarly, Sokol and Woods (59) found that the readiness of iron-starved bacteria to produce toxin A and elastase immediately upon being introduced into the chronic lung infection model in rats resulted in more tissue damage. Even though establishment of these infections was independent of colonization, the damage by cells grown in iron was less severe. Each bacterium may have a different response in this assay; some may depend on where the infection is initiated. Colonization and infection of mucosal surfaces (anaerobic sites in the peritoneal cavity) or muscle may place different demands on the bacteria for iron.

### 7.3.3   Appearance of Bacteria Isolated from Infection; How Much Iron Do Bacteria Experience During Infection?

Iron injected to overload the nutritional immune systems of animals appears to enhance the growth and lethalities of many bacteria. Although this finding implies that bacteria may be starved for iron, there must be more direct experiments to analyze this form of nutritional deprivation. First of all, the growth rate of these bacteria should be slow. Maw and Meynell (60) carefully measured the growth kinetics of *S. typhimurium*, and determined generation times of 8–10 h during infection in comparison to 30 min in culture medium. A similar "sluggish" growth rate during infection was measured for *E. coli* in muscle (61). In some of these experiments no growth could be detected. These investigators determined that mammalian tissue exerted an effective bacteriostatic effect that aided in the clearance of bacteria in the first 3–4 h. Similar bacteriostatic effects were measured against *S. typhimurium* in the intestine (62). On the other hand, studies measuring the growth rate of an avirulent vaccine strain of *V. cholerae* in the small intestine revealed an apparent generation time of 65 min (63). More rapid generation times were also found by Hooke et al. (64). Generation times of 33 and 20 min were found for temperature-sensitive mutants of *E. coli* and *P. aeruginosa*, respectively, in the peritoneal cavities of mice (64). This same trend was also supported by the 32- and 30-min generation times found for strains of *P. aeruginosa* in the lungs of different strains of mice (65).

These recent studies are disturbing because they indicate little or no bacteriostasis exerted by the animals. At present, there is no explanation for these more rapid growth rates and how these values should be compared with the values determined in the 1960s and 1970s (60–62). Although these bacterial strains were grown on trypticase soy broth, which is rich in iron (64), it is uncertain how this pretreatment would affect the bacteria. Iron supply during the growth of bacteria for inocula has been discussed as an important factor determining the initial fate of infections by *P. aeruginosa* (58, 59). Iron might be internalized and allow generations of growth unhindered by nutritional immunity. However, iron-replete cells were incapable of even brief colonization during studies of corneal infections. Iron may also affect bacteria injected into different mammalian ecologies (lung versus peritoneal cavity versus cornea) quite differently, and this raises important clinical questions. For example, where was the origin of the bacteria and what were their histories with regard to iron supply? For a patient in the intensive care unit of a hospital, it may be pertinent to understand the relative growth capabilities of bacteria originating from different sources such as intestinal carriage by staff as opposed to those growing on porcelain surfaces of a nearby sink.

Although these in vivo growth rates appear to be of iron-replete bacteria, other investigators have found infecting bacteria to be iron starved. Bacteria from a wide range of genera respond to iron deprivation in culture medium with remarkable changes in the composition of the cell envelope proteins (66, 67). These changes in protein composition have been detected by polyacrylamide gel electrophoresis of detergent-solubilized outer membranes. The proteins that appear in the outer membranes during iron deprivation have usually been referred to as iron-regulated outer membrane proteins and in most cases their exact functions have not yet been determined. Recently, bacteria harvested directly from infections have been submitted to these same types of analyses. Griffiths et al. (68), found that *E. coli* harvested from the peritoneal cavities of infected guinea pigs demonstrated iron-regulated proteins in the outer membrane. Remarkably, Brown et al. (69) isolated, with no subculturing, *P. aeruginosa* from the lungs of patients with cystic fibrosis and revealed their outer membrane protein profiles to be those of iron-starved bacteria. Several additional reports (70, 71) have found that the outer membranes isolated from *K. pneumoniae* and *Proteus vulgaris*, harvested without subculture from urinary tract infections, also expressed the outer membrane proteins of iron starved bacteria. The sera from these patients also indicated immune responses against the iron-regulated proteins (70).

Because bacteria isolated directly from infections demonstrated characteristics similar to bacteria being starved for iron in culture media, it is important to consider the resistance of these bacteria in response to antibacterial mechanisms. Along with alterations in the outer membrane proteins (66), iron-limited bacteria have altered sensitivities to antibiotics (72–74). The host's immunoglobulin response to these iron-regulated proteins may be important in inhibiting iron acquisition (74). Iron deprivation has also been linked to the production of many different exopolysaccharides (16, 67). The nutritional control of both exopolysaccharides and lipopolysaccharides affects sensitivities of bacteria to phagocytosis (79–81) and to complement-mediated killing (82–84). These polysaccharides may also decrease the adherence of the bacterial cells (75, 76) or they may act as adhesins (77, 78). Iron supply also controls the production of extracellular proteins involved in the destruction of host tissues (57, 58, 85–88). All these changes caused by iron status during infection necessitate compensatory changes in the host's immune response to these new characteristics. Therefore these iron-controlled characteristics may determine some aspects of the virulence of bacteria.

### 7.3.4   Direct Effects of Iron on the Host

Injected iron may have many effects other than saturating transferrin. Interpretations of bacterial responses to iron are prone to error because of a lack of detailed studies on host–pathogen interactions. There have been many informal suggestions that iron overloads the reticuloendothelial system. Although one investigation found no evidence of blockade, there appeared to be direct compromise to kidney defense mechanisms (89). In addition to gross effects of iron, such as the lesions appearing in the kidneys (89), there have also been reports of more subtle changes important to the compromise of defense mechanisms. Investigators have detected the inhibition by iron of the phagocytic ability of monocytes for *L. monocytogens* (90). Iron and iron-containing proteins inhibited the phagocytosis and killing of *S. aureus* by polymorphonuclear leukocytes (91, 93). Iron appears to have an immediate effect on bacterial survival, whereas iron-containing compounds, such as hemoglobin, have a delayed effect in promoting survival (94). Iron apparently affected T-lymphocyte surface markers (95) and general lymphocyte migration (97). Iron would also affect the participation of transferrin and lactoferrin in the complement-mediated bactericidal activity that has been detected (97).

Therefore the concentration of iron in serum and the transferrin pool can have direct effects on bacterial nutrition and can control bacterial physiology. In turn this physiology, during infection, can affect not only the sensitivity of bacteria to defense mechanisms and antibiotics, but also the production of toxins and mediators of host damage. Yet with regard to host tissue, iron can also directly inhibit antibacterial mechanisms. Therefore it is very difficult to determine, on the basis of lethality studies based upon injections of iron, the exact importance of iron to bacterial virulence.

## 7.4 EXAMPLES OF MECHANISMS FOR BACTERIAL ACQUISITION OF IRON DURING INFECTION

Although the host animal appears to add excessive complexity to the analysis of bacterial virulence, a review of some mechanisms that bacteria may use to obtain iron from host tissues may clarify the relationship between iron and virulence. If pathogenic bacteria have evolved in response to selective pressures to obtain iron during infection, then there should be obvious bacterial mechanisms that can be described as contributing to bacterial virulence. These mechanisms are organized here under examples of bacterial pathogenicity, and ranked in approximate order of their increasing invasiveness or ecological obligation to mammalian tissue. This is done because it is important to determine whether or not iron acquisition mechanisms have evolved to fit precise ecological niches within the human.

### 7.4.1  Extracellular Parasites

#### 7.4.1.1  *E. coli (Other Than Enteroinvasive Strains)*

*7.4.1.1.1  Siderophores.* The most investigated mechanism of bacterial acquisition of iron is the use of siderophores; these are explained in detail in Chapter 5. *E. coli* is one of the best examples of a siderophore-producing bacterium and frequently serves as a model system. Siderophores, as defined by C. E. Lankford (98), are microbial products that bind iron in soluble organic chelates and present the iron to the bacterial envelope in a form suitable for active transport. There are different chemical forms that are based on either hydroxamate or catechol ligands (98). Each siderophore found in a bacterial species presumably requires specific cell receptors to provide favorable ferrisiderophore binding and iron transport. Enterochelin was the first siderophore to be isolated from this bacterium (99). Animal experiments in which enterochelin was injected together with *E. coli*, an example of both a Class I and Class IV pathogen (41), revealed that this siderophore increased virulence (100). Experiments involving siderophore injections must be interpreted differently from those involving iron overload. The siderophores are usually injected in the iron-free form so that any aid they give to the bacteria must be mediated through the mobilization of iron from host iron-binding proteins. Therefore, the increased virulence indicates that the siderophore is capable of stimulating bacterial growth by mobilizing iron from transferrin and implies bacterial aggressiveness for iron during infection. However, these experiments did not measure siderophore production during infection, nor toxicity by injected siderophore; for example, there may be other potential effects on host systems (phagocytosis, complement-mediated killing, immunoglobulin synthesis) that have not been measured.

In vitro experiments have confirmed a relatively facile removal of iron from transferrin (101) by enterochelin. However, later studies indicated that enterochelin had several inadequacies for in vivo growth; it was considerably less effective during growth studies in serum or during infections because it tends to bind to serum albumin (102), thereby becoming ineffective and also immunogenic (103). Antibodies formed to the hapten siderophore also rendered the iron-binding compound ineffective for iron transport (103). Catechol siderophores with ester bonds, such as enterochelin, also experience rapid hydrolysis in serum.

Another siderophore, aerobactin (104–106) has been found in certain *E. coli* strains that are "invasive" (107). These strains are more like the Class I pathogen (a K1 type in this instance) used by Payne and Finkelstein. Aerobactin proved to be stable in serum and nonimmunogenic, and formed surprisingly effective ternary complexes with iron and transferrin during active removal of iron to form ferriaerobactin (108). This is an excellent example of a bacterium producing a factor that actively binds to transferrin and somehow modifies the ligand structure of the protein so that iron is mobilized and bound by aerobactin for bacterial utilization. Therefore, although the iron-binding coefficient of aerobactin is lower than that of transferrin, it removes iron readily (108). Aerobactin was more effective at a concentration 500-fold lower than enterochelin in promoting growth (109). Although aerobactin and the specific transport mechanism for iron from ferric aerobactin were originally associated with *E. coli* strains carrying the Col V "virulence" plasmid, these characteristics have since been found in a wide variety of strains, coded by either plasmid or chromosomal genes (109, 110). Based on the structural organization of the two different siderophore gene clusters, convincing arguments (109) have been put forward to support the superior activity of aerobactin under the environmental conditions of mammalian infections.

Although the activity of aerobactin in iron mobilization explains the invasive character of these strains in comparison to normal Class IV strains, there are theoretical problems in the explanation of siderophore activity during infections. It is difficult to understand how bacteria in an inflamed tissue lesion can produce sufficient siderophore to support their tremendous growth during septicemia; sometimes $10^6$ bacteria per milliliter are recovered from blood. During the lethality experiments that have been discussed, siderophores can be injected into the bloodstream of animals at concentrations above the $K_m$ of the bacterial transport process [1 $\mu M$ in the case of enterochelin (111)]. Although enterochelin has been found in tissue during experimental infections (112), concentrations in blood that could explain fulminant septicemia have not been determined. Therefore the finding by Stuart et al. (104) that aerobactin is carried by the bacterium in a cell-bound state may indicate that the siderophore could work at short range. A single collision between an *E. coli* cell carrying cell-bound aerobactin and a transferrin molecule could lead to successful ternary complex formation, ferriaerobactin formation, and short-range transport of iron from ferriaerobactin. This perspective of siderophore activity may more easily explain rapid growth rates than explanations involving extracellular siderophores and diffusion of ferrisiderophores over millimeters or centimeters in well-mixed environments. A similar proposal was made by Kochan et al. (113) for the competitive action of cell-bound enterochelin with transferrin.

It may also be important to consider that bacterial products that are normally excreted, such as exotoxin A by *P. aeruginosa*, may, under conditions of membrane perturbation, be expressed as a cell-bound enzyme (114). Although toxin A excretion involves a mechanism of holoenzyme processing at the cell surface, a phenomenon more complex than the excretion of a small siderophore, future research must determine the in vivo expression of siderophores and exactly how they function for iron delivery.

Another area needing more research is the host's immune response to siderophore function. For example, normal human sera was found to contain antibodies against the enterochelin transport apparatus on the cell surface (74); even if iron could be successfully mobilized from transferrin by enterochelin, transport would be severely impeded. The antibody class implicated in this inhibition was IgA, a fact that brought attention to the inhibition of the processes of colonization and invasion of epithelial surfaces. Other researchers found that an immune response against colitose in lipopolysaccharide (116) inhibited enterochelin production. The mechanism of an antibody–carbohydrate complex on the cell surface in the inhibition of either siderophore synthesis or release remains unknown.

*7.4.1.1.2 Hemolysin.* The mechanisms of virulence endowed to *E. coli* strains by the Col V plasmid (116) involve factors in addition to aerobactin synthesis and iron transport. Indeed, the overall picture of virulence in *E. coli* (116) appears to be quite complex. Many strains carrying the Col V plasmid also produce an hemolysin (110). A high percentage of *E. coli* strains isolated from nonenteric infections express hemolytic activity (117–120). These strains also demonstrated enhanced lethalities when injected into either embryonated eggs (121) or rats and mice (122, 123). The connection between hemolysin activity and the iron nutrition of the bacteria is through bacterial utilization of released hemoglobin. Although some investigators have warned that hemoglobin had no effect on the lethality of certain *E. coli* strains (45), hemoglobin increases the growth of *E. coli* in tissue by dramatic proportions (124). Hemoglobin has been implicated as an important bacterial stimulant in other experimental infections as well (1, 50). In addition, the heme released during mammalian cell lysis is possibly an even more accessible form of iron (125) than hemoglobin. Recently, Lebek and Gruenig (126) found that hemolysin production is under control by the iron concentration in the medium. Soluble iron salts inhibited hemolysin production in strains carrying plasmid- or chromsomal-borne hemolysin genes. Although most strains were stimulated to produce even more hemolysin when iron was withheld from the bacteria by iron chelators, several strains either did not respond or excreted less hemolysin.

Although there is a good deal of evidence that hemolysin activity can provide iron to the invasive *E. coli* strains, there is the problem of cell lysis at great distances from infecting bacteria. Just as there has been a suggestion that aerobactin may reside on the cell surface, hemolysin has also been found in a cell-bound form (120). The hypothesis of close-range hemolysis for an invading bacterium is made more attractive by the ability of many invasive strains of *E. coli* to agglutinate human erythrocytes (117, 118). Binding and lysis of erythrocytes at close range could be important to bacteria because hemoglobin and heme are bound by other serum proteins and cleared rapidly from circulation.

Haptoglobin, present in serum, binds free hemoglobin and acts as a bacteriostatic agent against *E. coli* provided with hemoglobin as an iron source (127). Haptoglobin has also been observed to provide an antibacterial function during infections (128). Likewise, heme will not exist long as a free compound in serum because hemopexin (129), another serum glycoprotein, will bind this iron source and render it unusable by bacteria. These phenomena of iron release, iron-compound binding, and bacterial acquisition of iron from the iron-binding protein indicate a need for much more research. These important defense mechanisms may also be undergoing alterations during infection, just as the transferrin-bound iron moves rapidly during infection.

Another important consideration is that hemolysins also serve as general cytotoxic agents, capable of lysing many different types of cells (119, 120). The cells lysed by this activity would release an iron storage compound, ferritin. Although the phenomenon has not been studied adequately, enterochelin appeared to mobilize iron rapidly from this protein (131). Direct, siderophore-independent iron utilization of ferritin iron by *E. coli* has not been characterized sufficiently. Because each ferritin molecule might contain approximately 3000 iron atoms, this protein appears to be an excellent iron source. Serum ferritin, occuring in a glycosylated form, is different from intracellular ferritin and increases in the serum during infection (132). Little is known about these forms of ferritin and their use by bacteria as iron sources. Therefore, even though hemolysin is a virulence factor that causes direct harm to host cells, its contribution to iron acquisition by *E. coli* remains to be determined.

### 7.4.1.2 Klebsiella Species

*7.4.1.2.1 Siderophores.* There appears to be widespread association between plasmid-mediated aerobactin production and virulence (133, 134) among enteric bacteria. *Klebsiella pneumoniae* is used here as an example of an enteric that synthesizes enterochelin but, like invasive *E. coli* strains, appears to depend upon aerobactin to support invasiveness (133). Both *E. coli* and *K. pneumoniae* are obligate extracellular parasites that take opportunity of the compromised host in disease production. The pathogenicity of these opportunists has been associated with capsule types, the $K_1$ and $K_2$ types being particularly pathogenic in *K. pneumoniae* strains (133, 135), which are thought to be involved in bacterial survival in the host. Although all of the invasive $K_1$ and $K_2$ capsule-bearing strains produce enterochelin, there has been a correlation between aerobactin production and virulence (133). Therefore, growth in the host appears to be determined by this particular siderophore, which actively removes iron from transferrin. The prevalence of aerobactin production throughout the enterics is probably due to the spread of the plasmids carrying the aerobactin genes and the positive selection endowed on these strains by aerobactin's activity (133). Other related strains have been found to possess the same traits of aerobactin production and aerobactin-mediated iron uptake via similar outer membrane receptors (134).

Another species, *K. aerogenes*, produces only enterochelin under iron starvation (137). Although this species might be expected to be like Class IV pathogenic *E. coli* (41), these two bacteria behave differently during the stress of iron deprivation. Williams et al. (136) found that *E. coli* depleted its intracellular stores of iron before responding to the low external concentrations. However, under the same conditions *K. aerogenes* responded almost immediately with the appearance of outer membrane proteins characteristic of iron-starved cells. This finding stresses the importance of individualistic bacterial behaviors and control mechanisms during infection.

### 7.4.1.3 *Pseudomonas aeruginosa and Other Genera*

*7.4.1.3.1 Siderophores.* Although Payne and Finkelstein classified this bacterium as a Class I pathogen (41), it is an opportunist that produces a multitude of virulence factors capable of harming the host (58, 85). Unlike the examples taken from the enteric bacteria, there has been no association of invasive strains with capsule types or other virulence characteristics. Almost all strains appear to produce two prominent siderophores, pyochelin (a phenolate) (137, 138) and pyoverdin (a hydroxamate) (139, 140). Pyoverdin is produced as a group of related pigments (141) in a manner similar to the mycobactins of *Mycobacteria* (142), an example to be discussed below. Although pyochelin enhanced the lethality of *P. aeruginosa* when injected together with bacteria into mice (143), pyoverdin production (144) and activity (145) appeared to be the major factors allowing bacterial growth in human serum containing transferrin. This example is similar to *E. coli* in that the hydroxamate class of siderophore (pyoverdin and aerobactin) has proven to be the more significant growth-promoting factor in serum. However, pyoverdin is not coded by plasmid-borne genes (146, 147). Both pyochelin and pyoverdin stimulate bacterial growth in culture media containing transferrin, but only pyoverdin can be produced in adequate amounts to support growth in serum (144, 145). Therefore, all of the examples of bacteria that produce two siderophores simultaneously in culture media prefer production of the hydroxamate siderophore during infection. The phenolate siderophores probably fulfill positive selective roles in other environments.

*7.4.1.3.2 Iron Reduction Compounds.* Pyocyanin, the blue pigment of blue pus disease (148, 149), has been implicated in the reduction of Fe(III) to Fe(II) resulting in the release of iron from transferrin (150). This general reductive mechanism of iron release has been previously studied, and may be the manner in which host cells remove iron from transferrin (151). There are also transport mechanisms found in other bacteria for ferrous iron (152). This mechanism might occur naturally in ecologies low in oxygen and having acidic pH. Iron transport in *Streptococcus mutans* appears to be due to a membrane-bound enzyme capable of reducing iron before transport (153). A notably different system has been found in *Listeria monocytogenes* in which a large, 8,000–10,000 Da, extracellular compound has been implicated in the reduction and release of iron from transferrin (154). This is our first example of a facultative intracellular parasite. Although the investigators implicated reduction as a mechanism of acquisition in vitro (154), it would be most interesting to determine whether this mechanism was effective during both intracellular and extracellular growth when the bacteria had contact with transferrin.

*7.4.1.3.3 Exopolysaccharides.* There is evidence suggesting that the growth of *P. aeruginosa* during infection may be dramatically different from that observed in culture medium. This different mode of growth may affect nutrition, interactions with host defense mechanisms, and the mechanisms leading to septicemia. The most dramatic demonstration of altered growth and physiology occurs in the isolation of mucoid *P. aeruginosa* strains from patients with cystic fibrosis (155). The mucoid phenotype is very labile and generally nonmucoid variants accumulate after isolation on culture medium (156). The alginate slime, which accounts for the mucoid behavior, cannot be correlated with any of the more popular virulence mechanisms. The slime also had no apparent association with the nutritional supply to the bacteria during infection (157). However, in vitro studies indicated that alginate production was a more stable characteristic when cells were grown in low iron concentrations (158). Brown et al. (58) also demonstrated that mucoid bacteria, isolated directly from cystic fibrosis patients, have outer membrane protein profiles similar to those of bacteria starved for iron. These iron starvation proteins are recognized as antigens by the infected cystic fibrosis patients (159).

In addition to iron control of alginate production, low iron concentrations allow the synthesis of a biosurfactant, rhamnolipid, which is a nonenzymatic hemolysin (160) and cytolitic factor (120). Although it is not understood why these compounds are formed, the acidic polysaccharides, such as alginate slime, might help trap cations compounds such as iron.

*7.4.1.3.4 Glycocalyx (Capsule) and its Effect on the Mode of Growth.* According to Costerton et al. (161), the alginate slime has been associated with an entirely different mode of growth, the microcolony. Nutrient limitation appeared to force *P. aeruginosa* into alginate production, a characteristic that could be maintained over generations through iron deprivation in the lung (162). This mode of growth has been associated with slower growth rates, lower amounts of exoenzyme synthesis (157), and chronic infections (163). The alginate matrix, or glycocalyx, is an adhesive that cements the colony together to form a biofilm that is stuck to the tissue surface (164). Bacteria, encased in alginate, are less exposed to the host's phagocytic cells, proteins (immunoglobulins as well as transferrin), and antibiotics (162). The exopolysaccharides of *P. aeruginosa* have been implicated in attachment to host cells (77, 161). This mode of growth may be most important for an opportunistic pathogen, because the compromised state of the host may change by the hour. Under conditions of increased iron (greater degree of host compromise), increased replication rates by the bacteria may lead to the production of more cells not bearing alginate, called "swarmers," capable of leaving the microcolony and invading the bloodstream (161, 163). These swarmer cells may either form new microcolonies, owing to ecological stress, or may lead to increasing septicemia. Although the swarmer cell leads to septicemia, it is also the mode most readily cleared by the host (161). Therefore the available iron concentration may control the course of the infection by controlling the physiology of the infecting bacteria. More research is needed to determine the role of alginate in disease and to substantiate iron control over the growth behavior of *P. aeruginosa* and many other bacteria during infections.

### 7.4.1.4  Vibrio Species

*7.4.1.4.1 Lack of Effect by Siderophores.* *Vibrio cholerae* is a pathogen residing in a different ecological niche from that of the bacteria considered previously. These cells attach to the epithelial surface of the small intestine and exhibit no invasiveness. They produce a phenolate siderophore, vibriobactin (165, 166), and express outer membrane proteins typical of iron-starved bacteria when isolated directly from infection (167, 168). When iron starvation was relieved during infection by the administration of iron, both bacterial growth and disease were enhanced (169).

However, it has recently been determined that vibriobactin does not enhance the pathogenicity of *V. cholerae* in the infant mouse model (170). Vibriobactin may have ecological roles outside the host. Mutants incapable of transporting the ferrisiderophore colonized and caused the same disease as the wild-type strains. This phenomenon has been broadly interpreted to indicate that these noninvasive bacteria may grow at the expense of other iron compounds on the epithelial surface. Mucin has been suggested as one of these possible compounds because it carries iron (54, 55).

Other *Vibrio* species that have more invasive properties appear to depend upon siderophore production for pathogenicity. One of the best examples of siderophore-mediated virulence is that of the invasive fish pathogen *Vibrio anguillarum* (171); this disease has been directly related with the plasmid-mediated production of a siderophore, anguibactin, and its associated iron transport mechanism. Although there are other factors controlling invasiveness, anguibactin allows bacterial growth and the expression of the other virulence factors. In one of the most important demonstrations of siderophore effectiveness, Wolf and Crossa (171) demonstrated growth-promoting concentrations of this siderophore in the kidney and blood of infected salmon. In addition, these concentrations could sustain bacterial strains that could not produce anguibactin, but were otherwise virulent. Obviously, this siderophore is a virulence factor.

In another interesting example, *Vibrio vulnificus*, a hemolytic species is known to produce a fatal human septicemia. These bacteria appear to utilize hemoglobin as an iron source following lysis of erythrocytes (172). However, unlike the example in *E. coli*, the presence of haptoglobin did not decrease the growth capability of the *V. vulnificus* (172).

### 7.4.1.5   Neisseria meningitidis and N. gonorrhoeae

*7.4.1.5.1   Characteristics of Iron Acquisition.* Although these two species are discussed together because their iron acquisition mechanisms are so similar, their pathogenic characteristics are different. *N. meningitidis* is an extracellular parasite noted for causing invasive septicemias and meningitis. However, *N. gonorrhoeae* is a facultative intracellular parasite demonstrating limited invasiveness, typically for columnar epithelial cells of the genitourinary tract. For *N. gonorrhoeae*, there are invasive strains that are known to cause disseminated gonococcal infection, the so-called DGI strains (173). Among the urogenital, noninvasive strains, there are also morphological correlations between colony type and virulence. Types 1 and 2 of the four total colony types of *N. gonorrhoeae* are known to be virulent. Iron controls this expression to some degree because the reversion of type 4 to virulent and stable type 1 colonies was accomplished by elevating the iron concentration of culture media (174). These bacteria may need more iron because cells of colony types 1 and 2 were found to contain less iron than cells of colony types 3 and 4 (175).

Earlier, Payne and Finkelstein (41) had found that type 1 and 2 colony types were Class II pathogens, capable of obtaining iron from embryonated eggs except under conditions of iron restriction. Colony types 3 and 4 were

Class III pathogens, incapable of competing for iron and being totally dependent upon exogenous iron for growth. DGI strains of *N. gonorrhoeae* were Class I pathogens. Although *N. meningitidis* strains were Class I pathogens, these bacteria demonstrated iron-controlled growth in mice and responded with increased lethality in mice injected with iron (176).

### 7.4.1.5.2 Iron Acquisition Directly from Transferrin.

Additional investigations indicated that *N. meningitidis* was absolutely dependent upon the amount of iron bound to transferrin at the start of the infection. Iron dextran was injected into mice to control the amount of iron saturation of transferrin in the mice (177). The *N. meningitidis* grew and used that amount, but could obtain no more when that supply was exhausted. The iron on transferrin was not being replaced in the infected mice, therefore the infection was under control of the iron concentration. Although there have been some indications that free or cell-bound siderophores might be involved in this process of iron acquisition (178), recent analyses have detected no siderophore production by either *N. gonorrhoeae* (179, 180) or *N. meningitidis* (181).

All species appeared to have high-affinity uptake mechanisms for iron chelated to citrate during in vitro studies, but no other ferrisiderophores or iron salts supplied iron to these organisms (182, 183). Most importantly, Mickelsen and Sparling (183) found that all meningococci and gonococci utilized iron directly from transferrin in its normal state of 25% iron saturation. Although these pathogens utilized the mammalian proteins as iron sources, the commensal *Neisseria* species do not and suffer growth inhibition. However, lactoferrin added to the growth assays in place of transferrin (184) was utilized by all of the meningococci, 53% of the gonococci, and 24% of the commensal isolates. Therefore the pathogenic species appeared to have a specific mechanism for utilizing iron from transferrin, but there was no relationship between virulence and the utilization of iron from lactoferrin. It was suggested, just as with *V. cholerae* infections, that *Neisseria* use mucin or some other iron-containing compound rather than lactoferrin during colonization of mucosal surfaces (182, 184).

Iron acquisition directly from transferrin is an important research topic. *N. meningitidis* possesses a high-affinity transport mechanism utilizing an outer membrane receptor that binds both saturated and iron-free transferrin (185). The same conditions that enhanced the lethality of *N. meningitidis* in experimental animals (186), that is, growing cells for inocula under acid pH and iron starvation conditions, also yielded the most active bacteria for iron uptake in vitro (185). Although a few candidate polypeptides have been detected (181, 187), no single outer membrane protein involved in transferrin binding and uptake has been identified. One of the most promising iron-regulated outer membrane proteins has been found to occur in a highly conserved form throughout many pathogenic and commensal species of *Neisseria* (186). Yet according to the data on iron utilization from transferrin, only the pathogenic *Neisseria* species should possess binding activity. Although this protein may not be the one responsible for either transferrin binding or iron removal from transferrin, it appears to be important to pathogenesis and has been recognized widely as a dominant antigen by patients with infections.

### 7.4.1.6 Haemophilus influenzae

*7.4.1.6.1 Transferrin Binding.* This extracellular parasite has limited invasiveness for tissues around the site of colonization, but can cause septicemia and meningitis in certain age groups of humans. All of the virulent, type b isolates from human infections utilized transferrin as an iron source, whereas none of the *Haemophilus parainfluenzae* strains could (189). The lack of utilization by *H. parainfluenzae* has been correlated with its lack of invasiveness (189). Eighty-one percent of the nontypable *H. influenzae* strains isolated from human respiratory tracts used transferrin. Although all of the meningococci and some of the gonococci utilized lactoferrin, none of the Haemophilus species or strains could use this source (189). Although bacteria clearly used transferrin as an iron source, there were no obvious changes in the outer membrane protein profile when the cells were placed under iron starvation (189).

The characteristic indicated by the name of this genus, blood loving, has been recently investigated. *H. influenzae* appears capable of acquiring iron from hemoglobin, myoglobin, and heme (190) regardless of the presence of haptoglobin and hemopexin. Therefore, although the bacterium has no mechanism of lysing erythrocytes, once the heme-iron compounds are present, they can be utilized.

### 7.4.2  Facultative Intracellular Parasites

### 7.4.2.1  Salmonella

*7.4.2.1.1 Facultative Intracellular Parasites.* *Salmonella* is a genus comprising facultative intracellular parasites. Serotypes of *Salmonella enteritidis* parasitize the epithelial layers of the small intestine with limited invasiveness, whereas *Salmonella typhi* parasitizes monocytes and causes invasive septicemias. The diseases determined by these parasites are gastroenteritis and typhoid fever, respectively. However, the typhimurium serotype of *S. enteritidis* (referred to as *S. typhimurium* in most research) has been used as a model infection in rodents because it mimics the typhoid fever of humans.

*7.4.2.1.2 Siderophore-independent Pathogenicity.* Payne and Finkelstein characterized this a Class I pathogen because it did not need exogenous iron to grow and kill embyonated eggs (41). *Salmonella* species produce a catechol siderophore identical to that of *E. coli* strains, although it has been given a different name, enterobactin instead of enterochelin (191). Yancey et al. (192) demonstrated that enterobactin injections into mice challenged with *Salmonella typhimurium* dramatically increased the growth and lethality of the bacteria. Injection of enterobactin-defective mutants yielded significant reductions in lethality from wild-type strains, but both strains responded with significant increases in lethality when enterobactin was injected with the bacteria (192). These results could also be reproduced in serum and in transferrin with the same growth responses (103, 192). In addition, antibody against enterobactin found in normal human sera inhibited the growth of *S. typhimurium* in serum (103). However, a more recent report suggested that these results are incorrect. Benjamin et al. (193) found that a siderophore-defective mutant demonstrated the same virulence as wild type whether injected intraperitoneally or intravascularly. These authors used the same bacterial strains as Yancey et al. (192), finding that the original enterobactin-defective strain was leaky, but that there were no virulence differences between the original strains or between the original strain and a solidly enterobactin-defective mutant. The use of different breeds of mice is probably pertinent to the differences between the results of Yancey et al. (192) and Benjamin et al. (193). The fact that Benjamin et al. (193) used several inbred and out-bred lines of experimental mice lends credence to their conclusion that *S. typhimurium* does not utilize siderophore-mediated iron acquisition during intracellular growth. The new theory of enterobactin effectiveness indicates that the siderophore would be used during extracellular growth. Therefore, it might be imagined that breeds of mice with certain defects in phagocytosis or cell-mediated immunity might be more likely to allow enterobactin-mediated effects on extracellular bacterial growth. The new theory (193) is also in keeping with the findings that enterobactin, if produced during infection, will have a short half-life in serum (102, 108).

### 7.4.2.2 Shigella Species

*7.4.2.2.1 Facultative Intracellular Parasites.* *Shigella* species are facultative intracellular parasites having limited invasiveness for the epithelial cells of the colon. *S. flexneri* is an example of the domestic, endemic variety, and *Shigella dysenteriae* is the tropical and epidemic species. These two species were characterized by Payne and Finkelstein (41) as being Class II pathogens, being normally virulent for embyonated eggs, but susceptible to any decrease in the iron saturation. These investigators also included the interesting property of Congo Red binding by the bacterial colonies on plating media. They found that the Congo Red-negative strain, ranked in Class III as being unable to grow in embryonated eggs without added iron, was different from its Class II, wild-type parent. The loss of Congo Red binding has been studied recently and is associated with the loss of virulence (194).

*7.4.2.2.2 Siderophore-independent Pathogenicity.* Many *Shigella* species produce aerobactin (195). However, the existence of this siderophore could not be correlated to intracellular growth because the epidemic species causing the most severe disease, *S. dysenteriae*, lacked the capability to produce aerobactin (195). In addition, transposon-induced mutants of *S. flexneri* lacking aerobactin-mediated iron transport demonstrated the same virulence characteristics of invasiveness and capability to produce keratoconjunctivitis (Sereny positive) (196). Therefore, siderophore production does not appear to be related to the intracellular acquisition of iron. Alternatively, it was theorized that aerobactin might be important in colonization of the epithelial surface and obtaining iron from lactoferrin (196).

*7.4.2.2.3 Congo Red Binding.* Congo Red staining of bacterial colonies on plating media was developed by Surgalla and Beesely (197) to differentiate virulent strains of *Yersinia pestis* from those that had lost virulence for experimental animals. Virulence of *S. flexneri* strains isolated from a human could be correlated with colony type and a change in these colony types during cultivation on laboratory media. Avirulent, opaque colonies arose from the normally virulent, translucent colonies at a frequency of one colony in every $10^4$–$10^5$ bacteria. Avirulence has been characterized by mouse lethality assay, lack of invasiveness for cultured human cells, and lack of positive character in the Sereny assay. When these characteristics were studied carefully, it was found that avirulent variants lost the ability to adsorb Congo Red and had lost a 140-MDa plasmid (198). However, there appeared to be several different factors on the lost plasmid. A transductant with restored pigmentation in the presence of Congo Red did not also regain virulence in the Sereny assay. Therefore, it appeared that loss of Congo Red adsorption was only one event leading to loss of virulence, and that there were other genes also necessary for virulence (198, 199).

Because there has been an historical relationship between Congo Red binding and iron metabolism, nurtured by research on *Yersinia pestis*, it is most interesting that Daskaleros and Payne have recently found (200) that Congo Red binding can be correlated with hemin binding and transport. However, this phenomenon may have nothing to do with iron acquisition in the intracellular environment. These investigators found that both Congo Red binding cells (Crb+) and Crb− cells utilized hemin as iron sources, but the Crb− cells could not invade HeLa cells. Their conclusion was that Crb+ cells with hemin bound to hypothetical receptors could invade cells better than cells without hemin on their surfaces. However, the presence of several virulence characteristics on the 140-MDa plasmid is apparent, and several genes controlling or coding for invasiveness and hemin binding may be closely linked (198, 199). This system cannot be viewed simply. For example, recent cloning experiments have yielded transformed cells that could not adsorb Congo Red and could not yield positive Sereny assays, but could invade epithelial cells (201).

*7.4.2.2.4 Contact Hemolysin.* Another activity associated with the 140-MDa plasmid is a "contact hemolysin," so named because activity can be observed only through centrifugally assisted contact between bacteria and erythrocytes (202). This factor is thought to be responsible for the rapid penetration by bacteria through the phagocytic vacuole. Once penetration is completed, the bacteria could replicate freely in the cytoplasm. The potential relationship of this factor to iron metabolism might be in the progression of the bacteria from the nutritionally arid phagosome to the cytoplasm where sources of ferritin and other iron-containing compounds would be located. However, it will require a great deal of research to separate the invasiveness of these pathogens from other characteristics that allow extracellular and intracellular growth.

### 7.4.2.3 Yersinia Species

*7.4.2.3.1 Congo Red Binding.* *Yersinia pestis* was the first bacterial colony shown to adsorb Congo Red (197). Pigmentation in *Y. pestis* is denoted by P or Pgm and is defined by the appearance of red colonies on Congo Red agar or brown colonies on heme-containing medium. Adsorption or binding of heme and Congo Red has been associated with virulence (203). The derivation of the non-pigmented strains possessing all other known virulence factors led to the derivation of the EV vaccine strains and the realization that these cells regained lethality in experimental animals when injected with iron (204). In addition to Congo Red binding, Wake et al. (205) found that siderophore production correlated well with pigmentation. Crude siderophore extracts also enhanced the lethality of Pgm mutants during infections. Although Perry and Brubaker (206) confirmed finding a similar factor, they could not corroborate its activity during competition with more efficient iron chelators (e.g., conalbumin). Although growth of other species, *Y. enterocolitica* and *Y. pseudotuberculosis*, was stimulated by other bacterial siderophores (aerobactin, enterochelin, schizokinen, and desferal), iron-starved *Y. pestis* would not use these sources. All *Yersinia* species could use hemin, even the Pgm mutants, but they did not turn brown. Therefore it appears that pigmentation was not a characteristic of the transport of hemin, but had something to do with either the removal of iron and hemin from protein ligands or with the storage of iron (206). Following the development of a more appropriate medium to assay growth in low iron medium, growth differences between Pgm+ and Pgm− bacteria have been detected (207). Not only did the Pgm− cells have a greater demand for iron, but they converted into osmotically stable spheroplasts when incubated under iron starvation conditions. A collection of findings with *Y. pestis* appear to be similar to the picture emerging with *S. flexneri*. Pigmentation has something to do with the acquisition of iron intracellularly, but there is another, perhaps closely linked locus, that allows cytoplasmic entry and intracellular growth. Closely linked genes confuse the analysis of iron acquisition by these intracellular parasites. The pathogenesis by the other *Yersinia* species is different from that of *Y. pestis*, and no growth differences have been detected between Pgm+ and Pgm− strains. These strains are also different in that they must survive within other non-macrophage, phagocytic cells. Attention is being directed to the proteins of the outer membrane in bacteria grown under different iron concentrations, and investigators have found two iron-regulated proteins that have been associated with virulence demonstrated by species other than *Y. pestis* (208, 209).

### 7.4.2.4 *Mycobacterium Species*

*7.4.2.4.1 Facultative Intracellular Parasites.* This discussion ends with the bacterium in which investigations of siderophores and siderophore effects on lethality were initiated. *Mycobacterium tuberculosis* is a facultative intracellular parasite typically causing chronic lung disease. However, in some hosts it can produce a fulminating disease ending in miliary tuberculosis and widespread caseating lesions. Owing to the virulence and the prolonged generation time of *M. tuberculosis*, other *Mycobacteria* species have been used for in vitro studies.

*7.4.2.4.2 Cell-bound Siderophore Production.* Mycobacteria produce a complex series of compounds called mycobactins, comprised of salicyl rings and hydroxamate iron-binding moieties (142). These bacteria were found to be very fastidious after isolation from the disease state, and the "essential factor" (142) that allowed growth in culture medium was identified as lipid-soluble mycobactin. Media were developed to assay concentrations of these growth factors and also to demonstrate that these factors were vital to the growth of *Mycobacteria* species in serum and transferrin-containing media (210, 211). The first demonstration that bacterial factors could help feed bacteria during infection was by Wheeler and Hanks (212). This was an amazing demonstration of an exogenous factor affecting the growth of intracellular bacteria (212, 213). The cell-bound feature of mycobactins appeared to be important to pathogenicity, because those strains that released mycobactins were less virulent (211). Although cell-bound siderophores may be important to bacteria obtaining iron during infection owing to theoretical problems of diffusion of ferrisiderophores over large distances of well-mixed fluids, active transport in vitro appeared to depend upon soluble iron-binding factors called exochelins (214). These factors were predominantly collections of different salicyl compounds (215), but in some cases, had some specificities for particular species of *Mycobacterium* (216). There may be several different forms of exochelin-mediated iron transport including exochelin-mycobactin exchange (216, 217). Current studies have determined some of the structural differences between mycobactins (218). However, much more research is needed on the role of iron acquisition and transport in the intracellular ecology. It is essential to understand extracellular and cell-bound siderophore functions mediating iron mobilization and iron transport in both the extracellular and intracellular ecologies.

## 7.5  CONCLUSIONS

Iron and iron-containing compounds stimulate bacterial lethality during infections. However, host–parasite interactions are so complex and ill understood that few conclusions can be drawn from these studies. Bacterial virulence with respect to iron acquisition is also difficult to determine. At this point in human knowledge, it appears that pathogens occupying either intracellular ecologies or attachment sites at epithelial surfaces obtain iron for growth by unknown mechanisms. In addition, these mechanisms are apparently so highly evolved and integrated into the physiology of the pathogens that, like those in *Shigella* and *Yersinia* species, they are very difficult to discern.

So far, there are two cases in which iron-related virulence factors may be defined for bacteria. Anguibactin allows the growth and pathogenicity of *V. anguillarum*. This siderophore is a virulence factor because it is absolutely required for disease production. Although it is not as well defined, I anticipate that aerobactin will soon be defined as a virulence factor for numerous enteric bacteria. Although these bacteria are largely opportunists, their virulence or their capability to take advantage of the compromised host's defense mechanisms appears to depend upon production of aerobactin.

Therefore the only examples in which iron acquisition mechanisms appear to be obvious virulence factors are for bacteria with the least evolutionary adaptation to the mammalian environment. Possibly, increased evolutionary experience allows bacteria to find mechanisms for iron acquisition other than competition with transferrin. Poorly adapted bacteria, or opportunists, are forced to compete with the iron-binding proteins of the host. However, with increased study, iron-acquisition mechanisms may be discovered in highly evolved pathogens such as *Salmonella, Shigella,* and *Mycobacteria.* They may be similar to the mechanisms demonstrated by *Neisseria* species, involving direct binding of host iron-containing compounds.

Many experiments in my own research laboratory have begun on growth and clearance assays in animals using the opportunistic pathogen *P. aeruginosa*. The amount of apparent bacteriostasis produced by the animal has always been an obvious and powerful defense mechanism. However, removing the serum from that animal and attempting to observe bacteriostasis in vitro has often been disappointing. Usually, although there may be some retardation of the growth rate, the bacterial growth curve is surprisingly rapid. Therefore, although our investigations tend to isolate factors for precise study, an entire understanding must depend upon integration of our knowledge of the isolated factors back into the complexity of defense mechanisms operative in the animal. From our studies with *P. aeruginosa* it is obvious that we do not yet understand all of the bacteriostatic mechanisms against bacterial growth during infections in animals or humans.

## ACKNOWLEDGMENTS

The research discussed that was done in my laboratory was supported by U.S. Public Health Service Grant AI 13120 from the National Institutes of Health.

## REFERENCES

1. Bullen, J. J. 1981. The significance of iron in infection. Rev. Infect. Dis. *3*:1127.
2. Weinberg, E. E. 1984. Iron withholding: a defense against infection and neoplasia. Physiol. Rev. *64*:65.
3. Weinberg, E. D. 1986. "Iron as a factor in disease development in animals," in T. R. Swinburne, Ed. *Iron, Siderophores, and Plant Diseases*. Plenum, New York, p. 203.
4. Barclay, R. 1985. The role of iron in infection. Med. Lab. Sci. *42*:166.
5. van Asbeck, B. S., and J. Verhoef. 1983. Iron and host defense. Eur. J. Clin. Microbiol. *2*:6.
6. Finkelstein, R. A., C. V. Sciortino, and M. A. McIntosh. 1983. Role of iron in microbe–host interactions. Rev. Infect. Dis. *5*:S759.
7. Kochan, I. 1977. "Role of siderophores in nutritional immunity and bacterial parasitism," in E. D. Weinberg, Ed., *Microorganisms and Minerals*. Dekker, New York. 1977.
8. Miles, A. A. 1955. "The meaning of pathogenicity," in *Mechanisms of Microbial Pathogenicity*, Cambridge University Press, New York, p. 1.
9. Weinberg, E. D. 1974. Iron and susceptibility to infectious disease. Science. *184*:952.
10. Holmberg, C. G., and C. B. Laurell. 1947. Investigation in serum copper. I. Nature of serum copper and its relation to the iron-binding proteins in human serum. Acta. Chem. Scand. *1*:944.
11. Schade, A. L. 1963. Significance of serum iron for the growth, biological characteristics, and metabolism of *Staphylococcus aureus*. Biochem. Z. *338*:140.
12. Martin, C. M. 1962. Relation of transferrin to serum bacteriostatic activity in agammaglobulinemic and other patients. Am. J. Med. Sci. *244*:334.
13. Masson, P. L., J. F. Heremans, and C. Dive. 1966. An iron-binding protein common to many external secretions. Clin. Chim. Acta *14*:735.
14. Aisen, P., and I. Listowsky. 1980. Iron transport and storage proteins. Ann. Rev. Biochem. *49*:357.
15. Lestas, A. N. 1976. The effect of pH upon human transferrin: selective labelling of the two iron-binding sites. Br. J. Haematol. *32*:341.

16. Freter, R., and G. W. Jones. 1983. Models for studying the role of bacterial attachment in virulence and pathogenesis. Rev. Infect. Dis. *5*:S647.

17. Mims, C. A. 1976. In *The Pathogenesis of Infectious Disease*. Academic, London, p. 36.

18. Welsh, J. K., and J. T. May. 1979. Anti-infective properties of breast milk. J. Ped. *94*:1.

19. Bullen, C. L., and A. T. Willis. 1971. Resistance of the breast-fed infant to gastroenteritis. Br. Med. J. *3*:338.

20. Goldman, A. S. 1973. Host resistance factors in human milk. J. Ped. *82*:1082.

21. Spik, G., B. Brunet, C. Mazurier-Dehaine, G. Fontaine, and J. Montreuil. 1982. Characterization and properties of the human and bovine lactotransferrin extracted from the faeces of newborn infants. Acta Paediatr. Scand. *71*:979.

22. Spitznagel, J. K., F. G. Dalldorf, M. S. Leffell, J. D. Folds, I. R. H. Welsh, M. H. Cooney, and L. E. Martin. 1974. Character of azurophil and specific granules purified from human polymorphonuclear leukocytes. Lab. Invest. *30*:774.

23. Bortner, C. A., R. D. Miller, and R. R. Arnold. 1986. Bactericidal effect of lactoferrin on *Legionella pneumophila*. Infect. Immun. *51*:373.

24. Arnold, R. R., M. Brewer, and J. J. Gauthier. 1980. Bactericidal activity of human lactoferrin: sensitivity of a variety of microorganisms. Infect. Immun. *28*:893.

25. Arnold, R. R., J. E. Russell, W. J. Champion, M. Brewer, and J. J. Gauthier. 1982. Bactericidal activity of human lactoferrin: differentiation from the stasis of iron deprivation. Infect. Immun. *35*:792.

26. Oseas, R., H. H. Yang, R. L. Baehner, and L. A. Boxer. 1981. Lactoferrin: a promoter of polymorphonuclear leukocyte adhesiveness. Blood *57*:939.

27. Masson, P. L., J. F. Heremans, and E. Schonne. 1969. Lactoferrin, an iron-binding protein in neutrophilic leukocytes. J. Exp. Med. *130*:643.

28. Abrusco, D. R., and R. B. Johnston. 1981. Lactoferrin enhances hydroxyl radical production by human neutrophils, neutrophil particulate fraction, and an enzymatic generating system. J. Clin. Invest. *67*:357.

29. Griffiths, E., and J. Humphreys. 1977. Bacteriostatic effect of human milk and bovine colostrum on *Escherichia coli*: importance of bicarbonate. Infect. Immun. *15*:396.

30. Ward, C. G., J. S. Hammond, and J. J. Bullen. 1986. Effect of iron compounds on antibacterial function of human polymorphs and plasma. Infect. Immun. *51*:723.

31. Menkin, V. 1956. "The role of the hydrogen iron concentration and the cytology of an exudate. Glycolysis in the inflammation. Some aspects of the chemistry of exudates," in *Biochemical Reactions in Inflammation*. Charles C Thomas, Springfield, p. 66.

32. Guttenberg, T. J., B. Haneberg, and T. Jorgensen. 1984. Lactoferrin in relation to acute phase proteins in sera from newborn infants with severe infections. Eur. J. Pediatr. *142*:37.

33. Venge, P., T. Foucard, J. Henriksen, L. Hakansson, and A. Kreuger. 1984.

Serum-levels of lactoferrin, lysozyme, and myeloperoxidase in normal, infection-prone, and leukemic children. Clin. Chim. Acta. *136*:121.

34. Torrance, J. D., R. W. Charlton, M. O. Simon, S. R. Lynch, and T. H. Bothwell. 1978. The mechanism of endotoxin-induced hypoferraemia. Scand. J. Haematol. *21*:403.

35. Ballantyne, G. H. 1984. A rapid drop in serum iron concentration as a host defense mechanism. Am. Surg. *50*:405.

36. Kochan, I. 1973. The role of iron in bacterial infections, with special consideration of host-tubercle bacillus interaction. Curr. Top. Microbiol. *60*:1.

37. Cartwright, G. E., M. A. Lauritsen, S. Humphreys, P. J. Jones, I. M. Merril, and M. M. Wintrobe. 1946. The anemia of infection. II. The experimental production of hypoferremia and anemia in dogs. J. Clin. Invest. *25*:81.

38. Letendre, E. D., and B. E. Holbein. 1984. Mechanism of impaired iron release by the reticulendothelial system during the hypoferremic phase of experimental *Neisseria meningitidis* infection in mice. Infect. Immun. *44*:320.

39. Letendre, E. D., and B. E. Holbein. 1984. Ceruloplasmin and regulation of transferrin iron during *Neisseria meningitidis* infections in mice. Infect. Immun. *45*:133.

40. Pryjma, J., T. Herman, J. Zebrak, J. Gawel, S. Herman, and A. Scislicki. 1985. Studies of bronchial secretion. The influence of inflammatory response and bacterial infection. Ann. Aller. *54*:60.

41. Payne, S. M., and R. A. Finkelstein. 1978. The critical role of iron in host-bacterial interaction. J. Clin. Invest. *61*:1428.

42. Schade, A. L., and L. Caroline. 1944. Raw hen egg white and the role of iron in growth inhibition of *Shigella dysenteriae, Staphylococcus aureus, Escherichia coli,* and *Saccharomyces cerevisiae.* Science *100*:14.

43. Schade, A. L., and L. Caroline. 1946. An iron binding component in human blood plasma. Science *104*:340.

44. Miles, A. A., P. L. Khimji, and J. Maskell. 1978. The variable response of bacteria to excess ferric iron in host tissues. J. Med. Microbiol. *12*:17.

45. Maskell, J. P., and A. A. Miles. 1984. The variable response of bacteria to free haemoglobin in the tissues. J. Med. Microbiol. *18*:377.

46. Sawatzki, G., F. A. Hoffmann, and B. Kubanek. 1983. Acute iron overload in mice: pathogenesis of *Salmonella typhimurium* infection. Infect. Immun. *39*:659.

47. Jones, R. L., C. M. Petersen, R. W. Grady, T. Kumbaraci, A. Cerami, and J. Graziano. 1977. Effect of iron chelators and iron overload on *Salmonella* infection. Nature *267*:63.

48. Bullen, J. J., and H. J. Rogers. 1969. Bacterial iron metabolism and immunity to *Pasteurella septica* and *Escherichia coli.* Nature *224*:380.

49. Al-Sultan, I., and I. D. Aitken. 1984. Promotion of *Pasteurella hemolytica* infection in mice by iron. Res. Vet. Sci. *36*:385.

50. Bullen, J. J., L. C. Leigh, and H. J. Rogers. 1968. The effect of iron compounds on the virulence of *Escherichia coli* for guinea-pigs. Immunology *15*:581.

51. Forseberg, C. M., and J. J. Bullen. 1972. The effect of passage and iron on the virulence of *Pseudomonas aeruginosa* J. Clin. Pathol. *25*:65.

52. Cox, C. D., 1979. Passage of *Pseudomonas aeruginosa* in compromised mice. Infect. Immun. *26*:118.

53. Ford, A., and J. P. V. Haghor. 1976. An investigation of alternatives to gastric mucin or virulence-enhancing agents in the cholera vaccine potency assay. J. Biol. Stand. *4*:353.

54. Archibald, F. S., I. W. DeVoe. 1978. Iron in *Neisseria meningitidis*: minimum requirements, effects of limitation, and characteristics of uptake. J. Bacteriol. *136*:35.

55. Calver, G. A., C. P. Kenny, and G. Lavergne. 1976. Iron as a replacement for mucin in the establishment of meningococcal infection in mice. Can. J. Microbiol. *22*:832.

56. Mellencamp, M. W., M. A. McCabe, and I. Kochan. 1981. The growth-promoting effect of bacterial iron for serum-exposed bacteria. Immunol. *43*:483.

57. Henderson, L. C., S. Kadis, W. L. Champman. 1978. Influence of iron on *Corynebacterium renale*-induced pyelonephritis in a rat experimental model. Infect. Immun. *21*:540.

58. Woods, D. E., P. A. Sokol, and B. H. Iglewski. 1982. Modulating effect of iron on the pathogenesis of *Pseudomonas aeruginosa* mouse corneal infections. Infect. Immun. *35*:461.

59. Sokol, P. A., and D. E. Woods. 1984. Relationship of iron and extracellular virulence factors to *Pseudomonas aeruginosa* lung infections. J. Med. Microbiol. *18*:125.

60. Maw, J., and G. G. Meynell. 1968. The true division and death rates of *Salmonella typhimurium* in the mouse spleen determined with the superinfecting phage P22. Br. J. Exp. Pathol. *49*:597.

61. Polk, H. C., and A. A. Miles. 1973. The decisive period in the primary infection of muscle by *Escherichia coli*. Br. J. Exp. Pathol. *54*:99.

62. Meynell, G. G., and T. V. Subbaiah. 1963. Antibacterial mechanisms of the mouse gut. I. Kinetics of infection by *Salmonella typhimurium* in normal and streptomycin-treated mice studied with abortive transductants. Br. J. Exp. Pathol. *44*:197.

63. Sigel, S. P., R. A. Finkelstein, and C. D. Parker. 1981. Ability of an avirulent mutant of *Vibrio cholerae* to colonize in the infant mouse upper bowel. Infect. Immun. *32*:474.

64. Hooke, A. M., D. V. Sordelli, M. C. Cerquetti, and A. J. Vogt. 1985. Quantitative determination of bacterial replication in vivo. Infect. Immun. *49*:424.

65. Sordelli, D. V., M. C. Cerquetti, and A. M. Gooke. 1985. Replication rate of Pseudomonas aeruginosa in the murine lung. Infect. Immun. *50*:383.

66. Neilands, J. B. 1982. Microbial envelope proteins related to iron. Ann. Rev. Microbiol. *36*:285.

67. Brown, M. R. W., and P. Williams. 1985. The influence of environment on envelope properties affecting survival of bacteria in infections. Ann. Rev. Microbiol. *39*:527.

68. Griffiths, E., P. Stevenson, and P. Joyce. 1983. Pathogenic *Escherichia coli* express new outer membrane proteins when growing in vivo. FEMS Micobiol. Lett. *16*:95.

69. Brown, M. R. W., H. Anwar, and P. A. Lambert. 1984. Evidence that mucoid *Pseudomonas aeruginosa* in the cystic fibrosis lung grows under iron-restricted conditions. FEMS Microbiol. Lett. *21*:113.

70. Shand, G. H., H. Anwar, J. Kadurugamuwa, M. R. W. Brown, S. H. Silverman, and J. Melling. 1985. In vivo evidence that bacteria in urinary tract infection grow under iron-restricted conditions. Infect. Immun. *48*:35.

71. Lam, C., F. Turnowsky, E. Schwarzinger, and W. Neruda. 1984. Bacteria recovered without subculture from infected human urines expressed iron-regulated outer membrane proteins. FEMS Microbiol. Lett. *24*:255.

72. Turnowsky, F., M. R. W. Brown, H. Anwar, P. H. Lambert. 1983. Effect of iron limitation of growth rate on the binding of penicillin G to the penicillin binding proteins of mucoid and non-mucoid strains of *Pseudomonas aeruginosa* FEMS Microbiol. Lett. *17*:243.

73. Kadurugamuwa, J. J., H. Anwar, M. R. W. Brown, and O. Zak. 1985. Effect of subinhibitory concentrations of cephalosporins on surface properties and siderophore production in iron-depleted *Klebsiella pneumoniae*. Antimicrobial Agent. Chemother. *27*:220.

74. Brown, M. R. W., and P. Williams. 1984. Influence of substrate limitation and growth phase on sensitivity to antimicrobial agents. J. Antimicrobial Chemother. *15*(Suppl A):7.

75. Moore, D. G., and C. F. Earhart. 1981. Specific inhibition of *Escherichia coli* ferrienterochelin uptake by normal human serum immunoglobulin. Infect. Immun. *31*:631.

76. Craven, D. E., M. S. Peppler, C. E. Frasch, L. F. Mocca, P. P. McGrath, and G. Washington. 1980. Adherence of isolates of *Neisseria meningitidis* from patients and carriers to human buccal epithelial cells. J. Infect. Dis. *142*:556.

77. Anderson, B., B. Eriksson, E. Falsen, A. Fogh, L. A. Hanson, D. Nylen, H. Peterson, and C. S. Eden. 1981. Adhesion of *Streptococcus pneumoniae* to human pharyngeal epithelial cells in vitro: differences in adhesive capacity among strains isolated from subjects with otitis media, septicemia, meningitis or from healthy carriers. Infect. Immun. *32*:311.

78. Ramphal, R., and G. B. Pier. 1985. Role of *Pseudomonas aeruginosa* mucoid exopolysaccharide in adherence to tracheal cells. Infect. Immun. *47*:1.

79. Sutherland, I. W. 1983. Microbial expopolysaccharides. Their role in microbial adhesion in aqueous systems. Crit. Rev. Microbiol. *10*:173.

80. Bartell, P. F. 1983. Determinants of the biologic activity of surface slime in experimental *Pseudomonas aeruginosa* infections. Rev. Infect. Dis. *5*:S871.

81. Peterson, P. K., Y. Kim, D. Schmeling, M. Lindemann, J. Verhoef, and P. G. Quie. 1978. Complement-mediated phagocytosis of *Pseudomonas aeruginosa* J. Lab. Clin. Med. *92*:883.

82. Ogata, R. T. 1982. Factors determining bacterial pathogenicity. Clin. Physiol. Biochem. *1*:145.

83. Traub, W. H. 1977. Further studies on the susceptibility of *Serratia marcescens* to the bactericidal activity of human serum. Exp. Cell Biol. *45*:184.

84. Morse, S. A., C. S. Mintz, S. K. Sarafian, L. Bartenstein, M. Bertram, and M. A. Apicella. 1983. Effect of dilution rate on lipopolysaccharide and serum

resistance of *Neisseria gonorrhoeae* grown in continuous culture. Infect. Immun. *41*:74.

85. Anwar, H., M. R. W. Brown, and P. A. Lambert. 1983. Effect of nutrient depletion on sensitivity of *Pseudomonas cepacia* to phagocytosis and serum bactericidal activity at different temperatures. J. Gen. Microbiol. *129*:2021.

86. Bjorn, M. J., P. A. Sokol, and B. H. Iglewski. 1979. Influence of iron on yields of extracellular products in *Pseudomonas aeruginosa* cultures. J. Bacteriol. *138*:193.

87. Pappenheimer, A. J., and S. J. Johnson. 1936. Studies in diphtheria toxin production. I. The effect of iron and copper. Br. J. Exp. Pathol. *17*:335.

88. McCardell, B., A. M. Madden, and J. T. Stanfield. 1986. Effect of iron concentration on toxin production in *Campylobacter jejuni* and *Camplyobacter coli*. Can. J. Microbiol. *32*:395.

89. Fletcher, J., and E. Goldstein. 1970. The effect of parenteral iron preparations on experimental pyelonephritis. Br. J. Exp. Pathol. *51*:280.

90. Van Asbeck, B. S., H. A. Verbrugh, B. A. van Oost, J. J. M. Marx, G. W. Imhof, and J. Verhoef. 1982. *Listeria monocytogenes* meningitis and decreased phagocytosis associated with iron overload. Br. Med. J. *284*:542.

91. Van Asbeck, B. S., J. J. M. Marx, A. Struyvenberg, J. H. van Kats, and J. Verhoef. 1984. Effects of iron(III) in the presence of various ligands on the phagocytic and metabolic activity of human polymophonuclear leukocytes. J. Immunol. *132*:851.

92. Gladstone, G. P., and E. Walton. 1971. Effect of iron and haematin on the killing of staphylococci by rabbit polymorphs. Br. J. Exp. Pathol. *52*:452.

93. Bullen, J. J., and S. N. Wallis. 1977. Reversal of the bactericidal effect of polymorphs by a ferritin–antibody complex. FEMS Microbiol. Lett. *1*:117.

94. Ward, C. G., J. S. Hammond, and J. J. Bullen. 1986. Effect of iron on antibacterial function of human polymorphs. Infect. Immun. *51*:723.

95. Nishiya, K., M. DeSousa, E. Tsoi, J. J. Bognacki, and E. De Harven. 1980. Regulation of expression of a human lymphoid cell surface marker by iron. Cell. Immunol. *53*:71.

96. DeSousa, M. 1978. Lymphoid cell positioning: A new proposal for the mechanism of control of lymphoid cell migration. Symp. Soc. Exp. Biol. *32*:393.

97. Griffiths, E. 1975. Effect of pH and haem compounds on the killing of *Pasteurella septica* by specific antiserum. J. Gen. Microbiol. *88*:345.

98. Lankford, C. E. 1973. Bacterial assimilation of iron. Crit. Rev. Microbiol. *2*:273.

99. O'Brien, I. G., and F. Gibson. 1979. The structure of enterochelin and related 2, 3-dihydroxybenzoylserine conjugates from *Escherichia coli*. Biophys. Biochim. Acta. *215*:393.

100. Rogers, H. J. 1973. Iron binding catechols and virulence in *Escherichia coli*. Infect. Immun. *7*:445

101. Carrano, C. J., and K. N. Raymond. 1979. Ferric ion sequestering agents. 2. Kinetics and mechanism of iron removal from transferrin by enterochelin and synthetic tricatechols. J. Am. Chem. Soc. *101*:5401.

102. Konopka, K., and J. B. Neilands. 1984. Effect of serum albumin on siderophore-mediated utilization of transferrin iron. Biochem. *23*:2122.

102. Moore, D. G., R. J. Yancey, C. E. Lankford, and C. R. Earhart. 1980. Bacteriostatic enterochelin-specific immunoglobulin from normal human serum. Infect. Immun. 27:418.

104. Stuart, S. J., K. T. Greenwood, and R. J. K. Luke. 1980. Hydroxamate-mediated transport of iron controlled by Col V plasmids. J. Bacteriol. 143:35.

105. Warner, P. J., P. H. Williams, A. Bindereif, and J. B. Neilands. 1981. Col V plasmid-specified aerobactin synthesis by invasive strains of Escherichia coli. Infect. Immun. 33:540.

106. Braun, V. 1981. Escherichia coli cells containing the plasmid Col V produce the iron ionophore aerobactin. FEMS Microbiol. Lett. 11:225.

107. Williams, P. H. 1979. Novel iron uptake system specified by Col V plasmids: an important component in the virulence of invasive strains of Escherichia coli. Infect. Immun. 26:925.

108. Konopka, K., A. Bindereif, and J. B. Neilands. 1982. Aerobactin-mediated utilization of transferrin iron. Biochem. 21:6503.

109. Williams, P. H., and N. H. Carbonetti. 1986. Iron, siderophores, and the pursuit of virulence: independence of the aerobactin and enterochelin iron uptake systems in Escherichia coli. Infect. Immun. 51:942.

110. Valvano, M. A., R. P. Silver, and J. H. Crosa. 1986. Occurrence of chromosome- or plasmid-mediated aerobactin iron transport systems and hemolysin production among clonal groups of human invasive strains of Escherichia coli K1. Infect. Immun. 52:192.

111. Frost, G., and H. Rosenberg. 1973. The inducible citrate-dependent iron transport system in Escherichia coli K12. Biophys. Biochim. Acta. 330:90.

112. Griffiths, E., and J. Humphreys. 1980. Isolation of enterochelin from peritoneal washings of guinea pigs lethally infected with Escherichia coli. Infect. Immun. 28:286.

113. Kochan, I., J. T. Kvach, and T. I. Miles. 1977. Virulence associated acquisition of iron in mammalian serum by Escherichia coli. J. Infect. Dis. 135:623.

114. Lory, S., P. C. Tai, and B. D. Davis. 1983. Mechanism of protein excretion by gram-negative bacteria: Pseudomonas aeruginosa exotoxin A. J. Bacteriol. 156:695.

115. Fitzgerald, S. P., and H. J. Rogers. 1980. Bacteriostatic effect of serum: role of antibody to lipopolysaccharide. Infect. Immun. 27:302.

116. Selander, R. K., T. K. Korhanen, V. Vaisanen-Rhen, P. H. Williams, E. Pattison, and D. A. Caugant. 1986. Genetic relationship and clonal structure of strains of Escherichia coli causing neonatal septicemia and meningitis. Infect. Immun. 52:213.

117. Green, C. P., and V. L. Thomas. 1981. Hemagglutination of human type O erythrocytes, hemolysin production, and serogrouping of Escherichia coli isolates from patients with acute pyelonephritis, cystitis, and asymptomatic bacteriuria. Infect. Immun. 31:309.

118. Minshew, B. H., J. Jorgensen, G. W. Counts, and S. Falkow. 1978. Association of hemolysin production, hemagglutination of human erythrocytes and virulence for chicken embryos of extraintestinal Escherichia coli isolates. Infect. Immun. 20:50.

119. Cavalieri, S. J., G. A. Bohach, and I. S. Snyder. 1984. *Escherichia coli* hemolysin: characteristic and probable role in pathogenicity. Microbiol. Rev. *48*:326.

120. Smith, H. W. 1963. The haemolysins of *Escherichia coli*. J. Pathol. Bacteriol. *85*:197.

121. Purcell, C. J., and R. A. Finkelstein. 1966. Virulence of *Escherichia coli* strains for chick embryos. J. Bacteriol. *91*:1410.

122. Welsh, R. A., E. P. Dellinger, B. Minshew, and S. Falkow. 1981. Hemolysin contributes to virulence of extraintestinal *Escherichia coli* infections. Nature (London) *294*:665.

123. van den Bosch, J. F., L. Embody, and I. Ketyi. 1982. Virulence of hemolytic strains of *Escherichia coli* in various animal models. FEMS Microbiol. Lett. *13*:427.

124. Bornside, G. H., P. J. Vouis, and I. Cohn. 1968. Haemoglobin and *Escherichia coli*: a lethal intraperitoneal combination. J. Bacteriol. *95*:1567.

125. Linggood, M. A., and P. L. Ingram. 1982. The role of alpha hemolysin in the virulence of *Escherichia coli* for mice. J. Med. Micro. *15*:23.

126. Lebek, G., and H-M. Gruenig. 1985. Relation between the hemolytic property and iron metabolism in *Escherichia coli*. Infect. Immun. *50*:682.

127. Eaton, J. W., P. Brandt, and J. R. Mahony. 1982. Haptoglobin: a natural bacteriostat. Science *215*:691.

128. Owen, J. A., R. Smith, R. Padayi, and J. Martin. 1964. Serum haptoglobin in disease. Clin. Science *26*:1.

129. Muller-Eberhard, V., and H. H. Lien. 1975. Hemopexin, the heme-binding serum beta-glycoprotein. La Ricerca in Clinica e in Laboratorio *5*:275.

130. Bhakdi, S., N. Mackman, J-M. Nicaud, and I. B. Holland. 1986. *Escherichia coli* hemolysin may damage target cell membranes by generating transmembrane pores. Infect. Immun. *52*:63.

131. Tidmarsh, G. F., P. E. Kebba, and L. T. Rosenberg. 1983. Rapid release of iron from ferritin by siderophores. J. Inorg. Biochem. *18*:161.

132. Birgegqard, G. 1980. The source of serum ferritin during infection. Studies with concanavalin A-Sepharose absorption. Clin. Sci. *59*:385.

133. Nassif, X., and P. J. Sonsonetti. 1986. Correlation of the virulence of *Klebsiella pneumoniae* K1 and K2 with the presence of a plasmid encoding aerobactin. Infect. Immun. *54*:603.

134. Krone, W. J. A., G. Komingstein, F. K. deGraf, and B. Oudega. 1985. Plasmid-determined cloacin DF13-susceptibility in *Enterobacter cloacae* and *Kelbsiella edwardsii*, identification of the cloacin DF13/aerobactin outer membrane receptor proteins. Antonie van Leuwenhoek J. Microbiol Serol. *51*:203.

135. Mizuta, K., M. Ohta, M. Mori, T. Hasegawn, I. Nakashima, and N. Kato. 1983. Virulence for mice of K strains belonging to the O1 group: relationship to their capsular (K) types. Infect. Immun. *40*:56.

136. Williams, P., M. R. W. Brown, and P. A. Lamber. 1984. Effect of iron deprivation on the production of siderophores and outer membrane proteins in *Klebsiella aerogenes*. J. Gen. Microbiol. *130*:2357.

137. Cox, C. D., and R. Graham. 1979. Isolation of an iron-binding compound from *Pseudomonas aeruginosa.* J. Bacteriol. *137*:357.

138. Cox, C. D., K. L. Rinehart, M. L. Moore, and J. C. Cook. 1981. Pyochelin: novel structure of an iron-chelating growth promoter for *Pseudomonas aeruginosa.* Proc. Natl. Acad. Sci. *78*:4256.

139. Cox, C. D., and P. Adams. 1985. Siderophore activity of pyoverdin for *Pseudomonas aeruginosa.* Infect. Immun. *48*:130.

140. Wendenbaum, S., P. Demange, A. Dell, J. M. Meyer, and M. A. Abdallah. 1983. The structure of Pyoverdine Pa, the siderophore of *Pseudomonas aeruginosa.* Tetrahedron Lett. *24*:4877.

141. Brisket, G., K. Faraz, and H. Budzikiewicz. 1985. Siderophore von pyoverdintyp aus *Pseudomonas aeruginosa* [1]. A. Naturforsch. *41*:497.

142. Snow, G. A. 1970. Mycobactin: iron chelating growth factors from *Mycobacteria.* Bacteriol. Rev. *34*:99.

143. Cox, C. D. 1982. Effect of pyochelin on the virulence of *Pseudomonas aeruginosa.* Infect. Immun. *36*:17.

144. Ankenbauer, R., S. Sriyosachati, and C. D. Cox. 1985. Effects of siderophores on the growth of *Pseudomonas aeruginosa* in human serum and transferrin. Infect. Immun. *49*:132.

145. Sriyosachati, S., and C. D. Cox. 1986. Siderophore-mediated iron acquisition from transferrin by *Pseudomonas aeruginosa.* Infect. Immun. *52*:885.

146. Ankenbauer, R., L. F. Hanne, C. D. Cox. 1986. Mapping of mutations in *Pseudomonas aeruginosa* defective in pyoverdin production. J. Bacteriol. *167*:7.

147. Hohnadel, D., D. Haas, and J. M. Meyer. 1986. Mapping of mutations affecting pyoverdine production in *Pseudomonas aeruginosa.* FEMS Microbiol. Lett. *36*:195.

148. Turner, J. M., and A. J. Messenger. "Occurrence, biochemistry, and physiology of phenazine pigments," In A. H. Rose and D. W. Tempest, Eds., Adv. Microb. Physiol. *27*:221.

149. Gessard, C. 1882. On the blue and green coloration that appears on bandages. C. R. Seances Acad. Sci. Paris. *94*:536.

150. Cox, C. D. 1986. Role of pyocyanin in the acquisition of iron from transferrin. Infect. Immun. *52*:263.

151. Kojima, N., and G. W. Bates. 1979. The reduction and release of iron from $Fe^{3+}$ transferrin $CO_3^{2-}$. J. Biol. Chem. *254*:8847.

152. Bezkorovainy, A., N. Topouzian, and R. Miller-Catchpole. 1986. Mechanisms of ferric and ferrous iron uptake by *Bifidobacterium bifidum* var. pennsylvanicus. Clin. Physiol. Biochem. *4*:150.

153. Evans, S. L., J. E. L. Arceneaux, B. R. Byers, M. E. Martin, and H. Aranha. 1986. Ferrous iron transport in *Streptococcus mutans.* J. Bacteriol. *168*:1096.

154. Cowart, R. E., and B. G. Foster. 1985. Differential effects of iron on the growth of *Listeria monocytogenes*: minimum requirements and mechanism of acquisition. J. Infect. Dis. *151*:721.

155. May, J. R., N. C. Herrick, and D. Thompson. 1972. Bacterial infection in cystic fibrosis. Arch. Dis. Child. *47*:908.

156. Govan, J. R. W. 1975. Mucoid strains of *Pseudomonas aeruginosa*: the influence of culture medium on the stability of mucus production. J. Med. Microbiol. *8*:513.

157. Ohman, D. E., and A. M. Chakrabarty. 1982. Utilization of human respiratory secretions by mucoid *Pseudomonas aeruginosa* of cystic fibrosis origin. Infect. Immun. *37*:662.

158. Boyce, J. R., and R. V. Miller. 1982. Selection of nonmucoid derivatives of mucoid *Pseudomonas aeruginosa* is strongly influenced by the level of iron in the culture medium. Infect. Immun. *37*:695.

159. Anwar, H., M. R. W. Brown, A. Day, and P. H. Weller. 1984. Outer membrane antigens of mucoid *Pseudomonas aeruginosa* isolated directly from the sputum of a cystic fibrosis patient. FEMS Microbiol. Lett. *24*:235.

160. Guerra-Santos, L., O. Kappeli, and A. Fiechter. 1984. *Pseudomonas aeruginosa* biosurfactant production in continuous culture with glucose as carbon source. Appl. Environ. Microbiol. *48*:301.

161. Costerton, J. W., J. Lam, K. Lam, and R. Chan. 1983. The role of the microcolony mode of growth in the pathogenesis of *Pseudomonas aeruginosa* infections. Rev. Infect. Dis. *5*:S867.

162. Ombaka, E. A., R. M. Cozens, and M. R. W. Brown. 1983. Influence of nutrient limitation of growth on stability and production of virulence factors of mucoid and nonmucoid strains of *Pseudomonas aeruginosa*. Rev. Infect. Dis. *5*:S880.

163. Costerton, J. W. 1984. The etiology and persistence of cryptic bacterial infections: a hypothesis. Rev. Infect. Dis. *6*:S608.

164. Costerton, J. W., R. T. Irvin, and K. J. Cheng. 1981. The bacterial glycocalyx in nature and disease. Ann. Rev. Microbiol. *35*:299.

165. Payne, S. M., and R. A. Finkelstein. 1978. Siderophore production by *Vibrio cholerae*. Infect. Immun. *20*:310.

166. Griffiths, G. L., S. P. Sigel, S. M. Payne, and J. B. Neilands. 1984. Vibriobactin, a siderophore from *Vibrio cholerae*. J. Biol. Chem. *259*:383.

167. Sciortino, C. V., and R. A. Finkelstein. 1983. *Vibrio cholerae* expresses iron-regulated outer membrane proteins in vivo. Infect. Immun. *42*:990.

168. Sigel, S. P., and S. M. Payne. 1982. Effect of iron limitation on growth, siderophore production, and expression of outer membrane proteins of *Vibrio cholerae*. J. Bacteriol. *150*:148.

169. Payne, S. M., and R. A. Finkelstein. 1978. The critical role of iron in host-bacterial interactions. J. Clin. Invest. *61*:1428.

170. Sigel, S. P., J. A. Stoebner, and S. M. Payne. 1985. Iron-vibriobactin transport system is not required for virulence of *Vibrio cholerae*. Infect. Immun. *47*:360.

171. Wolf, M. K., and J. H. Crosa. 1986. Evidence for the role of a siderophore in promoting *Vibrio anguillarum* infections. J. Gen. Microbiol. *132*:2949.

172. Helms, S. D., J. D. Oliver, and J. C. Travis. 1984. Role of heme compounds and haptoglobin in *Vibrio vulnificus* pathogenicity. Infect. Immun. *45*:345.

173. Payne, S. M., and R. A. Finkelstein. 1975. Pathogenesis and immunology of experimental gonococcal infection: role of iron in virulence. Infect. Immun. *12*:1313.

174. Odugbemi, T. O., and S. Hafiz. 1978. The effects of iron chelators on the colonial morphology of *Neisseria gonorrhoeae*. J. Gen. Microbiol. *104*:165.

175. Odugbemi, T. O., and B. Dean. 1978. Iron contents of different colonial types of *Neisseria gonorrhoeae*. J. Gen. Microbiol. *104*:161.

176. Holbein, B. E. 1980. Iron-controlled infection with *Neisseria meningitidis* in mice. Infect. Immun. *29*:886.

177. Archibald, F. S., and I. W. DeVoe. 1978. Iron in *Neisseria meningitidis*: minimum requirements, effects of limitation, and characteristics of uptake. J. Bacteriol. *136*:35.

178. Holbein, B. E. 1981. Enhancement of *Neisseria meningitidis* infections in mice by addition of iron bound to transferrin. Infect. Immun. *34*:120.

179. Yancey, R. J., and R. A. Finkelstein. 1981. Siderophore production by pathogenic *Neisseria* spp. Infect. Immun. *32*:600.

180. Norrod, P., and R. P. Williams. 1978. Growth of *Neisseria gonorrhoeae* in media deficient in iron without detection of siderophores. Current Microbiol. *1*:281.

181. West, S. E. H., and P. F. Sparling. 1985. Response of *Neisseria gonorrhoeae* to iron limitation: alterations in expression of membrane proteins without apparent siderophore production. Infect. Immun. *47*:388.

182. Archibald, F. S., and I. W. DeVoe. 1980. Iron acquisition by *Neisseria meningitidis* in vitro. Infect. Immun. *27*:322.

183. Mickelsen, P. A., and P. F. Sparling. 1981. Ability of *Neisseria gonorrhoeae*, *Neisseria meningitidis*, and commensal *Neisseria* species to obtain iron from transferrin and iron compounds. Infect. Immun. *33*:555.

184. Mickelsen, P. A., E. Blackman, and P. F. Sparling. 1982. Ability of *Neisseria gonorrhoeae*, and *Neisseria meningitidis*, and commensal *Neisseria* species to obtain iron from lactoferrin. Infect. Immun. *35*:915.

185. Simonson, C., D. Brener, and I. W. DeVoe. 1982. Expression of a high-affinity mechanism for acquisition of transferrin iron by *Neisseria meningitidis*. Infect. Immun. *36*:107.

186. Brener, D., I. W. DeVoe, and B. E. Holbein. 1981. Increased virulence of *Neisseria meningitidis* after in vitro iron-limited growth at low pH. Infect. Immun. *33*:59.

187. Mietzner, T. A., G. H. Luginbuhl, E. C. Sandstrom, and S. A. Morse. 1984. Identification of an iron-regulated 37,000 dalton protein in the cell envelope of *Neisseria gonorrhoeae*. Infect. Immun. *45*:410.

188. Mietzner, T. A., R. C. Barnes, Y. A. JeanLouis, W. M. Shafer, and S. A. Morse. 1986. Distribution of an antigenically related iron-regulated protein among the *Neisseria* spp.. Infect. Immun. *51*:60.

189. Herrington, D. A., and P. F. Sparling. 1985. *Haemophilus influenzae* can use human transferrin as a sole source for required iron. Infect. Immun. *48*:248.

190. Stull, T. L. 1987. Protein sources of heme for *Haemophilus influenzae*. Infect. Immun. *55*:148.

191. Pollack, J. R., and J. B. Neilands. 1970. Enterobactin, an iron transport compound from *Salmonella typhimurium*. Biochem. Biophys. Res. Commun. *38*:889.

192. Yancey, R. J., S. A. L. Breeding, and C. E. Lankford. 1979. Enterochelin (enterobactin): virulence factor for *Salmonella typhimurium*. Infect. Immun. *24*:174.

193. Benjamin, W. H., C. L. Turnbough, B. S. Posey, and D. E. Briles. 1985. The ability of *Salmonella typhimurium* to produce the siderophore enterobactin is not a virulence factor in mouse typhoid. Infect. Immun. *50*:392.

194. Maurelli, A. T., B. Blackmon, and R. Curtiss. 1984. Loss of pigmentation in *Shigella flexneri* 2a is correlated with loss of virulence and virulence-associated plasmid. Infect. Immun. *43*:397.

195. Lawlor, K. M., and S. M. Payne. 1984. Aerobactin genes in *Shigella* spp. J. Bacteriol. *160*:266.

196. Lawlor, K. M., P. A. Daskaleros, R. E. Robinson, and S. M. Payne. 1987. Virulence of iron transport mutants of *Shigella flexneri* and utilization of host iron compounds. Infect. Immun. *55*:594.

197. Surgalla, M. J., and E. D. Beesley. 1969. Congo red agar plating medium for detecting pigmentation in *Pasteurella pestis*. Appl. Microbiol. *18*:834.

198. Sasakawa, C., K. Kamata, T. Sakai, S. Y. Murayama, S. Makino, and M. Yoshikawa. 1986. Molecular alteration of the 140-megadalton plasmid associated with loss of virulence and Congo Red binding activity in *Shigella flexneri*. Infect. Immun. *51*:470.

199. Sakai, T., C. Sasakawa, S. Makino, K. Kamata, and M. Yoshikawa. 1986. Molecular cloning of a genetic determinant for Congo Red binding ability which is essential for the virulence of *Shigella flexneri*. Infect. Immun. *51*:461.

200. Daskaleros, P. A., and S. M. Payne. 1987. Congo red binding phenotype is associated with hemin binding and increased infectivity of *Shigella flexneri* in the HeLa cell model. Infect. Immun. *55*:1393.

201. Maurelli, A. T., B. Baudry, H. D'Hauteville, T. L. Hale, and P. J. Sansonetti. 1985. Cloning of plasmid DNA sequences involved in invasion of HeLa cells by *Shigella flexneri*. Infect. Immun. *49*:164.

202. Sansonetti, P. J., A. Ryter, P. Clerc, A. T. Maurelli, and J. Mounier. 1986. Multiplication of *Shigella flexneri* with HeLa cells: Lysis of the phagocytic vacuole and plasmid-mediated contact hemolysis. Infect. Immun. *51*:461.

203. Jackson, S., and T. W. Burrows. 1956. The pigmentation of *Pasteurella pestis* on defined medium containing haemin. Br. J. Exp. Pathol. *37*:570.

204. Jackson, S., and T. W. Burrows. 1956. The virulence-enhancing effect of iron on non-pigmented mutant of virulent strains of *pasteurella pestis*. Brit. J. Exp. Pathol. *37*:577.

205. Wake, A., M. Misawa, and A. Matsui. 1975. Siderochrome production by *Yersinia pestis* and its relation to virulence. Infect. Immun. *12*:1211.

206. Perry, R. D., and R. R. Brubaker. 1979. Accumulation of iron by Yersiniae. J. Bacteriol. *137*:1290.

207. Sikkema, D. J., and R. R. Brubaker. 1987. Resistance to pesticin, storage of iron, and invasion of HeLa cells by Yersiniae. Infect. Immun. *55*:572.

208. Carniel, E., D. Mazigh, and H. H. Mollaret. 1987. Expression of iron-regulated proteins in *Yersinia* species and their relation to virulence. Infect. Immun. *55*:277.

209. Portnoy, D. A., H. Wolf-Watz, I. Bolin, A. B. Beeder, and S. Falkow. 1984. Characterization of common virulence plasmids in *Yersinia* species and their role in the expression of outer membrane proteins. Infect. Immun. *43*:108.

210. Golden, C. A., I. Kochan, and D. R. Spriggs. 1974. Role of mycobactin in the growth and virulence of tubercle bacilli. Infect. Immun. *9*:34.

211. Kochan, I., D. L. Cahall, and C. A. Golden. 1971. Employment of tuberculostasis in serum-agar medium for the study of production and activity of mycobactin. Infect. Immun. *4*:130.

212. Wheeler, W. C., and J. H. Hanks. 1965. Utilization of external growth factors by intracellular microbes: *Mycobacterium paratuberculosis* and wood pigeon *Mycobacteria*. J. Bacteriol. *89*:889.

213. Hanks, J. H. 1966. Host-dependent microbes. Bacteriol. Rev. *30*:114.

214. Macham, L. P., and C. Ratledge. 1975. A new group of water-soluble iron-binding compounds from *Mycobacteria*: The exochelins. J. Gen. Microbiol. *89*:379.

215. Ratledge, C., L. P. Macham, K. A. Brown, and B. J. Marshall. 1974. Iron transport in *Mycobacterium smegmatis*: a restricted role for salicylic acid in the extracellular environment. Biochim. Biophys. Acta. *372*:39.

216. Stephenson, M. C., and C. Ratledge. 1980. Specificity of exochelins for iron transport in three species of *Mycobacteria*. J. Gen. Microbiol. *116*:521.

217. Kochan, I. 1977. "Siderophores in nutritional immunity and bacterial parasitism," in E. D. Weinberg, Ed., *Microorganisms and Minerals*. Dekker, New York. pp. 251–288.

218. Barclay, R., D. F. Ewing, and C. Ratledge. 1985. Isolation, identification, and structural analysis of the mycobactins of *Mycobacterium avium*, *Mycobacterium intracellulare*, *Mycobacterium scrofulaceum*, and *Mycobacterium paratuberculosis*. J. Bacteriol. *164*:896.

# CHAPTER 8

# Minerals and Bacterial Spores

ROBERT E. MARQUIS

Department of Microbiology and Immunology
University of Rochester
Rochester, New York

## Contents

## 8.1  INTRODUCTION

One of the most striking compositional differences between vegetative bacterial cells and endospores derived from them is in mineral content. Generally the chief mineral in vegetative cells is potassium, which serves as counterion for excess negative charges in cell polymers such as RNA, DNA, and proteins. In addition, potassium is the major osmolite for maintenance of the positive turgor pressure required for metabolism, growth, and cell division. Its level in the cytoplasm rises and falls in response to increases and decreases in environmental osmolality, and bacteria generally have multiple transport systems for potassium regulated by a complex system sensitive to turgor (1, 2). The K within vegetative cells, including that serving as counterion for polymers, appears to be highly mobile and able to move in high-frequency electrical fields (3). Spores, on the other hand, are calcified cells. Calcium may make up some 3% or more of the cell dry weight (4). The Ca of the spore is largely immobilized, especially in the core or pro-

**247**

toplast, and spores have extremely low electrical conductivity, even at frequencies as high as 50 MHz (5). The high levels of calcification of spores have been related directly to heat resistance and to dormancy (6). However, recent work has indicated that all of the minerals in spores, except perhaps for Na, contribute to increased heat resistance (7). Thus total mineralization, as well as specific mineralization with Ca, can contribute to resistance to heat damage. However, it is clear that heat resistance of spores, and possibly also dormancy, has multiple bases. For heat resistance, a so-called inherent component can be defined in relation to molecular stabilities of spore biopolymers at high temperatures. Thus thermophiles produce more heat-resistant spores, on average, than do mesophiles and psychrophiles (8). Extrinsic resistance is then superimposed on inherent resistance by the spore state, largely owing to dehydration of the spore core, but also owing to mineralization.

Despite its general title, this chapter focuses on bacterial endospores, mainly because they have been extensively studied over many decades and are noted for extreme dormancy and extreme resistance to heat. Moreover, their industrial and medical importance is major in that multibillion-dollar industries have been built for their destruction in food, sterile supplies, fermentation media, and a host of other commodities. Other bacterial spores are generally also more mineralized than the vegetative cells from which they arise and are more resistant to desiccation, and often to heat and to other noxious agents. Examples include arthrospores of the actinomycetes, exospores of methane-oxidizing bacteria, *Azobacter* cysts, and myxospores. For more information on mineralization and resistance of these forms, reference should be made to the recent literature, for example, the general book by Dworkin (9) or more specific articles, such as that of Salas et al. (10).

Endospores are formed by members of the eubacterial genera *Bacillus, Clostridium, Sporolactobacillus, Desulfotomaculum, Thermoactinomyces,* and possibly members of a few other genera, such as *Oscillospira* (11). The process of sporulation has been studied in great physiological and genetic detail for certain members of the genus *Bacillus*. The process is triggered by nutrient depletion, generally of carbon or nitrogen, and involves production of new sigma factors with resultant reading of spore genes rather than vegetative genes (12). Thus sporulation can be considered to have so-called global regulation, with many genes becoming derepressed at once. Sporulation begins only after growth has stopped for cultures in the commonly used media formulated specifically for nearly synchronous induction of sporogenesis. In addition, the process can be carried out endotrophically with cells already committed to sporulation removed from growth media and suspended in simple salts solution (13), or in a microcycle with germinated spores and no intervening vegetative phase (14). The process of sporulation is commonly divided into stages from 0, the vegetative stage, to VII, the stage of release of free spores during sporangial lysis.

In stage II, the cell undergoes an unusual, asymmetric division to form a large and a small compartment separated by a septum. The smaller cell becomes the spore, and the larger becomes the sporangial or mother cell. The sporangial cell then engulfs the smaller cell by a process involving synthesis of new membrane but minimal synthesis of wall. After engulfment is complete, the forespore or prespore is now within the sporangial cytoplasm and has two enveloping membranes. Its original membrane is right-side-out, and the membrane derived from engulfment is inside-out.

Then, mainly during stage IV, cortical peptidoglycan is laid down between the two forespore membranes. The thin layer of peptidoglycan immediately surrounding the spore core seems to be of the vegetative type and may be a remnant of wall synthesized during engulfment. However, the greatly thickened, more peripheral layer is of cortical peptidoglycan. It has a low degree of peptide cross-linking, has muramyl residues with only an L-alanyl substituent instead of a tetra- or pentapeptide, and has about half of the muramyl residues without substituent peptides but with a δ-muramyl lactam (4). The cortical peptidoglycan has a higher, net negative charge than does vegetative peptidoglycan and is more contractile because of its low degree of cross-linking (15). However, we have recently found that this open structure may be due to damage during isolation and that the cortical peptidoglycans of intact spores may be much more highly cross-linked.

Coat layers are deposited on the surface of the outer membrane during stages III–V. The coat proteins are synthesized by the sporangial cell and are linked on the forespore surface by disulfide bonds. They appear to confer resistance to chemicals but are not involved in any major way in heat resistance. Spores decoated chemically retain full heat resistance, and spores formed from cells with genetic defects for coat formation are fully heat resistant (16). In contrast, any upset in cortex formation results in heat-sensitive spores, even if the cells become fully refractile. Many spores also have a chemically complex exosporium external to the coats, but its function has not been clearly defined.

During stage IV, the forespore starts to become mineralized, mainly with calcium but also with other minerals. The process involves a new, high-affinity calcium transport system of the sporangial cell, which acts to move Ca into the sporangial cytoplasm rather than out of the cell as vegetative transport systems for Ca do. The concentrated Ca then moves passively into the forespore. At approximately the same time, dipicolinic acid (DPA) is synthesized and concentrated within the forespore. However, it appears that DPA accumulation by the forespore occurs somewhat later than Ca uptake, and there are still unresolved problems regarding movements of charge equivalents during mineralization. The forespore becomes refractile during stage V, indicating a high level of dehydration of the core. Heat resistance is acquired only very late in sporulation, in stage VI, and a maturation process may occur after full mineralization before development of heat resistance. The final stage of sporulation involves lysis of the sporangial cell and release of a spore with a dehydrated, mineralized protoplast in a state of essentially complete dormancy with a high degree of resistance to heat and resistance to a variety of other noxious agents.

To get back to the vegetative state, the spore must germinate. The return to the vegetative state is commonly viewed in terms of a number of phases— activation, triggering or initiation, germination proper, and outgrowth. Heat resistance is lost early in the process, at about the time Zn is realeased (17). Calcium, other minerals, and DPA also are released, apparently somewhat after the loss of heat resistance. The spore swells and becomes phase dark, presumably owing to breakdown of the cortical peptidoglycan with resultant uptake of water as spore turgor is diminished. Mineral cations can act as germinants for some spores. However, even for spores that respond only to organic germinants, mineral cations still have major influences on both the rate and extent of germination (18).

This brief overview is meant to give a context to the more extended review of spore mineralization that follows.

## 8.2   MINERALIZATION DURING SPORULATION

A curious aspect of sporogenesis is the engulfment of the forespore that follows asymmetric cell division, in essence the phagocytosis of one pro-karyotic cell by another. The forespore then has a double membrane. The outer, forespore membrane has reversed polarity, as indicated by the bio-chemical studies of Wilkinson et al. (19). Isolated forespores hydrolyze ex-ogenously added ATP, whereas vegetative cells or protoplasts do not. Thus the $F_1$ or hydrolytic portions of the ATPases of the outer membrane are oriented outward into the sporangial cytoplasm. This reversed polarity ap-parently upsets osmotic and ion balances for the forespore and results in loss of minerals, predominantly potassium. Determinations of the mineral contents of isolated forespores (20) revealed extremely low levels of K, Na, Ca, Mg, and Mn. The total ionic equivalents for the mineral ions of fore-spores were only 0.12 $\mu$eq/mg cell dry weight, compared with values of 2.35 and 0.88 for mature spores and sporulating cells, respectively. This loss of mineral ions from forespores is accompanied by a loss of water. Volumes of isolated forespores of *B. megaterium* determined by the dextran-exclusion method (20) were only 2.8–3.4 mL per g dry weight when the cells were in media with osmolality approximately equal to that of the sporangial cyto-plasm. Thus the degree of dehydration approached that of the mature spore, which was found to have a dextran-impermeable volume of 2.6 mL per g dry weight, or well below the value of 7.3 mL per g for vegetative cells of this particular organism. When sporulating cells are viewed with the phase microscope, the forespores appear dark in a lighter cytoplasm. In other words, the overall refractive index of the forespores is greater than that of the sporangial cytoplasm, indicating a higher solids content and a lower water content. The results of direct observation with the phase microscope then confirm the conclusions based on determinations of dextran-impermeable volumes.

Forespores are osmotically sensitive when isolated shortly after engulfment and swell or shrink in response to changes in environmental osmolality. They become progressively less sensitive as the peptidoglycan cortex is laid down. It seems that the initial dehydration of the forespore is due to loss of mineral ions and that this dehydrated state is then stabilized by the formation of the thick, elastic cortex. Forespores have been found to be less responsive to changes in environmental osmolality than are vegetative protoplasts (19), and this diminished responsiveness can be interpreted readily in terms of low levels of osmotically active solutes in forespores. In fact, the potassium levels within forespores were found to be remarkably low, only about 0.01 $\mu$mol mg$^{-1}$ dry weight (20). This amount of potassium is not even sufficient to act as counterion for fixed, negative charges of cell polymers. Forespores can take up K if the medium level is raised. For example, in a set of experiments, we found that the K level in forespores incubated with gentle shaking at 25°C in 10% (w/v) sucrose solution could be increased to as high as 0.51 $\mu$mol mg$^{-1}$ protein if 10 m$M$ NADH was also added to the suspension. Addition of 10 m$M$ glucose did not enhance uptake. However, addition of 5 m$M$ ATP resulted in a dramatic drop in intracellular K level to as low as 0.03 $\mu$mol mg$^{-1}$ protein. Thus the hydrolytic activities of the ATPase of the outer membrane appear to be associated with movement of K out of the cell. These activities are also associated with acidification of the cell and presumably with protonation of anionic groups on biopolymers.

As shown diagrammatically in Figure 8.1, the ATPases of both the inner and outer forespore membranes would act to acidify the cortical space. This acidification would be severe because the cortical space is small and because protons would flow into it initially from both the forespore and the sporangial cytoplasms. The acidification would extend in time to the forespore cytoplasm because of the diminished metabolic capacity of the compartment resulting from dehydration, solute depletion, and lack of oxygen. Acidification itself would further diminish metabolic capacity.

Overall, there appear to be three bases for initial dehydration of the forespore. The first has to do with movement of free K$^+$ out of the forespore associated with the reversed workings of the outer membrane. Then the second would be related to acidification of the forespore with additional loss of K$^+$ associated with titration of anionic groups on polymers. The third should be relatively minor and related to the turgor pressure within the sporangial cell. Sporangial turgor pressure would be in the range of 1–2 MPa as indicated by measured contents of small solutes, mainly K. This pressure would be opposed by the elasticity of the cell wall at the outer face of the sporangial protoplast. However, it would not be opposed by any restraining structure between the forespore membranes prior to cortex formation. Therefore the forespore compartment would be compressed, much as gas

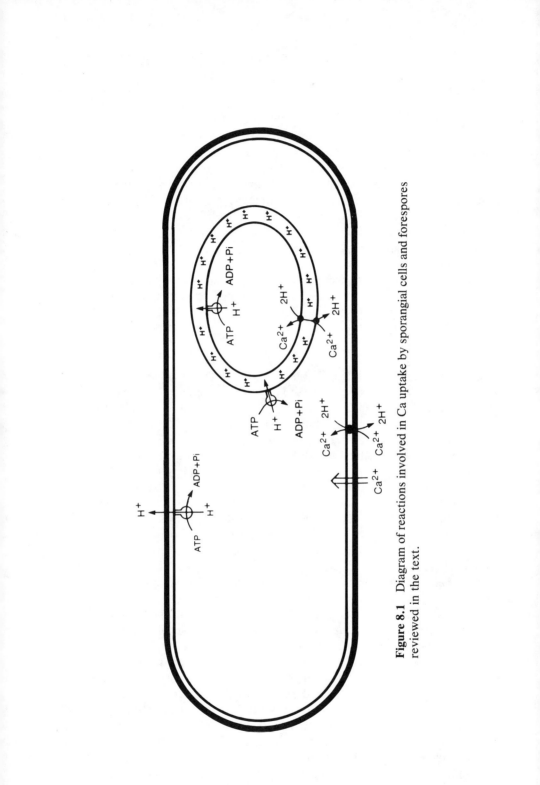

**Figure 8.1** Diagram of reactions involved in Ca uptake by sporangial cells and forespores reviewed in the text.

vacuoles are in gas-vacuolate bacteria. However, the forespore is filled with water and so would not collapse as readily as do gas vacuoles. The reduction in water activity ($a_w$) within forespores owing to turgor of the sporangial cell would be only about 0.012 if the turgor was 1.5 MPa. In contrast, dehydration due to loss of K would be major, and this dehydration is clearly reflected in the dark phase microscopic image of forespores and their low dextran-impermeable volumes per gram dry weight (20). Moreover, acidification of the forespore not only contributes to K loss but also sets the stage for subsequent mineralization. The acidification is indicated by increased movements of protons into forespores after addition of ATP to forespore suspensions.

The cortical peptidoglycan is synthesized in the acidified environment between the two membranes. In *B. subtilis*, it appears to involve penicillin-binding protein 3 (PBP3), which also serves for synthesis of vegetative peptidoglycan, and a new PBP5 is synthesized during sporogenesis (21, 22). The function of the cortical peptidoglycan seems to be to stabilize the initial state of dehydration of the forespore protoplast. After completion of the thick envelope of elastic, cortical peptidoglycan, any movement of water into the forespore would be resisted. Forespores with well-developed cortices become osmotically insensitive.

During normal vegetative growth and up to stage III of sporulation, the levels of Ca in sporangial cells are low, even in sporulation media supplemented with Ca. In fact, bacterial cells move Ca out of the cytoplasm by means of Ca-transporting ATPases (23) or by means of DCCD-sensitive, proton-translocating ATPases coupled to a Ca/proton antiporter (24). However, especially in stages IV–VI of sporulation, sporangial cells take up large amounts of Ca and certain other minerals, including Mn, Mg, Zn, Fe, and even K. Early work by Silver and colleagues (25–27) and by Bronner et al. (28) was reviewed by Silver, who proposed that Ca uptake by sporangial cells involves a Ca/H$^+$ antiporter and that movement of the Ca from the sporangial cytoplasm to the forespore involves Ca/H$^+$ antiport or symport with DPA. Ellar and colleagues (29–33) studied the process in detail to determine possible mechanisms. They found that Ca uptake by the sporangium was active or coupled to metabolism with an apparent $K_m$ of 31 $\mu M$; and it was saturable, specific for Ca, and sensitive to inhibitors of respiration. The inhibitor carbonyl cyanide–*p*-(trifluoromethoxy)phenylhydrazone at a concentration of 1 $\mu M$ completely inhibited uptake of Ca by stage-V protoplasts of sporulating cells of *B. megaterium* KM but inhibited respiration by only about 12%. Thus it appeared that an energized membrane was required for uptake. The inhibitor of proton-translocating ATPases, DCCD or dicyclohexylcarbodiimide, did inhibit Ca uptake but less so than respiration, and so there was no clear indication if uptake involved a Ca-ATPase or a Ca/H$^+$ antiport system acting in conjunction with a proton-translocating ATPase. Subsequent experiments (33) with the ionophores nigericin and valinomycin, with arsenate, and with ATPase inhibitor efrapeptin led to the conclusion "that calcium is transported across the membrane via an antiport system in exchange for one or more protons." Recently, Kusaka and Matsushita (34) have characterized a Ca uniporter of *B. subtilis* in membrane vesicles prepared from cells in the exponential phase of batch culture. The system, which depends on the magnitude of the membrane potential, had been described earlier by De Vrij et al. (35). It is not known if this system for Ca uptake operates during sporogenesis. Bacterial Ca transport systems have recently been reviewed by Rosen (36).

Calcium uptake by isolated forespores proved to be passive and insensitive to inhibitors. It had a high $K_m$ value of 2.1 m$M$ (32). In essence, it appeared that Ca was transported actively into the sporangial cytoplasm to levels of 3–9 m$M$ and was taken up passively by the forespore. Although Ca movement into the forespore appeared in the experiments of Ellar and colleagues to be passive, it still could be related to acidification of the forespore as shown in Figure 8.1. Thus the transport of Ca into the sporangial cell would involve the new or augmented transport system appearing at stage III. Presumably, there would remain a system for moving Ca back out of the cell, shown here as a Ca/H$^+$ antiporter. The total system for movement of Ca would then be similar to that of mitochondria, which are noted for being able to concentrate Ca and for being able to regulate cellular Ca levels in cells. Ca would flow into the sporangial cell rapidly but flow out into the medium slowly. The outer membrane of the forespore would act to concentrate Ca into the cortical space by means of a Ca/H$^+$ antiporter. The Ca would then move into the forespore protoplast in exchange for protons previously accumulated. Thus the initial acidification of the forespore would serve for later Ca uptake.

There is still question about the role of DPA in Ca uptake by forespores. DPA is synthesized at about the time of Ca uptake by the forespore. However, generally DPA synthesis is slightly later than Ca uptake. For example, the data presented by Gorman et al. (37) for sporulation of *B. subtilis* show clearly that the forespores had taken up nearly all of the Ca they were going to take up before any DPA was detected. Also, Seto-Young and Ellar (33) found that inhibitors of Ca uptake were variable in their effects on DPA synthesis, and they concluded that DPA is not involved in the primary uptake mechanism for Ca. In essence, it seems that movement of Ca into the forespore depends mainly on previous acidification rather than on any symport with DPA. In fact, Ca uptake would reduce acidification of the forespore, and if the forespore compartment were then at a more alkaline pH value than the sporangial cytoplasm, DPA would move readily into the forespore because it is a weak acid with $pK_a$ values of about 2.1 and 4.6. This uptake of DPA could then result in precipitation of Ca–DPA–polymer complexes and subsequent further uptake of DPA and possibly further osmotic dehydration to yield the fully refractile, dense spore.

Hanson et al. (38) were able to isolate DPA-less spores of *B. cereus* with full resistance to heat, and subsequently, Dring and Gould (39) independently isolated a similar DPA-less variant. The isolations required two steps—isolation first of a DPA-less mutant sensitive to heat and subsequent isolation of a heat-resistant variant of the mutant organism. The DPA-less spores contained less Ca and Mn than normal spores of this bacterium. In our own experience with spores demineralized by acid extraction, Ca and DPA can go their separate ways. Thus it is possible to demineralize completely spores, say, of *B. megaterium* without loss of DPA. The spores become heat sensitive, and heat resistance is restored when the spores are remineralized with base titration in the presence of Ca. Moreover, with some batches of spores, we have been able to obtain more than 90% depletion of DPA by extending the demineralizing period. When these DPA-depleted spores are remineralized, they can regain full heat resistance.

Decalcified spores are more heat resistant than are vegetative cells or forespores, and DPA could contribute to this resistance. Balassa et al. (40) isolated DPA-deficient spores of *B. subtilis* that were heat sensitive and became heat resistant when they accumulated DPA. However, other changes may have occurred in conjunction with DPA uptake. Overall, there are still open questions regarding the roles of DPA in heat resistance, even though it is clear that DPA is not absolutely required for full resistance.

Spores concentrate mineral ions other than $Ca^{2+}$. For example, Eisenstadt et al. (41) found that sporulating cells of *B. subtilis* W23 developed a system for concentrating Mn from the medium, initially into an exchangeable form but later into a form not exchangeable with radioactive Mn added exogenously. Presumably, the system is mainly in the protoplast membrane of the sporangial cells, as is the Ca-uptake system of stage-III sporulating cells.

Later in the process of sporulation, the forespore becomes phase-gray and then refractile. The refractility viewed with the ordinary positive, phase-contrast microscope is due to an increase in cell refractive index beyond that of the forespore. Presumably this increase is associated with further dehydration and with accumulation of minerals and DPA. Normally, uptake of minerals and DPA would be accompanied by an osmotic uptake of water. However, these materials probably precipitate within the spore cytoplasm and so become osmotically inactive. Moreover, the thick, cortical peptidoglycan layer would resist water movement into the cell. Recently Beaman and Gerhardt (16) have found that remineralization of demineralized spores is accompanied by dehydration of the core. Thus the contribution of mineralization to heat resistance may be partly due to associated dehydration. However, minerals can also protect against dry-heat damage, as shown by the data of Alderton and Snell (42) and by recent data from our laboratory. Thus there appears to be a protective effect of mineralization independent of dehydration.

After forespores have become calcified and have taken up DPA, there is a maturation process before full heat resistance is acquired about which little is known. In fact, there is a possibility that maturation is an artifact associated with imperfect synchrony in sporulating suspensions or that it is simply due to a change in environmental conditions as the spore is released from the sporangial cell into the environment.

## 8.3 MANIPULATION OF MINERAL CONTENT AND RESISTANCE

One of the most direct ways to manipulate the mineral contents of spores is by changing the mineral composition of the media used for growth and sporulation. A number of defined media have been developed for sporulation studies with specified mineral contents. Slepecky and Foster (43) used a defined medium for growth and sporulation of *B. megaterium* ATCC 19213 to investigate the effects of varying mineral concentrations from the minimal amounts required for sporulation to maximal amounts permitting growth. They found, for example, that the minimum level of Ca for sporulation was about 0.40 mg L$^{-1}$ (0.01 m$M$) and that the spores grown in this low-Ca medium had only 0.69% Ca (172.5 µmol Ca g$^{-1}$ dry weight). The maximal level tested was 722 mg L$^{-1}$ (18.05 m$M$), and spores from this high-Ca medium had 3.04% Ca (760 µmol Ca g$^{-1}$ dry weight), that is, an increase of some 441%. Comparable increases after manipulation of medium levels of Mn, Zn, and Co were 433, 575, and 350%, respectively. Even larger percentage increases were found for Ni and Cu because they were not required for growth or sporulation but did become incorporated into spores when added to the medium. Added Co also was not required for sporulation or growth but the medium used contained contaminating Co. The total capacity of the spores to incorporate minerals appeared to be limited in that increased incorporation of Ca resulted in reduced incorporation of other minerals. The level of Ca in the spores could be related directly to heat resistance, but accumulation of Zn, Mn, Ni, or Co resulted in reduced resistance, possibly because of lowered Ca content, except for the spores with increased Co content, which did not have reduced Ca content. Differences in mineralization had no effect on resistance to ultraviolet irradiation, phenol, or desiccation.

Subsequently, Aoki and Slepecky (44, 45) found that increased incorporation of Mn into spores of *B. megaterium* ATCC 19213 or *Bacillus fastidiosus* resulted in increased heat resistance. Moreover, the *B. megaterium* spores grown in a medium with a high level of Mn had increased resistance to ultraviolet irradiation and to X–rays. Manganese incorporation did not affect incorporation of Ca or DPA in any discernible way.

Foerster and Foster (46) used a procedure for endotrophic sporulation to obtain spores of *B. megaterium* QM B1551 and *Bacillus cereus* T with Ca, Sr, or Ba as the major mineral. In this procedure, cells committed to sporulation were removed from culture and suspended in deionized water. The cells could then complete the process of sporulation depending only on sporangial cell materials. Endotrophically formed spores had been found by

Black et al. (47) to be deficient in Ca and DPA and heat sensitive, but not sensitive to phenol or gamma radiation. However, these defects could be corrected if calcium salts were added to the deionized water used. Foerster and Foster (46) found that addition of $CaCl_2$, $SrCl_2$, or $BaCl_2$ resulted in formation of Ca, Sr, or Ba salt forms of the spores. The Sr and Ba forms contained only minimal amounts of Ca. They were somewhat resistant to heat, but Ca appeared to be required for full resistance. However, it was found also that the populations of Sr spores and Ba spores contained two subpopulations each—one very sensitive to heat and the other as resistant as fully calcified spores. This type of heterogeneity is difficult to interpret because nearly all spore populations have some highly resistant cells, and the so-called "tailing" phenomenon of killing curves often indicates a more resistant subpopulation, although increased resistance may actually be acquired during the heating process rather than during sporulation. One possible interpretation is that the amount of Ca in the Sr or Ba spores is unevenly distributed so that the spores with higher levels of Ca and lower levels of Sr or Ba are the more heat resistant.

Manipulation of the mineral contents of spores through alteration of the environmental levels of minerals is limited by the minimal requirements of the minerals for growth or sporulation and by toxicities of the mineral salts at higher concentrations. Even for endotrophic sporulation, these limits are only somewhat expanded, although endotrophic sporulation does allow for better control of mineral content. Alderton and Snell (48) developed procedures to bring about mineral exchange by means of acid–base titration of fully mature spores isolated free of sporangial cells. The procedures involved initial acid titration to displace mineral ions and then back-titration with chosen bases in the presence of chosen salts to produce remineralized forms. Initially, acid titrations generally involved mild exposures to pH values of about 4.0 with heating, but subsequently, more severe procedures were carried out to obtain more demineralization with titration to pH values as low as 1.0. Heat sensitivities of exchanged spores have been assessed in a number of laboratories, and data are presented, for example, in papers by Alderton and colleagues (49–51), by Rode and Foster (52), by Ando and Tsuzuki (53), and by Bender and Marquis (7). In all cases, demineralized spores showed markedly increased sensitivities to heat, and remineralized spores could regain the full resistance of the native spores, especially when the procedures involved remineralization with Ca. For example, we found that the $D$ value for a batch of native spores of *Bacillus stearothermophilus* ATCC 7953 at 123°C was about 1.0 min. The $D$ value here refers to the time required for 90% killing of the test population of spores during exponential death. Thus $D$ refers to the time for a so-called decade reduction in viability during which the $\log_{10}$ of the count of survivors is reduced by 1. For vegetative cells, this same $D$ value of 1.0 min was obtained with heating at only about 68°C. For spores totally demineralized by means of acid titration, a $D$ value of 1.0 min was obtained at a heating temperature of some 102°C, whereas for spores from the same preparation remineralized with Ca, the temperature at which a *D* value of 1.0 min was obtained was again 123°C. It is apparent then that spores are much more heat resistant than vegetative cells, that demineralized spores are more heat sensitive than native spores but significantly less heat sensitive than vegetative cells, and that remineralization of the spores with Ca results in complete restoration of the resistant state of the native spore.

The tolerance of spores to demineralizing procedures is truly amazing. In the past few years, we have been able to take advantage of the basic procedures developed by Alderton and colleagues for ion exchange to produce salt forms of a variety of organisms with closely controlled and assayed mineral contents. Each organism has required a different procedure to achieve the desired results, but we have managed to design specific procedures for organisms ranging from the relatively heat-sensitive spores of *B. megaterium* ATCC 19213 to the highly resistant spores of *B. stearothermophilus* ATCC 7953. In a typical procedure, say, for *B. megaterium* ATCC 19213, the spores in thick suspensions are titrated with HCl solution to a pH value of 2.0. The titration may take some hours because, as the spores become demineralized, the pH value of the suspension rises, and more acid must then be added to maintain the pH value of the suspension at 2.0. Finally, the cells are heated briefly at 60°C to achieve full demineralization. This last step is the most sensitive in that the demineralized spores have become sensitive to heat, and a prolonged exposure to 60°C will result in reduction in viability of the population. With care, however, it is possible on a regular basis to obtain complete demineralization of the spores with no reduction in viability of samples subsequently plated directly onto complex media. The cells are truly demineralized, and assays of ashed spores by atomic absorption spectrophotometry indicate almost no Ca, Mn, Mg, or K. Often the demineralized spores we prepared did appear to contain some Na, but the Na was from contaminating sources and could be reduced if the procedures were carried out with plastic vessels. The demineralized spores, or H-spores, were fully viable, yielded normal colonies on agar medium, and therefore must have retained the ability to germinate. The resistance of the spores to acidification is generally much greater than that of vegetative cells of the same species. Vegetative cells of *B. megaterium* ATCC 19213 are killed rapidly when the pH value of thick suspensions is reduced to 3.0. Presumably, the acid resistance of spores is related to the dormant, dehydrated state of the protoplast so that any changes in membranes, ribosomes, or enzymes caused by exposure to acid environments are fully reversible. The recent work of Beaman and Gerhardt (16) indicates that demineralization increases the state of hydration of the spore protoplast, but the cell is still markedly less hydrated than are vegetative cells in aqueous suspensions. Earlier work of Rajan et al. (54) indicated that Ca-form spores of *Clostridium botulinum* 33A actually had higher water contents than H-form spores at relative humidities below about 50%, but the opposite was true at higher relative humidities.

Presumably, when spores are exposed to media sufficiently acid to bring about complete demineralization, the interior of the spore must be at a pH value close to that of the environment. Determinations of the pH within dormant *Bacillus* spores by Setlow and Setlow (55) and by Swerdlow et al. (56) by use of weak-base probes and by NMR procedures indicated that the value for dormant spores was about 6.5 and that this value rose rapidly to about 7.5 during germination. However, it seems that there could not be a $\Delta$pH across the spore membranes when the medium pH value is as low as 2.0. Moreover, the loss of minerals from the core of the spores indicates that charged species can move across the membranes. The heating to 60°C required for complete demineralization of spores of *B. megaterium* ATCC 19213 could affect membrane permeability to protons, but it is not required for all organisms. For example, spores of *B. subtilis* niger are relatively acid sensitive, but they can be demineralized totally by titration of suspensions to a pH value of 4.0 without heating. Spores of *B. cereus* T are generally more acid sensitive and will not tolerate titration even to a pH value of 4.0 without loss of refractility.

Movements of DPA during demineralization are largely independent of movements of minerals. For example, we found that native spores of *B. subtilis* niger contained 306 nmol DPA $mg^{-1}$ dry weight. Measured mineral contents, in terms of nmol $mg^{-1}$ dry weight, were Ca, 420; Mg, 301; Mn, 990; K, 280, and Na, 180. Demineralized spores were prepared by titration to a pH of 4.0. There was no loss of DPA, but the mineral contents were reduced to Ca, 17; Mg, 26; Mn, 29; K, 17; and Na, 50 nmol $mg^{-1}$. The demineralized spores showed the expected increase in heat sensitivity. Thus for native spores, the temperature at which a *D* value of 1 min was obtained was 100.3°C, but for the demineralized spores it was 87.2°C. When the Na form of the spores was prepared, the DPA content was reduced to only 53 nmol $mg^{-1}$. If these sodium spores were remineralized with Ca, heat resistance of the native state was regained, even though the resultant spores were markedly deficient in DPA. In effect, heat resistance does not appear to be related to DPA content but does appear to be related to calcification or mineralization.

Demineralized spores can be remineralized with a variety of minerals. The remineralization process involves back-titration, usually to a pH value of about 8.0, usually with brief heating at 60°C. The base used for the back-titration may be that of the desired mineral, for example, KOH to obtain the K form of the spores, or it may be NaOH in the presence of $CaCl_2$ to obtain the Ca form. In the latter procedure, advantage is taken of the higher affinity of spores for divalent cations than for monovalent cations. This same difference in affinity was noted by Crosby et al. (57) for demineralization of spores of *B. megaterium*. They subjected spores to extraction first with a 0.02 *M* solution of EDTA (ethylenediamine tetraaacetate) at a pH value of

5.5, and then to extractions with HCl solutions at pH values of 2.5, 1.75, and 1.3. Potassium was easily removed, even with just water washing, whereas Ca was removed mainly only after treatment at a pH value of 1.3. In fact, even with the acid treatment, the spores retained about 10% of their Ca. Washing with water and EDTA solution easily removed Zn and Mg also, as well as part of the Mn. However, about 70% of the Mn was as difficult to extract as the Ca. Also part of the Fe was easily extracted, but another part, about 40%, was difficult to extract.

With the remineralizing procedures we used (7), it was possible to obtain salt forms of spores with little mixing of minerals. Thus the capacity of each of the chosen minerals to stabilize against heat damage could be assessed without interference from other minerals. In the hierarchy determined with spores of *B. megaterium*, *B. subtilis*, and *B. stearothermophilus*, Ca was most effective, Mn was only slightly less effective, and Mg and K were somewhat less effective still. Sodium appeared to be completely ineffective, and the Na forms of the spores were essentially as heat sensitive as the H forms. However, it was clear from the results that minerals other than Ca were effective for stabilizing spores against heat damage. Previously, Murrell and Warth (6) had used 19 types of spores of *Bacillus* organisms to develop a correlation between Ca content and resistance. Overall, their data indicate that there was an approximately 30-fold increase in $D$ value (at 100°C) for each 1% increase (% dry weight) in Ca content. They found an inverse correlation for heat resistance and Mg content, but presumably this inverse correlation arose because of decreased Ca content associated with increased Mg content. Certainly Mg was effective in our experiments in increasing the heat resistance of demineralized–remineralized spores, even though it was somewhat less effective than Ca (7).

The capacities of spores to be remineralized are presumably related to their contents of anionic groups, primarily in proteins and nucleic acids. Thus demineralization would involve substitution of protons for mineral counterions, and remineralization would be the reverse. As indicated, DPA may or may not be involved depending on whether or not it has been retained or lost during remineralization. There is also the possibility that minerals could precipitate in inorganic complexes or mixed organic/inorganic complexes in the spores as suggested by Rajan et al. (54) and also by others. Inorganic complexes appear to be involved also in the excess capacities of spores to take up Mn relative to other minerals. The excess is probably due mainly to binding and oxidation of the type described by Rosson and Nealson (58) for spores of a marine *Bacillus*. The oxidized mineral is deposited on the surfaces of the spores, on the exosporium or outer coats, and is not likely to contribute to heat resistance. However, the oxidized Mn may serve as a nucleation site for deposit of the mineral in the environment of the ocean floor or elsewhere in the biosphere.

Minerals were found (7) to be more effective in protecting spores at lower killing temperatures than at higher ones. An example is presented in Figure

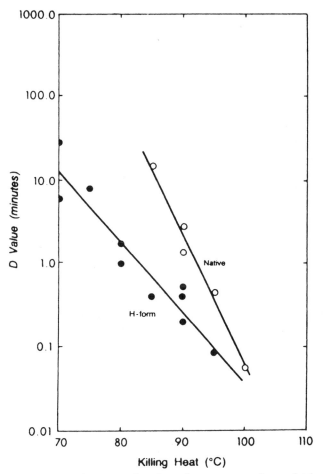

**Figure 8.2** Plots of $D$ values as a function of temperature for moist heat killing of native and demineralized, H-spores of *B. megaterium* ATCC 19213. The figure is part of one of the figures in the paper by Bender and Marquis (7).

8.2 for native and demineralized, H-form spores of *B. megaterium* ATCC 19213. The slope of the line relating log $D$ value to the killing temperature for the native spores is greater than that for the H-form spores, and it appears that the lines would intersect at a temperature slightly over 100°C. Presumably, at the temperature of intersection, mineralization would not contribute to stabilizing spores against heat damage. In addition, the relationship between the degree of remineralization and the protective effect varies with killing temperature. For example, spores of *B. stearothermophilus* ATCC 7953 had maximal resistance to damage by heating at 121°C when they had taken up only about 0.4 $\mu$mol Ca mg$^{-1}$ dry weight, and further remineralization did not result in any increase in the maximal $D$ value of about 4 min.

However, protection against damage caused by 115°C increased with increasing remineralization up to a maximum $D$ value of some 16 min with uptake of about 0.6 μmol Ca mg$^{-1}$ dry weight.

Minerals seem to be more important in the natural resistance of some spores than of others. *B. megaterium* ATCC 19213 and *B. subtilis* niger both are mesophiles, and there is little difference in the heat sensitivities of their vegetative forms (7). In addition, we found only small differences in the sensitivities of H-form spores of the organisms to heat. However, native, mineralized spores of *B. subtilis* were found to be markedly more resistant to heat than spores of *B. megaterium*. The difference appeared to be related to the greater mineralization of *B. subtilis* spores. Both types of native spores had about the same Ca content, some 0.42–0.45 μmol Ca mg$^{-1}$ dry weight. However, *B. subtilis* spores had much more Mn (0.99 versus 0.16 μmol mg$^{-1}$) and also more Mg (0.30 versus 0.15 μmol mg$^{-1}$) and K (0.28 versus 0.10 μmol mg$^{-1}$).

Vegetative cells of the thermophilic *B. stearothermophilus* were more resistant to heat than vegetative cells of the mesophiles, and this difference was apparent also in H-form spores prepared from the organisms. The differences were even greater for native spores, possibly because spores of the thermophile were highly calcified with about 0.74 μmol Ca mg$^{-1}$. Thus the very high resistance of spores of *B. stearothermophilus* appeared to have multiple bases, including greater dehydration of the spore protoplast (16).

Mineralization also has major effects on resistance to dry heat. For example, Alderton and Snell (42) found that demineralized spores of *B. stearothermophilus* NCA 1518 could be killed by dry heat at 105°C with a $D$ value of 3.17 min. The $D$ value for native spores at 105°C was found to be 26.8 min, and for spores demineralized and remineralized with Ca, it was 20.3 min. We have obtained similar results for *B. subtilis* niger but found that mineralization had little effect on resistance to spores of *B. megaterium* ATCC 19213 to dry heat.

Mineralization does not appear to have major effects on resistance to chemicals such as phenol (43, 47), hypochlorite (59), or as we have found in collaborative work with Dr. Patrick McCormick of Sybron Corporation, ethylene oxide.

Mineralization or calcification does not appear to play a major role in the resistance of spores to ionizing radiation (47, 60), although Aoki and Slepecky (45) did find that spores containing higher levels of Mn were more resistant to both X-rays and ultraviolet radiation. Mineralization has been related to resistance to ultraviolet radiation by a number of workers, but the protective effect seems to be due primarily to DPA rather than to minerals (60–62).

Mineralization does appear to affect the sensitivities of spores to the germinating action of hydrostatic pressure (63). Bacterial spores respond in an unusual way to compression in that they commonly are relatively resistant to the adverse effects of high pressures, in the kilobar range, yet may be killed by lower pressures in the centibar range. The bases for these peculiar responses have been worked out by Gould and Sale (64, 65) in Britain and by Australian workers (66–68). The lower pressures cause the spores to germinate, and it is the germinated forms that are killed under pressure. Higher pressures inhibit germination, and the ungerminated, dormant spores remain immune to the adverse effects of pressure. There is a wide range of responsiveness to pressure among different types of spores, and this variability has hampered efforts to develop pressure devices for sterilization. Bender and Marquis (63) determined a hierarchy of resistance of the salt forms of *B. megaterium* ATCC 19213 to the germinating action of pressure with H > K > Ca, Mg, Na > native. The resistance of the H form was such that germination was not induced even at 1020 bar.

Unfortunately, the study of the resistances of the various salt forms of spores to heat or other damaging agents has not yielded a very clear view of the possible mechanisms of stabilization due to mineralization. The results of Beaman and Gerhardt (16) suggest that part of the increased stabilization against heat damage is due to dehydration associated with mineralization. However, because mineralization also increases resistance to dry heat, there must be additional mechanisms. Certainly, there appears to be no readily discernible pattern in the hierarchy of stabilizing potential, other than that divalent cations are more effective than monovalent cations. However, stabilizing potential does not appear to be correlated with either crystal radii of the mineral ions or hydrated radii. Moreover, because DPA does not seem to be required for stabilization, the peculiarities of DPA–mineral complexes described, for example, by Chung et al. (69) do not seem pertinent. It is clear that stabilizing potentials can be defined, but they must be defined in relation to some particular temperature because mineralization is more effective in protecting against heat damage at lower than at higher temperatures.

## 8.4 LOCATION AND PHYSICAL STATE OF MINERALS IN SPORES

As one might expect, the minerals in spores are located mainly, but not exclusively, in the core or protoplast. Scherrer and Gerhardt (70) were the first to use electron-probe, X ray microanalysis to determine that calcium is located primarily in the core of *Bacillus* spores, and Ando (71) subsequently extended the findings to spores of *Clostridium perfringens*. Later, with more advanced instrumentation, Stewart et al. (72) analyzed mineral distributions in individual spores of *B. cereus* T and a DPA-less variant in freeze-dried cryosections and concluded that essentially all of the Ca, Mg, and Mn were localized in the core. Johnstone et al. (73) applied the procedure to study distributions of elements in spores of *B. megaterium* KM. Their data indicated that Ca, K, Mg, and Mn were concentrated in the core, whereas Na was throughout the cell, and Zn was concentrated in the coats.

Nishihara et al. (74) used ashed spores of *B. megaterium* QM B1551 and ATCC 19213 and found that Ca and Mg were concentrated in the core. However, minerals were detected also in the coats, especially with the QM B1551 strain, which has thick, prominent coats. The minerals were detected in the cortex also, but the region did not appear to be as highly mineralized as the core and coats. Acid demineralized spores were examined also. They were not very different from native spores. However, they were titrated only to a pH value of 4, and the extent of Ca loss was small, only some 25% of the total.

The physical states of minerals within spores have been assessed with a number of techniques. Early on Windle and Sacks (75) used electron paramagnetic resonance techniques to determine that Mn(II) and Cu(II) in spores of *Bacillus* and *Clostridium* were bound. Later Johnstone et al. (76) interpreted results obtained with similar techniques as indications that Mn(II) in *Bacillus* spores was in a crystalline lattice within the cells. Unfortunately, as indicated above, Mn is often precipitated on the surfaces of spores, and this precipitated mineral could have been responsible for a major part of the observed spectra. However, they had previously found (73) that Mn was nearly entirely in the core of spores of *B. megaterium* KM.

Dielectric techniques have proved to be very useful in gaining detailed information on the physical states of minerals in each of the main compartments of spores, although the techniques require large masses of spores in thick suspensions and give only average values for conductivity. The initial determinations of Carstensen et al. (77) indicated that spores of *B. cereus* T had remarkably low conductivities, even at high frequencies, and so all of the minerals within the cells appeared to be immobilized. Details of the procedures used have been presented previously (20, 78, 79). Conductivities and dielectric constants of cells in thick suspensions were assessed over a range of frequencies, from about 1 to 200 MHz. In typical experiments, measurements are carried out with suspensions and then with supernatant fluids obtained after centrifugations. By use of relationships developed initially by James Clerk Maxwell, we could then calculate the effective, homogeneous conductivities and dielectric constants of the cells themselves on the basis of the measured values and the volume fractions of the suspensions occupied by the cells. The latter were estimated in terms of the dextran-impermeable volumes with use of Dextran 2000, which consists of molecules too large to penetrate the porous structure of the cell wall or the spore coats. At low frequencies, the cell membrane is an effective insulator, and the only conductive structures of the cell are those exterior to the membrane. For vegetative cells of Gram-positive bacteria, the cell wall may have relatively high conductivity because of the large number of charged groups in the peptidoglycan network. For example, cell walls of *Micrococcus luteus* have ion exchange capacities as great as 3.54 meq $g^{-1}$ dry weight (80), and cells of this organism were found (3) to have conductivities for current of

1592 Hz of 0.27 S m$^{-1}$, even though protoplasts had almost undetectable conductivity. (A 0.1 $M$ NaCl solution has a conductivity of about 1 S m$^{-1}$).

At higher frequencies, generally about 50 MHz, the cell membrane is capacitatively short-circuited, and all of the mobile ions in the cell, including those in the cytoplasm, participate in current conduction. The conductivity of the cytoplasm, or of the region within the cell membrane, can be estimated by subtracting the low-frequency conductivity from the high-frequency value. For vegetative cells the cytoplasmic conductivity has been found to be about one-third of the expected value based on assays of electrolytes and on their mobilities in dilute solutions. For example, cells of *Enterococcus hirae* ATCC 9790 had measured conductivities in media of low ionic strength of 0.90 S m$^{-1}$ compared with a predicted value of 3.08 S m$^{-1}$. Comparable values for cells of *M. luteus* ATCC 4698 were 0.68 and 2.06 S m$^{-1}$ (3). Spores suspended in media of low ionic strength had conductivities one order of magnitude lower than the measured conductivities for vegetative cells. For example, conductivities for spores of *B. megaterium* ATCC 19213 and *B. cereus* T were 0.09 and 0.02 S m$^{-1}$, respectively (79). The lower-than-expected conductivities of vegetative cells appear to be due to the high viscosity of the cytoplasm and to deviations from chemical ideality in the concentrated solution of the cytoplasm. However, the measured values for spores are so low in relation to mineral contents that the most reasonable interpretation is that the electrolytes are precipitated. However, because the spore interior is more dehydrated than that of a vegetative cell, there is still the possibility that the mobilities of the electrolytes are sharply curtailed without occurrence of actual precipitation.

Spores are cytologically more complicated than vegetative cells of most Gram-positive bacteria. Carstensen et al. (79) found that the high-frequency conductivity of intact spores of *B. megaterium* ATCC 19213 was due mainly to movements of ions within the cortical space. When the spores were de-coated chemically with resultant removal of the outer membrane, the cell conductivity was increased somewhat. Moreover, the characteristic frequency for the transition from high to low dielectric constant was shifted markedly to lower values. This shift was interpreted in terms of the coatless spores having much lower internal conductivities than the spores with coats. In other words, the core appeared to have much lower conductivity than the cortex. The conductivity of the cortical region was estimated to be about 0.13 S m$^{-1}$ whereas that of the core was estimated to be only about 0.01 S m$^{-1}$. Moreover, the results indicated that the coat–outer membrane complex of the spore was a dielectrically effective membrane and that this membrane could be effectively removed by the decoating procedures.

It was of interest to find that the entire spore of *B. cereus* T, including the cortex, had such low conductivity in view of the theory of Gould and Dring (81) for heat resistance involving an expanded, osmoregulatory cortex with a high level of mobile, osmotically active counterions. Spores of *B. megaterium* ATCC 19213 do have high levels of mobile ions in the cortex, as indicated by conductivity determinations. Moreover, high conductivity values for the cortices of intact spores seem to be common, based on determinations with spores of *Bacillus sphaericus* ATCC 9602, *B. subtilis* niger, and *B. stearothermophilus* ATCC 7953. However, *B. cereus* T is clearly different, and the low conductivity of the cortex can be related to the recent findings in our laboratory of a tight molecular structure for cortical peptidoglycans in intact spores. The high conductivities of cortices of other spores are presumably due to trapped co-ions. Gould and Dring found that coat-defective spores were sensitized to heat by high concentrations of salts of multivalent cations and that the increasing order of effectiveness for sensitization was $Sr^{2+}$, $Ca^{2+}$, $Mg^{2+}$, and $La^{3+}$. Salts of monovalent cations were not effective. Gould and Dring interpreted their data, including data obtained with *B. cereus* T, in terms of an expanded cortex acting to dehydrate the core. Contraction of the cortex would then lead to core expansion. Actually, the original theory for heat resistance based on cortical contractility was that of Lewis et al. (82), in which a contracted cortex was viewed as squeezing water from the core. However, at present it is not possible to decide which, if either, theory is the more useful, or if the theory of Warth (83), in which the cortex is viewed as expanding anisotropically, has merit. There seems little doubt that the cortex is important for heat resistance and that spores with damaged coats can be sensitized to heat with divalent cations. However, at this time, there is need for direct measurements of the state of contraction of cortical peptidoglycans in intact spores or decoated spores.

## 8.5  MINERALS AND GERMINATION

Minerals may be involved in a number of ways in the germination process. Clearly, to return to the vegetative state, spores must become decalcified and must take up $K^+$. It is important also to get rid of toxic minerals such as Mn, which is mutagenic. Mineral ions may act directly as germinants for some spores or may modify the process. Rode and Foster (84) proposed that ions are the inducing agents of germination and that nonionic compounds only augment the activities of ions. Organic ions are more often effective as germinants than are inorganic ions, as shown by the extensive cataloging of germination requirements and modifiers by Foerster and Foster (85). Demineralized spores have been found (63, 86) to germinate poorly in response to specific germinants, such as L-alanine and inosine. However, even totally demineralized H-spores will germinate if placed in complex media. Presumably the process involves an initial ion exchange to replenish cell minerals and then germination. H-spores germinated more readily when they were suspended in potassium phosphate buffer than when they were suspended in water at a pH value of 6.8 (63). The germination of H-spores of *C. perfringens* S40 was found (87) to require Ca and to be stimulated by monovalent cations. Ando and Tsuzuki (53) determined that the most probable basis for the increased heat sensitivities of H-spores of *C. perfringens* was sensitization of the germination apparatus, and heat-damaged H-spores could be recovered by use of lysozyme. However, Bender and Marquis (7) were unable to recover heat-damaged H-spores of *Bacillus* strains by use of lysozyme, and so the basis for sensitization must be different for these organisms.

It seems that germination in many spore populations can be amplified once started by Ca–DPA released from germinating cells. Riemann and Ordal (88) first discerned that Ca–DPA serves as a germinant for spores of a variety of *Bacillus* and *Clostridium* species. Fleming and Ordal (89) proposed a mechanism for Ca–DPA-induced germination involving disruption of Ca–DPA complexes in the spore compartments. They had concluded that ion effects on germination must involve physicochemical rather than catalytic mechanisms because of the wide range of ionic species supporting germination and the relatively high ionic strengths required for maximal rates of germination. Ca–DPA could affect cortical tonus, but it might also trigger cortex lytic enzymes. However, degradation of the cortex is not thought to be one of the initial reactions in germination. Moreover, the recent findings of Nakatani et al. (90) for germination of spores of *B. megaterium* ATCC 12872 by $CdCl_2$ indicate that cortex lysis does not even occur in this type of germination. Of course, there is always the possibility that loosening of the cortical structure is all that is required for germination and that the degree of loosening required can occur without loss of cortical fragments into the suspending medium. The findings of Sacks (18) with coatless spores of *C. perfringens* 8-6 and of Nakatani et al. (91) with decoated, ion exchanged spores of *B. megaterium* ATCC 19213 indicate that coats are not required for the involvement of mineral cations in germination, and presumably, then, the outer membrane also is not required.

Mineral release during germination occurs in a sequence. Johnstone et al. (92) germinated spores of *B. megaterium* KM with 1 m$M$ L-alanine in 50 m$M$ KCl solution without heat activation and followed release of minerals and DPA in the first minutes after triggering. Release of DPA, Ca, and Zn was detected immediately after addition of germinant. Mg was released only after a lag of about 1 min, and Mn was released still later after a lag of about 3 min. Cortex hydrolysis did not begin until about 2 min after germinant addition, and the rise in ATP pool did not begin until after about 4 min. Johnstone et al. proposed that release of Zn was involved in the triggering reaction resulting in commitment to germinate since both phenomena showed similar kinetics. The site of the triggering reaction is thought to be the inner membrane, as reviewed, for example, by Keynan (93), and the receptor for germinants appears to have allosteric binding sites. However, the exact reactions involved are not defined, and the proposed bases for any modulation by mineral ions are speculative. Moreover, it appears that many of the changes in germination may be reversible prior to outgrowth; at least phase-dark spores can regain refractility (94). Clearly, future research on the effects of minerals on heat stabilization and on germination must be in the direction of molecular information, and the new techniques of molecular genetics should be of major help. However, there still is need for work on basic physiology and biochemistry to provide information on just what is being stabilized against heat damage, what is the triggering reaction for germination, and what are the roles of the cortical peptidoglycan in heat resistance and in germination.

## ACKNOWLEDGMENTS

The contributions of Gary R. Bender to the work in our laboratory on spores and mineralization are acknowledged with pleasure, as are the general encouragement and advise of Philipp Gerhardt over many years. The work was supported by award number DAALO3-86-K-0075 from the U.S. Army Research Office.

## REFERENCES

1. W. Epstein and L. Laimins, Potassium transport in *Escherichia coli*: Diverse systems with common control by osmotic forces, Trends Biochem. Sci. *5*, 21–23 (1981).

2. F. M. Harold, *The Vital Force: A Study of Bioenergetics*, Freeman, New York, 1986.

3. R. E. Marquis and E. L. Carstensen, Electric conductivity and internal osmolality of intact bacterial cells, J. Bacteriol. *113*, 1198–1206 (1973).

4. A. D. Warth, Molecular structure of the bacterial spore, Adv. Microbial Physiol. *17*, 1–45 (1978).

5. R. E. Marquis, E. L. Carstensen, G. R. Bender, and S. Z. Child, "Physiological biophysics of spores," in G. J. Dring, D. J. Ellar, and G. W. Gould, Eds., *Fundamental and Applied Aspects of Bacterial Spores*, Academic, London, 1985, pp. 227–240.

6. W. G. Murrell and A. D. Warth, "Composition and heat resistance of bacterial spores," in L. L. Campbell and H. O. Halvorson, Eds., *Spores III*, American Society for Microbiology, Ann Arbor, MI, 1965, pp. 1–24.

7. G. R. Bender and R. E. Marquis, Spore heat resistance and specific mineralization, Appl. Environ. Microbiol. *50*, 1414–1421 (1985).

8. A. D. Warth, Relationship between the heat resistance of spores and the optimum and maximum growth temperatures of *Bacillus* species, J. Bacteriol. *134*, 699–705 (1978).

9. M. Dworkin, *Developmental Biology of the Bacteria*, Benjamin/Cummings, Reading, MA, 1985.

10. J. A. Salas, J. A. Guijarro, and C. Hardison, "Metal ion content of *Streptomyces* spores: high calcium content as a feature of *Streptomyces*," in G. J. Dring, D.

J. Ellar, and G. W. Gould, Eds., *Fundamental and Applied Aspects of Bacterial Spores*, Academic, London, 1985, pp. 341–350.

11. J. Grain and J. Senaud, *Oscillospira guillermondii*, bactérie du rumen: Etude ultrastructurale du trichome et de sporulation, J. Ultrastr. Res. *55*, 228–244 (1976).

12. E. Freese and J. Heinze, "Metabolic and genetic control of bacterial sporulation," in A. Hurst and G. W. Gould, Eds., *The Bacterial Spore*, Vol. 2, Academic, London, 1983, pp. 102–172.

13. W. A. Hardwick and J. W. Foster, On the nature of sporogenesis in some aerobic bacteria, J. Gen. Physiol. *35*, 907–927 (1952).

14. M. Mychajlonka, A. M. Slee, and R. A. Slepecky, "Requirements for microcycle sporulation in outgrowing *Bacillus megaterium* cells," in P. Gerhardt, R. N. Costilow, and H. L. Sadoff, Eds., *Spores VI*, American Society for Microbiology, Washington, DC, 1975, pp. 434–440.

15. R. E. Marquis, G. R. Bender, E. L. Carstensen, and S. Z. Child, "Electrochemical and mechanical interactions in *Bacillus* spore and vegetative mureins," in R. Hakenbeck, J-V. Höltje, and H. Labischinski, Eds., *The Target of Penicillin*, Walter de Gruyter, Berlin, 1983, pp. 43–48.

16. T. C. Beaman and P. Gerhardt, Heat resistance of bacterial spores correlated with protoplast dehydration, mineralization, and thermal adaptation, Appl. Environ. Microbiol. *52*, 1242–1246 (1986).

17. K. Johnstone, G. S. A. B. Stewart, I. R. Scott, and D. J. Ellar, Zinc release and the sequence of biochemical events during triggering of *Bacillus megaterium* KM spore germination, Biochem. J. *208*, 407–411 (1982).

18. L. E. Sacks, Influence of cations on lysozyme-induced germination of coatless spores of *Clostridium perfringens* 8–6, Biochim. Biophys. Acta *674*, 118–127 (1981).

19. B. J. Wilkinson, J. A. Deans, and D. J. Ellar, Biochemical evidence for the reversed polarity of the outer membrane of the bacterial forespore, Biochem. J. *152*, 561–569 (1975).

20. R. E. Marquis, G. R. Bender, E. L. Carstensen, and S. Z. Child, Dielectric characterization of forespores isolated from *Bacillus megaterium* 19213, J. Bacteriol. *153*, 436–442 (1983).

21. J. A. Todd and D. J. Ellar, Alteration in the penicillin-binding profile of *Bacillus megaterium* during sporulation, Nature *300*, 640–643 (1982).

22. C. E. Buchanan and S. L. Neyman, Correlation of penicillin-binding protein composition with different functions of two membranes in *Bacillus subtilis* forespores, J. Bacteriol. *165*, 498–503 (1986).

23. H-S. Houng, A. R. Lynn, and B. P. Rosen, ATP-driven calcium transport in membrane vesicles of *Streptococcus sanguis*, J. Bacteriol. *168*, 1040–1044 (1986).

24. S. V. Ambudkar, G. W. Zlotnick, and B. P. Rosen, Calcium efflux from *Escherichia coli*. Evidence for two systems. J. Biol. Chem. *259*, 6142–6146 (1984).

25. E. Eisenstadt and S. Silver, "Calcium transport during sporulation in *Bacillus subtilis*," in H. O. Halvorson, R. Hanson, and L. L. Campbell, Eds., *Spores V*, American Society for Microbiology, Washington, DC, 1972, pp. 425–433.

26. S. Silver, K. Toth, and H. Scribner, Facilitated transport of calcium by cells and subcellular membranes of *Bacillus subtilis* and *Escherichia coli*, J. Bacteriol. *122*, 880–885 (1975).

27. S. Silver, "Calcium transport in microorganisms," in E. D. Weinberg, Ed., *Microorganisms and Minerals*, Dekker, New York, 1978, pp. 49–103.

28. F. Bronner, W. C. Nash, and E. E. Golub, "Calcium transport in *Bacillus megaterium*," in P. Gerhardt, R. N. Costilow, and H. L. Sadoff, Eds., *Spores VI*, American Society for Microbiology, Washington, DC, 1975, pp. 356–361.

29. J. M. La Nauze, D. J. Ellar, G. Denton, and J. A. Postgate, "Some properties of forespores isolated from *Bacillus megaterium*" in A. N. Barker, G. W. Gould and J. Wolf, Eds., *Spore Research 1973*, Academic, London, 1974, pp. 41–46.

30. C. Hogarth and D. J. Ellar, Calcium accumulation during sporulation of *Bacillus megaterium* KM, Biochem. J. *176*, 197–203 (1978).

31. C. Hogarth and D. J. Ellar, Energy-dependence of calcium accumulation during sporulation of *Bacillus megaterium* KM, Biochem. J. *178*, 627–632 (1979).

32. D. J. Ellar, "Spore specific structures and their function," in R. Y. Stanier, H. J. Rogers, and J. B. Ward, Eds., *Relations between Structure and Function in the Prokaryotic Cell*, Cambridge University Press, 1978, pp. 295–325.

33. D. L. T. Seto-Young and D. J. Ellar, Studies of calcium transport during growth and sporulation, Microbios *30*, 191–208 (1981).

34. I. Kusaka and T. Matsushita, Characterization of a $Ca^{2+}$ uniporter for *Bacillus subtilis* by partial purification and reconstitution into phospholipid vesicles, J. Gen. Microbiol. *133*, 1337–1342 (1987).

35. W. De Vrij, R. Bulthuis, E. Postma, and W. N. Konings, Calcium transport in membrane vesicles of *Bacillus subtilis*, J. Bacteriol. *164*, 1294–1300 (1985).

36. B. P. Rosen, Bacterial calcium transport, Biochim. Biophys. Acta *906*, 101–110 (1987).

37. S. P. Gorman, E. M. Scott, and E. P. Hutchinson, Emergence and development of resistance to antimicrobial chemicals and heat in spores of *Bacillus subtilis*, J. Appl. Bacteriol. *57*, 153–163 (1984).

38. R. S. Hanson, M. V. Curry, J. V. Garner, and H. O. Halvorson, Mutants of *Bacillus cereus* strain T that produce thermoresistant spores lacking dipicolinate and have low levels of calcium, Can. J. Microbiol. *18*, 1139–1143 (1972).

39. G. J. Dring and G. W. Gould, Reisolation of the *B. cereus* T DPA-negative heat resistant spore mutant of Hanson et al., Spore Newsletter *8*, 130–131 (1981).

40. G. Balassa, P. Milhaud, E. Raulet, M. T. Silva, and J. C. F. Sousa, A *Bacillus subtilis* mutant requiring dipicolinic acid for the development of heat-resistant spores, J. Gen. Microbiol. *110*, 365–379 (1979).

41. E. Eisenstadt, S. Fisher, C-L. Der, and S. Silver, Manganese transport in *Bacillus subtilis* W23 during growth and sporulation, J. Bacteriol. *113*, 1363–1372.

42. G. Alderton and N. Snell, Chemical states of bacterial spores and dry heat resistance, Appl. Environ. Microbiol. *17*, 745–749 (1969).

43. R. Slepecky and J. W. Foster, Alterations in metal content of spores of *Bacillus megaterium* and the effects on some spore properties, J. Bacteriol. *78*, 117–123 (1959).

44. H. Aoki and R. A. Slepecky, Inducement of a heat shock requirement for germination and production of increased heat resistance in *Bacillus fastidiosus* spores by manganous ions, J. Bacteriol. *114*, 137–143 (1973).

45. H. Aoki and R. Slepecky, "The formation of *Bacillus megaterium* spores having increased heat and radiation resistance and variable heat shock requirements due to manganous ions," in A. N. Barker, G. W. Gould, and J. Wolf, Eds., *Spore Research 1973*, Academic, London, 1974, pp. 93–102.

46. H. F. Foerster and J. W. Foster, Endotrophic calcium, strontium, and barium spores of *Bacillus megaterium* and *Bacillus cereus*, J. Bacteriol. *91*, 1333–1345 (1966).

47. S. H. Black, T. Hashimoto, and P. Gerhardt, Calcium reversal of the heat susceptibility and dipicolinate deficiency of spores formed "endotrophically" in water, Can. J. Microbiol. *6*, 213–224 (1960).

48. G. Alderton and N. Snell, Base exchange and heat resistance in bacterial spores, Biochem. Biophys. Res. Commun. *10*, 139–143 (1963).

49. G. Alderton, P. T. Thompson, and N. Snell, Heat adaptation and ion exchange in *Bacillus megaterium* spores, Science *143*, 141–143 (1964).

50. G. Alderton and N. Snell, Bacterial spores: Chemical sensitization to heat, Science *163*, 1212–1213 (1969).

51. G. Alderton, J. K. Chen, and K. A. Ito, Heat resistance of the chemical resistance forms of *Clostridium botulinum* 62A spores over the water activity range of 0 to 0.9, Appl. Environ. Microbiol. *40*, 511–515 (1980).

52. L. J. Rode and J. W. Foster, Quantitative aspects of exchangeable calcium in spores of *Bacillus megaterium*, J. Bacteriol. *91*, 1589–1593 (1966).

53. Y. Ando and T. Tsuzuki, Mechanism of chemical manipulation of heat resistance of *Clostridium perfringens* spores, J. Appl. Bacteriol. *54*, 197–202 (1983).

54. K. S. Rajan, R. Jaw, and N. Grecz, Role of chelation and water binding of calcium in dormancy and heat resistance of bacterial endospores, Bioinorg. Chem. *8*, 477–491 (1978).

55. B. Setlow and P. Setlow, Measurements of the pH within dormant and germinated bacterial spores, Proc. Natl. Acad. Sci. USA *77*, 474–476 (1980).

56. B. M. Swerdlow, B. Setlow, and P. Setlow, Levels of $H^+$ and other monovalent cations in dormant and germinating spores of *Bacillus megaterium* QM B1551, J. Bacteriol. *148*, 20–29 (1981).

57. W. H. Crosby, R. A. Greene, and R. A. Slepecky, "The relationship of metal content to dormancy, germination and sporulation in *Bacillus megaterium*," in A. N. Barker, G. W. Gould, and J. Wolf, Eds., *Spore Research 1971*, Academic, London, 1971, pp. 143–160.

58. R. A. Rosson and K. H. Nealson, Manganese binding and oxidation by spores of a marine *Bacillus*, J. Bacteriol. *151*, 1027–1034 (1982).

59. S. P. Gorman, E. M. Scott, and E. P. Hutchinson, Hypochlorite effects on spores and spore forms of *Bacillus subtilis* and on a spore lytic enzyme, J. Appl. Bacteriol. *56*, 295–303 (1984).

60. A. S. Kamat and D. S. Pradhan, Involvement of calcium in dipicolinic acid in the resistance of *Bacillus cereus* BIS-59 spores to u.v. and gamma radiations, Int. J. Radiat. Biol. *51*, 7–18 (1987).

61. N. Grecz, T. Tang, and H. A. Frank, Photoprotection by dipicolinate against inactivation of bacterial spores with ultraviolet light, J. Bacteriol. *113*, 1058–1060 (1973).

62. G. R. Germaine and W. G. Murrell, Effect of dipicolinic acid on the ultraviolet radiation resistance of *Bacillus cereus* spores, Photochem. Photobiol. *17*, 145–154 (1973).

63. G. R. Bender and R. E. Marquis, Sensitivity of various salt forms of *Bacillus megaterium* spores to the germinating action of hydrostatic pressure, Can. J. Microbiol. *28*, 643–649 (1982).

64. G. W. Gould, "Mechanisms of resistance and dormancy," in A. Hurst and G. W. Gould, Eds., *The Bacterial Spore*, Vol. 2, Academic, London, 1984, pp. 173–209.

65. G. W. Gould and A. J. H. Sale, "Role of pressure in the stabilization and de-stabilization of bacterial spores," in M. A. Sleigh and A. G. Macdonald, Eds., *The Effects of Pressure on Organisms*, Academic, New York, 1972, pp. 147–157.

66. J. G. Clouston and P. A. Wills, Initiation of germination and inactivation of *Bacillus pumilus* spores by hydrostatic pressure, J. Bacteriol. *97*, 684–690 (1969).

67. J. G. Clouston and P. A. Wills, Kinetics of initiation of germination of *Bacillus pumilus* spores by hydrostatic pressure, J. Bacteriol. *103*, 140–143 (1970).

68. W. G. Murrell and P. A. Wills, Initiation of *Bacillus* spore germination by hydrostatic pressure: Effect of temperature, J. Bacteriol. *129*, 1272–1280 (1977).

69. L. Chung, K. S. Rajan, E. Merdinger, and N. Grecz, Coordinative binding of divalent cations with ligands related to bacterial spores, Biophys. J. *11*, 469–482 (1971).

70. R. Scherrer and P. Gerhardt, Location of calcium within *Bacillus* spores by electron probe X-ray microanalysis, J. Bacteriol. *112*, 559–568 (1972).

71. Y. Ando, Some properties of ionic forms of spores of a *Clostridium perfringens* strain, Japan J. Bacteriol. *31*, 713–717 (1976).

72. M. Stewart, A. P. Somylo, A. V. Somylo, H. Shuman, J. A. Lindsay, and W. G. Murrell, Distribution of calcium and other elements in cryosectioned *Bacillus cereus* T spores determined by high resolution scanning electron probe X-ray microanalysis, J. Bacteriol. *143*, 481–491 (1980).

73. K. Johnstone, D. J. Ellar, and T. C. Appleton, Location of metal ions in *Bacillus megaterium* spores by high resolution electron probe X-ray microanalysis, FEMS Microbiol. Lettr. *7*, 97–101 (1980).

74. T. Nishihara, T. Ichikawa, and M. Kondo, Location of elements in ashed spores of *Bacillus megaterium*, Microbiol. Immunol. *24*, 495–506 (1980).

75. J. J. Windle and L. E. Sacks, Electron paramagnetic resonance of manganese (II) and copper (II) in spores, Biochim. Biophys. Acta *66*, 173–179 (1963).

76. K. Johnstone, G. S. A. B. Stewart, M. D. Barratt, and D. J. Ellar, An electron paramagnetic resonance study of the manganese environment within dormant spores of *Bacillus megaterium*, Biochim. Biophys. Acta *714*, 379–391 (1982).

77. E. L. Carstensen, R. E. Marquis, and P. Gerhardt, Dielectric study of the phys-

ical state of electrolytes and water within *Bacillus cereus* spores, J. Bacteriol. *107*, 106–113 (1971).

78. E. L. Carstensen and R. E. Marquis, "Dielectric and electrochemical properties of bacterial cells," in P. Gerhardt, R. N. Costilow, and H. L. Sadoff, Eds., *Spores VI*, American Society for Microbiology, Washington, DC,. 1975, pp. 563–571.

79. E. L. Carstensen, R. E. Marquis, S. Z. Child, and G. R. Bender, Dielectric properties of native and decoated spores of *Bacillus megaterium*, J. Bacteriol. *140*, 917–928 (1979).

80. L-T. Ou and R. E. Marquis, Electrochemical interactions in cell walls of gram-positive cocci, J. Bacteriol. *101*, 92–101 (1970).

81. G. W. Gould and G. J. Dring, Heat resistance of bacterial endospores and concept of an expanded osmoregulatory cortex, Nature (London), *258*, 401–405 (1975).

82. J. C. Lewis, N. S. Snell, and H. K. Burr, Water permeability of bacterial spores and the concept of a contractile cortex, Science *132*, 544–545 (1960).

83. A. D. Warth, "Mechanisms of heat resistance," in G. J. Dring, D. J. Ellar, and G. W. Gould, Eds., *Fundamental and Applied Aspects of Bacterial Spores*, Academic, London, 1985, pp. 209–225.

84. L. J. Rode and J. W. Foster, Ions and the germination of spores of *Bacillus cereus* T, Nature (London) *194*, 1300–1301 (1962).

85. H. F. Foerster and J. W. Foster, Response of *Bacillus* spores to combinations of germinative compounds, J. Bacteriol. *91*, 1168–1177 (1966).

86. L. J. Rode and J. W. Foster, Influence of exchangeable ions on germinability of bacterial spores, J. Bacteriol. *91*, 1582–1588 (1966).

87. Y. Ando, "Germination of *Clostridium perfringens* spores: A proposed role for ions," in H. S. Levinson, A. L. Sonenshein, and D. J. Tipper, Eds., *Sporulation and Germination*, American Society for Microbiology, Washington, DC, 1981, pp. 240–242.

88. H. Riemann and Z. J. Ordal, Responses of *Bacillus subtilis* spores to ionic environments during sporulation and germination, J. Bacteriol. *88*, 1529–1537 (1964).

89. H. P. Fleming and Z. J. Ordal, Responses of *Bacillus subtilis* spores to ionic environments during sporulation and germination, J. Bacteriol. *88*, 1529–1537 (1964).

90. Y. Nakatani, I. Tanida, T. Koshikawa, M. Imagawa, T. Nishihara, and M. Kondo, Collapse of cortex expansion during germination of *Bacillus megaterium* spores, Microbiol. Immunol. *29*, 689–699 (1985).

91. Y. Nakatani, K. Tani, M. Imagawa, T. Nishihara, and M. Kondo, Germinability of coat-lacking spores of *Bacillus megaterium*, Biochem. Biophys. Res. Commun. *128*, 728–732 (1985).

92. K. Johnstone, G. S. A. B. Stewart, I. R. Scott, and D. J. Ellar, Zinc release and the sequence of biochemical events during triggering of *Bacillus megaterium* KM spore germination, Biochem. J. *208*, 407–411 (1982).

93. A. Keynan, "Spore structure and its relations to resistance, dormancy, and

germination,'' in G. Chambliss and J. C. Vary, Eds., *Spores VII*, American Society for Microbiology, Washington, DC 1978, pp. 43–53.

94. H. S. Levinson and F. E. Feenerry, ''Reversion of phase-dark germinated spores of *Clostridium perfringens* Type A to refractility,'' in H. S. Levinson, A. L. Sonenshein, and D. J. Tipper, Eds., *Sporulation and Germination*, American Society for Microbiology, Washington, DC, 1981, pp. 228–231.

# CHAPTER 9

# How Cell Walls of Gram-Positive Bacteria Interact with Metal Ions

RONALD J. DOYLE

Department of Microbiology and Immunology
University of Louisville
Louisville, Kentucky

## Contents

## 9.1 INTRODUCTION: NATURE OF THE INTERACTION BETWEEN CELL WALLS OF GRAM-POSITIVE BACTERIA AND METAL IONS

In Gram-positive bacteria, the cell wall is a solvent-exposed organelle that may offer the first encounter between a bacterium and a molecule in its environment. The wall constitutes a relatively high content of cellular dry weight, up to 40–50% in bacilli, staphylococci, and streptococci. Most cell walls of Gram-positive bacteria contain reasonably large amounts of peptidoglycan and an anionic polymer, such as a teichoic or a teichuronic acid. In *Bacillus subtilis,* there is an approximately equal amount of peptidoglycan and teichoic acid in cell walls obtained from cultures in phosphate-sufficient growth media (1). As far as is known, all walls of Gram-positive bacteria

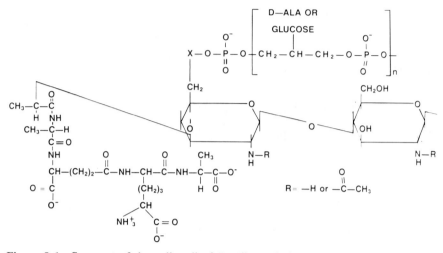

**Figure 9.1** Segment of the cell wall of *Bacillus subtilis* 168. The structure reveals both positively and negatively charged sites. The teichoic acid portion may contain a D-alanine residue in place of the α-D-glucose as shown. The "X" represents the linkage between a muramic acid residue and a teichoic acid polymer.

are negatively charged in media capable of supporting growth (2–5). It is traditional to view the teichoic (or teichuronic) acid as an "accessory" polymer of the cell wall, but this is erroneous because these polyelectrolytes are always found covalently bound to the peptidoglycan portion of the wall. It is certain, however, that the walls contain positive charges, along with the more numerous negative charges. Figure 9.1 shows a segment of the cell wall structure of *B. subtilis* 168. Anionic sites include carboxylate (from peptidoglycan) and phosphate (from teichoic acid). Positively charged sites are exclusively ammonium, from D-alanine (teichoic acid), amino sugar (glycan), and diaminopimelic acid (peptide portion of peptidoglycan). These are the charges that mediate the interaction between cell walls and metal ions.

Many cell surface enzymes require metal ions for activity, such as autolysins (in *B. subtilis*) (6), teichoic acid synthetases, phospholipid-synthesizing enzymes, and peptidoglycan synthetases (reviewed by Hughes et al., 7). The surface-associated glucan-binding lectin of *Streptococcus cricetus* requires $Mn^{2+}$ for expression of activity (8). Cytoplasmic enzymes frequently require monovalent or divalent cations. For example, the phosphoglycerate phosphomutase of *Bacillus subtilis* also requires $Mn^{2+}$ for activity (9). The cations required for protein function or enzyme activity must first pass through the cell wall in order to reach their sites near the membrane or in the cytoplasm. The initial interaction of metal ion with cell wall and the subsequent passing of the ion to the membrane suggested that the wall

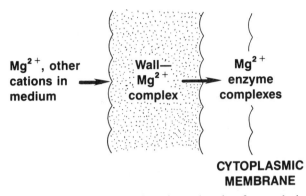

**Mg²⁺, other
cations in  →
medium**

**Wall—
: Mg²⁺ :
complex**

**Mg²⁺
enzyme
complexes**

**CYTOPLASMIC
MEMBRANE**

**Figure 9.2**  Model depicting the transfer of metal cation from solution to wall and to membrane.

was a type of ion exchange resin (see Fig. 9.2). This view was first promoted by the Newcastle group of Archibald, Baddiley, Hancock, Hughes, and colleagues (10–16).

There are several attractive features about the wall–ion exchange concept; these are discussed below. It must be pointed out, however, that the metal–wall–membrane concept was derived largely from the ability of teichoic acid to sequester metal ions. It is known now that peptidoglycan also contributes significantly to the ability of cell walls to complex with cations (17–20).

The transport of metal ions into the cytoplasm of bacteria represents a different level of complexity. In Chapter 3 Sprott provides a review of the means by which bacteria maintain ion gradients in membranes (largely $K^+$ ion). Strategies for the transport of $K^+$, $Mg^{2+}$, and $Ca^{2+}$ are now becoming better understood (21), but the transport of $Mn^{2+}$, $Ni^{2+}$, $Zn^{2+}$, and other transition metals are not so well-defined. If these ions enter the cell as charged cations, then they must first penetrate the relatively thick cell wall, dissociate from the wall, then reassociate with transporter molecules, only to be liberated in the cytoplasm. Some bacteria, including several members of the genus *Bacillus*, possess surface arrays (S-layers) external to the peptidoglycan layer which may also have the ability to complex with metal ions (22). The ultimate incorporation of metal ions into membrane or cytoplasmic proteins may therefore involve several distinct kinetic steps.

For years, textbooks have emphasized that bacterial cell walls are rigid. Work based largely in the laboratory of Marquis in the 1970s has led to a reevaluation of the concept of a rigid cell wall. It is known now that walls are flexible, having the ability to expand and contract depending on ionic conditions and pH. Metal ions can cause a contraction in cell walls, giving rise to more dense structures (23–25). This is because repulsive charges have been effectively neutralized by the cations. In this regard, the teichoic acid of *B. subtilis* behaves as a rigid rod in distilled water, but as a random coil polyelectrolyte in salt solution (26). Divalent cations, such as $Mg^{2+}$, may also serve to cross-link teichoic acid molecules, possibly via coordination of phosphate residues from two teichoic acid molecules with a single $Mg^{2+}$ aquo-ion. The importance of expansion/contraction of walls has been emphasized recently in the reports of Koch and colleagues. It has been shown that when exponential bacteria lose their turgor pressure, then the cells reduce their volumes (27, 28). Earlier papers by Koch et al. (29, 30) established that cell wall responded to surface stress, and that surface stress played a role in maintenance of cell morphology and cell division. The role that divalent ions could have in maintaining turgor or wall shape is unclear. Jurado et al. (31) found that $Sr^{2+}$ ion induced gross morphological alterations in *B. stearothermophilus*. Some *B. subtilis* mutants grow as rods in high concentrations (0.8 *M*) of sodium chloride, but as spheres in low ionic strength media (32). Other mutants of *B. subtilis* assume a normal rod-shaped morphology when $Mg^{2+}$ ion is added at sufficient quantities (33). At present, it is thought that physical forces govern the shapes of bacteria (30). It seems unlikely that the sequestering of ions by the bacterial surface could lead to shape determination or to changes in morphology.

## 9.2 DISTRIBUTION OF CHARGE IN THE CELL WALL OF GRAM-POSITIVE BACTERIA

Weiss (34) provided an early study on the surface charge of *B. subtilis*. It was found that cell-bound penicillinase behaved as if it were at a lower pH than the bulk medium, suggesting that the cell surface was protonated. Several studies have shown that the surfaces of Gram-positive bacteria have low isoelectric values (2, 3, 5) reflecting contributions from teichoic and teichuronic acids. There is considerable evidence to support a view that negative charges are concentrated on the outer face of the cell wall, although the wall matrix contains teichoic acid. Burger (35) found that lysozyme-solubilized walls of *B. subtilis* could bind more anti-teichoic acid antibody

---

**Figure 9.3** Binding of cationized ferritin (CF) to cell walls of *Bacillus subtilis*. (*a*) Thin section of a polar cap joined to cylindrical wall stained with cationized ferritin. Only the outer surface of the wall adsorbed the cationic probe. Bar = 100 nm. (*b*) High magnification of a thin section of cylindrical wall, which clearly shows asymmetric distribution of CF. The arrow points to CF. Bar, 100 nm. (*c*) Thin section of cylindrical wall containing a septum (arrows) that has been treated with CF. Unlike the previous thin sections, this sample was not contrasted with uranyl or lead salts,

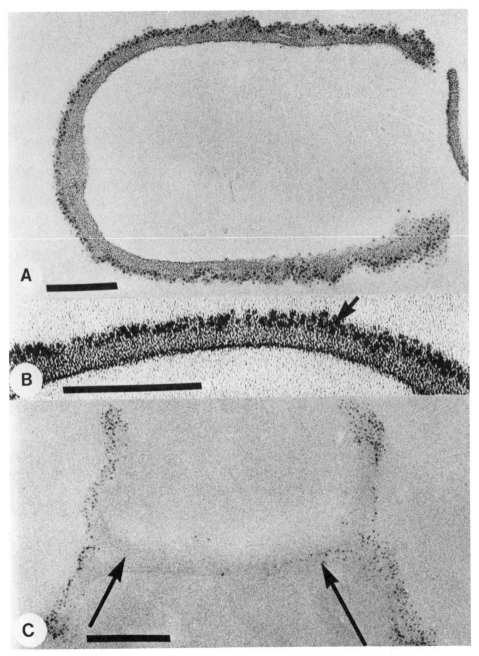

so that the CF probe is more apparent. Very little CF was adsorbed on the septum, whereas the outer surface of the cylindrical wall was labeled. Bars = 100 nm. See Ref. 37 for experimental details. Reprinted by permission of the authors and the American Society for Microbiology (Ref. 37).

than the intact walls. Doyle et al. (36) observed that autolysis or enzymic hydrolysis by lysozyme released concanavalin A-reactive teichoic acids from cell walls of *B. subtilis* 168. They suggested that about one-half of the teichoic acids were surface-exposed and available for interaction with the lectin and about one-half were embedded in the wall matrix. The matrix teichoic acids became lectin-reactive only upon solubilization of the walls by enzymes.

Recently Sonnenfeld et al. (37) have observed that when cationized ferritin (CF) was added to suspensions of *B. subtilis* cell walls, the CF bound strongly to the outer wall face. Electron microscopic examination of CF-treated *B. subtilis* walls revealed that poles and side wall, but not septa, were capable of binding the CF (Fig. 9.3). Presumably, the CF complexed with the most electronegative sites on the wall surface. Autolysis of the walls prior to their interaction with CF resulted in the binding of the label on both wall faces. When very dilute CF was used, it was observed that the poles contained an area that had an especially high affinity for the CF (38). This area appeared to be a "tuft" very near the tip of the cell pole. It was suggested that the wall is laid down in such a manner as to orient the anionic polymers away from the cell membrane and toward the solvent. Previously, Garland et al. (39) observed that gold–concanavalin A tended to bind to the outer surface of *Streptococcus faecalis* 8191. Ruthenium red, however, was able to bind to all regions of the wall, suggesting that teichoic acids were in the wall matrix. Umeda et al. (40) found that CF tended to bind more strongly to the outer part of the cell wall of *Staphylococcus aureus* than to the inner wall face. This binding gave rise to the impression that the wall was smooth on its inner face, but serrated or textured on its outer face. The general conclusion to be reached on the distribution of charge in Gram-positive walls is that more electronegative sites are on the outer surfaces than on the inner surfaces. Work from Beveridge's laboratory has provided strong evidence to show that all portions of the cell wall contain anionic groups (41–49). At present, it is unclear how the asymmetric distribution of charges could influence metal binding and subsequent uptake of metal ions from solution.

## 9.3  METHODS FOR THE MEASUREMENT OF METAL BINDING TO THE CELL WALL

The methods for the qualitative and quantitative determination of cell wall–metal ion interactions are no different from those employed for the study of metal ions with proteins or other polymers. In some respects, however, it is easier to study wall–metal complexes than metal–protein complexes because the walls are insoluble and can be readily separated from unreactive metal ions. Metal–wall interactions have been studied by use of electron microscopy (42, 44, 48), electron spin resonance (49), conductivity (50), equilibrium dialysis (16, 17, 19), centrifugation (51, 52), electron scattering (14), acid–base titrations (51, 52), volume changes (25), and autoradiography (53). In several reports, wall–metal ion mixtures have been centrifuged, decanted, and washed. The wall residue is then analyzed for metal content. This technique is convenient and simple, yet suffers from a major short-coming. The association between metal ion and cell wall is generally quite low, on the order of $10^3$–$10^4$ $M^{-1}$. If, for example, a 1-mg sample of cell wall in a 1-ml volume is centrifuged and washed twice with 5–10 ml water or buffer, there would be considerable loss of metal in the washings owing to dissociation reactions. Equilibrium dialysis largely circumvents this loss of bound metal. At equilibrium, the outside of the dialysis bag contains the unbound (U) metal, whereas the inside of the bag contains both bound (B) and unbound metal. A plot of $B/U$ versus $B$ (Scatchard plot) can be used to obtain association constants ($K_a$) and numbers of metal reactive sites, $n$. Figure 9.4 shows the results of typical equilibrium dialysis experiments for

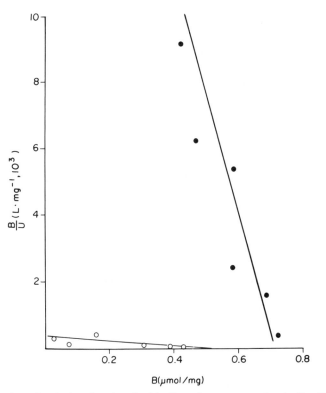

**Figure 9.4**  Scatchard plot showing the binding of manganous ion to *Bacillus subtilis* cell walls. The closed circles represent unmodified cell wall, whereas the open circles represent a mildly acid hydrolyzed wall sample depleted of acetyl groups.

the binding of $Mn^{2+}$ to *B. subtilis* cell walls. It is generally convenient to run several samples at once, employing a range of metal ion concentrations. Equilibrium dialysis is versatile in that various buffers, salts, competing ions, and so on may be included. Major shortcomings of the method include the facts that at least 40–48 h is required to attain equilibrium and there is a requirement for very many concentrations of metal ion.

## 9.4    METAL ION BINDING SITES IN THE CELL WALL OF *BACILLUS SUBTILIS*

It is assumed that the carboxylate and phosphate groups of the cell wall would be potential metal binding sites. Methods are available for chemically modifying or removing these electronegative groups so that their role in metal complex formation can be assessed (Figure 9.5). For example, ammonium groups can be neutralized (by acetic anhydride), removed (deamination by nitrous acid), or converted into negative sites (by use of succinic anhydride). Carboxylate groups can be neutralized or converted into positively charged sites by water-soluble carbodiimides and ethanolamine or ethylenediamine, respectively. In addition, teichoic acids may be removed by dilute base, resulting in a phosphorus-free wall preparation. Furthermore, mild acid hydrolysis removes some of the acetyl groups from *N*-acetylhexosamines of the glycan portion of the wall, creating new ammonium group sites (the wall is also partially hydrolyzed, but only the insoluble portion is used for studies on metal ion binding). It is clear then that the functional groups of the wall may be modified in such a manner as to remove ionic residues or change the charge distribution. These walls are valuable in assessing the chemical basis for the specificity of cell wall–metal ion complex formation. Table 9.1 summarizes some results on the binding of $Mn^{2+}$, $Ca^{2+}$, and $Na^{2+}$ to unmodified and chemically modified cell walls of *B. subtilis*

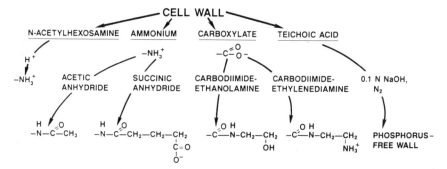

**Figure 9.5**    Modification of charge distribution on Gram-positive bacterial cell walls.

TABLE 9.1  Metal Ion Complex Formation with Chemically Modified Cell Walls of *Bacillus subtilis*[a]

| Modifying Agent | Mn²⁺ | | Ca²⁺ | | Na⁺ | |
|---|---|---|---|---|---|---|
| | $n$[b] | $K_a$[c] | $n$ | $K_a$ | $n$ | $K_a$ |
| None, control walls | 0.74 ± 0.16 | 52 ± 11 | 0.75 ± 0.15 | 40 ± 8 | 0.83 ± 0.04 | 3.9 ± 0.1 |
| Acetic anhydride | 0.98 ± 0.13 | 60 ± 8 | 1.0 ± 0.30 | 37 ± 17 | 1.1 ± 0.20 | 9.0 ± 2 |
| Succinic anhydride | 1.0 ± 0.20 | 67 ± 22 | 1.1 ± 0.30 | 47 ± 6 | 1.3 ± 0.26 | 3.8 ± 2 |
| Ethanolamine carbodiimide | 0.72 ± 0.14 | 25 ± 6 | 0.75 ± 0.42 | 36 ± 24 | 0.3 ± 0.10 | 15 ± 3 |
| Ethylenediamine carbodiimide | 0.27 ± 0.10 | 17 ± 4 | 0.1 ± 0.1 | 1.2 ± 0.18 | 0.03 ± 0.03 | 1 ± 1 |
| Sodium hydroxide–extracted. Phosphorus-free walls | 0.69 ± 12 | 75 ± 11 | 0.61 ± 0.18 | 18 ± 7.9 | 0.48 ± 0.17 | 6.3 ± 3.4 |
| Mild acid hydrolysis of wall | 0.11 ± 0.08 | 11 ± 7 | 0.1 ± 0.1 | 0.3 ± 0.2 | ND[d] | ND |

[a] Some of the data were taken from Refs. 17 and 19.
[b] Micromoles per milligram cell wall.
[c] $M^{-1} \times 10^{-3}$.
[d] ND, not determined.

168 (see also Fig. 9.4). The data show three general trends: (1) Introduction of positive charges in the wall greatly reduce the $K_a$ and the $n$ (number of sites). This is seen by comparing the binding of the control walls with carbodiimide–ethylenediamine and mildly acid hydrolyzed walls. In contrast, when walls were acetylated to neutralize the ammonium groups, there was usually a rise in both $K_a$ and $n$ values. (2) Succinoylation increased $n$ values but did not change association constants. (3) Removal of phosphorus resulted in a reduction of $n$ without a change in $K_a$ for any of the metal ions. It seems certain then that teichoic acid and peptidoglycan contribute to the ability of the cell wall of *B. subtilis* to complex with metal (17, 19). In other experiments using unmodified walls, the sequence $Mn^{2+} = Ni^{2+} = Ca^{2+} > Na^+ = Li^+$ for the $K_a$ has been reported (19). It is probable that the cell walls of other Gram-positive bacteria behave similarly to metal ions. Ou et al. (51), on the basis of acid–base titrations of streptococcal walls, concluded that carboxylate groups were involved in complex formation with metal ions. Galdiero et al. (54), however, suggested that the wall of *S. aureus* interacted with monovalent cations by a mechanism different from divalent cations.

## 9.5 REGULATION OF COMPLEX FORMATION BETWEEN CELL WALLS AND METAL IONS

There may be several levels for regulation of cation–wall interactions. Unfortunately, the literature reveals very little about ion–wall regulatory mechanisms. The results with chemically modified walls show that the higher the ratio of ammonium to carboxylate or phosphate, the lower the extent of complex formation with cations. It is therefore possible that the cell can modulate metal binding by regulating the insertion of ammonium groups. In *B. subtilis*, it is known that the glycan hexosamines are not fully acetylated (55). The glucosamine is approximately 71% N-acetylated, whereas the muramic acid is approximately 67% N-acetylated. A small change in the degree of N-substitution could result in a much greater change in metal binding to the wall (Table 9.1). It is likely that if N-acetylation is a regulatory reaction in controlling metal–wall interactions, the acetylation step would occur during wall precursor synthesis. This is because wall, once inserted, is pushed farther and farther away from the cell membrane during growth (this has been referred to as the inside-to-outside growth; see Ref. 1 for review). Even though *B. subtilis* possesses a deacetylase (56), it seems remote that this enzyme would be far removed from the plasma membrane. Studies are needed on cell walls from metal-sufficient and metal-limiting cultures to confirm that N-acetylation may be important in cation recognition by Gram-positive bacteria.

In *B. subtilis*, as well as in most other bacteria, there is an efflux of protons from the cells during growth. Usually, $H^+$ is exchanged for $K^+$ to maintain

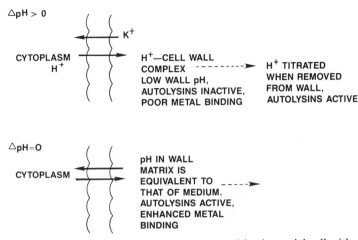

**Figure 9.6**   Schematic representation of a Gram-positive bacterial cell with and without a protonmotive force imposed across the cytoplasmic membrane.

electroneutrality. Work from the laboratory of Marquis (52, 57) has shown that the wall binds protons in preference to metal cations. This suggests that the wall may be a sink or reservoir for protons. A protonated wall would have very little tendency to bind metal cations. It is known that dissipation of the protonmotive force results in uncontrolled autolysis in *B. subtilis*, but that the lysis can be arrested by imposing an artificial energized state on the plasma membrane (58). The energized membrane appears to play a role in regulating autolysins in bacilli. Figure 9.6 depicts a cell with and without proton gradients in its membrane. The energized cell would have very little tendency to sequester metals, whereas the depolarized cell would be able to complex with cations. It should be pointed out that most studies on wall–metal ion complexes have been derived from use of isolated cell walls and not from metabolizing bacteria. Figure 9.7 shows the results of lowering the pH on the ability of *B. subtilis* cell walls to bind the $Mn^{2+}$–aquo ion (19). As predicted from the studies of Marquis et al. (25, 57), it is seen that high hydrogen ion concentrations reduce the association (but not the numbers of combining sites) between the $Mn^{2+}$ and the cell walls. Weiss (34) reported an indirect means of determining the surface pH values of exponentially growing *B. subtilis*. When constitutive penicillinase activity was determined as a function of pH, it was found that the cell wall-bound enzyme behaved as if it were at a lower pH than soluble enzyme. In addition, Kemper et al. (59) recently found that the inducible levansucrase was inactive until it was secreted into the medium. The levansucrase activity was very low while it was traversing the cell wall, possibly because of a low pH in the wall. It should be pointed out that the pH of the wall when saturated

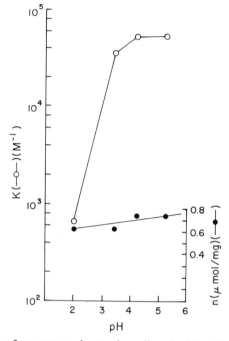

**Figure 9.7**   Binding of manganous ion to the cell wall of *Bacillus subtilis* at different hydrogen ion concentrations. Taken from Ref. 19. Reprinted by permission of the authors and the American Society for Microbiology (Ref. 19).

with protons would be dictated by the pHs of the carboxylates and the secondary phosphate groups. If the pH of the wall of a metabolizing bacterium is low, it would present some difficulties in the cell being able to acquire cations. A cation would unlikely be able to diffuse through a relatively thick positively charged wall matrix. Some bacteria may have a means to circumvent this low pH wall barrier. For example, divalent cations may enter cells as chelates of carboxylic acids or as complexes with peptides. Haavik (60) showed that bacitracin enhanced the toxicity of divalent cations in *B. licheniformis*, but the toxicity could be reduced by excess $Mg^{2+}$. Haavik speculates, "The function of the bacitracin peptides may be to extract essential divalent cations from 'waiting sites' on the surface of the cells and transfer the cations to the transport mechanisms in the cytoplasmic membrane." When complexed, the cation would be effectively neutralized and therefore able to diffuse through the cell wall.

In any discussion about the interaction between bacterial cell surfaces and metal ions it must be emphasized that the surfaces are dynamic. For example, during exponential growth of *B. subtilis*, at least 50% of the wall is lost into the medium during each cell division (1). This loss of wall is termed turnover, but the shed wall components are not reutilized or recycled. The inside-to-outside wall growth of cell cylinders assures that newly inserted wall materials are always pushed away from the plasma membrane toward the cell periphery. The interaction between metal ions and wall components on the very outer surface would not appear to provide any benefit to the cell. The surface-associated cations would probably be returned to the growth medium in the form of a soluble wall–metal ion complex as wall is turned over. An insoluble wall–cation complex serving as a cation exchanger would therefore seem remote, unless the cations were first sequestered or neutralized with nonwall compounds prior to their interaction with the cellular surface. Cell wall turnover has been reported in a number of bacteria, including members of the genera *Bacillus, Lactobacillus, Listeria, Staphylococcus, Escherichia, Neisseria,* and *Salmonella* and others (61).

The restrictive influence of D-alanine on the binding of cations to cell walls has been documented by several reports (10, 13, 16). When D-Ala is esterified to the teichoic acid, an ammonium group is introduced into the chain. This is probably another level of regulation for the binding of metal ions by bacteria. Growth of Gram-positive bacteria in high sodium chloride concentrations results in cells with walls containing reduced amounts of D-Ala in their teichoic acids. These D-Ala-deficient walls bind $Mg^{2+}$ ions much better than D-Ala containing walls (10, 16). In addition, when cells are grown in relatively low pH ranges the walls contain more esterified D-Ala than walls from cells grown at near-neutral pH (10). These low-pH walls bind $Mg^{2+}$ less well than walls from neutral cultures (10). When *B. coagulans* was grown at 55°C, its wall contained less D-Ala and bound $Mg^{2+}$ to a greater extent than did walls from a 37°C culture (31). Lambert et al. (16) showed that the removal of D-Ala from a *S. aureus* wall preparation did not result in a change of the affinity of the walls for $Mg^{2+}$. These de-esterified walls did however exhibit an increase in the number of combining sites. The results with D-Ala, coupled with those obtained from the modification of ammonium groups, clearly reveal that positive charges in the wall profoundly influence cell wall–metal ion complex formation. It is not certain that a bacterium would synthesize D-Ala containing teichoic acids solely in order to regulate metal uptake. The D-Ala may influence other cellular processes, such as autolysin activity. The loss of metal binding upon insertion of D-Ala in the teichoic acid may be a tangential consequence of some unrelated function of the D-Ala moiety.

Growth of Gram-positive bacteria in high salt concentrations also results in an increase in the amount of wall-bound teichoic acid (62, 63). Heptinstall et al. (12) found that these walls had an increased capacity to bind $Mg^{2+}$. Moreover, growth of cells in reduced $Mg^{2+}$ gives rise to cells with walls containing high amounts of phosphorus. These walls also bind more $Mg^{2+}$ than walls from Mg-sufficient cultures. The higher amounts of teichoic acid incorporated in the wall seems to be an evolutionary adaptation to reduced $Mg^{2+}$ in the environment. The versatility of Gram-positive bacteria in response to changes in their growth media is remarkable. Most Gram-positive cells, when cultured in limiting phosphorus, synthesize a peptidoglycan-associated teichuronic acid. The teichuronic acids maintain a net negative surface charge, and at the same time, are capable of complexing with metal ions (11). In fact, the $K_a$ of $Mg^{2+}$ for teichoic acid walls of *B. subtilis* W23 is very similar to that for teichuronic acid walls of the same bacterium (11). Metal ion binding seems to be tightly coupled with high ratios of negative to positive charges.

Another possibility for the modulation of numbers of charges in the cell wall is the cross-linking reaction. When diaminopimelic acid is cross-linked to a terminal D-Ala (Fig. 9.1), there is a loss of both a positive and negative charge. In keeping with the above discussion, the loss of the positive charge may greatly enhance metal binding. As far as is known, no studies on metal binding have been performed on walls of the same chemotype with variable degrees of cross-linking.

## 9.6   METAL ION-WALL INTERACTIONS IN PERSPECTIVE

It now seems clear that the chemistry of the cell wall–metal ion interaction is far better understood than the regulation of charges in the cell wall. The signals that dictate cross-linking or amino sugar substitution (acetylation for many bacteria) remain unidentified. It is unfortunate that no studies have appeared, other than those involving D-alanine, describing metal uptake, cell wall cross-linking, and amino sugar content. This would appear to be a particularly critical area for examination, because bacteria are important in metal transformations and may be effective in reducing heavy metal contamination of the environment.

Archibald (64) has recently emphasized that the wall, because of its ionic character, contributes to the homeostasis of bacterial growth. Archibald reviewed the role of the wall as a putative donor of $Mg^{2+}$ for cellular processes. Before the role of the wall can be better defined in the sequestration of metal ions from the environment, it will be necessary to study cation binding and uptake during the bacterial cell cycle. Careful analyses of wall constituents as a function of the cell cycle should reveal information about subtle differences in positive charges that could mediate large changes in metal binding.

If it is accepted that the energized membrane plays a role in the regulation of autolysins (58), then energized membrane also must be coupled to metal ion binding by cell walls, because walls of many Gram-positive bacteria are shed into the medium during growth. The relationship between walls, metal ions, and membranes is further complicated by the extrusion of protons as a result of metabolic processes. If the wall is protonated during division, there may be little tendency to bind metals by the bacterial surface. It may be possible to determine wall pH in situ by use of appropriate indicator dyes.

The in vitro studies have shown many times that the walls of Gram-positive bacteria have a reasonably high affinity for cations. Furthermore, in many cases, there is a pronounced selectivity for the metals. In addition, many membrane and cytoplasmic enzymes require $Mg^{2+}$ or trace metals for activity. It seems compelling to conclude that the wall serves to bind these metal ions and serve them up to the enzymes. What is lacking is in vivo studies describing the kinetics and mechanism of cation transfer from medium to wall to membrane (or cytoplasm). These studies will require methods that have not been employed in the past.

## ACKNOWLEDGMENTS

Work in the author's laboratory related to *Bacillus* cell walls has been supported by the National Science Foundation PCM 78-08903. The author thanks former students T. H. Matthews and E. M. Sonnenfeld for help with some of the experiments.

## REFERENCES

1. R. J. Doyle and A. L. Koch, The functions of autolysins in the growth and division of *Bacillus subtilis*. CRC Crit. Reviews Microbiol. *15*, 169–222 (1987).

2. A. M. James, The electrical properties and topochemistry of bacterial cells. Adv. Colloid Interface Sci. *15*, 171–221 (1982).

3. V. P. Harden and J. O. Harris, The isoelectric point of bacterial cells. J. Bacteriol. *65*, 198–202 (1953).

4. R. Neihof and W. H. Echols, Physicochemical studies of microbial cell walls. 1. Comparative electrophoretic behavior of intact cells and isolated cell walls. Biochim. Biophys. Acta *318*, 22–32 (1973).

5. D. V. Richmond and D. J. Fisher, The electrophoretic mobility of microorganisms. Adv. Microb. Physiol. *9*, 1–27 (1973).

6. H. J. Rogers, C. Taylor, S. Rayter, and J. B. Ward, Purification and properties of autolytic endo-β-N-acetylglucosaminidase and the N-acetylmuramyl-L-alanine amidase from *Bacillus subtilis* strain 168. J. Gen. Microbiol. *130*, 2395–2402 (1984).

7. A. H. Hughes, I. C. Hancock, and J. Baddiley, The function of teichoic acids in cation control in bacterial membranes. Biochem. J. *132*, 83–93 (1973).

8. D. Drake, K. G. Taylor, and R. J. Doyle, Expression of the glucan-binding lectin

of *Streptococcus cricetus* requires manganous ion. Infect. Immun. *56*, 2205–2207 (1988).

9. N. Vasantha and E. Freese, The role of manganese in growth and sporulation of *Bacillus subtilis*. J. Gen. Microbiol. *112*, 329–336 (1979).

10. A. R. Archibald, J. Baddiley, and S. Heptinstall, The alanine ester content and magnesium binding capacity of walls of *Staphylococcus aureus* H grown at different pH values. Biochim. Biophys. Acta *291*, 629–634 (1973).

11. J. E. Heckels, P. A. Lambert, and J. Baddiley, Binding of magnesium ions to cell walls of *Bacillus subtilis* W23 containing teichoic acid or teichuronic acid. Biochemical J. *162*, 359–365 (1977).

12. S. Heptinstall, A. R. Archibald, and J. Baddiley, Teichoic acids and membrane function in bacteria. Nature *225*, 519–521 (1970).

13. A. Hurst, A. Hughes, M. Duckworth, and J. Baddiley, Loss of D-alanine during sublethal heating of *Staphylococcus aureus* s6 and magnesium binding during repair. J. Gen. Microbiol. *89*, 277–284 (1975).

14. J. Baddiley, I. C. Hancock, and P. M. A. Sherwood, X-Ray photoelectron studies of magnesium ions bound to the cell walls of Gram-positive bacteria. Nature *243*, 43–45 (1973).

15. P. A. Lambert, I. C. Hancock, and J. Baddiley, The interaction of magnesium ions with teichoic acid. Biochem. J. *149*, 519–524 (1975).

16. P. A. Lambert, I. C. Hancock, and J. Baddiley, Influence of alanyl ester residues on the binding of magnesium ions to teichoic acids. Biochem. J. *151*, 671–676 (1975).

17. T. H. Matthews, R. J. Doyle, and U. N. Streips, Contribution of peptidoglycan to the binding of metal ions by the cell wall of *Bacillus subtilis*. Curr. Microbiol. *3*, 51–53 (1979).

18. M. K. Rayman and R. A. MacLeod, Interaction of $Mg^{2+}$ with peptidoglycan and its relation to the prevention of lysis of a marine pseudomonad. J. Bacteriol. *122*, 650–659 (1975).

19. R. J. Doyle, T. H. Matthews, and U. N. Streips, Chemical basis for selectivity of metal ions by the *Bacillus subtilis* cell wall, J. Bacteriol. *143*, 471–480 (1980).

20. B. D. Hoyle and T. J. Beveridge, Metal binding by the peptidoglycan sacculus of *Escherichia coli* K-12, Can. J. Microbiol. *30*, 204–211 (1984).

21. B. P. Rosen and S. Silver, Eds., *Ion Transport in Prokaryotes*, Academic Press, New York, 1987.

22. F. Galdiero, M. A. Tufano, M. T. Berlingieri, and L. Sommese, Ion-binding properties of S-layer proteins from *Bacillus subtilis*, Microbiologica (Italy) *5*, 371–376 (1982).

23. L.-T. Ou and R. E. Marquis, Coccal cell wall compactness and the swelling action of denaturants. Can. J. Microbiol. *18*, 623–629 (1972).

24. L.-T. Ou and R. E. Marquis, Electromechanical interactions in cell walls of Gram-positive cocci. J. Bacteriol. *101*, 92–101 (1970).

25. R. E. Marquis, Salt-induced contraction of bacterial cell walls, J. Bacteriol. *95*, 775–781 (1968).

26. R. J. Doyle, M. L. McDannel, U. N. Streips, D. C. Birdsell, and F. E. Young,

Polyelectrolyte nature of bacterial teichoic acids. J. Bacteriol. *118*, 606–615 (1974).

27. A. L. Koch and M. F. S. Pinette, Nephelometric determination of turgor pressure in growing Gram-negative bacteria. J. Bacteriol. *169*, 3654–3663 (1987).

28. A. L. Koch, S. L. Lane, J. A. Miller, and D. G. Nickens, Contraction of filaments of *Escherichia coli* after disruption of cell membrane by detergent. J. Bacteriol. *169*, 1979–1984 (1987).

29. A. L. Koch, M. L. Higgins, and R. J. Doyle, The role of surface stress in the morphology of microbes. J. Gen. Microbiol. *128*, 927–945 (1982).

30. A. L. Koch, The surface stress theory of microbial morphogenesis. Adv. Microb. Physiol. *24*, 301–366 (1983).

31. A. S. Jurado, A. C. Santana, M. S. DaCosta, and V. M. C. Madeira, Influence of divalent cations on the growth and morphology of *Bacillus stearothermophilus*. J. Gen. Microbiol. *133*, 507–513 (1987).

32. D. Karamata, M. McConnell, and H. J. Rogers, Mapping of *rod* mutants of *Bacillus subtilis*. J. Bacteriol. *111*, 73–79 (1972).

33. H. J. Rogers, P. F. Thurman, C. Taylor, and J. N. Reeve, Mucopeptide synthesis by *rod* mutants of *Bacillus subtilis*. J. Gen. Microbiol. *85*, 335–350 (1974).

34. L. Weiss, The pH value at the surface of *Bacillus subtilis*. J. Gen. Microbiol. *32*, 331–340 (1963).

35. M. M. Burger, Teichoic acids: antigenic determinants, chain separation, and their location in the cell wall. Proc. Natl. Acad. Sci. USA *56*, 910–917 (1966).

36. R. J. Doyle, M. L. McDannel, J. R. Helman, and U. N. Streips, Distribution of teichoic acid in the cell wall of *Bacillus subtilis*. J. Bacteriol. *122*, 152–158 (1975).

37. E. M. Sonnenfeld, T. J. Beveridge, A. L. Koch, and R. J. Doyle, Asymmetric distribution of charge on the cell wall of *Bacillus subtilis*, J. Bacteriol. *163*, 1167–1171 (1985).

38. E. M. Sonnenfeld, T. J. Beveridge, and R. J. Doyle, Discontinuity of charge on cell wall poles of *Bacillus subtilis*, Can. J. Microbiol. *31*, 875–877 (1985).

39. J. M. Garland, A. R. Archibald, and J. Baddiley, An electron microscopic study of the location of teichoic acid and its contribution to staining reactions in walls of *Streptococcus faecalis* 8191. J. Gen. Microbiol. *89*, 73–86 (1975).

40. A. Umeda, Y. Ueki, and K. Amako, Structure of the *Staphylococcus aureus* cell wall determined by the freeze-substitution method. J. Bacteriol. *169*, 2482–2487 (1987).

41. T. J. Beveridge and W. S. Fyfe, Metal fixation by bacterial cell walls, Can. J. Earth Sci., *22*, 1893–1898 (1985).

42. T. J. Beveridge and R. G. E. Murray, Sites of metal deposition in the cell wall of *Bacillus subtilis*. J. Bacteriol. *141*, 876–887 (1980).

43. T. J. Beveridge and R. G. E. Murray, Uptake and retention of metals by cell walls of *Bacillus subtilis*, J. Bacteriol. *127*, 1502–1518 (1976).

44. T. J. Beveridge, J. D. Meloche, W. S. Fyfe, and R. G. E. Murray, Diagenesis of metals chemically complexed to bacteria: laboratory formation of metal phosphates, sulfides, and organic condensates in artificial sediments, Appl. Environ. Microbiol. *45*, 1094–1108 (1983).

45. T. J. Beveridge and J. A. Davies, Cellular responses of *Bacillus subtilis* and *Escherichia coli* to the Gram stain, J. Bacteriol. *156*, 846–858 (1983).

46. F. G. Ferris, W. S. Fyfe and T. J. Beveridge, Metallic ion binding by *Bacillus subtilis*: implications for the fossilization of microorganisms, Geology, *16*, 149–152 (1988).

47. T. J. Beveridge, C. W. Forsberg, and R. J. Doyle, Major sites of metal binding in *Bacillus licheniformis* walls. J. Bacteriol. *150*, 1438–1448 (1982).

48. T. J. Beveridge, "Wall ultrastructure: how little we know," Chapter 1 in P. Actor, L. Daneo-Moore, M. L. Higgins, M. R. J. Salton, and G. D. Shockman, Eds., *Antibiotic Inhibition of Bacterial Cell Surface Assembly and Function*, American Society for Microbiology, Washington, D.C., 1988, pp. 3–20.

49. F. G. Ferris and T. J. Beveridge, Binding of a paramagnetic metal cation to *Escherichia coli* K-12 outer membrane vesicles. FEMS Microbiol. Letts. *24*, 43–46 (1984).

50. E. L. Carstensen and R. E. Marquis, Passive electrical properties of microorganisms. III. Conductivity of isolated bacterial cell walls. Biophys. J. *8*, 536–548 (1968).

51. L.-T. Ou, A. N. Chatterjee, F. E. Young, and R. E. Marquis, The physiology of teichoic acid-deficient staphylococci. Can. J. Microbiol. *19*, 1393–1399 (1973).

52. R. E. Marquis, N. Porterfield, and P. Matsumura, Acid-base titration of streptococci and the physical states of intracellular ions. J. Bacteriol. *114*, 491–498 (1973).

53. B. Zamani, B. D. Knezek, S. L. Flegler, E. S. Beneke, and F. B. Dazzo, Autoradiographic method to screen for soil microorganisms which accumulate zinc. Appl. Environ. Microbiol. *49*, 137–142 (1985).

54. F. Galdiero, M. Lembo, and M. A. Tufano, Affinity of various cations for *Staphylococcus aureus* cell wall. Experientia *24*, 34–36 (1968).

55. G. F. Zipperle, Jr., J. W. Ezzell, Jr., and R. J. Doyle, Glucosamine substitution and muramidase susceptibility in *Bacillus anthracis*. Can. J. Microbiol. *30*, 553–559 (1984).

56. C. J. Bates and C. A. Pasternak, Further studies on the regulation of amino sugar metabolism in *Bacillus subtilis*. Biochem. J. *96*, 147–154 (1965).

57. R. E. Marquis, K. Mayzel, and E. L. Carstensen, Cation exchange in cell walls of Gram-positive bacteria, Can. J. Microbiol. *22*, 975–982 (1976).

58. L. K. Jolliffe, R. J. Doyle, and U. N. Streips, The energized membrane and cellular autolysis in *Bacillus subtilis*. Cell *25*, 753–763 (1981).

59. M. A. Kemper, A. L. Koch, and R. J. Doyle, Cell wall pH may regulate extracellular enzymes in *Bacillus subtilis* (submitted).

60. H. I. Haavik, On the role of bacitracin peptides in trace metal transport by *Bacillus licheniformis*. J. Gen. Microbiol. *96*, 393–399 (1976).

61. R. J. Doyle, J. Chaloupka, and V. Vinter, Turnover of cell walls in microorganisms, Microbiol. Rev. *52*, 554–567 (1988).

62. J. L. Meers and D. W. Tempest, The influence of growth-limiting substrate and

medium NaCl concentration on the synthesis of magnesium-binding sites in the walls of *Bacillus subtilis var. niger*. J. Gen. Microbiol. *63*, 325–331 (1970).

63. D. C. Ellwood and D. W. Tempest, Effects of environment on bacterial cell wall content and composition. Adv. Microb. Physiol. *7*, 83–117 (1972).

64. A. R. Archibald, Bacterial cell wall structure and the ionic environment. FEMS Symposium No 44, Bath University Press, 1988, pp. 159–173.

# CHAPTER 10

# Metallic Ion Interactions with the Outer Membrane of Gram-Negative Bacteria

F. GRANT FERRIS*

Department of Geology
University of Western Ontario
London, Ontario, Canada

## Contents

## 10.1 INTRODUCTION

The cell walls of Gram-negative and Gram-positive bacteria differ fundamentally with respect to design. One of the major differences is that Gram-

---

* Nova Husky Research Corp., Calgary, Alberta, Canada

negative cells possess an outer membrane that consists of lipid and protein arranged in a planar two-dimensional bilayer matrix (1, 2). This highly specialized structure, which resides outside a monolayer of peptidoglycan, not only physically separates the cell body from the external environment, but also serves as a selective permeability barrier that controls the access of solutes and other external agents to the plasma membrane (3, 4).

The outer membrane is essentially held together by noncovalent forces that arise from the amphipathic nature of the constituent membrane lipids; by adopting a bilayer format in an aqueous milieu, the lipids achieve a minimum free energy conformation with their hydrophobic fatty acid chains buried in the membrane interior (5). The hydrophilic polar head groups of the lipids, which contain anionic phosphoryl and carboxyl groups, therefore remain exposed to the external environment and effectively determine the reactivity of the cell surface (1, 4). Consequently, the outer membrane interacts efficiently with metal cations in aqueous solution (6–8). This chapter centers on the structural dependence, site specificity, and physicochemical implications of metallic ion interactions with the outer membrane. The chemistry and molecular organization of the outer membrane are also briefly reviewed to provide a framework for discussion.

## 10.2   OUTER MEMBRANE CHEMISTRY

Although early electron microscopic studies revealed the outer membrane as a distinct component of the Gram-negative cell envelope (9, 10), detailed chemical analyses were hindered by an inability to obtain outer membrane preparations free of contaminating plasma membrane. The original method of separating the outer membrane from other components of the cell envelope was developed by Miura and Mizushima (11, 12). Cells of *Escherichia coli* were disrupted by the osmotic lysis of sphaeroplasts formed by ethylenediaminetetraacetate (EDTA)–lysozyme treatment, and the membranes were then separated by isopycnic sucrose density gradient centrifugation. However, because EDTA was known to extract components from the cell envelope of Gram-negative bacteria (13), the Miura–Mizushima procedure was modified to avoid the perturbing effects of this metal chelator. Instead of using EDTA-lysozyme lysis, intact cells were disrupted by physically shearing the bacteria in a French pressure cell (14, 15). Although this method frequently results in a poor recovery of the plasma membrane owing to its extensive fragmentation into small vesicles (16), it remains the preferred technique for outer membrane isolation (2, 17).

### 10.2.1   Biochemical Composition

The major molecular constituents of the Gram-negative outer membrane are phospholipids, lipopolysaccharide (LPS), and proteins (1, 2). The actual amounts of these various components can vary substantially, depending on the growth conditions and organism involved (18). However, the outer membrane usually contains between 20 and 25% phospholipid, 30% LPS, and 45–50% protein by weight (1).

The principal phospholipids in the outer membrane are phosphatidylethanolamine, phosphatidylglycerol, and diphosphatidylglycerol (19). High levels of lysophosphatidylethanolamine have been reported in the *E. coli* outer membrane (20). This is now believed to be an artifact, however, caused by a partial degradation of phosphatidylethanolamine by lysophospholipase enzymes associated with the outer membrane (2). The predominant species is usually phosphatidylethanolamine, which can account for 75–95% of the total phospholipid content of the membrane (21). Approximately equal proportions of phosphatidylglycerol and diphosphatidylglycerol make up most of the remainder, but only trace amounts of lysophosphatidlyethanolamine are normally found (2, 19).

The chemical structure of LPS is complex, and highly variable (22–25). A hydrophobic region, called lipid A, is covalently attached to a hydrophilic core polysaccharide which is usually substituted by the O-antigen, a polymer of repeating sugar units. The lipid A backbone consists of a $\beta$-1,6-linked disaccharide of $N$-hydroxymyristoyl-D-glucosamine which is $O$-acylated by $\beta$-hydroxymyristic acid and short-chain ($C_8$–$C_{14}$) fatty acids (26, 27). Phosphoryl or pyrophosphoryl substituents are located at the reducing terminus of the disaccharide, which is additionally phosphorylated at the 4' position (25). Substoichiometric amounts of ethanolamine or 4-aminoarabinose can be attached to LPS by means of a diester linkage through the 4'-phosphate (23).

The core polysaccharide of LPS, which is highly conserved among most Gram-negative bacteria, usually contains the unique sugars 3-deoxy-D-mannooctulosonate (2-keto-3-deoxyoctonate, KDO) and L-glycero-D-mannoheptose (heptose) (23, 28). A number of more common sugars, such as D-glucose, D-galactose, and $N$-acetylglucosamine, complete the core polysaccharide chain (2). The KDO residues, which afford free carboxyl groups, and heptose regions of the core polysaccharide may also contain phosphorylethanolamine and phosphoryl substituents, respectively (23).

Various lengths of the O-antigen are possible, and this component of LPS can consist of none to more than 40 repeating oligosaccharide subunits, each containing three to six sugar residues (29, 30). A large diversity of sugars has been found in O-antigen subunits. These include neutral sugars, uronic acids, and amino sugars. Moreover, each repeating unit can be further substituted by phosphate groups, amino acids, or O-acetyl groups (2). Consequently, the composition of the subunits within the O-antigen shows extreme diversity, even within a single species, and this property is used in O-serotyping, an immunological technique that can be used to identify different organisms or strains of single species (31, 32).

The protein complement of the outer membrane is strongly influenced by growth conditions, but typically consists of a limited number of proteins that tend to be present in high copy number (2, 3). As a class of proteins, outer membrane polypeptides share a number of unusual physical and chemical properties. These include a high proportion (ca. 40–50%) of nonpolar amino acids and β-structure in the native state, resistance to denaturation by detergents, and a strong tendency toward self-assembly (33). The outer membrane is also deficient in enzyme activity compared to the plasma membrane. However, small amounts of lipase, protease, and peptidoglycan hydrolytic enzymes have been detected in isolated outer membrane preparations (34–36).

## 10.2.2 Elemental Composition

A wide range of metallic ions are indigenous to the outer membrane of Gram-negative bacteria. The predominant metallic species under normal conditions are sodium, magnesium, and calcium (6–8, 37). These metal cations usually occur in the outer membrane at concentrations in the range of 0.04–0.10 $\mu$mol mg$^{-1}$ dry weight. Minor element components present at significant but lower levels (ca 0.001–0.007 $\mu$mol mg$^{-1}$ dry weight) include potassium, manganese, iron, aluminum, and zinc (7, 8). Trace amounts of other transition and rare-earth metals have also been found in isolated outer membrane preparations (6).

Quantitative elemental analyses accomplished by plasma emission spectroscopy show that the metallic ion content of isolated LPS generally tends to parallel that of intact outer membrane (7). However, the levels of magnesium and calcium associated with the outer membrane are typically enriched compared to the plasma membrane (Table 10.1). This enrichment of divalent cations in the outer membrane has been attributed to the presence

**TABLE 10.1 Elemental Composition of Plasma Membrane, Outer Membrane, and Lipopolysaccharide Isolated from *Escherichia coli***

| | Metal-to-Phosphorus Molar Ratio[a] | | |
|---|---|---|---|
| Metal | Plasma Membrane | Outer Membrane | Lipopoly-saccharide |
| Na | ND[b] | ND[b] | 0.09 |
| Mg | 0.15 | 0.45 | 0.43 |
| Ca | 0.03 | 0.09 | 0.12 |
| Fe | 0.006 | 0.009 | 0.01 |
| Al | 0.006 | 0.009 | 0.02 |
| Zn | 0.001 | 0.001 | 0.002 |

[a] Average of four isolates.
[b] ND, not determined.
*Source:* Ref. 7.

of LPS, which not only provides multiple sites for metallic ion interactions, but also exhibits a high affinity for both magnesium and calcium (38–40).

There are two principal factors that control the salt condition of the outer membrane, the chemical structure of LPS and the ionic composition of the medium in which cells grow. For example, LPS extracted from wild-type *E. coli* strains contained more magnesium and less calcium than LPS from a heptose-deficient mutant (7). Similarly, higher magnesium levels are observed in LPS isolated from bacteria grown in a medium rich in phosphate and magnesium (7). Because the extent to which LPS is phosphorylated is sensitive to the phosphate content of growth media (41), this later situation may also be partly related to a change in LPS chemistry.

## 10.3 MOLECULAR ORGANIZATION OF THE OUTER MEMBRANE

The recognition of an abundance of lipid in the Gram-negative cell envelope and early electron micrographs of thin sections suggested a type of bilayer molecular organization for the outer membrane (9, 10). Eventually, structural analyses using X-ray diffraction confirmed this (42, 43); other biophysical techniques, for example, freeze-fracture electron microscopy, nuclear magnetic resonance (NMR), and electron spin resonance (ESR), have since resolved the architectual features of the outer membrane to the molecular level.

### 10.3.1 The Lipid Matrix

The phospholipids and LPS of the outer membrane are arranged in a molecular bilayer format where the fatty acid chains or the lipids are oriented approximately perpendicular to the plane of the membrane (42–44). The lipid components are, however, asymmetrically distributed between the two halves of the outer membrane (Fig. 10.1). Labeling studies using ferritin conjugated to O-antigen specific antibodies have shown that the LPS is found almost exclusively in the outer half of the membrane (45). In contrast, the phospholipids of the outer membrane are not readily accessible to exogenously added cyanogen bromide-activated dextran and therefore must reside in the inner half of the membrane (46).

Further evidence for the segregation of lipid components into separate faces of the outer membrane comes from ESR studies. Based on the exchange broadening of ESR line widths, Nikaido and co-workers (47) concluded that the phospholipids occupy a domain completely separate from LPS. However, the digestion of the peptidoglycan layer with lysozyme caused a mixing of phospholipid and LPS in the outer membrane (45). Indeed, it seems that the asymmetry of the lipid bilayer of the outer membrane is relatively unstable and is maintained at least partially by the presence of an intact underlying peptidoglycan sacculus.

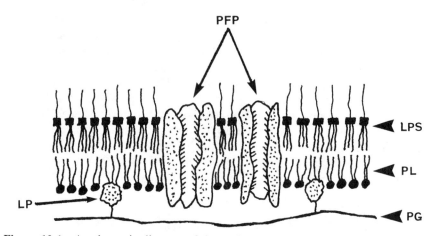

**Figure 10.1**   A schematic diagram of the molecular architecture of the outer membrane. LPS, lipopolysaccharide; PL, phospholipid; PG, peptidoglycan; LP, lipoprotein; PFP, pore-forming proteins.

Measurements from X-ray diffraction patterns obtained from isolated LPS indicate that the hydrocarbon tails of this molecule are more rigid, and in closer proximity than those of their phospholipid counterparts (48). In ESR experiments with artificial mixed bilayers, where the LPS interdigitates among phospholipid molecules, a significantly lower fluidity was observed than in bilayers of phospholipids alone (47, 49). Deuterium NMR procedures applied to intact outer membrane vesicles have provided similar results (50, 51). The lipid matrix of the outer membrane can therefore be visualized as a more rigid and ordered structure than most phospholipid membranes.

### 10.3.2   Protein Topology

The bilayer matrix formed by the phospholipids and LPS of the outer membrane constitutes a molecular continuum into which the proteins of the outer membrane are embedded. Some polypeptides, such as the Omp F and Omp C proteins of *E. coli* or protein F of *Pseudomonas aeruginosa*, span the bilayer (i.e., are intrinsic proteins), whereas others, such as the outer membrane lipoprotein of the Enterobacteriaceae, are confined to one side of the membrane (i.e., extrinsic proteins) (1–3).

Although extraction of *E. coli* with 2% SDS at 70°C solubilizes the plasma membrane and most of the outer membrane (52), the external surface of the insoluble peptidoglycan sacculus remains covered with protein arranged in a periodic two-dimensional lattice of three- and sixfold symmetry (53). The addition of high concentrations of NaCl causes the dissociation of the hexagonal array, suggesting that the protein is anchored to the peptidoglycan through ionic salt bridges. The significance of these findings to the situation has been questioned, however, for similar arrays have been observed in vesicles formed from *E. coli* LPS, Omp F, and magnesium in the absence of peptidoglycan (54). Thus the formation of the hexagonal lattice, at least in vitro, does not require a peptidoglycan template and depends only on the presence of LPS, suitable divalent metallic ions, and strong protein–protein interactions (33).

It is now well established that the hexagonal lattice of protein observed in association with peptidoglycan extracted from *E. coli* consists of either Omp F or Omp C trimers, which form aqueous pores through the outer membrane (2, 3, 17). The exclusion limit for the diffusion of hydrophilic solutes through these pores in the *E. coli* outer membrane is near 600 D, which corresponds to a channel diameter of approximately 1.0 nm (2). Most members of the Enterobacteriaceae have pores of a similar size in their outer membranes. In contrast, the major pore-forming polypeptide of *P. aeruginosa* (protein F) forms channels with a diameter near 2.2 nm which permits the passage of molecules almost six times larger than those excluded by the outer membrane of enteric bacteria (55). Porin proteins from other non-enteric bacteria also form rather large pores, suggesting that the Enterobacteriaceae are unique in producing very narrow channels through the outer membrane (2).

The lipoproteins of enteric bacteria bear acyl substituents at the amino terminus which anchor the polypeptide to the outer membrane (1, 56). In *E. coli*, approximately one-third of the lipoprotein molecules of the outer membrane are covalently attached at the carboxyl terminus to the peptidoglycan (57). The outer membrane of other Gram-negative bacteria is not, however, always covalently bound to the peptidoglycan through a lipoprotein. For example, the lipoproteins of *P. aeruginosa* are noncovalently associated with the peptidoglycan (58). The nature of this association is not yet understood, but probably involves both hydrophobic and ionic interactions.

### 10.3.3  The Polymeric Nature of the Outer Membrane

The lateral diffusion of biological membrane components is usually interpreted in terms of the Singer and Nicolson fluid mosaic model (59). In the context of this model, molecules should be able to intermix and diffuse over large distances in the membrane. These concepts alone are not, however, in accord with experimental evidence that indicates that the major molecular constituents of the outer membrane are comparatively immobile and do not freely intermix (47, 49).

To explain the difference between the fluid mosaic model and outer membrane data, Schindler and co-workers (60) adopted an approach that incorporates the concept of diffusion in a polymeric network. Their model suggests that the random thermal motion of diffusing monomers within the plane of a membrane would tend to be inhibited by the formation of intramembranous macromolecular complexes (i.e., polymeric domains) of monomeric component molecules. Anything that would tend to increase the size of the polymeric domains, such as the formation of LPS–protein complexes, would therefore be expected to restrict the movement of monomers within the plane of the membrane (60).

When outer membrane proteins are incorporated into LPS–phospholipid vesicles, the diffusion coefficient for LPS is reduced (60). Similarly, the addition of calcium to aqueous dispersions of isolated LPS decreases the degree of motional freedom available to the molecules (61). By extrapolating these findings to freeze-etching data, which reveals large intramembranous macromolecular complexes of LPS and protein (1, 2), the outer membrane of Gram-negative bacteria can be visualized as a complex polymeric fluid mosaic.

## 10.4   OUTER MEMBRANE INTERACTIONS WITH METALLIC IONS

The outer membrane is capable of binding a wide range of metallic ions including members of the alkali, alkaline earth, transition, and rare earth series (6–8, 37). These metal cations are generally regarded as important accessory components that function to stabilize the molecular architecture of the outer membrane. Presumably, metallic ions bound by the outer membrane reduce charge repulsion between highly anionic constituent molecules, bridge adjacent molecules of LPS and (or) protein, and help anchor the outer membrane to the underlying fabric of the peptidoglycan (1, 2, 17, 33).

Exactly how important the metal-binding capacity of the outer membrane is to the vitality of Gram-negative bacteria is difficult to ascertain. Certainly the structural continuity and, therefore, the discriminatory molecular sieving properties of the outer membrane depend on the presence of bound metallic ions. For example, potent metal chelators, such as EDTA, scavenge outer membrane-bound metal and cause a concomitant release of up to half of the total LPS (62). Consequently, EDTA-treated cells are typically more susceptible to hydrolytic enzymes and antibiotics that are normally excluded by the outer membrane (62, 63).

Other nonstructural functions for outer membrane bound metallic ions exist, but these are not well understood. Sometimes autolysis is induced when rapidly growing cells are exposed to EDTA (64, 65), suggesting perhaps that metal cations complexed by the outer membrane play an active role in the regulation of autolytic enzymes. In addition, calcium displaced from the outer membrane during infection by bacteriophage T4 and T5 caused a transient depolarization of the plasma membrane, and a concomitant uptake of the phage nucleic acid (66). The implication is that a selective desorption of metal cations from the outer membrane could be used to convey information to the protoplast about events at the cell surface. Furthermore, in natural environments, the outer membrane could immobilize toxic heavy metals and prevent their penetration to sensitive internal sites (67). Alternatively, the ability of the outer membrane to bind metallic ions could concentrate metal cations essential to the metabolic processes of the cell from more dilute surroundings (1).

### 10.4.1 Structural Dependence on Metal Cations

Based primarily on biochemical information derived from studies with metal chelators, Leive (62) proposed that calcium was the principal metal cation responsible for the stabilization of LPS in the lipid domain of the outer membrane. This hypothesis has been confirmed by data from a recent investigation which shows that EDTA-modified outer membrane from *E. coli* is not only deficient in LPS but also in calcium (8). Of the other predominant metallic species normally found in the outer membrane, only magnesium was slightly reduced by the chelator, whereas sodium appeared to be completely unaffected (Table 10.2).

At least two interpretations for the more efficient extraction by EDTA of calcium from the outer membrane, compared with that of magnesium, are possible. The first is that outer membrane-bound calcium is readily accessible to EDTA, whereas outer membrane-bound magnesium is hidden within LPS-protein complexes and is not available (7, 54). Alternatively, it is possible that the strength of magnesium binding to the outer membrane is greater than that of calcium. Because EDTA is a potent chelator of both calcium and magnesium, and extracts both of these cations from isolated LPS (7), the first possibility is favored. In this context, LPS in the calcium

**TABLE 10.2. Metal Content of Native and EDTA-modified Outer Membrane**

| Metal | Metal Content (nmol metal mg$^{-1}$ dry wt OM)[a,b] | | Amount of Metal Removed by EDTA Treatment[c] (nmol mg$^{-1}$ dry wt OM) |
|---|---|---|---|
| | Native | EDTA | |
| Na | $91.0 \pm 8.0$ | $87.0 \pm 4.0$ | 4.0 |
| K | $1.0 \pm 0.4$ | $1.0 \pm 0.4$ | 0 |
| Mg | $57.0 \pm 4.0$ | $43.0 \pm 2.0$ | 14.0 |
| Ca | $93.0 \pm 16.0$ | $54.0 \pm 6.0$ | 39.0 |
| Mn | $2.0 \pm 0.2$ | $2.0 \pm 0.2$ | 0 |
| Fe | $7.0 \pm 1.0$ | $4.0 \pm 3.0$ | 3.0 |

[a] Plus or minus standard deviations derived from 8–10 estimations per sample.
[b] The high sodium content of the outer membrane preparations presumably reflects the use of sodium buffers during the isolation procedure.
[c] These figures were obtained by subtracting the values in column two from the corresponding values in column one.

*Source:* Ref. 8, with permission of the *Canadian Journal of Microbiology.*

salt form probably represents a unique physicochemical subfraction that is more prone to co-extraction from the outer membrane than LPS and magnesium (8).

The effects of calcium on the molecular organization of isolated LPS have been studied using electron microscopy, ESR, and $^{31}$P-NMR (39, 61, 68). The results of these investigations show that calcium is capable of stabilizing LPS in a lipid bilayer conformation. In contrast, other metallic ions, for example, sodium or magnesium, are not as competent as calcium in accommodating bilayer structures (68). Presumably, these differences arise because the metallic ions differ in their abilities to neutralize or bridge between repulsive anionic groups in the core polysaccharide and lipid A regions of LPS (69, 70).

Because sodium and magnesium seem to be unable to stabilize LPS in a bilayer conformation, understanding the structural roles of these metal cations is more difficult. With sodium, the available evidence suggests that it is mostly confined to areas devoid of EDTA-extractable LPS (Table 10.2), such as the phospholipid domain, where electrostatic repulsion between molecules may not need to be as stringently controlled; that is, the cross-sectional charge density in the polar region of a phospholipid [one anionic group per $0.5$ nm$^2$ (71)] is approximately three to four times less than that of LPS [one anionic group per $0.15$ nm$^2$ (72)]. The situation with magnesium is, however, quite different.

Coughlin and co-workers (7) found that LPS–protein complexes from *E. coli* are richer in magnesium than isolated outer membrane. This suggests that magnesium ions participate in the formation of LPS–protein, protein–protein, and protein–peptidoglycan complexes. With the exception of protein–peptidoglycan interactions, the principal cohesive forces within these macromolecular complexes are believed to be derived from noncovalent hydrophobic bonds (33). For this reason, the specific role of magnesium in complex formation probably originates through entropy effects, that is, by restricting the degrees of interaction of water with molecules in the complexes (73). These effects may be partially related to the tertiary structures adopted by the molecules of the complexes in the presence of magnesium (54).

The loss of over 40% of the outer membrane bound calcium during EDTA treatment must increase the electrostatic repulsion between anionic groups of the constituent outer membrane molecules (Table 10.2). Repulsive forces that arise between like charges are known to impose certain limitations on how close the individual components of a membrane can approach each other (73), and the conformational change that results in the release of LPS from the outer membrane can be readily visualized in terms of this destabilization process. In order to maximize the allowable spacing between repulsive anionic groups, small vesicular structures with a high degree of surface curvature are formed (Fig. 10.2). This type of macromolecular packing is clearly not compatible with the more planar native outer membrane and

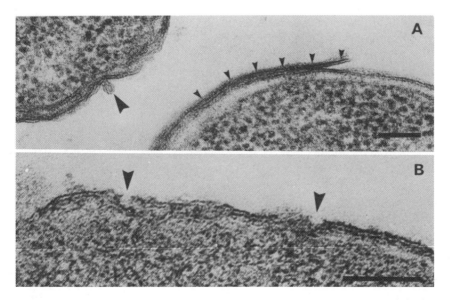

**Figure 10.2** Thin-section profiles of EDTA-treated cells; (*a*) A small vesicle (large arrow) and area of superimposed outer membrane (small arrows); (*b*) lesions in the outer membrane (indicated by arrows). Illustrated Bar = 100 nm.

therefore these domains are released from the cell surface as vesicles into the menstruum. As a result, lesions and regions of superimposed outer membrane are formed (Fig. 10.2).

The action of EDTA is enhanced when used in conjunction with tris(hydroxymethyl)aminomethane (Tris) buffers (74, 75). This large organic cation is also capable of disrupting the outer membrane alone, if used in moderately high concentrations (76). The disruptive effects of Tris are probably related to its ability to interact with LPS and displace divalent metallic ions (7).

The outer membrane is also sensitive to other organic polycations (77, 78). For example, polymyxin B (an acylated polycationic-peptide antibiotic) causes small outer membrane vesicles to form (79, 80). Similarly, highly electropositive aminoglycoside antibiotics, such as gentamicin, compete with and displace divalent cations from the outer membrane, thereby disturbing its integrity (37, 81). In each of these situations, it is the structural dependence of the outer membrane on metal cations that facilitates the perturbing effects of these antibiotics.

## 10.4.2 Metal Binding Assays

The binding of metallic ions by the outer membrane of Gram-negative bacteria is generally perceived as an electrostatic phenomenon mediated by interactions between the soluble metal cations and fixed anionic groups at the hydrophilic surfaces of the membrane (1, 17). However, the structural and compositional complexity of the outer membrane implies that a single metallic species would not be capable of interacting in the same way with all parts of the membrane; it would depend on the local outer membrane chemistry (8). Moreover, because different metallic ions possess distinct physical and chemical properties (82), there is no reason to expect that all cations interact with the outer membrane in the same way. In this context, differences in the metal binding capacity of native and EDTA-modified (LPS deficient) outer membrane preparations provide valuable information concerning the preferred intermolecular sites of metal coordination among the component membrane molecules (8).

If metal cation binding involved little more than electrostatic interactions, EDTA-modified outer membrane would be expected to bind fewer cations than native outer membrane, regardless of the metallic species, simply because of the reduced LPS content (i.e., the reduced availability of anionic sites) of the membrane. However, this is not always observed because monovalent cations such as sodium and potassium are bound by EDTA-modified outer membrane just as well as they are bound by native outer membrane (Table 10.3). In contrast, multivalent cations show a reduced level of binding to EDTA-modified outer membranes (8). These results agree well with the fact that monovalent cations are generally preferred by widely spaced sites (e.g., the phosphoryl groups of phospholipids), whereas multivalent cations are preferred by closely opposed sites (e.g., the phosphoryl or carboxyl groups of LPS) (83). These are essentially electrical field strength effects

**TABLE 10.3.   Metal Bound to Native and EDTA-modified Outer Membrane**

| Metal | Bound Metal (nmol metal mg$^{-1}$ dry wt OM)[a,b] | | Decrease in Binding due to EDTA Treatment[c] (nmol mg$^{-1}$ dry wt OM) |
|---|---|---|---|
|  | Native | EDTA |  |
| Na | 200.0 ± 20.0 | 196.0 ± 16.0 | 4.0 |
| K | 1.0 ± 0.1 | 1.0 ± 0.1 | 0 |
| Mg | 84.0 ± 10.0 | 22.0 ± 6.0 | 62.0 |
| Ca | 185.0 ± 35.0 | 103.0 ± 16.0 | 82.0 |
| Mn | 355.0 ± 24.0 | 142.0 ± 12.0 | 213.0 |
| Fe | 541.0 ± 98.0 | 344.0 ± 73.0 | 197.0 |

[a] Plus or minus standard deviations derived from 8–10 estimations per sample.

[b] The background levels of the metals in the OM preparations (Table 10.2) have been subtracted so as to reflect the actual quantities of metallic ions bound by the membranes.

[c] These figures were obtained by subtracting the values in column two from the corresponding values in column one.

*Source:* Ref. 8, with permission of the *Canadian Journal of Microbiology.*

that reflect the high anionic charge density of LPS and its high affinity for multivalent metal cations (38–40).

Of the monovalent cations, sodium binds to outer membrane extremely well, much better than potassium (Table 10.3). The sodium ion has the smaller ionic radius of these two cations (82), and it is tempting to speculate that the observed differences in binding are a function of ionic size. Although this interpretation is correct in a sense, it fails to address the fact that the radius of the hydrated potassium ion is actually smaller than that of hydrated sodium ions. However, potassium also has a lower hydration energy than sodium (82), so the total free energy difference for the binding of the potassium ion would be less than that of the sodium ion. In this context, the uptake and retention of sodium by the outer membrane is favored (8).

Most multivalent cations are bound by the outer membrane in amounts related to their respective valencies, ionic radii, hydrated radii, and hydration energies (8). This is in agreement with the concepts outlined above, and explains the observed binding concentration series of iron > manganese > calcium (Table 10.3). Magnesium, however, provides an interesting exception to this trend. This metal cation has a small ionic radius, and an extremely high hydration energy, so the free energy difference for magnesium binding should be large (82, 83). Consequently, some type of compensation for the strong interactions between the ion and water molecules must be made for magnesium to bind. In this view, when magnesium is bound it must be very tightly attached to a select number of sites capable of overcoming strong ion–water interactions. Possibly these sites are contained within LPS–protein complexes (7, 54), and are not readily accessible to the aqueous environment. Supportive of this point of view is the observation that EDTA is capable of extracting calcium from the outer membrane with relative ease, but not magnesium (8).

An interesting feature associated with the binding of ferric iron and other heavy metal ions to bacterial cell wall components is the formation of insoluble metal hydroxide precipitates (84, 85). These metal hydroxide precipitates are typically visible in transmission electron micrographs of outer membrane preparations reacted within various trivalent metal salt solutions (Fig. 10.3). Most trivalent cations are unstable in aqueous solution (82), and hydroxide formation probably arises from the hydrolysis of water molecules upon the binding of the metallic ions.

## 10.4.3 Site Specificity of Metallic Ion Binding

The most abundant reactive electronegative sites in the outer membrane capable of binding metal cations are the phosphoryl groups of LPS and phospholipids (7, 8). A convenient technique that can be used to detect and monitor the phosphoryl groups of lipids in biological membranes is $^{31}$P-NMR. Because the natural abundance of the $^{31}$P isotope is 100%, no artificial labeling or chemical modifications are required and, as such, the technique is

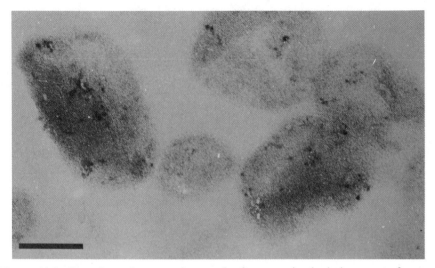

**Figure 10.3** Low-dose electron micrograph of an unstained whole mount of membrane vesicles reacted with trivalent europium ions. The electron contrast is provided by europium ions bound to the outer membrane vesicles. Small electron dense hydroxide precipitates are also visible in the membrane fabric. Bar = 100 nm.

nonperturbing (86). Thus membranes can be studied in their native state. Furthermore, the inherent sensitivity of NMR to paramagnetic metal cations can be used to describe interactions between the phosphoryl groups of lipids and metallic ions in greater detail; by virtue of their unpaired electrons, paramagnetic metal cations possess a large electronic magnetic moment (87, 88). Consequently, any nuclei in the immediate vicinity of a paramagnetic cation experiences a large local field fluctuation, which in turn gives rise to paramagnetic shifts and broadening of NMR spectra.

The effect of europium ions (a trivalent paramagnetic lanthanide) on the position and shape of $^{31}$P-NMR spectra obtained with outer membrane from *E. coli* has been investigated (85). An increase in the molar ratio of exogenously added europium ions to outer membrane phosphorus resulted in a progressive upfield shift in resonance position, and extensive broadening of the spectra (Fig. 10.4). This confirmed that the phosphoryl groups of LPS and phospholipid are the major sites for metallic ion interactions within the outer membrane (85). However, the extent of the broadening caused by europium binding to outer membrane was greater than that reported in similar studies using model phospholipid vesicles (89). This difference was attributed to the presence of LPS, which contains approximately 75% of the total phosphorus in the outer membrane of *E. coli* (85).

There are two possible explanations for the increased degree of broadening observed in the outer membrane-europium $^{31}$P-NMR spectra. First, the formation of salt bridges between adjacent molecules, most likely LPS,

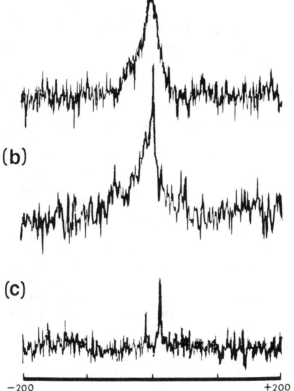

**(a)**

**(b)**

**(c)**

−200                                    +200

**Figure 10.4**   161.98-MHz $^{31}$P-NMR spectra of outer membrane vesicles in the presence of several concentrations of $Eu^{3+}$; europium to phosphorus mole ratios of (a) 1:4, (b) 1:2, and (c) 1:1. As the $Eu^{3+}$ concentration was increased, the spectra were broadened and shifted to the right (85). (With permission of *FEMS Microbiology Letters*.)

could severely restrict molecular motion within the outer membrane and cause an increase in the chemical shift anisotropy (width) of the spectrum (86). In accord with this concept are the data of van Alphen and co-workers (61), who found that calcium ions were capable of producing extensive broadening in $^{31}$P-NMR spectra of aqueous dispersions of isolated LPS. Second, if the exchange rate between the bound and free europium ions was very slow (i.e., high affinity interactions), relaxation times and therefore spectral broadening would be increased (87, 88). Certainly the ability of the outer membrane to bind metallic ions from aqueous solution (6–8) and the very high affinity of LPS for divalent metallic ions (38–40) favor the later situation.

It has been reported that the KDO-carboxyl groups in the core polysaccharide and certain phosphoryl groups in the lipid A backbone form a specific site for high-affinity interactions between LPS and divalent metallic ions (38). These authors based their conclusions on the absence of high affinity binding for calcium and magnesium in lipid A derivatives of whole LPS from *Salmonella typhimurium*; that is, the removal of the core polysaccharide compromised the ability of lipopolysaccharide to interact strongly with divalent cations. However, data from recent $^{31}$P-NMR studies using paramagnetic manganese as a probe for divalent metal cation binding indicate that the high affinity of LPS for divalent cations is related more to the polyanionic nature of the entire molecule, rather than a specific grouping of negatively charged sites (90). In this investigation, a loss of intensity from all resonance peaks was observed when high-resolution $^{31}$P-NMR spectra of lipopolysaccharide were obtained in the presence of manganese, indicating that each phosphoryl group contributed to the high affinity of lipopolysaccharide for divalent metallic ions (Fig. 10.5).

The importance of the phosphoryl groups to high affinity binding of divalent metal cations is further emphasized by a similar loss of spectral intensity owing to $Mn^{2+}$ of all resonance peaks from LPS with chemically neutralized KDO-carboxyl groups (90). Biochemical analyses of the chemically modified LPS also showed that at least two of the three KDO–carboxyl groups were internally cross-linked to closely opposed phosphorylethanolamine substituents (Fig. 10.6). This argues in favor of a situation where, under normal circumstances, only one carboxyl group is available for metal cation interactions because the remaining two are screened by the close proximity of endogenous amino groups (23, 24, 90).

Conformational energy calculations and X-ray diffraction studies show that the KDO-trisaccharide of LPS is tightly packed and rests against the lipid A backbone (91). Certainly, this type of molecular conformation would be possible if, as the $^{31}$P-NMR data suggest, two of the three anionic carboxyl groups interact electrostatically with internal cationic amino groups (7, 90). The remaining carboxyl group would therefore be free to bind exogenous metal cations and, by forming salt bridges to lipid A phosphoryl groups, the KDO-trisaccharide would be further compacted (90).

### 10.4.4 Effects on Surface Hydrophobicity

The diffuse double layer theory of counterion binding to charge surfaces, such as the outer membrane, predicts that, immediately adjacent to the site bound ions, there will be a layer of water molecules that are coordinated by virtue of their electrostatic dipoles (71, 92). The absolute order of the water molecules in this hydration layer of course depends on the nature of the charged surface, as well as the quantity and chemical character of the bound counterions. Because of this water molecules in the bulk aqueous phase are restricted in the ways that they can interact with the hydrated surface. Such

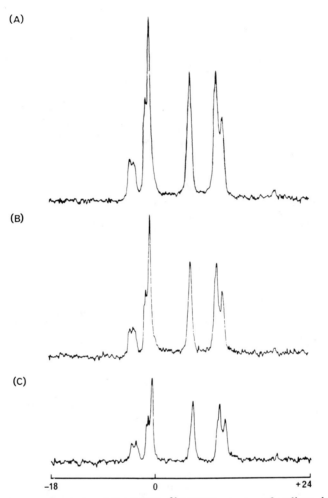

**Figure 10.5** High-resolution 161.98-MHz $^{31}$P-NMR spectra of sodium dodecyl sulfate-solubilized lipopolysaccharide in the absence (a) and presence (b and c) of several concentrations of $Mn^{2+}$; the manganese to phosphorus mole ratios were (b) 1:10000 and (c) 1:3300 (90). (With permission of the *Canadian Journal of Microbiology*.)

increases in the degree of local order of liquid water should result in a decrease of solvent entropy, and accordingly, an increase in the interfacial free energy (hydrophobicity) of the surface (73, 93).

Because LPS is a highly polar molecule compared to phospholipid, and resides predominantly on the exterior surface of the outer membrane (22, 45), cells exposed to the metal chelator EDTA should become more hydrophobic than untreated control cells (94, 95). In a biphasic system of dextran and polyethyleneglycol, this increase in cell surface hydrophobicity is re-

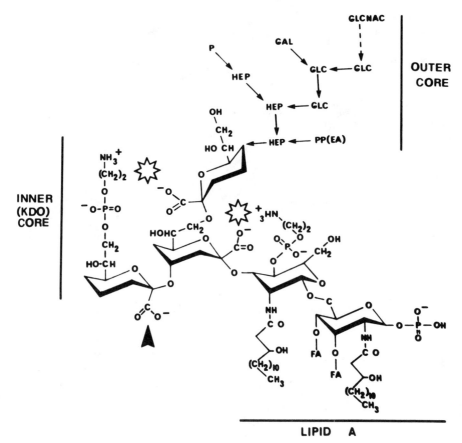

**Figure 10.6**   The molecular structure of isolated *Escherichia coli* K-12 LPS showing a possible arrangement (suggested by space-filling models) for the covalent attachment of exogenously added glycine ethyl ester (arrow) and internal cross-linking (stars) after carbodiimide activation of the 2-keto-3-deoxyoctonate (KDO) carboxyl groups. Under normal conditions, only the 2,4-linked KDO-carboxyl (arrow) would be free for metallic ion interactions because the remaining two carboxyl groups would be screened by the cationic amine groups of closely opposed phosphorylethanolamine substituents at the 4'-position of lipid A and the 7(8)-position of the 2,4-linked KDO residue (90). (With permission of the *Canadian Journal of Microbiology*.)

vealed by an increase in the phase partition coefficient of the cells (Table 10.4) (8). This increase in interfacial free energy, as exhibited by EDTA-treated cells, essentially occurs because of the loss of molecular components (LPS) capable of hydrogen bonding to the liquid water lattice (73). In addition, an exposure of cells to aqueous metal salt solutions before phase partitioning also increases cell surface hydrophobicity in an order related to the quantity of metal bound by the outer membrane, and the hydration energy and valence of the cation (8). These phase partitioning results are

TABLE 10.4   **Partition Coefficients of Cells Exposed to EDTA and/or Aqueous Metal Salt Solutions Before Phase Partitioning in a Biphasic System of 7% (w/v) Dextran T500 and 4% (w/v) Polyethyleneglycol 20000**

| Metal | Partition Coefficient $(K)^{a,b}$ | |
| | Control | EDTA |
| --- | --- | --- |
| — | 0.20 | 0.37 |
| Na | 0.18 | 0.24 |
| Mg | 1.13 | 0.88 |
| Ca | 0.68 | 0.69 |
| Mn | 1.43 | 0.75 |

$^a$ $K$ = $OD_{600}$ PEG phase/$OD_{600}$ Dextran phase.
$^b$ Figures represent averages of triplicate samples prepared from three separate 1-L cultures; the standard deviations are all less than ±15%.
Source: Ref. 8, with permission of the *Canadian Journal of Microbiology*.

interesting because they suggest that the surface hydrophobicity of Gram-negative bacteria is affected not only by the quantity and chemical character of LPS but also by the salt condition of the outer membrane. This is a particularly provocative finding because the hydrophobicity of the cell surface is known to influence outer membrane permeability, and cell–cell or cell–substrate adhesion (94, 95).

### 10.4.5   Influence on Molecular Bonding Profiles

The outer membrane of *E. coli* is difficult to split by the freeze-etching technique (1). Normally when a membrane is subjected to mechanical rupture while in a frozen state, fractures form through the hydrophobic core because it represents the plane of lowest bond energy within the membrane (96, 97). If the strength of van der Waals forces (which must predominate in the hydrophobic domain of membranes) equals or exceeds the strength of polar interactions at the hydrophilic surfaces, the characteristic feature of an internalized fracture plane is lost and the membrane does not split (98). This latter situation must apply to the *E. coli* outer membrane because it is not usually labile to cleavage and therefore can be visualized as a tightly knit structure of uniform bond energy across the lipid bilayer (1).

A number of biophysical studies have shown that the acyl chains of LPS are more rigid and in closer proximity to each other than those of their phospholipid counterparts (47–49). Because the strength of van der Waals forces between nonpolar groups are distance dependent, and are strongest over short distances (98), LPS should contribute to the maintenance of a

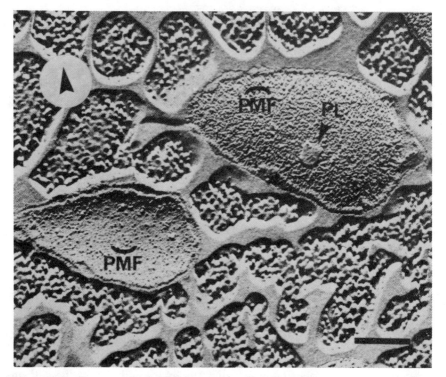

**Figure 10.7** Freeze-etched EDTA-treated cells. The concave plasma membrane fracture (PMF) is evident in the cell to the left. A single plateau (PL) that reaches into the convex outer membrane fracture can be seen on the convex plasma membrane fracture (PMF) of the cell to the right. Arrow indicates direction of platinum shadowing. Bar = 200 nm (8). (With permission of the *Canadian Journal of Microbiology*.)

high degree of internal bond energy within the outer membrane. Indeed, the small outer membrane fractures (plateaus) that are observed when EDTA-treated cells are subjected to freeze-etching (Fig. 10.7) suggest that some regions within the outer membrane are weakened by an extraction of LPS (8, 99).

Bayer and Leive (99) originally suggested that the outer membrane plateaus visible after EDTA treatment represent areas of newly inserted LPS. However, an alternative hypothesis has been presented based on the increased frequency of plateaus observed when EDTA-treated cells are exposed to sodium ions before freeze-etching (Fig. 10.8)(8). The metal binding capacity of outer membrane for monovalent cations such as sodium does not appear to be strongly affected by LPS, so this metal must bind to other molecules, most probably phospholipids (8). Although the precise nature of the interactions between sodium ions and phospholipids is not known, the

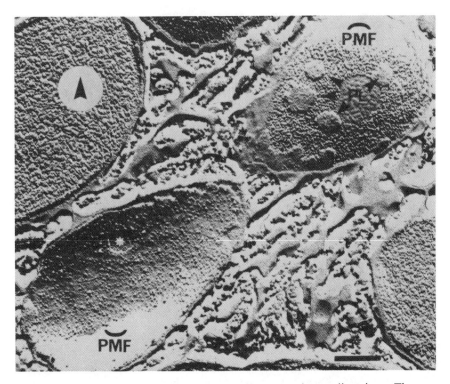

**Figure 10.8**  Freeze-etched EDTA-treated cells exposed to sodium ions. The concave plasma membrane fracture (P̂MF) is evident in the cell on the lower left. At one area, the fracture has broken through the plasma membrane toward the outer membrane (∗). The convex plasma membrane fracture (P̌MF) of the cell on the upper right is studded with plateaus (PL) that reach into the convex outer membrane fracture plane. Arrow indicates direction of platinum shadowing. Bar = 200 nm (8). (With permission of the *Candian Journal of Microbiology*.)

cation tends to increase membrane fluidity (100). When phospholipids are in a fluid state, their hydrocarbon tails are more loosely packed and, as a result, the strength of the van der Waals forces within the membrane is reduced (98, 101). For these reasons, it is possible that the outer membrane plateaus are areas of phospholipids that were originally destabilized by the loss of LPS, and that their increased occurrence following an exposure of EDTA-treated cells to sodium is a result of the fluidizing effects of this metal cation on the outer membrane phospholipids (100). In this view, these outer membrane plateaus are believed to represent discrete regions of increased phospholipid fluidity (8).

The frequency and extent of outer membrane cleavage can also be increased by exposing cells to divalent metal cations before freeze-etching (8). These metallic ions, in contrast to monovalent cations, bind predominantly

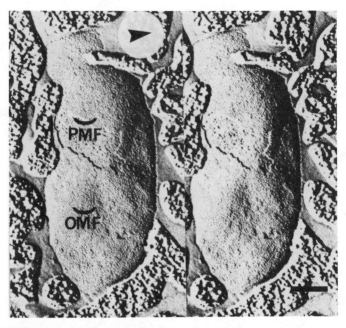

**Figure 10.9** Stereo pair of concave fractures through the plasma membrane (PMF) and outer membrane (OMF) of a control cell exposed to magnesium ions before freeze-etching. Arrow indicates direction of platinum shadowing. Bar = 200 nm (8). (With permission of the *Canadian Journal of Microbiology*.)

to LPS and the acyl chains of this molecule, unlike those of phospholipids, are not influenced to the same extent by metal cation binding (48). In addition, the binding of divalent metallic ions by the outer membrane appears to potentiate an increase in the interfacial free energy (hydrophobicity or rigidity) of water molecules immediately adjacent to the membrane surface (8). Taken together, these concepts suggest that the strength of the polar interactions at the outer membrane–water interface can be increased by the binding of divalent metal cations without an alteration in the internal bond energy of the membrane; that is, a plane of weak bond energy is formed that runs through the hydrophobic core. This type of change in the bond energy profile of the membrane therefore favors the formation of fracture planes through the hydrocarbon core (Fig. 10.9)(8).

## 10.5 CONCLUSIONS

There are several conclusions that can be made concerning interactions between metallic ions and the outer membrane of Gram-negative bacteria. First, because of its structural complexity, the outer membrane can be expected to exhibit a certain degree of selectivity with regard to the types of metal cations that are used to steady the molecular architecture of the membrane. For example, calcium ions are noticeably more effective than magnesium ions in stabilizing LPS in a bilayer conformation (68). Second, it has been established that interactions between the outer membrane and metallic ions conform to certain basic thermodynamic principles that govern the cation selectivity of biological membranes (8, 83). Thus the structural roles of metal cations associated with the outer membrane must be coupled to the physical properties of both the component membrane molecules and the metal cations themselves. Third, the salt condition of the outer membrane, which can be manipulated by the organism through alterations in the chemistry and charge characteristics of the constituent membrane molecules (7), is at least partially responsible for determining how the outer membrane interacts with its aqueous environment.

With the above conclusions in mind, it can be appreciated that the outer membrane metal cation requirements of different Gram-negative bacteria probably vary. Similarly, the metal cation requirements of outer membrane from a single species probably differ, depending on the growth conditions and the physiological status of the cells involved. Ultimately, it should depend on the native environment, and the selective pressures experienced by a microorganism. Moreover, recent evidence suggests that the physico-chemical roles of metal cations extend beyond the structural level; metallic ions are known to influence outer membrane permeability profoundly (3), and may regulate autolytic enzymes (64, 65) or signal the protoplast about events at the cell surface (66). Indeed, the ability of the outer membrane to interact strongly with metallic ions is, in the end, envisioned to facilitate cellular growth, and to couple the protoplast more effectively to its environment.

## ACKNOWLEDGMENTS

The author's work has been made possible by a Postdoctoral Fellowship from the Natural Sciences and Engineering Research Council of Canada.

## REFERENCES

1. T. J. Beveridge. Ultrastructure, chemistry, and function of the bacterial wall. *Int. Rev. Cytol. 72*, 229 (1981).
2. D. Lugtenberg and L. van Alphen. Molecular architecture and functioning of the outer membrane of *Escherichia coli* and other gram-negative bacteria. *Biochim. Biophys. Acta, 737*, 51 (1983).
3. R. E. W. Hancock. Alterations in outer membrane permeability. *Ann. Rev. Microbiol. 38*, 237 (1984).

4. F. G. Ferris and T. J. Beveridge. Functions of bacterial cell surface structures. *BioScience 35*, 172 (1985).

5. M. K. Jain, "Nonrandom lateral organization in bilayers and biomembranes," in R. C. Aloia, Ed., *Membrane Fluidity in Biology (Concepts of Membrane Structure Vol. 1)*, Academic, New York, 1983, p. 1.

6. B. Hoyle and T. J. Beveridge. Binding of metallic ions to the outer membrane of *Escherichia coli. Appl. Environ. Microbiol. 46*, 749 (1983).

7. R. T. Coughlin, S. Tonsager, and E. J. McGroarty. Quantitation of metal cations bound to membranes and extracted lipopolysaccharide from *Escherichia coli. Biochemistry 22*, 2002 (1983).

8. F. G. Ferris and T. J. Beveridge. Physicochemical roles of soluble metal cations in the outer membrane of *Escherichia coli* K-12. *Can. J. Microbiol. 32*, 594 (1986).

9. R. G. E. Murray, P. Steed, and H. E. Elson. The location of the mucopeptide in sections of the cell wall of *Escherichia coli* and other gram-negative bacteria. *Can. J. Microbiol. 11*, 547 (1965).

10. P. Steed and R. G. E. Murray. The cell wall and cell division of gram-negative bacteria. *Can. J. Microbiol. 12*, 263 (1966).

11. T. Miura and S. Mizushima. Separation by density gradient centrifugation of two types of membranes from spheroplast membranes of *Escherichia coli* K-12. *Biochim. Biophys. Acta 150*, 159 (1968).

12. T. Miura and S. Mizushima. Separation and properties of outer and cytoplasmic membranes in *Escherichia coli. Biochim. Biophys. Acta 193*, 263 (1969).

13. L. Leive. Release of lipopolysaccharide by EDTA treatment of *E. coli. Biochem. Biophys. Res. Commun. 21*, 290 (1965).

14. C. A. Schnaitman. Protein composition of the cell wall and cytoplasmic membrane of *Escherichia coli. J. Bacteriol. 104*, 890 (1970).

15. J. Koplow and H. Goldfine. Alterations in the outer membrane and cell envelope of heptose-deficient mutants of *Escherichia coli. J. Bacteriol. 117*, 527 (1974).

16. N. C. Jones and M. J. Osborn. Translocation of phospholipids between the outer and inner membranes of *Salmonella typhimurium. J. Biol. Chem. 252*, 7405 (1977).

17. H. Nikaido and T. Nakae. The outer membrane of gram-negative bacteria. *Adv. Microb. Physiol. 20*, 163 (1979).

18. M. R. W. Brown and P. Williams. The influence of environment on envelope properties affecting the survival of bacteria in infections. *Ann. Rev. Microbiol. 39*, 527 (1985).

19. J. E. Cronan, "Phospholipid synthesis and assembly," in M. Inouye, Ed., *Bacterial Outer Membranes: Biogenesis and Functions*, Wiley, New York, 1979, p. 35.

20. D. A. White, W. J. Lennarz, and C. A. Schnaitman. Distribution of lipids in the wall and cytoplasmic membrane subfractions of *Escherichia coli. J. Bacteriol. 109*, 686 (1972).

21. E. J. J. Lugtenberg and R. Peters. Distribution of lipids in cytoplasmic and outer membranes of *Escherichia coli. Biochim. Biophys. Acta 441*, 38 (1976).

22. A. J. Wicken and K. W. Knox. Bacterial cell surface amphiphiles. *Biochim. Biophys. Acta 604*, 1 (1980).

23. M. J. Osborn. "Biosynthesis and assembly of the lipopolysaccharide of the outer membrane," in M. Inouye, Ed., *Bacterial Outer Membranes: Biogenesis and Functions*, Wiley, New York, 1979, p. 15.

24. P. Prehm, G. Schmidt, B. Jann, and K. Jann. The cell wall lipopolysaccharide of *Escherichia coli* K-12. Structure and acceptor site for O-antigen and other substituents. *Eur. J. Biochem. 70*, 171 (1976).

25. M. R. Rosner and H. Khorana. Structure of the lipopolysaccharide from an *Escherichia coli* heptose-less mutant II. The application of $^{31}$P-NMR spectroscopy. *J. Biol. Chem. 254*, 5918.

26. G. B. Pier, R. B. Markham, and D. Eardley. Correlation of the biological responses of C3H/HEJ mice to endotoxin with the chemical and structural properties of the LPS from *Pseudomonas aeruginosa* and *Escherichia coli*. *J. Immun. 127*, 184 (1981).

27. S. G. Wilkinson. Composition and structure of LPS from *Pseudomonas aeruginosa*. *Rev. Infect. Dis. 5*, s941 (1983).

28. A. M. Kropinski, B. Jewell, J. Kuzia, F. Milazzo, and D. Berry. Structure and function of *Pseudomonas aeruginosa* lipopolysaccharide. *Antibiot. Chemother. 36*, 58 (1985).

29. R. C. Goldman and L. Leive. Heterogeneity of antigenic side chain length in lipopolysaccharide from *Escherichia coli* 0111 and *S. typhimurium* LT2. *Eur. J. Biochem. 107*, 145 (1980).

30. E. T. Palva and P. M. Makela. LPS heterogeneity in *S. typhimurium* analyzed by SDS-PAGE. *Eur. J. Biochem. 107*, 137 (1980).

31. I. Orskov, F. Orskov, B. Jann, and K. Jann. Serology, chemistry, and genetics of O and K antigens of *Escherichia coli*. *Bacteriol. Rev. 41*, 667 (1977).

32. J. Y. Homa. Designation of the thirteen O-group antigens of *Pseudomonas aeruginosa*. An amendment for the tentative proposal in 1976. *Jap. J. Exp. Med. 52*, 317 (1982).

33. M. J. Osborn and H. C. P. Wu. Proteins of the outer membrane of gram-negative bacteria. *Ann. Rev. Microbiol. 34*, 369 (1980).

34. M. J. Osborn, J. E. Gander, E. Parisi, and J. Carson. Mechanism of assembly of the outer membrane of *Salmonella typhimurium*. Isolation and characterization of cytoplasmic and outer membrane. *J. Biol. Chem. 247*, 3962 (1972).

35. C. Zwinsinski, T. Date, and W. Wickner. Leader peptidase is found in both the inner and outer membrane of *Escherichia coli*. *Eur. J. Biochem. 256*, 3593 (1981).

36. H. Wolf-Watz and S. Normack. Evidence for a role of *N*-acetylmuramyl-L-alanine amidase in septum separation in *Escherichia coli*. *J. Bacteriol. 128*, 580 (1976).

37. N. L. Martin and T. J. Beveridge. Gentamicin interaction with *Pseudomonas aeruginosa* cell envelope. *Antimicrobial Agents Chemother. 29*, 1079 (1986).

38. M. Schindler and M. J. Osborn. Interactions of divalent cations and polymyxin B with lipopolysaccharide. *Biochemistry 18*, 4425 (1979).

39. R. T. Coughlin, C. R. Caldwell, A. Haug, and E. J. McGroarty. A cationic

electron spin resonance probe used to analyze cation interactions with lipopolysaccharide. *Biochem. Biophys. Res. Commun. 100*, 1137 (1981).

40. S. M. Strain, S. W. Fesik, and I. M. Armitage. Structure and metal-binding properties of lipopolysaccharides from heptose-less mutants of *Escherichia coli* studied by $^{13}$C and $^{31}$P nuclear magnetic resonance. *J. Biol. Chem. 258*, 13466 (1983).

41. M. R. Rosner, H. G. Khorana, and A. C. Satterthwait. The structure of lipopolysaccharide from a heptose-less mutant of *Escherichia coli* K-12. *J. Biol. Chem. 254*, 5918 (1979).

42. A. Forge, J. W. Costerton, and K. A. Kerr. Freeze-etching and X-ray diffraction of the isolated double tract layer from the cell wall of a gram-negative pseudomonad. *J. Bacteriol. 113*, 445 (1973).

43. P. Overath, M. Brenner, T. Gulik-Krzywicki, E. Shechter, and L. Letellier. Lipid phase transitions in cytoplasmic and outer membranes of *Escherichia coli*. *Biochim. Biophys. Acta 389*, 358 (1975).

44. E. Burnell, L. van Alphen, A. Verkleij, B. De Kruijff, and B. Lugtenberg. $^{31}$P nuclear magnetic resonance and freeze-fracture electron microscopy studies on *Escherichia coli* III. The outer membrane. *Biochim. Biophys. Acta 597*, 518 (1980).

45. P. F. Muhlradt and J. R. Golecki. Asymmetrical and artifactual reorientation of lipopolysaccharide in the outer bilayer of *Salmonella typhimurium*. *Eur. J. Biochem. 51*, 343 (1975).

46. L. van Alphen, B. Lugtenberg, R. van Boxtel, and K. Verhoef. Architecture of the outer membrane of *Escherichia coli* K-12 I. Action of phospholipase A$_2$ and C on wild type strains and outer membrane mutants. *Biochim. Biophys. Acta 466*, 257 (1977).

47. H. Nikaido, Y. Takeuchi, S.-I. Ohnishi, and T. Nakae. Outer membrane of *Salmonella typhimurium*. Electron spin resonance studies. *Biochim. Biophys. Acta 465*, 152 (1977).

48. G. Emmerling, U. Henning, and T. Gulik-Krzywicki. Order-disorder transition of hydrocarbon chains in lipopolysaccharide from *Escherichia coli*. *Eur. J. Biochem. 78*, 503 (1977).

49. S. Rottem and L. Leive. Effect of variations in lipopolysaccharide on the fluidity of the outer membrane of *Escherichia coli*. *J. Biol. Chem. 252*, 2077 (1977).

50. J. H. Davis, C. P. Nichol, G. Weeks. and M. Bloom. Study of the cytoplasmic and outer membranes of *Escherichia coli* by deuterium nuclear magnetic resonance. *Biochemistry 18*, 2103 (1979).

51. C. P. Nichol, J. H. Davis, G. Weeks, and M. Bloom. Quantitative study of the fluidity of *Escherichia coli* membranes using deuterium nuclear magnetic resonance. *Biochemistry 19*, 45 (1980).

52. J. P. Rosenbusch. Characterization of the major envelope protein from *Escherichia coli*. Regular arrangement in the peptidoglycan and unusual dodecyl sulfate binding. *J. Biol. Chem. 254*, 5918 (1974).

53. A. D. Steven, B. ten Heggeler, R. Muller, J. Kistler, and J. P. Rosenbusch. Ultrastructure of a periodic protein layer in the outer membrane of *Escherichia coli*. *J. Cell Biol. 72*, 292 (1977).

54. H. Yamada and S. Mizushima. Stimulation of the binding of outer membrane proteins O-8 and O-9 to the peptidoglycan layer of *Escherichia coli* K-12. *Eur. J. Biochem. 103*, 209 (1980).

55. R. Benz and R. E. W. Hancock. Properties of the large ion permeable pores formed from protein F of *Pseudomonas aeruginosa* in lipid bilayer membranes. *Biochim. Biophys. Acta 646*, 298 (1981).

56. V. Braun. Covalent lipoprotein from the outer membrane of *Escherichia coli*. *Biochim. Biophys. Acta 415*, 335 (1975).

57. I. Hindennach and U. Henning. The major proteins of the *Escherichia coli* outer cell envelope membrane. Preparative isolation of all major membrane proteins. *Eur. J. Biochem. 59*, 207 (1975).

58. R. E. W. Hancock, R. T. Irvin, J. W. Costerton, and A. M. Carey. *Pseudomonas aeruginosa* outer membrane peptidoglycan associated proteins. *J. Bacteriol. 145*, 628 (1981).

59. S. J. Singer and G. L. Nicolson. The fluid mosaic model of the structure of cell membranes. *Science 175*, 720 (1972).

60. M. Schindler, M. J. Osborn, and D. E. Koppel. Lateral mobility in reconstituted membranes: comparisons with diffusion in polymers. *Nature* (London) *283*, 346 (1980).

61. L. van Alphen, A. Verkleij, E. Burnell, and B. Lugtenberg, $^{31}$P nuclear magnetic resonance and freeze-fracture electron microscopy studies on *Escherichia coli* II. Lipopolysaccharide and lipopolysaccharide complexes. *Biochim. Biophys. Acta 597*, 505 (1980).

62. L. Leive. The barrier function of the gram-negative envelope. *Ann. NY Acad. Sci. 235*, 109 (1974).

63. R. A. Scudamore, T. J. Beveridge, and M. Goldner. Outer membrane penetration barriers as components of intrinsic resistance to beta-lactam and other antibiotics in *Escherichia coli* K-12. *Antimicrobial Agents Chemother. 15*, 182 (1979).

64. J. van Heijenoort, M. Leduc, Y. van Heijenoort, and R. Kasra, "Autolysis of *Escherichia coli*: induction and control," in R. Hakenbeck, J.-V. Höltje, and H. Labischinski, Eds., *The Target of Penicillin*, Walter de Gruyter, Berlin, 1983, p. 191.

65. M. Leduc, R. Kasra, and J. van Heijenoort. Induction and control of the autolytic system of *Escherichia coli*. *J. Bacteriol. 152*, 26 (1982).

66. L. Lettelier, and B. Labedan. Involvement of envelope bound calcium in the transient depolarization of the *Escherichia coli* cytoplasmic membrane induced by bacteriophage T4 and T5 adsorption. *J. Bacteriol. 157*, 789 (1984).

67. T. J. Beveridge. "Mechanism of the binding of metallic ions to bacterial walls and the possible impact on microbial ecology," in C. A. Reddy and M. J. Klug, Eds., *Current Perspectives in Microbial Ecology*, American Society for Microbiology, Washington, DC, 1984, p. 601.

68. R. T. Coughlin, A. Haug, and E. J. McGroarty. Physical properties of defined lipopolysaccharide salts. *Biochemistry 22*, 2007 (1983).

69. J. S. D'Arrigo. Screening of membrane surface charges by divalent cations: an atomic representation. *Am. J. Physiol. 235*, c109 (1978).

70. S. McLaughlin, G. Szabo, and G. Eisenman. Divalent ions and the surface potential of charged phospholipid membranes. *J. Gen. Physiol. 58*, 667 (1971)

71. S. McLaughlin. Electrostatic potentials at membrane-solution interfaces. *Current topics in membranes and transport 9*, 71 (1977).

72. P. F. Mühlradt. Topology of outer membrane assembly in *Salmonella. J. Supramol. Structure. 5*, 103 (1976).

73. C. Tanford. *The Hydrophobic Effect. Formation of micelles and biological membranes*, 2nd ed., Wiley, New York, 1980.

74. M. C. Goldschmidt and O. Wyss. The role of Tris in EDTA toxicity and lysozyme lysis. *J. Gen. Microbiol. 47*, 421 (1967).

75. R. E. W. Hancock, V. J. Raffle, and T. I. Nicas. Involvement in the outer membrane in gentamicin and streptomycin uptake and killing in *Pseudomonas aeruginosa. Antimicrobial Agents Chemother. 19*, 777 (1981).

76. R. T. Irvin, T. J. MacAlister, and J. W. Costerton. Tris-(hydroxymethyl)-aminomethane buffer modifiication of the *Escherichia coli* outer membrane. *J. Bacteriol. 145*, 1397 (1981).

77. M. Vaara and T. Vaara. Polycations sensitize enteric bacteria to antibiotics. *Antimicrobial Agents Chemother. 24*, 107 (1983).

78. M. Vaara and T. Vaara. Polycations as outer membrane disorganizing agents. *Antimicrobial Agents Chemother. 24*, 114 (1983).

79. H. E. Gilleland and R. G. E. Murray. Ultrastructural study of polymyxin-resistant isolates of *Pseudomonas aeruginosa. J. Bacteriol. 125*, 267 (1976).

80. R. G. Schindler and M. Teuber. Action of polymyxin B on bacterial membranes—morphological changes in cytoplasm and in outer membrane of *Salmonella typhimurium* and *Escherichia coli* B. *Antimicrobial Agents Chemother. 8*, 95 (1975).

81. S. G. Walker and T. J. Beveridge. Amikacin disrupts the cell envelope of *Pseudomonas aeruginosa* ATCC 9027. *Can. J. Microbiol., 34*, 12 (1988).

82. F. A. Cotton and G. Wilkinson. *Advanced Inorganic Chemistry. A Comprehensive Text*, 3rd ed., Wiley, New York, 1972.

83. J. M. Diamond and E. M. Wright. Biological membranes: the physical basis of ion and nonelectrolyte selectivity. *Ann. Rev. Physiol. 31*, 581 (1969).

84. T. J. Beveridge and R. G. E. Murray. Uptake and retention of metals by cell walls of *Bacillus subtilis. J. Bacteriol. 127*, 1502 (1976).

85. F. G. Ferris and T. J. Beveridge. Binding of a paramagnetic metal cation of *Escherichia coli* K-12 outer membrane vesicles. *FEMS Microbiol. Lett. 24*, 43 (1984).

86. J. Seelig and A. Seelig. Lipid conformation in model and biological membranes. *Quart. Rev. Biophys. 13*, 19 (1980).

87. D. R. Burton. "Paramagnetic ions as relaxation probes in biological systems," in I. Bertini and R. S. Drago, Eds., *ESR and NMR of paramagnetic species in biological and related systems*, D. Reidel, Dordrecht, 1980, p. 151.

88. T. L. James, "NMR studies of biomolecular interactions," in *Nuclear Magnetic Resonance in Biochemistry*, Academic, New York, 1975, p. 173.

89. M. F. Brown and J. Seelig. Ion induced changes in headgroup conformation of lecithin bilayers. *Nature* (London) *269*, 721 (1977).

90. F. G. Ferris and T. J. Beveridge. Site specificity of metallic ion binding in *Escherichia coli* K-12 lipopolysaccharide. *Can. J. Microbiol. 32*, 52 (1986).

91. H. Labischinski, G. Barnickel, H. Bradaczek, D. Naumann, E. T. Rietschel, and P. Giesbrecht. High state order of isolated bacterial lipopolysaccharide and its possible contribution to the permeation barrier property of the outer membrane. *J. Bacteriol. 162*, 9 (1985).

92. A. M. James. The electrical properties and topochemistry of bacterial cells. *Adv. Colloid Interface Sci. 15*, 171 (1982).

93. P. A. Albertsson, *Partitioning of Cell Particles and Macromolecules*, 2nd ed., Wiley, New York, 1971.

94. K.-E. Magnusson, O. Stendahl, C. Tagesson, L. Edebo, and G. Johansson. The tendency of smooth and rough *Salmonella typhimurium* bacteria and lipopolysaccharide to hydrophobic and ionic interactions as studied in aqueous polymer two-phase systems. *Acta Pathol. Microbiol. Scand. Sec. B 84*, 212 (1977).

95. K.-E. Magnusson, J. Davies, T. Grundstrom, E. Kihlstrom, and S. Normack. Surface charge and hydrophobicity of *Salmonella, E. coli*, and gonococci in relation to their tendency to associate with animal cells. *Scand. J. Infect. Dis. Suppl. 25*, 135 (1980).

96. D. Branton. Fracture faces of frozen membranes. *Proc. Natl. Acad. Sci. USA 55*, 1048 (1966).

97. P. P. DaSilva and D. Branton. Membrane splitting in freeze-etching. Covalently bound ferritin as a membrane marker. *J. Cell Biol. 45*, 598 (1970).

98. F. S. Sjostrand. The interpretation of pictures of freeze-fractured biological material. *J. Ultrastruct. Res. 69*, 378 (1979).

99. M. E. Bayer and L. Leive. Effect of ethylenediaminetetraacetate upon the surface of *Escherichia coli*. *J. Bacteriol. 130*, 1364 (1977).

100. J. Eibl. "The effect of the proton and of monovalent cations on membrane fluidity," in R. C. Aloia, Ed., *Membrane Fluidity in Biology (Vol. 2, General Principles)*, Academic, New York, 1983, p. 217.

101. D. Chapman. "Biomembrane fluidity: the concept and its development," in R. C. Aloia, Ed., *Membrane Fluidity in Biology (Vol. 2, General Principles)*, Academic, New York, 1983, p. 5.

# CHAPTER 11

# Interactions Between Metal Ions and Capsular Polymers

GILL G. GEESEY

Department of Microbiology
California State University
Long Beach, California

LARRY JANG

Department of Chemical Engineering
California State University
Long Beach, California

## Contents

## 11.1  INTRODUCTION

Many different types of bacteria elaborate a capsule or slime layer as their outermost envelope component. Among its many functions, the capsule serves as a buffer between the environment and the cell. The capsule may prevent some substances such as antibiotics and biocides in the environment from contacting the cell surface, yet at the same time concentrate growth-limiting nutrients from the surrounding environment for subsequent transport into the cell.

Of the various dissolved substances that exist in aquatic habitats, metal ions are unique in that over a rather narrow concentration range, their status can change from an essential growth-promoting element to a toxin. Bacteria must therefore maintain tight control over the level of metal to which they are exposed in habitats with widely fluctuating dissolved metal concentrations.

One of the two main mechanisms of metal accumulation by bacteria involves nonspecific binding of the metal to the cell surface, capsule, and extracellular slime layer (1). Capsules possess features that suggest that they act as effective modulators of metal ion concentration at the cell surface, scavenging metals from solution when their concentrations are low and serving as impermeable barriers when metals exist at toxic levels in the surrounding environment.

Besides the influence exopolymer–metal interactions have on cell survival, the binding of metals by bacterial capsular material also has an impact on ecological and geochemical processes. Recent evidence suggests that the complexation of metal ions by capsular polymers may even contribute to corrosion reactions that have significant economic consequences. Before these broader implications of capsular–metal interactions can be clearly understood, more accurate information is needed on the thermodynamic and kinetic properties of the complexes that are formed.

The physical and chemical properties of bacterial capsule and slime polymers promote unique associations with metals. The tendency for many bacterial exopolymers to exist in a colloidal or gel-like state in the presence of metal ions results in the establishment of a multiple phase system. Consequently, classical approaches that describe equilibrium conditions for simple molecules or other polyelectrolytes in single-phase sytems must be modified in order to obtain useful thermodynamic stability constants that apply to the range of conditions over which bacterial–metal interactions occur.

In this chapter, interactions between metals and capsular polymers are described in terms of the chemical reactions that are involved as well as the consequences of such interactions to the bacterial cell and to the surrounding environment. Although the discussion focuses on the aquatic environment, many of the processes described apply to soil, plant, and animal systems as well. Finally, an approach is presented for the determination of "intrinsic" stability constants that takes into consideration the unique features of bacterial exopolymer–metal interactions.

## 11.2 THE BACTERIAL CAPSULE

The vast majority of bacteria observed in aquatic habitats, including the marine environment, possess an envelope structure characteristic of Gram-negative cells. The capsule, which is usually a polysaccharide with a repeating sequence of two to six sugar subunits (2), is anchored to the bacterial outer membrane. In some instances, the oligosaccharide side chain of lipopolysaccharide in the outer membrane is believed to contribute to the capsular structure (3). Some bacteria elaborate capsules composed of two chemically distinct polysaccharides (4, 5). A protein component is often recovered during isolation of capsule preparations (6–8). Whether the protein performs any function in this exocellular location is not well understood at this time. Other products of cell metabolism, excreted by the bacteria and trapped by the exopolymer matrix, may also contribute to the overall chemical properties of the capsule.

Exopolymers exhibit a variety of associations with the cell surface. Some bacteria elaborate capsular exopolymers that are firmly bound to the cell surface. This type of association often enables the cell to establish a stable orientation with respect to its environment. Cell-bound exopolymers may extend from 0.1 to 10 $\mu$m from the cell surface into the surrounding environment, creating a buffer zone between the surface of the cell and the external environment (9, 10).

In some instances, the capsular polymers maintain a more transient association with the cell and take the form of what is commonly referred to as "slime." A portion or, in some cases, the bulk of the exopolymer sloughs into the surrounding menstruum. Different strains of the same bacterium may elaborate exopolymers that maintain different associations with the cell (11). There is some evidence from the medical field that overproduction of capsular polymer leads to sloughing. Production of slime has been shown to be controlled, to some extent, by the culture or environmental conditions (12). When both capsules and slimes are produced, the chemical compositions of their polysaccharides are usually similar (13, 14).

In aquatic and industrial fields, the term "slime" is often used to refer to a slippery or visible growth of microorganisms on surfaces. In this context, slime includes the microorganisms, the exopolymers, and any adsorbed material from the aqueous phase.

The network of polymers that makes up the capsule or slime forms a colloid or gel phase, depending on the nature of the surrounding environment. The volume enclosed by the capsule, hereafter referred to as the gel phase, generally contains greater than 99% water by weight. Aggregation of the exopolymers may occur under certain conditions resulting in the formation of visible flocs. The tendency for bacterial exopolymers to form a colloid or gel phase around the cell, which often results in biofilm or floc formation, suggests that these biomolecules possess properties that are different from those of other naturally occurring polymers.

## 11.3   EFFECTS OF METALS ON EXOPOLYMER PRODUCTION

Metals have been shown to influence the production of capsule and slime exopolymers. Various ions are known to be required as cofactors in polysaccharide synthesis. Wilkinson and Stark (15) demonstrated in cultures of *Enterobacter aerogenes* that polysaccharide was stimulated by Mg, K, and Ca ions. Later, Corpe (6) reported that polysaccharide production in *Chromobacterium violaceum* was enhanced in the presence of Fe and Ca ions.

The amount of Cr in the culture medium affected the yield and form of exopolymer produced by a coryneform bacterium isolated from Cr-polluted marine sediments (16). Exopolysaccharide production increased as more Cr(III) was added to the medium.

The morphology of the capsule of *Azotobacter chroococcum* was also affected by metal availability in the growth medium (17). Under Fe- or Mo-sufficient conditions, the capsule was condensed, whereas under deficient conditions the capsule appeared more diffuse and extensive.

The composition of alginate produced by cells of *Azotobacter vinlandii* is affected by Ca availability. Removal of Ca from the growth medium leads to an increase in the relative concentration of mannuronic acid in the exopolymer (18, 19).

It is evident that no generalizations can be made with respect to the effects metals and other cations have on bacterial capsule production. This likely reflects basic physiological differences between bacterial types. It may also reflect differences in the types and concentrations of metals in the environment in which the bacteria exist.

## 11.4   PROTECTION FROM METAL TOXICITY

The role of capsular polymers in the protection of bacterial cells from the toxic effects of metals was demonstrated by Bitton and Friehofer (20). Survival of *Klebsiella aerogenes* in a 0.85% NaCl solution containing 10 μg Cu or Cd mL$^{-1}$ was significantly greater for cells that produced capsules compared to mutants that lost their capsule-producing ability. It was further shown that capsule isolated from the competent strain enhanced the survival of the noncapsulated cells when added to the metal-containing solution. The capsule bound 0.02 and 0.01 μg Cu and Cd mg$^{-1}$ polysaccharide.

In another study, nonmucoid variants of a coryneform bacterium isolated from Cr-contaminated marine sediments were less tolerant to 156 μg Cr (III) mL$^{-1}$ than a mucoid wild-type strain (21). The mucoid strain accumulated significantly more Cr (III) than the nonmucoid strain. Greater than 80% of the metal was in the exopolymer. At 91 μg Cr (III) mL$^{-1}$ external concentration, the slime polymers from coryneform and Enterobacteriaceae isolates contained 1000 and 1943 μg Cr (III) g$^{-1}$ dry weight polymer, respectively. It appears from these and other studies conducted to date that bacteria that produce exopolysaccharides tolerate higher concentrations of metal than strains that produce little or no capsule or slime. The tolerance likely occurs as a result of a reduction in free metal ion concentration at the cell surface, in turn a result of metal ion complexation by sites on the exopolymer molecules.

## 11.5  BIOACCUMULATION OF METALS VIA BACTERIAL EXOPOLYMERS

Bacteria that exist in sediments attached to particles or as a biofilm on submerged surfaces depend on capsule and slime exopolymers to maintain their sessile nature. Consequently, the exopolymers are optimally positioned to interact with metal ions that approach these surfaces. Complexation of metals by biofilms has been suggested to play an important role in controlling toxic metal concentrations in the water phase (22).

Montgomery and Price (23) indicated that the largest net uptake of metals from a source of sewage pollution occurred in the fouling community of a model turtle grass mangrove ecosystem. In other studies, bacterial epiphytes were shown to be a major factor in contributing to the total Cr, Cu, Fe, Pb, and Zn of aquatic plants (24). Binding of Mo by extracellular polysaccharides produced by the epiphytic bacteria resulted in a reduction in the amount of that entering the plant (25).

Because sessile bacteria contribute a significant portion of the total living biomass in sediments and, in addition, are high in nutritive value, they are a preferred food source for many benthic organisms. Harvey and Luoma (26) presented evidence that bacteria contribute to the nutrition of the estuarine clam *Macoma balthica*. The clam did not appear to utilize exopolymer isolated from a slime-producing strain of *Pseudomonas atlantica*, however. Exopolymers did increase the biological availability of particle-bound Ag, Cd, and Zn when the metals were present at low concentrations

(27). At higher metal concentrations, the clams avoided exopolymer-adsorbed particles.

Patrick and Loutit (28) demonstrated that metals, initially concentrated by bacteria and passed on through oligochaete worms, eventually accumulated in fish. More recently, it was shown that the Cr content of the snail *Amphibola*, which was fed Cr-complexed bacterial polysaccharide, contained threefold higher levels of the metal than snails fed polysaccharide containing very low levels of Cr (29). Examination of body parts demonstrated that 61% of the Cr was associated with internal tissues and only 39% was adsorbed to the shell of the snail. It was further shown that polysaccharide with bound Cr was degraded more slowly than Cr-free polysaccharide by the heterotrophic sediment bacteria. It is evident from these studies that detritivores are capable of accumulating exopolymer-bound metals during their ingestion of the bacteria. The capsular and slime exopolymers excreted by sessile bacteria therefore provide a means of metal entry into the aquatic food chain.

## 11.6  PROPERTIES OF CAPSULAR POLYMERS RELEVANT TO METAL INTERACTIONS

That capsular polymers are most readily visualized by electron microscopy after staining with cationic dyes such as ruthenium red leads to the suggestion that they are acidic in nature (30). Chemical characterization of capsular and slime polysaccharide subunits from bacteria isolated from a variety of natural habitats indicates that they contain uronic acids and other substituted sugars that possess acidic functional groups. The density of acidic residues on the polymer chain may vary in different bacterial species. Some bacteria produce capsular polymers that contain only neutral sugar subunits whereas a few bacteria excrete capsules or slime composed entirely of uronic acids. The capsules of most bacteria examined to date contain from 5 to 25% uronic acids (31). Ketal-linked pyruvylated sugars also contribute acidic functional groups to capsular and slime polysaccharides (32–34). Unlike the ester-linked residues, ketals confer a negative charge on the polysaccharide similar to that of a uronic acid. Sialic acids, which refer to a series of substituted neuraminic acids, are found in the capsules of several bacterial genera (35, 36). These also contain free carboxyl groups which confer a net negative charge to the polymer. Although a variety of other functional groups have been identified in bacterial capsules and slimes, apart from hydroxyl residues, there is little information on their interactions with metal ions.

## 11.7  MECHANISMS OF METAL ION BINDING TO BACTERIAL EXOPOLYSACCHARIDES

Although different classes of biological molecules may be associated with bacterial exopolymers, the metal binding reactions considered here are restricted to those involving the polysaccharide component. Metals tend to form bonds with electron-donating groups in order to fill their outer electron shell. The most effective electron donor group associated with acidic capsule and slime polysaccharides is the carboxyl residue. Lone-pair electrons on carboxyl groups interact with the charge-compensating metal ions. Weak electron donors are also present on acidic and neutral polysaccharides in the form of oxygen atoms associated with the ether bond and hydroxyl residues on the sugar subunits (37).

On the basis of Rendelman's (38) interpretation of ion interactions with polysaccharides, metal binding by uncharged polysaccharides occurs as a result of coordination between the metal cation and oxyanion and hydroxyl groups on the donor molecule. The affinity exhibited by uncharged polysaccharides generally decreases with increasing ionic radius of metals.

The general metal–molecule interaction is an acid–base reaction:

$$M^{n+} + LH \rightarrow M^{n+}-L^{-1} + H^{+}$$

where the acid is represented by $H^{+}$, the metal ion by $M^{n+}$, and the base by $L^{-1}$. The binding of Cu ion to the capsule of a freshwater sediment bacterium (FRI) was shown to result in the displacement of protons that caused a shift in the $pK_a$ of the capsule from 4.90 to 4.05 (39). An observed decrease in the conditional stability constant for the Cu–capsule complex with decreased pH also suggests that there was competition between Cu ions and protons at the site of metal binding. Although no uronic acids were detected in the capsular material, the $pK_a$ value suggests the presence of carboxyl groups, possibly in the form of ketal-linked pyruvate residues (40). The release of protons by other acidic polysaccharides during exposure to increased concentrations of copper has also been reported (41).

Steiner (42) described four classes of ion binding by extracellular polymers based on the shape of the adsorption isotherms. The two most important classes were those that involved salt bridges with carboxyl groups on acidic polymers and those that involved weak electrostatic bonds with hydroxyl groups on neutral polymers. The "S-type" isotherm produced by complexes between metal ions and the capsule of *Zoogloea ramigera* 115 was proposed to involve primarily hydroxyl groups of the glucose subunits even though the polysaccharide contains free carboxyl groups on the ketal-linked pyruvate residues (43). This type of metal binding is believed to be the most important mechanism of metal removal in activated sludge.

Metal interactions with charged polysaccharides are controlled to some extent by linear charge density. In some cases, the affinity of an acidic polysaccharide for a cation increases with increasing charge density (44). Metal–polymer interactions are often stronger when the polymer exists as a gel than when dissolved in solution. This is likely due to an increase in charge density in the former. Such evidence supports the concept of "salt bridging," in which a polyvalent metal ion bonds to two anionic groups on separate polymer chains. The recent studies of Manzini et al. (45), which suggest that more than two uronate groups are complexed with each Cu ion, supports the contention that metal ions participate in intermolecular bonding. "Steric fit" thus becomes important and supports the evidence that the ionic radius of a metal frequently determines whether complexation will occur.

In general, carboxylated polysaccharides exhibit preferential binding to cations with large ionic radii. With few exceptions, carboxylated polyanions exhibit a higher selectivity for transition metals than the alkaline earth metals. In some instances, however, the affinity of Mg fluctuates relative to other cations in different anionic polysaccharides. In addition, selectivity coefficients may be different, depending on whether the polymer exists in solution or in a gel state (46). Affinity of alginic acid for the transition metals decreases in the order Cu > Ni, Co > Zn > Mn, which roughly follows the Irving–Williams order of decreasing complex stability.

Polyuronides (alginates and pectic substances) have been recognized for their metal-binding ability for over 100 years. Consequently, much of what is known about complexes formed between acidic polysaccharides and metal ions is based on studies with these substances. As early as 1825, Braconnot suggested that pectins might be used to treat heavy metal poisoning in humans owing to the insoluble complex that is formed (47).

Cozzi et al. (48) proposed that the stability and selectivity of complexes between alkaline earth ions and alginates is influenced by hydroxyl groups. It was shown that two hydroxyl groups on the uronate subunit are more stabilizing than one. The differences in affinity among alkaline earth cations such as Ca for polymannuronic, polygalacturonic, and polyguluronic acid regions of alginic acid were suggested to be due to variations in the positioning of the hydroxyl groups on the monomer subunits (49). The spacing of coordinating oxygen atoms in the polyanion therefore has a major influence on which cations will bind as well as their stability. In general, the more coordination bonds that are formed between the metal and the "ligand" or donor molecule, the greater the stability of the complex. The formation of stable complexes of metal ions with organic ligands usually involved both electrovalent (nonionic) and coordinate covalent bonding.

An "egg-box" model has been proposed for the structure of alginic acid in which a series of cavities that offer four oxygens for coordination with Ca ions exists in regions containing repeating sequences of guluronic acid (47, 50). Cooperative binding of the guluronic acid-rich regions with functional groups on other nearby polymer chains is necessary for the proposed configuration. It was further demonstrated that with polygalacturonic acid, fewer cavities are possible, most of which offered only three oxygen atoms for coordination, and with polymannuronic acid, only shallow cavities are formed. Blocks of polyguluronic acid have greater selectivity toward and stability with Ca and Sr than do repeating sequences of polygalacturonic and polymannuronic acids. Bacterial alginates exhibit a wide variation in the relative contribution of guluronic acid and mannuronic acid residues in the polymer molecule. It may be concluded from the preceding discussion that the mechanisms of cation binding by alginic acid and possibly other bacterial exopolysaccharides are different from those described for ion binding to classical polyelectrolytes.

Copper ions in solution displace Ca ions bound to alginic acid. A high selectivity for Cu over Ca is a characteristic feature of carboxylated polyanions, in general. The binding mechanism that is responsible for the higher affinity for Cu than Ca appears to be independent of free hydroxyl groups in the polymer and of the steric arrangement of the carboxyl groups (49).

Metal ions in solution are always fully coordinated or solvated by water molecules. When a metal ion becomes complexed by an organic ligand there is a displacement and reordering of water molecules: the number of water molecules displaced depends on the dimension and charge of the metal ion and on the size of the coordinated electron-donating group of the ligand. It was proposed that Cu ions have a larger ordering effect on the water molecules than Ca ions, and that the displacement of Ca by Cu on the polymer should be favored by the relatively large positive entropic change (49).

Order within the liquid subphase may also depend on the chemical properties of the capsule. In the case of M41 capsular polysaccharide of *Escherichia coli*, only the polyanions are ordered and the cations and water molecules behave like a liquid filling the spaces between polymer molecules (32). This is in contrast to alginic acid and hyaluronic acid where cations and most water molecules have well-defined positions and may determine gross configuration of the polymer chains fibers.

More recently, Manzini et al. (45) emphasized the importance of carboxyl groups in cupric ion binding. They suggested that an intimate interaction exists between copper ions and carboxyl groups on acidic polysaccharides. Cupric ion binding to a carboxyl group is electrovalent. In the case of polyuronates, the mode and extent of the interaction are believed to depend on several factors: the nature of the component sugars and their relative distribution in the chain, the magnitude of the overall electrostatic field, and the ratios of copper to polymer and of copper to simple supporting electrolyte.

Molybdenum binding by extracellular slimes of rhizosphere bacteria was investigated by Tan and Loutit (51). They determined that Mo was bound mainly by a passive process to the uronic acid-containing portion of the slime layer surrounding a *Pseudomonas* sp. Greater than 90% of the Mo associated with the cells was bound to the slime. The slime polysaccharide from *P. aeruginosa* was reported to bind Mo through the glucuronic acid subunit (52). Copper is also bound to this subunit as well. Glucuronic acid was found to contribute 32% of the total slime weight. Complexation occurred through the two oxygen atoms of the carboxyl group and the oxygens on the hydroxyl groups of C-3 and C-4 of the uronic acid molecule. As much as 97% of the total Mo concentrated by the cells was bound to the slime.

In summary, oxygen atoms of carboxyl and hydroxyl groups on the uronic acid subunits participate in the binding of metal ions by acidic capsular and slime polysaccharides. Oxygen atoms of hydroxyl groups on neighboring neutral sugars also contribute to the coordinate binding of metal ions that promotes the formation of stable complexes.

## 11.8 SELECTIVITY AND RELATIVE AFFINITY OF BACTERIAL EXOPOLYMERS FOR METAL IONS

Early investigations on the interactions of metal ions with bacterial exopolymers arose from studies on the effects of metal wastes on sewage treatment microorganisms. The floc-forming strain 115 of Z. ramigera was shown to remove significantly more dissolved Co, Cu, Fe, and Ni from solution than a strain that did not produce a gelatinous matrix around the cells (53). Young cultures of the floc-forming strain exhibited a lower affinity for Zn than older cultures that contained more exopolymer. Zinc binding by isolated exopolymer material was later confirmed.

Further studies with the floc-forming *Zoogloea* sp. suggested that uptake of metal ions was nonspecific, although no selectivity coefficients were provided (54). About 25% of the floc weight could be attributed to bound ions. The capacity of the floc to bind iron ions was enhanced by the presence of anions such as phosphate. Purified preparations of the exopolymer bound 3.9 mg (70 μmol) Fe, 3.5 mg (140 μmol) Mg, and 7.6 mg (190 μgmol) Ca per 50 mg dry weight polymer. Cobalt, Al, Mn, and Ni were bound to a lesser extent. The relative affinity of the cell-floc material for metal ions was determined to be Fe > Cu > Co > Ni (55). Because the exopolymers bind large quantities of water, Dugan (54) proposed that metal binding occurred through an exchange with polymer-bound water molecules and that the removal of water resulted in the observed flocculation that occurred in the presence of metals.

The combined polysaccharide species purified from the crude floc produced by cells of Z. ramigera 115 was reported to bind 0.25 μmol $Fe^{3+}$ $mg^{-1}$ polysaccharide (56). In view of the Fe binding capacity based on total polymer weight (1.4 μmol $mg^{-1}$) reported by Dugan (54) for this same bacterial strain, it appears that constituents other than polysaccharide are responsible for the bulk of the metal complexing ability of this capsular material.

More recent studies have demonstrated that flocs of Z. ramigera 115 absorbed a maximum of 3 mmol Cu $g^{-1}$ dry weight between pH 6 and 7 and a maximum of 1.8 mmol Cd $g^{-1}$ dry weight at pH 8 (57). In contrast to most polyanions, the Cu and Cd binding capacity of the floc material was not affected by changes in ionic strength. Repeated flocculation of a solution containing either copper or uranium with flocs of the exopolymer-producing bacterium resulted in a reduction in the total dissolved concentration of each metal to less than 0.1 and 0.0005 g $L^{-1}$, respectively. Essentially all of the

Cu and Cd complexed to the flocs was released by acidification at pH 4 and pH 3, respectively. These results suggest that the metals were complexed to carboxyl groups on the floc exopolymer via ionic bonding. No attempt was made to identify the site of metal interaction, however.

During toxicity studies of metals on marine bacteria, Corpe (7) found that extracellular polymers elaborated by cells of *P. atlantica* exhibited selectivity for Mg and Cu over Ca, Zn, Pb, Co, and Ni. No binding constants were reported for any of the polymer–metal complexes that formed. It was reported, however, that cells cultured in the presence of $5 \times 10^{-5} M$ copper contained no more of the metal than exopolymers from cells cultured under conditions in which no copper was added (besides that present in the nutrients added for growth). On the basis of these results, Corpe concluded that the concentration of metal by bacteria is not influenced by the amount of free metal in the surrounding medium. However, when the added copper concentration was increased to $4 \times 10^{-4} M$, the cell wall and extracellular polymer fractions contained significantly higher concentrations of the metal than wall and exopolymer preparations obtained from cells receiving no copper supplement. Others have demonstrated that the amount of metals bound by extracellular polymers increases with increasing free metal ion concentration (58). Thus there is some evidence to suggest that the amount of metal bound by these envelope components is controlled by the surrounding metal concentration.

In another study, metal uptake was compared between a capsule-producing and noncapsulated strain of *K. aerogenes* (59). Of the metals tested (Cu, Cd, Ni, Mn, Co), only Ni was accumulated to the same extent by both strains. All the other metals were concentrated to a greater extent by the capsule-producing strain. Six to 10 times more Cu and Cd were concentrated by the capsular polymers than was taken up by the cells themselves. In continuous cultures, a shift from cellular uptake to extracellular binding of Cu, Cd, and Mn was observed as the dilution rate was decreased. Metal removal from solution by the encapsulated strain was of the order Cu > Cd > Co > Mn > Ni. This affinity series is similar to that of *Z. ramigera* 115 flocs and to laboratory-scale activated sludge biomass.

The extraction of extracellular polymers from *K. aerogenes* reduced the capacity of the cells to adsorb Cd, Mn, Co, and Ni (58). Freundlich isotherms indicated that the relative affinities of metals for binding sites on the extracellular polymer followed the series Cd > Co > Ni > Mn. At $0.1$ mg L$^{-1}$ free Co, Cd, or Ni, the polymer was close to saturation at approximately 1 mg metal bound per gram of polymer.

The majority of studies conducted to date, therefore, demonstrate that bacterial exopolymers exhibit an affinity and selectivity for metal ions. Unfortunately, the type of quantitative information needed for comparison of the affinities of different microbial exopolymers for various metals is not often provided. Consequently, parameters such as binding strength, competition, and binding site density are largely unknown for complexes formed between bacterial expolymers and metals.

## 11.9    CONDITIONAL STABILITY CONSTANTS FOR CAPSULE–METAL COMPLEXES

The stabilities of metal complexes in solution are measured by equilibrium constants for their formation. Although stability constants have been determined for over 1500 organic compounds for a variety of metals, only a few have been reported to date for bacterial exopolysaccharide–metal complexes. Rudd et al. (60) obtained log $K_i$ values of 7.69, 5.16, 5.48, and 5.49 for Cu, Cd, Co, and Ni complexes, respectively, with *K. aerogenes* Type 64 capsule at the same polymer concentration at pH 6.3 over a metal concentration range of 0.2 $\mu$M to 0.1 m$M$. The number of binding sites per molecule (1.7 $\times$ 10$^6$ MW) ranged from 51 for Cd to 7 for Cu. The complexation capacity (mol g$^{-1}$ dry wt) was 4 $\times$ 10$^{-6}$ and 3 $\times$ 10$^{-5}$ for Cu and Cd, respectively. Only one type of binding site was available to each metal. They found an indirect correlation between the stability constant and the number of binding sites on the polymer molecule. When metals were added in combination to *K. aerogenes* capsule, only Co was reduced in overall binding. This suggests some specificity of binding sites. Other evidence suggested that only two distinct types of binding sites were available on the polymer, however. The capsule was reported to contain glucose, mannose, rhamnose, and glucuronic acid along with acetate and pyruvate residues.

The conditional stability constant for a complex formed between Cu ions and a capsular polysaccharide component from a freshwater sediment bacterium was found to be comparable to that of a complex formed between the metal and a humic acid preparation (39). Protein as well as polysaccharide fractions of the capsular material participated in Cu binding. A highly purified polysaccharide fraction exhibited a maximum binding capacity of 253 nmol Cu mg$^{-1}$ carbohydrate. Evaluation of infrared spectra of the complex formed between Cu and the polysaccharide capsular component suggested that the interaction occurred at a carboxyl residue. Experiments conducted at Cu concentrations, pH, and temperatures recorded in sediments from which the bacterium was isolated indicated that the exopolymers were capable of binding Cu under natural conditions. In view of these results, it is likely that bacterial exopolymers compete with other metal-complexing agents for metal ions in natural aquatic systems.

## 11.10    INFLUENCE OF METAL IONS ON THE PHYSICAL STATE OF EXOPOLYMERS

Interactions with certain metal ions cause many capsular and slime exopolymers to flocculate. Bridging between bacterial exopolymers and metals either as free cations or in the form of organic complexes or inorganic hydroxides promotes flocculation and rapid settlement of the bacteria and metal from solution (61). At very high metal concentrations (0.2 M) the extracellular polymer from one strain of *P. atlantica* formed water-insoluble precipitates with Fe, Cu, and Pb (7). Binding of metals causes some slime polymers to condense into gels. Brown and Lester (43) stated that in the presence of Cu(II) ions, all carboxylated polymers form gels. Cations such as Ca may also cause gel formation as in the case of alginic acid.

Coprecipitation was reported when metals were mixed with the purified polysaccharide fraction from the *Zoogloea* floc. Maximum polymer precipitation occurred in the presence of a 0.5 mM Fe(III) solution (56). Ferrous iron was about 50% as effective in this regard as Fe(III). Because binding of metal ions to the exopolymer promoted flocculation, it was proposed that the reaction could provide a means of separating the metal ions in a highly concentrated form from acid mine water (54).

Rudd et al. (60) compared the metal-binding capacity of colloidal and soluble forms of capsular polymer recovered from *K. aerogenes*. By a subtraction method, they determined that approximately five times more Ni complexed with the soluble form than with the colloidal form. More Cu, Cd, Mn, and Co were also complexed with the former. Accurate estimation of the metal-binding capacity of polymers that exist in a colloid or gel phase, however, requires a more rigorous approach than any used to date.

## 11.11 PROBLEMS DETERMINING EFFECTIVE CONCENTRATION OF POLYMER-BOUND METALS

Of all the problems associated with determining the interactions between microorganisms and metals, the inability to determine actual effective metal concentration at the site of complex formation is the most significant (62). Determination of thermodynamic properties such as stability constants and binding site density depend on accurate estimations of the concentrations or activities of interacting chemical species at the site of complex formation. In the case of capsular polymers, a variety of factors complicates efforts to obtain accurate estimates of the amount of metal that is bound. It has been demonstrated, for example, that the concentration of counterions in the vicinity of negatively charged reaction sites of polyanions is higher than their concentration in the bulk solution (63). When this electrostatic field component is ignored, metal-binding constants of polyanions such as microbial capsules and humic substances tend to vary with pH and ionic strength of the surrounding medium (39, 64).

A feature exhibited by many bacterial capsules that hinders estimation of metal concentrations at binding sites is their tendency to exist as highly hydrated gels. In this respect, capsular polymers are similar to ion exchange resins and when hydrated form two separate phases: a gel phase composed of a polymer subphase containing metal-binding sites that are surrounded by and in contact with a liquid subphase and a bulk liquid phase. Marinsky (65) showed that by assuming the existence of a hypothetical semipermeable membrane between the gel phase and the bulk liquid phase, a difference in water activity leads to an osmotic pressure that contributes to the free energy of ionization even when there is no acting electrostatic field. Just as there are differences in water activity, so there are differences in metal ion and other counterion activities between the two phases. The formation of colloids, gels, and insoluble precipitates with increased metal binding by capsular polymers suggests that volume changes must also be taken into account when estimating metal concentrations at the site of interaction.

Thus in addition to the molecular structure and density of the ligand's charged groups and the size, structure, and hydration state of the metal, which must be considered when evaluating the thermodynamic properties of most complexes formed between organic compounds and metals, it is necessary to take into account electrostatic field and osmotic pressure effects as well as volume changes when determining metal-binding properties of bacterial capsule and slime polymers. In view of these circumstances, activity values based on valid activity coefficients should be employed instead of concentration measurements when describing thermodynamic constants of complexes between metals and bacterial exopolymers.

## 11.12   DETERMINATION OF INTRINSIC STABILITY CONSTANTS FOR EXOPOLYMER–METAL COMPLEXES

Characterization and comparison of complexes formed between metals and various ligands that exist in aquatic systems are most effectively achieved through thermodynamic expressions such as stability constants and binding site density determinations. These expressions are commonly obtained from Scatchard, Langmuir, and Freundlich plots based on measurements of the quantity of free metal in solution, the ligand concentration, and the quantity of metal bound to the ligand under equilibrium conditions (41, 58). The constants derived from these various plots are typically "conditional" constants in that they reflect the characteristics of the metal–ligand interaction for those conditions under which the empirical data were obtained.

To be of value in assessing interactions between metal ions in the environment and surface components of microbial cells under the variety of conditions to which natural aquatic populations and even laboratory cultures are exposed, "intrinsic" binding constants should be obtained that are independent of environmental variables. Intrinsic binding constants may be obtained if all of the factors that influence free energy change at the site of ligand–metal interaction are taken into account.

From the information presented in the preceding sections, it is evident that the number of independent variables that affect metal–polymer interactions is very high. Nevertheless, it is possible to determine the contributions these factors make to the free energy of complex formation. The remainder of this chapter describes an experimental and mathematical approach that can be used to obtain intrinsic binding constants and binding site density for bacterial exopolymer–metal complexes.

### 11.12.1 Acid Dissociation Constant

The first step in determining conditional or intrinsic metal binding constants for anionic capsular polymers involves the estimation of the number of moles of acidic groups (potential metal-binding sites) on the polymer molecule ($A_t$). This is achieved by potentiometric titration of the capsular polymer with base. Acidic polymers should be in their fully protonated form at the beginning of the titration because the amount of base consumed is used to estimate the number of acidic groups on the polymer molecule. An independent method of estimating the concentration of acidic functional groups on the polymer should be carried out and compared with the titration data. For example, a uronic acid assay (66) could be used if this class of subunits was known to be the sole contributor of acidic groups on the polymer. If the source of acidic groups is not known, a tritium exchange approach could be applied (67). Although it is desirable to have the polymer completely hydrated at the beginning of the titration, many capsular polymers are sparingly soluble in water, particularly when all the acidic groups are protonated. As long as the base is accessible to all of the reaction sites on the polymer by the end of the titration, the total number of groups can be obtained.

Titration is performed at different ionic strengths ($I$) using a salt in which the anion does not form complexes with the metal cation being studied. Sodium nitrate and sodium perchlorate salts are often used to control ionic strength in solutions in which complexes between copper and organic molecules are to be characterized. At low $I$, equilibration times are sometimes very long, particularly near the end point of the reaction. Electrode sensitivity also tends to decrease at low $I$. Equilibration times may be prolonged even more if the polymer forms a viscous gel at the relatively high concentrations desired for titration. Nevertheless, it is important to perform the titration under these conditions if accurate $pK_a$ values are to be obtained.

The number of moles of total acidic groups neutralized at any point in the titration, $A^-$, is calculated from the expression:

$$A^- = \frac{10^{-pH} V_s}{\gamma_{H^+}} + m_{b,ac} \tag{1}$$

where $V_s$ is the volume of the bulk liquid phase, $\gamma_{H^+}$ is the activity coefficient of hydrogen ions in the bulk liquid phase, and $m_{b,ac}$ is the number of moles of base added at any point in the titration of the polymer. The end point of the reaction is defined as the point at which a plot of pH versus $m_{b,ac}$ shows a maximum slope. The degree of polymer ionization, $\alpha$, can be estimated at any point in the titration by the expression

$$\alpha = \frac{A^-}{A_t}$$

or                                                                                      (2)

$$\alpha = \frac{A^-}{m_{b,ep}}$$

where $A_t$ is number of moles of titratable groups on the polymer and is equal to the number of moles of base added to reach the end point in the titration, $m_{b,ep}$.

Initially, an apparent dissociation constant, $K_{HA}^{app}$, of the polymer is calculated on the basis of the measured activities of species in the bulk liquid phase according to the expression

$$K_{HA}^{app} = \frac{(H^+)(A^-)}{(HA)}$$

$$= \frac{(H^+)\alpha}{1 - \alpha}$$                                                     (3)

and

$$pK_{HA}^{app} = -\log K_{HA}^{app}$$

or

$$= pH - \log \frac{\alpha}{1 - \alpha}$$                                              (4)

The parentheses above and hereafter refer to activity, which is the product of the molar concentration and activity coefficient. Activity reflects "effective concentration" of all interacting species that are used to determine thermodynamic equilibrium constants. After the titration is performed at several different ionic strengths, a plot of $-\log K_{HA}^{app}$ versus $\alpha$ should yield a different slope for each $I$ (Fig. 11.1). $I$ should be set high enough in one of the titrations to yield a slope of zero and the resulting p$K$ value used later as a first approximation of the intrinsic dissociation constant, $K_{HA}^{int}$.

From Figure 11.1, it is evident that the difference between $K_{HA}^{int}$ and $K_{HA}^{app}$ varies with the degree of neutralization and with ionic strength. In thermodynamic terms, this deviation (conventionally denoted as $\Delta pK = pK_{HA}^{app} - pK_{HA}^{int}$) reflects the net change in free energy of ionization

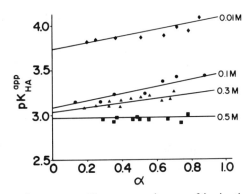

**Figure 11.1**  Plots of apparent $pK_{HA}$ versus degree of ionization of alginic acid in aqueous solutions of different concentrations of $NaNO_3$ as obtained from base titration experiments at 25°C.

contributed by the electrostatic field around the polymer molecule and that contributed by the difference in water activity across the hypothetical membrane which separates the gel phase from the bulk liquid phase (65).

The variation in $\Delta pK$ at different $\alpha$ and $I$ also reflects a change in gel phase volume or, more specifically, a change in the polymer subphase volume, where the ionization reactions occur. The polymer subphase volume may be accurately obtained using an iterative procedure that is applied to satisfy three simultaneous algebraic equations that calculate the number of moles of counterion bound electrostatically in the polymer subphase, ionic strength in the polymer subphase, and partitioning of the counterion activity between the polymer subphase and bulk liquid phase. Calculation of the intrinsic acid dissociation constant of capsular polymers depends on an accurate estimation of the polymer subphase volume at different $\alpha$.

One of the algebraic equations used to obtain the polymer subphase volume is based on the behavior of $Na^+$ formed during the titration of a salt-free solution of the capsular polymer with NaOH. Under these conditions, the activity of the $Na^+$ (counterion) in the bulk liquid phase (measured with a sodium electrode) can be used to calculate the sodium activity coefficient, $\gamma_{Na^+}$, from the expression

$$\gamma_{Na^+} = \frac{(Na^+)_{bp}}{C_{Na^+}}$$

where $(Na^+)_{bp}$ is the measured sodium ion activity in the bulk phase and $C_{Na^+}$ is the concentration of sodium ions present in the system (i.e., total number of moles of NaOH added/volume of the solution). In this case, the number of moles of NaOH added to the solution is approximately equal to $A^-$. In addition, $\phi_{P,Na}$, which is the practical osmotic coefficient of the free sodium ion in a salt-free solution containing the sodium form of the polymer, can be substituted for $\gamma_{Na^+}$ because the osmotic pressure is governed by the free, unbound $Na^+$ in a salt-free polyelectrolyte solution (68). $\phi_{P,Na}$ can therefore be determined from the expression

$$\phi_{P,Na} = \frac{[(Na^+)_{bp}]\,[V_t]}{A^-_{ionized}}$$

where $V_t$ is the total volume of the polymer suspension and the brackets here and in subsequent equations denote a grouping of mathematical terms.

The number of moles of sodium ion that are electrostatically bound to the polymer during titration with NaOH is obtained by subtracting the Na in the bulk phase from the total sodium in the system as described below

$$\overrightarrow{Na^+} = [1 - \phi_{P,Na}]\,A^- \tag{5}$$

where the arrow bar represents the gel polymer subphase. At each step of the titration, the change in $\phi_{P,Na}$ can be determined for each value of $\alpha$.

Just as Equation 5 provides a means to calculate the sodium activity in the polymer subphase from sodium ion measurements in the bulk liquid phase of an electrolyte-free system, it may also be used when $NaNO_3$ is added to the polymer suspension to adjust the ionic strength. According to the Boltzmann distribution theory, the electric potential reduces to a very low value in the gel liquid subphase and essentially to zero in the bulk liquid phase regardless of whether an electrolyte is present (68).

With $A^-$ and $(\overrightarrow{Na^+})$ calculated from Equations 1 and 5 and $V_p$ assigned some initial value that is less than the total solution volume, the first estimation of the polymer subphase ionic strength is obtained by the expression

$$\overrightarrow{I} = \frac{[\overrightarrow{Na^+} + A^-]}{2V_p} \tag{6}$$

where $V_p$ is the volume of the polymer subphase. If the estimation of $V_p$ is correct, the activity of sodium in the polymer subphase, $(Na^+)$, will equal the sodium activity in the bulk liquid phase multiplied by the deviation factor, $10^{\Delta pK}$, described earlier according to the expression

$$(\overrightarrow{Na^+}) = (Na^+)\,10^{\Delta pK} \tag{7}$$

where

$$(\overrightarrow{Na^+}) = \frac{\overrightarrow{Na^+}\,[\overrightarrow{\gamma}_{Na^+}]\overrightarrow{i}}{V_p} \tag{8}$$

and

$$(Na^+) = C_{Na^+}\, [\gamma_{Na^+}]_I$$

and

$$\Delta pK = pK_{HA}{}^{app} - pK_{HA}{}^{int}$$

The activity coefficient of sodium in the polymer subphase, $\gamma_{Na^+}$, is obtained from tabulated data (69) or from the expression

$$[\gamma_{Na^+}]_{\vec{I}} = \frac{[\gamma_{\pm NaCl}]^2_{\vec{I}}}{[\gamma_{\pm KCl}]_{\vec{I}}} \tag{9}$$

where $\gamma_{\pm NaCl}$ and $\gamma_{\pm KCl}$ are the mean activity coefficients of NaCl and KCl (70) at the ionic strength, $\vec{I}$, obtained from Equation 6. If Equation 7 cannot be satisfied, a new estimate of $V_p$ is obtained from the expression

$$V_p = \frac{[\vec{Na}^+]\,[\vec{\gamma}_{Na^+}]_{\vec{I}}}{[C_{Na^+}\,\gamma_{Na^+}]_I\, 10^{\Delta pK}} \tag{10}$$

which is obtained by substitution and rearrangement of Equation 8. The new estimate of $V_p$ is then substituted in Equation 6. Equations 6, 9, and 10 are iterated to generate second, third, . . . , $n$th improved estimations of $V_p$ until two successive trials provide values that are within acceptable limits.

Once an accurate polymer subphase volume is obtained at each $\alpha$ and $I$, the activity of sodium ion in the gel phase is calculated from Equation 8. Then from the Donnan equilibrium relationship (71, 72),

$$\vec{pH} = pH + \vec{pNa} - pNa$$

the hydrogen activity of the bulk liquid phase in Equation 4 is replaced by the actual hydrogen activity of the polymer subphase. The $pK_{HA}$ thus obtained should represent the $pK_{HA}{}^{int}$ at every point in the titration. In other words,

$$pK_{HA}{}^{int} = pK_{HA}{}^{app} + \vec{pNa} - pNa$$

The scheme presented above allows the ratio of sodium ion activity in the gel polymer subphase to sodium ion activity in the gel liquid subphase or bulk liquid phase, $(\vec{Na}^+)/(Na^+)$, to increase with decreasing ionic strength, a feature that cannot be taken into account by Manning's approach (73). In studies with ion exchange resins and alginate gels, Marinsky (71) was unable to predict the hydrogen ion activity in the gel polymer subphase from pH measurements in the bulk liquid phase without such a partition factor. Thus the scheme presented above takes into account any free energy change that occurs as a result of the transfer of counterions from the bulk liquid phase to the reaction sites on the capsular polymer molecules. Once the intrinsic acid dissociation constant for the capsular polymer has been determined, intrinsic stability constants for interactions between metal cations and the polymer molecule can be obtained by the approach described below. This same procedure can be used to describe interactions between metals and other polymers that exist as gels in their normal state of hydration.

### 11.12.2   Intrinsic Stability Constants

The interaction between a bivalent metal and a capsular polymer may involve the formation of one or more types of complexes, each with a characteristic intrinsic stability constant. The approach described below determines how many different complexes are formed and the intrinsic stability constant for each. Initially, it is assumed that a single monodentate complex is formed. If the conditions for this type of complex are met, then a single constant is derived. If the conditions are not met, then the data are subjected to an evaluation using expressions that assume the formation of a bidentate complex. It is also possible to evaluate a metal–polymer interaction that involves both types of complexes. The approach identifies the relative contribution of each type of complex and their respective stability constants. The method also determines the number of metal binding sites on the polymer molecule at different $\alpha$ and $I$.

An exopolymer suspension is prepared at the desired ionic strength and an estimation of the total titratable groups is estimated by uronic acid or tritium exchange assay as described above. Aliquots of a metal salt solution are added stepwise to the polymer suspension and the pH and metal ion activity monitored simultaneously until the equivalents of total metal ion added reaches a value that is no more than and preferably less than 5% of the total titratable groups present. The polymer suspension is then titrated with NaOH adjusted to the ionic strength of the polymer solution and the pH and metal ion activity are monitored with pH and ion specific electrodes until the end point is reached. The degree of polymer ionization, $\alpha$, is calculated from the expression

$$\alpha = \frac{A_t - HA - 2\vec{M}_{sb}}{A_t} \tag{11}$$

where $\vec{M}_{sb}$ is the number of moles of bivalent metal ion bound to the polymer, $HA$ is the number of moles of total undissociated functional groups on the polymer, and $A_t$ is the number of moles of total titratable functional groups on the polymer as described previously.

$\vec{M}_{sb}$ is determined as the total number of bivalent metal ions, $M_t^{2+}$, added minus the metal ions in the bulk liquid phase according to the expression

$$\vec{M}_{sb} = M_t^{2+} - \frac{(M^{2+})V_s}{[\gamma_{M^{2+}}]_I} \tag{12}$$

where $\gamma_{M^{2+}}$ is the activity coefficient of the free bivalent metal ion in the bulk liquid phase. The latter is determined from the expression

$$[\gamma_{M^{2+}}]_I = \frac{[\gamma_{\pm MCl_2}]_I^3}{[\gamma_{\pm KCl}]_{I^2}} \tag{13}$$

where the activity coefficients of the $MCl_2$ and KCl at a specific ionic strength can be obtained from published tables in the literature (70).

*HA* in Equation 11 is calculated as the total titratable functional groups on the polymer minus those groups neutralized by the added base and those groups ionized as a result of proton displacement by metal ions according to the expression

$$HA = A_t - \left[ m_{b,ac} + \frac{10^{-pH} V_s}{\gamma_{H^+}} \right] \tag{14}$$

where $m_{b,ac}$ refers to moles of base added during the titration.

**11.12.2.1 Monodentate Complexes.** When a monodentate complex is formed between a divalent metal and a polyanion the equilibrium reaction at the binding site may be defined as

$$M^{2+} + A^- = MA^+; \qquad \beta_{MA^+}{}^{int}$$

where $\beta_{MA^+}{}^{int}$ is the intrinsic stability constant of the monodentate complex. Coupling this reaction with the acid dissociation reaction

$$H^+ + A^- = HA; \qquad \beta_{HA}{}^{int} = [K_{HA}{}^{int}]^{-1}$$

yields

$$M^{2+} + 2HA = MA^+ + A^- + 2H^+; \qquad D_1$$

where

$$D_1 = \frac{(\vec{MA^+})(\vec{H^+})^2(\vec{A^+})}{(\vec{m^{2+}})(\vec{HA})^2} \tag{15}$$

$\overrightarrow{MA}^+$ refers to the bivalent metal ions that lose their hydration water and form complexes with specific functional groups on the polymer, and $M^{2+}$ refers to the electrostatically bound bivalent metal ions in the polymer subphase. $D_1$ can also be expressed as

$$D_1 = \frac{\beta_{MA^+}{}^{int}}{[\beta_{HA}{}^{int}]^2} \tag{16}$$

$\beta_{HA}{}^{int}$ is included in Equation 16 to account for effects due to changes in pH and $I$. In Equation 15, $(\overrightarrow{H}^+)^2/(\overrightarrow{M}^{2+})$ can be replaced by $(H^+)^2/(M^{2+})$ on the basis of the Donnan equilibrium expression described earlier. Because the polymer subphase volume cancels from the three terms $(\overrightarrow{MA}^+)$, $(\overrightarrow{A}^-)$, and $(\overrightarrow{HA})^2$, $D_1$ can be described in a form that contains the measurable terms

$$D_1 = \frac{(H^+)^2}{(M^{2+})} \times \frac{[\overrightarrow{MA}^+][A^-]}{[HA]^2} \tag{17}$$

where $(H^+)$ and $(M^{2+})$ are measured electrochemically. $\overrightarrow{MA}^+$ is the total number of moles of monodentate complex formed, which is assumed to equal the moles of metal that are bound to reaction sites on the polymer, $M_{sb}$, because most of the bivalent ions entering the polymer subphase are likely to be bound to ionized acid functional groups on the polymer. The total number of dissociated groups that are unoccupied, $A^-$, is defined by

$$A^- = \left[ m_{b,ac} + \frac{10^{-pH} V_s}{\gamma_{H^+}} \right] - MA^+$$

If only monodentate complexes are formed, $D_1$ will be constant at every value of $A^-/V_p$ in the titration. $A^-/V_p$ is an expression of $\alpha$ that has been adjusted for any volume changes that may have occurred in the polymer subphase.

**11.12.2.2 Bidentate Complexes.** A variation of $D_1$ with the amount of base, metal ion, or polymer added to the system indicates that all or part of the polymer-bound bivalent metal ions form a bidentate complex which is described by the equilibrium reaction

$$M^{2+} + 2A^- = MA_2; \qquad \beta_{MA_2}{}^{int}$$

and the overall reaction is described as

$$M^{2+} + 2HA = MA_2 + 2H^+; \qquad D_2$$

where

$$D_2 = \frac{\beta_{MA_2}{}^{int}}{[\beta_{HA}{}^{int}]^2} \tag{18}$$

or after substitution and rearrangement, $D_2$ can be described by

$$D_2 = \frac{(H^+)^2}{(M^{2+})} V_p \frac{\overrightarrow{MA_2}}{[HA]^2} \tag{19}$$

which, with the exception of $V_p$, consist of terms that can be measured. In Equation 19, $\overrightarrow{MA}_2$ is assumed to be equal to $\overrightarrow{M}_{sb}$.

When metal is introduced to the system, $V_p$ not only varies with pH and ionic strength, as demonstrated previously in the evaluation of the acid dissociation constant, but also with the amount of metal ion bound to the polymer. In the case of monodentate complex, the $V_p$ term cancels out of Equation 17 for the determination of $D_1$. This is not the case, however, in Equation 19 for the determination of $D_2$. Before describing the iterative procedure to determine $V_p$, it is necessary to consider the situation in which both monodentate and bidentate complexes contribute to a polymer–metal interaction, because it is unlikely that bidentate complexes are responsible for all of the interaction that occurs in aquatic environments or under the titration conditions described above, that is, when the equivalents of total metal ion present are equal to or less than 5% of the total titratable groups on the polymer (72).

### 11.12.2.3   *Monodentate and Bidentate Complexes.*

Where both monodentate and bidentate complexes contribute to the interaction between a capsular polymer and a bivalent metal ion, $\overrightarrow{MA}^+$ in Equation 17 is replaced by $\overrightarrow{M}_{sb}$, yielding

$$D_1{}' = \frac{(H^+)^2}{(M^{2+})} \frac{[\overrightarrow{M}_{sb}][A^-]}{[HA]^2} \tag{20}$$

where $\overrightarrow{M}_{sb}$ is defined as $[\overrightarrow{MA}^+ + \overrightarrow{MA}_2]$. Substituting Equations 17 and 19 into Equation 20 yields

$$D_1{}' = D_1 + \left[ D_2 \frac{A^-}{V_p} \right] \tag{21}$$

Similarly, by replacing $\overrightarrow{MA}_2$ with $\overrightarrow{M}_{sb}$, $D_2$ may be redefined as $D_2{}'$, where

$$D_2' = \frac{(H^+)^2}{(M^{2+})} \frac{[\vec{M}_{sb}] \, V_p}{[HA]^2} \tag{22}$$

or

$$D_2' = D_2 + \left[ D_1 \frac{V_p}{A^-} \right] \tag{23}$$

where $\vec{M}_{sb}$ and $HA$ in Equation 22 are determined from Equations 12 and 14, respectively.

Ideally, $D_1$ and $D_2$ should be obtained from the slope and intercept of plots of $D_1'$ versus $A^-/V_p$ and $D_2'$ versus $V_p/A^-$. Then substituting the values of $D_1$ and $D_2$ determined above and the experimentally obtained $\beta_{HA}^{int}$ (which is the reciprocal of the intrinsic acid dissociation constant determined previously) into Equations 16 and 18, the intrinsic stability constants for the monodentate complex, $\beta_{MA^+}^{int}$, and bidentate complex, $\beta_{MA_2}^{int}$, are obtained.

#### 11.12.2.4 Determination of the Relative Contribution of Monodentate and Bidentate Complexes.

By limiting the equivalents of metal added to the system to less than 5% of the total moles of titratable functional groups present, the likelihood of monodentate complex formation is maximized. This is necessary in order to minimize the possibilty of error when Equation 20 is used to determine $D_1$ (which assumes that the bulk of the interaction is due to monodentate complex formation) for cases in which bidentate complexes contribute significantly to the polymers interaction with a metal.

Once $D_1$ and $D_2$ have been calculated, the extent to which the bidentate complex $MA_2$ contributes to the polymer–metal interaction can be determined in a subsequent titration that places no limits on the amount of metal present. This is achieved by simultaneously solving Equations 17 and 19, where

$$\vec{M}_{sb} = \vec{MA}^+ + \vec{MA}_2 \tag{24}$$

and $\vec{M}_{sb}$ is obtained by subtracting the moles of free metal in the bulk liquid phase (measured electrochemically) from the total moles of metal added to the system.

It is also possible to determine the relationship between the actual number of binding sites that are occupied by metal ions and the potential number of metal binding sites on the polymer. Assuming that the moles of potential metal binding sites are equivalent to the moles of total titratable functional groups $A_t$, substitution of Equation 14 in Equation 20 or 22 reveals that the portion of available sites that are occupied by metal ions (defined as $\vec{M}_{sb}/A_t$) is influenced by the stability constant and $A_t$ in addition to pH and metal concentration. The average number of binding sites occupied per polymer molecule, $\overrightarrow{Mp}_{sb}$, can be defined as

$$\overrightarrow{Mp}_{sb} = \frac{\overrightarrow{M}_{sb}}{P}$$

where $P$ is the moles of polymer added to the titration solution. The binding site density can thus be determined for each type of complex that is formed at any pH or $I$.

### 11.12.2.5 Determination of Polymer Subphase Volume in the Presence of Metal Ions.
In the case of capsular polymers, accurate estimation of the amount of metal that is contained in the polymer subphase volume is complicated by the fact that the polymer volume changes with environmental conditions. Nevertheless, this difficulty can be overcome by modifying the iterative procedure that was applied to the solution of the three simultaneous equations described earlier. The equations used to estimate the effective polymer subphase volume when the polymer is titrated in the presence of metal ions are derived from those employed previously for the determination of the intrinsic acid dissociation constant. The equations are modified in order to account for the fact that both monovalent and divalent ions are present and because the latter not only interact electrostatically with the polymer but also form complexes with specific functional groups on the polymer molecule. Equation 6 is thus modified to

$$\overrightarrow{I} = \frac{4\overrightarrow{M}^{2+} + \overrightarrow{Na}^+ + A^- + \overrightarrow{MA}^+}{2V_p} \tag{25}$$

Assuming that the majority of metal–polymer complexes formed are monodentate under the initial conditions of the titration as discussed above, the last two terms of the numerator, $[A^- + \overrightarrow{MA}^+]$, may be replaced by $[A_t - HA]$ in Equation 14.

The moles of monovalent (sodium) ion, $\overrightarrow{Na}^+$, that interact electrostatically with the polymer, which was previously defined by Equation 5, is redefined as

$$\overrightarrow{Na}^+ = [A_t - HA - 2\overrightarrow{M}_{sb}] [1 - \phi_{P,Na}]$$

for bivalent metal ions that have a tendency to form strong complexes with the polymer. By substitution, then,

$$\overrightarrow{Na}^+ = [m_{b,ac} + \frac{10^{-pH}}{\gamma_{H^+}} - 2\overrightarrow{M}_{sb}] [1 - \phi_{P,Na}] \tag{26}$$

For a bivalent metal that forms weak complexes with the polymer, the term $2\vec{M}_{sb}$ must be modified to $2\vec{M}_{sb}[1 + \phi_{P,M}]$ to include the electrostatically bound component, which is negligible for strongly complexing metals. $\phi_{P,M}$ is the practical osmotic coefficient of the bivalent metal ion form of the polymer. Similar to $\phi_{P,Na}$, $\phi_{P,M}$ is determined by titration of electrolyte-free polymer with a metal hydroxide while measuring the activity of free metal ion. Dividing this activity by the moles of metal hydroxide added provides an estimate of $\phi_{P,M}$.

Because the terms $\vec{M}^{2+}$ and $V_p$ are not known, their values must be estimated in Equation 25, then using two nested iterative loops, more precise values are obtained as follows: If the estimated $V_p$ is correct, Equation 7 will be satisfied. If Equation 7 is not satisfied, Equation 10 is used to obtain an improved estimate of $V_p$ by the iterative procedure described previously except that Equation 25 is used in place of Equation 6. Each time an improved estimate of $V_p$ is generated, the algorithm enters an outer loop to determine whether the value of $\vec{M}^{2+}$ generated by the equation

$$\vec{M}^{2+} = \frac{[C_{M^{2+}} \gamma_{M^{2+}} 10^{2\Delta pK}]V_p}{[\vec{\gamma}_{M^{2+}}]\vec{i}} \tag{27}$$

equals the estimated value used in Equation 25, where

$$\gamma_{M^{2+}} = \frac{[\gamma_{\pm MCl_2}]^3 \vec{i}}{[\gamma_{\pm KCl}]^2 \vec{i}} \tag{28}$$

The new values of $V_p$ and $\vec{M}^{2+}$ generated in Equations 10 and 28, respectively, are substituted in Equation 25 and the iterative process continued until the values of $V_p$ and $\vec{M}^{2+}$ satisfy Equations 10 and 28. A computer program has been developed that accepts the measured titration data and, using the equations described above, provides the intrinsic binding constants for each type of metal–capsular polymer complex that is formed.

The importance of taking into account changes in ionic strength, polymer subphase volume, and competition of $H^+$ and $M^{2+}$ for binding sites when describing the interactions between metal ions and bacterial exopolymers may be illustrated by the interaction between alginic acid and cupric ions in Figures 11.2–11.4 below. A plot of $D_1'$ versus $A^-/V_p$ (Fig. 11.2) provides a series of data points that scatter around a $D_1$ value of $1 \times 10^{-3}$. The slope of the line does not permit an evaluation of $D_2$. However, a plot of $D_2'$ versus $V_p/A^-$ (Fig. 11.3) estimates $D_2$ to be $8 \times 10^{-5}$. The slope of the line in Figure 11.3 provides an additional estimate of $D_1$ and verifies the previous estimate of $1 \times 10^{-3}$ obtained from Figure 11.2. From these extrapolated values of $D_1$ and $D_2$ and a calculated $\beta_{HA}$ value of $1.26 \times 10^{-3}$, instinsic binding constants of 631 and 50.1 were obtained for $\beta_{MA^+}$ and $\beta_{MA_2}$, respectively.

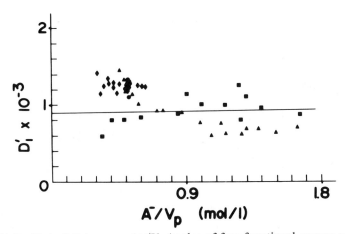

**Figure 11.2**  Plot of $D_1'$ versus $A^-/V_p$ (moles of free functional groups per liter of polymer subphase volume). Reaction mixture contains 0.0083 g alginic acid in 10 mL 0.1 $M$ NaNO$_3$(aq), ●; 0.0083 g alginic acid in 10 mL 0.01 $M$ NaNO$_3$(aq), ▲; 0.0400 g alginic acid in 10 mL 0.1 $M$ NaNO$_3$(aq), ◆; and 0.0400 g alginic acid in 10 mL 0.01 $M$ NaNO$_3$(aq), ■.

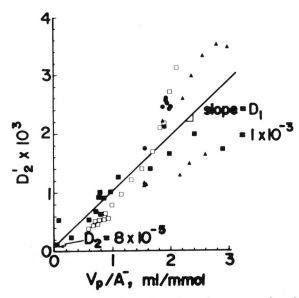

**Figure 11.3**  Plot of $D_2'$ versus $V_p/A^-$. Reaction mixture contains: 0.0883 g alginic acid in 10 mL 0.1 $M$ NaNO$_3$, ●; 0.0083 g alginic acid in 10 mL 0.01 $M$ NaNO$_3$, ▲; 0.040 g alginic acid in 10 mL 0.1 $M$ NaNO$_3$, □; and 0.040 g alginic acid in 10 mL 0.01 $M$ NaNO$_3$, ■.

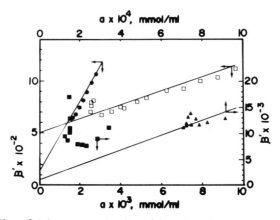

**Figure 11.4** Plot of $\beta_1'$ versus $a$ (moles of free functional groups/liter of solution volume). Conformational changes in and electric field effects around the polymer molecules are not taken into account by this expression. Reaction mixture contains 8.3 mg alginic acid in 10 mL 0.1 $M$ NaNO$_3$(aq), ●; 8.3 mg alginic acid in 10 mL 0.01 $M$ NaNO$_3$(aq), ▲; 40 mg alginic acid in 10 mL 0.1 $M$ NaNO$_3$(aq), □; 40 mg alginic acid in 10 mL 0.01 $M$ NaNO$_3$(aq), ■. Arrows indicate appropriate axis.

If pH effects and conformational changes are not taken into account, a plot of $\beta_1'$ versus $a$, where $a$ is the monomeric concentration of ionized ligand and $\beta_1'$, which is based on bulk liquid phase volume $V_s$, is defined as

$$\beta_1' = \frac{(M_{sb})}{(A^-)(M^{2+})} = \beta_1 + \beta_2 a$$

where

$$a = \frac{A^-}{V_s}$$

$$\beta_1 = \frac{(MA^+_{sb})}{(A^-)(M^{2+})} = \frac{[MA_{sb}]}{[A^-](M^{2+})}$$

$$\beta_2 = \frac{(MA_{2,sb})}{(A^-)^2 (M^{2+})} = \frac{[MA_{2,sb}] \, V_t}{[A^-]^2 (M^{2+})}$$

The values of $\beta_1'$ scatter over two orders of magnitude (Fig. 11.4) and, although a rough linear relationship may exist for values obtained from a particular set of conditions, no general correlation can be obtained if different experimental conditions are imposed. Comparison of Figures 11.2–11.4 demonstrates how data may be misinterpreted if critical features of the polymer–metal interaction are overlooked.

In summary, accurate assessment of the interactions between metal ions and bacterial capsules or other cell wall components requires knowledge of the effective concentration of the metal and other counterions at the site of complex formation. In the case of capsules, it is necessary to consider the possibility that more than one phase exists and that variation in pH, ionic strength, and metal concentration induce volume changes in the polymer subphase where the interactions take place. By taking into account these features of bacterial capsules and slimes, it is possible to obtain accurate estimates of the thermodynamic constants. The constants may then be used to predict how these microbial products compete with other metal-complexing agents in the bacterial cell and in the surrounding environment under the variety of conditions in which metal binding takes place. This approach should be useful in assessing the relative importance of microbial exopolymers in controlling the movement and fate of metals in natural systems.

## ACKNOWLEDGMENT

Support for the work presented in this chapter was provided by grants ECE-8521693, CES-8521693, and ECE-8701462 from the National Science Foundation.

## REFERENCES

1. G. M. Gadd and A. J. Griffiths. Microorganisms and heavy metal toxicity, Microb. Ecol., *4*, 303 (1978).

2. I. W. Sutherland. Biosynthesis of microbial exopolysaccharides. Adv. Microb. Physiol., *23*, 79 (1972).

3. J. W. Shands. Localization of somatic antigen in gram-negative bacteria using ferritin antibody conjugates. Ann. NY Acad. Sci., *133*, 292 (1966).

4. H. T. Flammann, J. R. Golecki, and J. Weckesser. The capsule and slime polysaccharides of the wild type and a phage resistant mutant of *Rhodopseudomonas capsulata* St. Louis. Arch. Microbiol., *139*, 38 (1984).

5. B. E. Christensen, J. Kjosbakken, and O. Smidsrod. Partial chemical and physical characterization of two extracellular polysaccharides produced by marine, periphytic *Pseudomonas* sp. strain NCMB 2021. Appl. Environ. Microbiol., *50*, 837 (1985).

6. W. Corpe. Factors influencing growth and polysaccharide formation by strains of *Chromobacterium violaceum*. J. Bacteriol., *88*, 1433 (1964).

7. W. A. Corpe. Metal-binding properties of surface materials from marine bacteria. Dev. Ind. Microbiol., *16*, 249 (1975).

8. J. L. Povoni, M. W. Tenney, and W. F. Echelberger. Bacterial exocellular polymers and biological flocculation. J. Water Pollut. Contr. Fed., *44*, 414 (1972).

9. I. Sutherland. "Bacterial exopolysaccharides—their nature and production," in I. Sutherland, Ed., *Surface carbohydrates of the procaryotic cell*, Academic, London, 1977, p. 27.

10. W. J. Cretney, R. W. MacDonald, C. S. Wong, D. R. Green, B. Whitehouse, and G. G. Geesey. "Biodegradation of a Chemically Dispersed Oil," in *Proceedings of the 1981 Oil Spill Conference*, Atlanta, GA, 1981, p. 37.

11. J. F. Wilkinson, J. P. Duguid, and P. N. Edmunds. The distribution of polysaccharide production in *Aerobacter* and *Escherichia* strains and its relation to antigenic character, J. Gen. Microbiol., *11*, 59 (1954).

12. A. G. Williams and J. W. T. Wimpenny. Exopolysaccharide production by *Pseudomonas* NCIB11264 grown in batch culture, J. Gen. Microbiol., *102*, 13 (1977).

13. G. H. Cohen and D. B. Johnstone. Extracellular polysaccharides of *Azotobacter vinlandii*, J. Bacteriol., *33*, 329 (1964).

14. A. Jeanes. *Encyclopedia of Polymer Science and Technology*, Vol. 4, Wiley-Interscience, New York, 1966, pp. 806–824.

15. J. F. Wilkinson and G. H. Stark. The synthesis of polysaccharide by washed suspensions of *Klebsiella aerogenes*, Proc. Roy. Physical Soc., Edinburgh, *25*, 35 (1956).

16. P. J. Bremer and M. W. Loutit. The effect of Cr(III) on the form and degradability of a polysaccharide produced by a bacterium isolated from a marine sediment, Mar. Environ. Res., *20*, 249 (1986).

17. N. F. Ferala, A. K. Champlin, and F. A. Fekete. Morphological differences in the capsular polysaccharide of nitrogen-fixing *Azotobacter chroococcum* B-8 as a function of iron and molybdenum starvation, FEMS Microbiol. Lett., *33*, 137 (1986).

18. I. Couperwhite and M. F. McCallum. The influence of EDTA on the composition of alginate synthesized by *Azotobacter vinlandii*, Arch. Microbiol., *97*, 73 (1974).

19. G. Annison and I. Couperwhite. Consequences of the association of calcium with alginate during batch culture of *Azotobacter vinlandii*, Appl. Microbiol. Biotechnol., *19*, 321 (1984).

20. G. Bitton and V. Friehofer. Influence of extracellular polysaccharide on the toxicity of copper and cadmium toward *Klebsiella aerogenes*, Microb. Ecol., *4*, 119 (1978).

21. J. Aislabie and M. W. Loutit. Accumulation of Cr(III) by bacteria isolated from polluted sediments, Mar. Environ. Res., *20*, 221 (1986).

22. K. M. Hsieh, L. W. Lion, and M. L. Schuler. Bioreactor for the study of defined interactions of toxic metals and biofilms, Appl. Environ. Microbiol., *50*, 1155 (1985).

23. J. R. Montgomery and M. T. Price. Release of trace metals by sewage sludge and the subsequent uptake by members of a turtle grass mangrove ecosystem, Environ. Sci. Technol., *13*, 546 (1979).

24. F. M. Patrick and M. W. Loutit. The uptake of heavy metals by epiphytic bacteria on *Alisma plantago-aquatica*, Water Res., *11*, 699 (1977).

25. T. E. Lee and M. W. Loutit. Effect of extracellular polysaccharides of rhizo-

sphere bacteria on the concentration of molybdenum in plants, Soil Biol. Biochem., *9*, 411 (1977).

26. R. W. Harvey and S. N. Luoma. The role of bacterial exopolymers and suspended bacteria in the nutrition of the deposit feeding chain, *Macoma balthica*, J. Mar. Res., *42*, 957 (1984).

27. R. W. Harvey and S. N. Luoma. Effects of adherent bacteria and bacterial extracellular polymers upon assimilation by *Macoma balthica* of sediment bound Cd, Zn, and Ag, Mar. Ecol. Prog. Ser., *22*, 281 (1985).

28. F. M. Patrick and M. W. Loutit. Passage of metals to freshwater fish from their food, Water Res., *12*, 395 (1978).

29. P. J. Bremer and M. W. Loutit. Bacterial polysaccharide as a vehicle for entry of Cr(III) to a food chain, Mar. Res., *20*, 235 (1986).

30. J. H. Luft. Ruthenium red and ruthenium violet. I. Chemistry, purification, methods of use for electron microscopy, and mechanisms of action, Anat. Rec., *171*, 347 (1971).

31. I. W. Sutherland. "Polysaccharides in the adhesion of marine and freshwater bacteria," in R. C. W. Berkeley, J. M. Lynch, J. Melling, and B. Vincent, Eds., *Microbial Adhesion to Surfaces*, Ellis Horwood, Chichester, United Kingdom, 1980, p. 329.

32. R. Moorhouse, W. T. Winter, S. Arnott, and M. E. Bayer. Conformation and molecular organization in fibers of the capsular polysaccharide from *Escherichia coli* M41 mutant, J. Mol. Biol., *109*, 373 (1977).

33. P. A. Sandford, J. E. Pittsley, C. A. Knutson, P. R. Watson, M. C. Cadmus, and A. Jeanes. "Variations in *Xanthomonas campestris* NRRL B 1459: characterization of xanthan products of differing pyruvic acid content," in P. A. Sandford and A. Laskin, Eds., *Extracellular Microbial Polysaccharides*, Am. Chem. Soc. Symp. Ser. No. 45, American Chemical Society, Washington, DC, 1977, p. 192.

34. C. D. Boyle and A. E. Reade. Characterization of two extracellular polysaccharides from marine bacteria, Appl. Environ. Microbiol., *46*, 392 (1983).

35. C. W. Dewitt and J. A. Rowe. Sialic acids (*N*,7-*O*-diacetylneuraminic acid and *N*-acetylneuraminic acid) in *Escherichia coli*. J. Bacteriol., *82*, 838 (1961).

36. T.-Y. Liu, E. C. Gotschlich, F. T. Dunne, and E. K. Jonnsen. Studies on the meningococcal polysaccharides. J. Biol. Chem., *246*, 4703 (1971).

37. A. E. Martell. "Principles of complex formation," in S. J. Faust and J. V. Hunter, Eds., *Organic Compounds in Aquatic Environments*, Dekker, New York, 1971, p. 239.

38. J. A. Rendleman. Metal–polysaccharide complexes—Part II, Fd. Chem. *3*, 127 (1978).

39. M. W. Mittleman and G. G. Geesey. Copper-binding characteristics of exopolymers from a freshwater sediment bacterium, Appl. Environ. Microbiol., *49*, 846 (1985).

40. R. M. Platt, G. G. Geesey, J. D. Davis, and D. C. White. Isolation and partial chemical analysis of firmly bound exopolysaccharide from adherent cells of a freshwater sediment bacterium, Can. J. Microbiol., *31*, 675 (1985).

41. H. Zunino and J. P. Martin. Metal-binding organic macromolecules in soil. 2.

characterization of the maximum binding ability of the macromolecules, Soil Sci., *123*, 188 (1977).

42. I. Steiner, D. A. McLaren, and C. F. Forster. The nature of activated sludge flocs, Water Res., *10*, 25 (1976).

43. M. J. Brown and J. N. Lester. Metal removal in activated sludge: the role of bacterial extracellular polymers, Water Res., *13*, 817 (1979).

44. M. B. Mathews. Trivalent cation binding of acid mucopolysaccharides, Biochim. Biophys. Acta, *37*, 288 (1960).

45. G. Manzini, A. Cesaro, F. Delben, S. Paoletti, and E. Reisenhofer. Copper(II) binding by natural ionic polysaccharides Part 1. Potentiometric and spectroscopic data, Bioelectrochem. Bioenerg., *12*, 443 (1984).

46. O. Smidsrod and A. Haug. Dependence upon the gel-sol state of ion exchange properties of alginates, Acta Chem. Scand., *26*, 2063 (1972).

47. R. Kohn. Ion binding on polyuronides-alginate and pectin. Pure Appl. Chem., *42*, 371 (1975).

48. D. Cozzi, P. G. Desideri, and L. Lepri. The mechanisms of ion exchange with alginic acid, J. Chromatogr., *40*, 130 (1969).

49. A. Haug and O. Smidsrod. Selectivity of some anionic polymers for divalent metal ions, Acta Chem., Scand., *24*, 843 (1970).

50. D. A. Rees. Polysaccharide gels, Chem. Ind., *19*, 630 (1972).

51. E. L. Tan and M. W. Loutit. Concentration of molybdenum by extracellular material produced by rhizosphere bacteria, Soil Biol. Biochem., *8*, 461 (1976).

52. S. Stojkovski, R. A. Magee, and J. Leisegang. Molybdenum binding by *Pseudomonas aeruginosa*, Aust. J. Chem., *39*, 1205 (1986).

53. B. A. Friedman and P. R. Dugan. Concentration and accumulation of metallic ions by the bacterium *Zoogloea*. Dev. Ind. Microbiol., *9*, 381 (1968).

54. P. R. Dugan. "Removal of mine water ions by microbial polymers," in Proc. 3rd Symp. on Coal Mine Drainage Research, Carnegie Mellon Institute, Pittsburgh, 1970, p. 279.

55. P. R. Dugan and H. M. Pickrum. "Removal of mineral ions from water by microbially produced polymers," in Proc. 27th Industrial Waste Conference, Purdue University, Lafayette, IN, 1972, p. 1019.

56. F. Ikeda, H. Shuto, T. Saito, T. Fukui, and K. Tomita. An extracellular polysaccharide produced by *Zoogloea ramigera* 115, Eur. J. Biochem., *123*, 437 (1982).

57. A. B. Norberg and H. Persson. Accumulation of heavy-metal ions by *Zoogloea ramigera*. Biotechnol. Bioeng., *26*, 239 (1984).

58. M. J. Brown and J. N. Lester. Role of bacterial extracellular polymers in metal uptake in pure bacterial cultures and activated sludge-I Effects of metal concentration, Water Res., *16*, 1539 (1982).

59. T. Rudd, R. M. Sterritt, and J. N. Lester. Mass balance of heavy metal uptake by encapsulated cultures of *Klebsiella aerogenes*, Microb. Ecol., *9*, 261 (1983).

60. T. Rudd, R. M. Sterritt, and J. N. Lester. Formation and conditional stability constants of complexes formed between heavy metals and bacterial extracellular polymers, Water Res., *18*, 379 (1984).

61. C. L. Brierley and G. R. Lanza. "Microbial technology for aggregation and dewatering of phosphate clay slimes: Implications on resource recovery," in R. L. Tate and D. A. Klein, Eds., *Soil Reclamation Processes*, Dekker, 1985, p. 243.

62. T. Duxbury. Ecological aspects of heavy metal responses in microorganisms, Adv. Microb. Ecol., *8*, 185 (1985).

63. J. A. Marinsky. Ion binding in charged polymers, Coordination Chem. Rev., *19*, 125 (1976).

64. J. A. Marinsky and M. M. Reddy. Proton and metal ion binding to natural organic polyelectrolytes-II. Preliminary investigation with a peat and a humic acid, Org. Geochem., *7*, 215 (1984).

65. J. A. Marinsky. An interpretation of the sensitivity of weakly acidic (basic) polyelectrolyte (cross-linked and linear) equilibria to excess neutral salt, J. Phys. Chem., *89*, 5294 (1985).

66. N. Blumenkrantz and G. Asboe-Hansen. New method for quantitative determination of uronic acids, Anal. Biochem., *54*, 484 (1973).

67. J. Evans and P. W. Albro. Microdetermination of carboxyl groups in fulvic acid and related polycarboxylates, Intern. J. Environ. Anal. Chem., *24*, 133 (1986).

68. A. Katchalsky, Z. Alexandrowicz, and O. Kedem. "Polyelectrolyte solutions," in B. E. Conway and R. G. Barradas, Eds., *Chemical Physics of Ionic Solutions*, Wiley, New York, 1966, p. 302.

69. J. Kielland. Individual activity coefficients of ions in aqueous solutions, J. Am. Chem. Soc., *59*, 1675 (1937).

70. R. A. Robinson and R. H. Stokes. *Electrolyte Solutions*, 2nd ed., *Butterworth Publications,* London, 1959, p. 481.

71. J. A. Marinsky, F.-G. Lin, and K. S. Chung. A simple method for classification of the physical state of colloid and particulate suspensions encountered in practice, J. Phys. Chem., *87*, 3139 (1983).

72. D. S. Gamble, J. A. Marinsky, and C. H. Langford. "Humic-trace metal ion equilibria in natural waters," in J. A. Marinsky and Y. Marcus, Eds., *Ion Exchange and Solvent Extraction*, Vol. 9, Dekker, New York, 1985, p. 373.

73. G. S. Manning. The molecular theory of polyelectrolyte solutions with applications to the electrostatic properties of polynucleotides, Quart. Rev. Biophys. II, *2*, 179 (1978).

# CHAPTER 12

# Applied Microbial Processes for Metals Recovery and Removal from Wastewater

CORALE L. BRIERLEY*, JAMES A. BRIERLEY**, and
MICHAEL S. DAVIDSON***

Advanced Mineral Technologies, Inc.
Golden, Colorado

## Contents

* VistaTech Partnership, Ltd. Salt Lake City, Utah
** Salt Lake City, Utah
*** Orange County Water District Fountain Valley, California

## 12.1   INTRODUCTION

It has long been known that microorganisms accumulate metals. Metals accumulation to support vital metabolic and reproduction functions has been extensively studied and reviewed (1). With increasing concern about toxic metals entering the food chain, researchers turned their attention to the role of microorganisms as the first step in bioaccumulation. However, in the past two decades microorganisms have been increasingly studied for the purpose of removing metals from waste or process solutions for waste treatment and resource recovery. This chapter

1. Reviews the mechanisms that microorganisms employ for removing metals from solution,
2. Traces the development of microbial technology for metals removal,
3. Examines the state of the art of this emerging technology, and
4. Explores the future of microbial metal removal systems in industrial applications.

## 12.2   REVIEW OF MECHANISMS USED BY MICROORGANISMS FOR METALS REMOVAL

There are five predominant mechanisms by which microorganisms facilitate removal of soluble metals from solution:

1. Volatilization
2. Extracellular precipitation
3. Extracellular complexing and subsequent accumulation
4. Binding to the cell surface
5. Intracellular accumulation

We only summarize these metals removal mechanisms in this chapter because they are discussed in greater detail in other chapters of this book.

### 12.2.1 Volatilization

Volatilization occurs when living microorganisms methylate metals. Biological methylation was first reported by Challenger (2, 3). He noted that, through the action of molds, organometals and organometalloids could be formed. It was proposed that methylation processes were a mechanism that organisms used for detoxification of their environment (4). The most well-known example of volatilization is the methylation of mercury, whereby the mercuric ion, Hg(II), is converted to methylmercury compounds such as dimethylmercury. Other metals, such as Se, Te, As, and Sn are also subject to volatilization by bacteria and fungi (5, 6).

Volatilization is important in metals transformation in the environment, particularly in soils and sediments (7). However, because of the toxicity of some methylated metals (6) and the difficulties in capturing volatilized metals, little research and development effort has been devoted to developing commercial processes employing this microbial mechanism of metals' transformation.

### 12.2.2 Extracellular Precipitation

Extracellular precipitation of metals occurs when microorganisms produce metabolic products that are excreted and result in the immobilization of metals. One of the bext examples of extracellular precipitation of metals is the production of hydrogen sulfide by the sulfate-reducing bacteria. These bacteria, which inhabit anaerobic environments such as bogs, anoxic soils, and sediments, oxidize organic matter and reduce sulfate to sulfide:

$$H_2SO_4 + 8(H) \rightarrow H_2S + 4H_2O$$

The $H_2S$ readily reacts with soluble heavy metals to form insoluble metal sulfide minerals. This biological reaction has reportedly been responsible for the formation of mineral deposits such as covellite (CuS) and sphalerite (ZnS) (7). Formation of $H_2S$ by the sulfate-reducing bacteria is responsible for removing soluble metals from metal-polluted waters. This biological reaction has been used to treat metal-contaminated streams and lakes. This application is detailed in Section 12.3.

### 12.2.3 Extracellular Complexing and Subsequent Accumulation

Some microorganisms generate chemicals that have a high binding efficiency for metals. Examples include the production of siderophore systems in bacteria (See Chapter 5) and generation of metal-binding polymers (See Chapters 9–11).

Many microorganisms synthesize chelating agents known as siderophores. These siderophores have very strong binding constants for ferric ions.

Siderophores are produced by microorganisms to facilitate uptake of iron into the cell (8). Iron-specific siderophores, which are catechol or hydroxamate derivatives, can be employed for removal of specific metals from solution. Reportedly, the catechol derivative can be modified by substituting electrophilic ions on the benzene ring. These substitutions include $Cl^-$, $Br^-$, NO, or $NO_2^-$. These substitutions draw electrons from the benzene ring, changing the binding capacity of the entire molecule. A microbial siderophore, or a synthetically manufactured siderophore, can therefore be chemically treated to yield a chelating agent that can reportedly bind metals from solution on a selective basis. This modification of siderophores has been the subject of a patent application (9). Selective capture of base metals, such as Cd, Cr, Cu Pb, Hg, Ni, and Zn, and of radioactive metals, including Co, Cs, Fe, Sr, Th, and U, using modified siderophore compounds has been reported (10). Application of this technology is described in greater detail in Section 12.4.

Bacterial extracellular polymers play an important role in the adsorption of metal ions from solution (11). This biologically-mediated mechanism of metals accumulation is most evident in activated sludge systems for biological wastewater treatment (11–14). Extracellular polymers that are important for metals removal in activated sludge are principally polysaccharide in nature. Ionic metals are removed from solution by adsorption to sites on bacterial extracellular polymers. However, physical entrapment by the extracellular polymers of precipitated or insoluble metals facilitates their removal as well (15). The use of bacterial polymers in commercial application for metals removal is discussed in greater detail below.

### 12.2.4   Binding to the Cell Surface

Microorganisms can accumulate metabolic and nonmetabolic metals by precipitating or binding the metals onto cell walls or cell membranes. Microbial walls are anionic owing to the presence of carboxyl, hydroxyl, phosphoryl, and other negatively charged sites. Cationic metals rapidly bind to these sites by an energy-independent reaction. Cell surface binding of metals by bacteria and fungi has been extensively studied and reviewed (1, 16).

*12.2.4.1  Bacterial Cell Walls.* Cell walls of *Bacillus subtilis*, which are complex polyanions, are likely sites for concentration of metal cations (17). The isolated cell walls possess select sites, such as diaminopimelic acid residues, which retain metals having atomic numbers greater than 11. Beveridge and Murray (17) demonstrated that the isolated cell walls have the greatest preference for Mg, Fe, Cu, Na, and K. Lesser amounts of Mn, Zn, Ca, Au, and Ni were accumulated. Small amounts of Hg, Sr, Pb, and Ag were also accumulated by the cell wall material. Some cell wall reactive sites also acted as nucleation sites for Au accumulation with formation of microscopic elemental Au crystals.

The Gram-positive bacteria are particularly suited for metal ion removal. The processes involved in metal binding by this group of bacteria have been extensively review by Hancock (18). Beveridge and Murray (19) suggested that carboxyl groups associated with *B. subtilis* cell wall polymers are the major site for metals accumulation with cell wall teichoic acids involved in the metal uptake function. Metal binding to the phosphoryl residues may be the basis for metal binding to teichoic acids of the *B. subtilis* cell wall (19). Amine groups did not appear to function in metals sorption (19).

Gram-negative microbes, specifically *Escherichia coli*, also exhibit metal-binding capacity. With this microbial group, metals deposition occurred at polar head group regions of the constituent membranes or along the peptidoglycan layer (21). It appeared that the lipopolysaccharide component of the cell wall was the site for binding divalent cations. In this case, the binding was to the phosphoryl substituents, and not to free carboxyl groups (20).

### 12.2.4.2  *Fungal Cell Walls.*

Fungal cell walls also adsorb a variety of different metal cations and anions (22–27). Like bacteria, both living and nonliving fungal biomass can accumulate heavy metals. Biosorption of metals by fungi has been studied with numerous metals. Extensive study has been undertaken using fungal biomass for U accumulation. The uptake of U by *Rhizopus arrhizus* is a three-phase process. The first stage involves the formation of a complex between the uranyl ions in solution and the nitrogen of the chitin in the fungal cell wall. In the second stage additional U is adsorbed by the three-dimensional network of the chitin around the uranyl–chitin complex formed in the first stage. The uranyl–chitin complex acts as a nucleation site. In the third stage of the adsorption process the uranyl ion–chitin complex hydrolyses, precipitating uranyl hydroxide within the chitin network. Research work with Cu adsorption using *R. arrhizus* has shown that a similar three-dimensional arrangement of chitin–metal ion complex is formed (28).

### 12.2.4.3  *Algal Cell Walls.*

Metal uptake by algal biomass has been intensively studied (29–33). Most of what is known regarding algal metal sorption has been determined from studies of freshwater species of *Chlorella*. However, at least one marine alga (seaweed) has been demonstrated to accumulate significant amounts of Co (approximately 17% of the dry weight present) (34). The ability of the eluted (nonliving) algal material to resorb additional Co was demonstrated for a total of five complete cycles. The algae biomass compared quite favorably with conventional ion exchange resins, suggesting the possibility for a commercial application.

As is the case with most biosorbant materials, the exact molecular mechanisms for metal–algae biomass interaction remain elusive. They are in all likelihood similar, if not identical, to those operating in metal–fungal, metal–bacterial, and metal–polymer interactions. Given the general reversibility of metal ion–algae biomass binding, the major operating mechanism is likely an electrostatic bond, that is, metal cations attracted to anionic sites in and on the biomass with metal anions being attracted to cationic biomass sites. Suggested functional groups in algae and other biomass materials include carboxyl, amide, hydroxyl, phosphate, amino, imidazole, thiol, and thioether moieties that are present in the proteins, carbohydrates, and lipids that compose the materials.

Algae genera showing significant metal sorption in the nonviable state include species of *Chlorella*, *Chlamydomonas*, and *Ulothrix*. *Chlorella vulgaris* and *Chlorella reguloris* have been the best studied owing to relative ease of maintenance, cultivation, and handling of the organisms. Freeze-dried *Chlorella* species exhibit some selectivity in metal ion accumulation from multicomponent aqueous solutions (pH 5.0 and 1 mmol of each respective ion). In decreasing order metals are bound selectively as shown (31):

$$UO_2^{2+} > Cu^{2+} > Zn^{2+} > Ba^{2+} = Mn^{2+} > Cd^{2+} = Sr^{2+}$$

Solution pH strongly influences metal binding by *Chlorella* preparations. A functional classification of metal ion affinity, as a function of pH, has been elucidated (31):

1. Metals that bind strongly at pH $\geq$ 5.0 and are eluted from *Chlorella* species at pH $\leq$ 2.0 include $Cd^{2+}$, $Cr^{3+}$, $Co^{2+}$, $Ni^{2+}$, $Zn^{2+}$, $Fe^{3+}$, $Be^{2+}$, $Al^{3+}$, $Cu^{2+}$, $Pb^{2+}$, and $UO_2^{2+}$.

2. Metal anions that bind strongly at pH $\leq$ 2.0 and not strongly at pH 5.0 include $PtCl_4^{2-}$, $CrO_4^{2-}$, and $SeO_4^{2-}$.

3. Metals that bind strongly but independent of solution pH include $Ag^+$, $Hg^{2+}$, and $AuCl_4^-$.

An interesting characteristic of algae metal sorption is that alkaline earth metal cations, such as $Mg^{2+}$ and $Ca^{2+}$ have little binding affinity (31).

The interaction between gold ionic species and *Chlorella* species biomass is complex (31, 32, 35). Both $Au^+$ and $Au^{3+}$ species are accumulated with high affinity (up to 10% of the algae by dry weight). Strong competing ligands such as mercaptoethanol, cyanide, and thiourea exert an inhibitory effect on algae Au sorption. Depending on pH and molarity, these ligands can remove (elute) Au from the biomass (36). Algae biomass also exhibits the ability to rapidly reduce $Au^{3+}$ to $Au^{2+}$ (35). Ultimately the $Au^{2+}$ is converted to the elemental ($Au^0$) state. The mechanisms responsible for these conversions are currently unknown.

### 12.2.4.4 Implications of Metal Binding to Cell Surfaces.

The high affinity of microbial cell walls for metals can have an impact on the transport of metals in the environment. Cell wall material can help to remove and concentrate soluble metal pollutants, either introducing the metals to the food chain or sequestering them to sediments (37). The cell wall can also be considered as a source material for functional removal or concentration of metals from wastewater. Metals bound to cell surfaces are easily removed by acid or by chelating agents. The commercial use of cell walls as binding material for metals and the subsequent recovery of these metals and reuse of the cell walls are discussed further in Section 12.4.

### 12.2.5  Intracellular Accumulation

Microbial cells can accumulate intracellularly both metabolically essential metals, such as Ca, K, Na, Fe, and Mg, as well as nonmetabolic metals (e.g., Ni, Cd, Co). Intracellular accumulation can be an energy-dependent function requiring active respiration by the microbial cell. Active uptake usually requires a specific transport system. Microorganisms have well-developed transport systems capable of accumulating metals against a concentration gradient (Chapter 3). When a metal is taken into the cell, ions of an equivalent charge are released by the cell (38). pH and the presence of other ions can substantially affect intracellular metal uptake. Uptake of specific metals usually occurs at an optimal pH value. For example, Ni uptake in *Neurospora crassa* occurs optimally at pH 4, whereas Zn uptake by *Neocosmospora vasinfecta* occurs optimally at pH 6.5. Hg, Co, Mg, Mn and Cu inhibited Cd binding by *Aureobasidium pullulans* (24).

## 12.3  LIVING SYSTEMS FOR METALS REMOVAL

Metals removal from water has been accomplished using biologically complex or "intact" ecosystems. Study of these systems is difficult owing to the complex array of interactions among the biota present (algae, bacteria, fungi, higher plants, and animals) and distribution of the biota (sediment-associated, surface-associated and water-suspended). The physical setting for living-system, metal-removal processes may either be natural or man-made. The natural-setting systems incorporate existing landforms such as ponds, streams, bogs, or marshy areas. The man-made systems employ purpose-built ditches and ponds with or without an underlying containment of clay, plastic sheeting, or other suitable material.

### 12.3.1  Natural-Setting Systems

One of the most well studied of the "natural-setting" systems for metals removal was the investigation by Jackson (39) of the removal of metals from mine wastes, which contaminated a lake in Canada. Mine and smelter wastes containing Zn, Cd, Cu, Hg, and Fe were discharged into surface waters, which were also the recipient of sewage from a nearby town. The algae growth promoted by the presence of sewage and other available nutrients acted as effective material for accumulating the heavy metals. When the algae died and sank through the water column, most metals became incorporated into the lake sediments through a mineralization process. This occurred when the algal biomass served as an organic substrate for the sulfate-reducing bacteria. These bacteria, as they oxidized the organic matter, produced $H_2S$, which reacted with the heavy metals to form metal sulfides such as ZnS, CdS, CuS, and FeS. It is believed that the Hg was converted to volatile dimethylmercury. Jackson (39) suggested that deliberate construction of impoundments with the addition of organic nutrients to stimulate algal growth and produce anaerobic sediments may be a low-cost mechanism for metals removal from contaminated water.

### 12.3.2   Purpose-Built Systems for Metals Removal

This section describes some systems that have been constructed for the purpose of using living biological systems for the removal of metals from contaminated waters. Of course, the most well-known and most frequently used systems for metals removal are sewage treatment facilities. The biological sludge present in these systems accumulates metals that are often present in industrial wastes discharged to publicly owned treatment works.

*12.3.2.1   Metals Removal by Publicly Owned Treatment Works.* Most publicly owned treatment works (POTW) use primary sedimentation to remove suspended solids from the influent. It is estimated that between 40 and 60% of the total metals (soluble and insoluble) concentration is removed with this process. Exceptions are Ni, which is 15–35% removed, and Mn, which is about 30% removed. Metals not removed by sedimentation pass into the biological treatment system, which is normally either an activated sludge or trickling filter system. Typical removal efficiencies for heavy metals in activated sludge range from 1 to 83% depending on the metal present. In general Ni, Mn, and Co removal is consistently low in activated sludge processing, whereas Cu, Pb, Cr, and Zn removal averages over 50%. The few studies that have been done on metals removal in trickling filters indicate about the same degree of metals removal occurs as observed in activated sludge systems (11). Sewage effluents are usually discharged to rivers and streams, which are often used for drinking water supplies. These effluents often contribute up to 35% of the volumetric flow of receiving rivers. Therefore, sewage effluents have a direct effect on water quality. A comparison of metals concentrations in sewage effluents and in river water with permissible metal concentrations in drinking water sources shows that POTW's are clearly having an impact on surface water quality (11).

In 1975 Dugan (40) detailed the bioflocculation and accumulation of metals by floc-forming microorganisms—the organisms present in sewage treatment plants. He reported that the metals are largely bound by the polymeric materials produced by the microorganisms, with little of the metal actually being accumulated by the organisms themselves. Dugan also described the flocculation of insoluble particles, including clay, other bacteria, and insoluble metals, by the abundant polymers produced by the microorganisms. The microorganisms he studied appeared to be related to the genera, *Zoogloea*, *Pseudomonas*, *Acetomonas*, *Acetobacter*, and *Gluconobacter*.

Extracellular polymers extracted from activated sludge were found to complex Cd, Ni, Mn, and Co. Saturation of activated sludge polymer binding sites occurred after the addition of 10 mg metal $L^{-1}$ for all metals studied except Mn, which was complexed to a very limited extent (41). Metals were removed by the activated sludge polymer to a concentration of 1 mg $L^{-1}$; however, removal below that concentration was minimal with the exception of Cd. The more soluble metals displayed the lowest metals removal. The age of sludge appeared to affect metals removal; as long as the activated sludge was less than 9 days old, its capacity for metals adsorption remained high (42).

Low concentrations of Cd, Co, U, and Zn strongly affected the growth of *Zoogloea ramigera* (43). However, selective adsorption of Cd, Cu, and U was accomplished by controlling the pH. Uptake of Cu was rapid and efficient by *Z. ramigera* with accumulation of 0.17 g Cu adsorbed per gram of biomass within 10 min (44); the concentration of Cu used in the experiment was 0.58 g $L^{-1}$ and the biomass concentration was 22 g $L^{-1}$. The pH values ranged from 4.45 to 3.25 and retention times for the biomass in the Cu solution ranged from 4 to 20 min (45). The presence of other cations in solution did affect the loading of *Z. ramigera* with Cu. Aluminum was more effective than Mg and Na in preventing Cu adsorption (13).

After loading *Z. ramigera* biomass with Cu and Cd the metals could be released from the flocculated particles by acid treatment. The stripped biomass was reexposed to the metals with subsequent loading of 0.323 g Cu $g^{-1}$ biomass and 0.223 g Cd $g^{-1}$ biomass. The acid treatment did not affect the metal binding capacity of the biomass (13).

### 12.3.2.2 *Meanders and Impoundments for Metals Removal.*

An example of successful application of the living system approach is the "meander" system operated by the Amax–Homestake Buick lead mine and mill located in the New Lead Belt District of southern Missouri (46, 47). Excess mine and mill water containing soluble Pb, Cu, Zn, Mn, Ni, Fe, and Cd that exits the mill tailings dam was passed through a series of man-made switchable channels (meanders) prior to discharge to a natural watercourse. The system supported a variety of single- and multi-cell algae such as species of *Chlorella*, *Oscillatoria*, *Cladophora*, *Spirogyra*, *Rhizoclonium*, and *Hydrodictyon* as well as the higher plants *Potomogeton* (pond weed) and *Typha* (cattail). The primary mechanisms of metal removal were reported to be entrainment of particulates and adsorption of soluble metals by the algae and plant biomass. System efficiency was stated to be in excess of 99% with the effluent meeting or exceeding federal guidelines for Fe, Pb, Cu, Ni, and Cd. Metal accumulation by algae was also noted in a "natural" (nonengineered) stream system receiving mine and mill water from the St. Joe–Fletcher operation, which is also situated in Missouri. The contribution made by bacterial metal accumulation in the overall purification process was not determined at the Missouri sites.

Another example of metal removal by an "engineered" living system was described by Brierley and others (48, 49). Wastewaters resulting from mining operations at a U mining and milling facility near Grants, New Mexico, were given primary treatment by conventional ion exchange resin to remove U followed by a secondary treatment with Ba to remove Ra. The water from the secondary treatment was then passed through a series of man-made "algae-ponds;" to lower further the U, Se, Ra, and Mo content (see Fig. 12.1). The predominant algae species present in the algae impoundments were *Spirogyra*, *Chara*, and *Oscillatoria*. Pond sediments contained sulfate-reducing bacteria thought to be *Desulfovibrio* and/or *Desulfotomaculum* species. Passage of mine water through the algae ponds resulted in lowering of U, Se, and Mo from initial concentrations of 5.8, 0.3, and 2.3 ppm, respec-

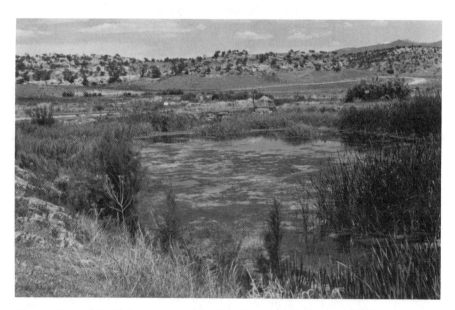

**Figure 12.1** This impoundment is an "engineered" living system for the removal of heavy metals from waters contaminated by mining activities. Accumulation of heavy metals by the algae present in the impoundment is responsible for purifying the water. Sulfate-reducing bacteria in the sediments further contribute to sequestering metals.

tively, to final concentrations of 0.8 ppm U, 0.01 ppm Se, and 0.8 ppm Mo in the treated effluent. Both physical entrainment of solids and adsorption of soluble metal ions by algae biomass were believed to be the primary water purification mechanisms operating in the ponds. Laboratory findings indicated that death of metal-laden algae and subsequent decay of the biomass in the pond sediment did not result in resolubilization of either U or Mo.

***12.3.2.3  The Wetlands Approach.*** Recently studies have indicated the potential for using naturally occurring or artifically constructed wetlands (bogs) containing plant/microbe systems to act as biofilters for metals present in acid mine drainage (50, 51). These wetland environments include mosses (*Sphagnum* and *Polytrichum*) cattails (*Typha*), bulrushes (*Scirpus*), and sedges (*Carex*), as well as various cyanobacteria (unidentified species). At a test site in Pennsylvania (51) Mn removals ranging from 69 to 90% were obtained over a 4-month period. Fe removal was less consistent over the test period ranging from negligible to 80%. Fe removal appeared related to a seasonal (temperature) effect with good efficiency (over 60% removal) obtained only during July and August (midsummer).

Metal uptake by *Sphagnum* is thought to occur by a cation exchange phenomenon exhibited by cell wall polyuronic acids. Other metal removal mechanisms thought to be occurring include precipitation by sulfide released by sulfate-reducing bacteria functioning in low-oxygen areas where Fe and Mn are present and bacterial oxidation (and precipitation) of Mn in areas of the wetlands with higher oxygen availability. With additional study and development it may be possible to render these wetland metal removal systems self-sustaining (50).

The use of living biological systems to remove heavy metals from mining/metallurgical wastewaters, although practical in selected applications, has significant limitations. The foremost of these limitations involves the problems inherent to

1. Maintaining the living systems in a viable, if not actively growing state in heavily polluted wastewaters;
2. Obtaining adequate contact of the living biomass with the wastewater stream;
3. Physical containment of the biomass within the treatment facility;
4. Disposal of nonviable (or excess) biomass containing heavy metals and a very high proportion of water; and
5. Seasonal effects on growth.

These limitations generally apply to the use of all proposed living biomass metal recovery systems including those based on higher plants, algae, fungi/yeasts, and bacteria.

### 12.3.2.4 Immobilized Living Systems.

Microbial cells can be colonized on support materials to form a biofilm. Rigid supports for biofilm development include glass, stainless steel wire, wood shavings, reticulated foams (52, 53), anthracite coal particles (54), string and wooden supports coated with alumina (55), and polyvinyl chloride (56). Biofilm growth is obtained by culturing microorganisms in the presence of the inert material.

When a mixed culture of denitrifying bacteria was attached to particles of anthracite coal and subjected to a U solution, biosorption of U was rapid. Saturation of the biosorbent with U was attained at a concentration of 140 mg U g$^{-1}$ dry cells. Using a countercurrent contacting device for continuous separation of U from a solution containing 25 mg U L$^{-1}$, U concentrations were reduced to 0.5 mg U L$^{-1}$ in an 8-min residence time (54).

Viable *Pseudomonas fluorescens* cells were immobilized on polyvinyl chloride granules and used for simultaneous denitrification and uptake of heavy metals. Cell loading was reported as 0.1–0.4 g dry weight per gram of plastic. With an influent feed rate of 1500 mL h$^{-1}$, Pb(NO$_3$)$_2$ was reduced from 1.0 mg to 0.05–0.1 mg L$^{-1}$ and ZnSO$_4$ concentration from 10 to 5 mg L$^{-1}$. Copper was reported to be highly toxic to the denitrifying bacterial population (56).

Living *Citrobacter* species immobilized on rigid supports including reticulated foams, stainless steel wire, and wood shavings were evaluated for U (uranyl ion) removal. The functional component of U accumulation by the *Citrobacter* species was identified as a surface-located phosphatase. With liberation of HPO$_4^{2-}$ metals (M) were precipitated extracellularly as MHPO$_4$. The best U recoveries and metal accumulation were achieved using a biofilm formed on reticulated foam. 90% U removal was attained and U precipitation was reported at 3.9 g U g$^{-1}$ dry weight of reticulated foam with *Citrobacter* species biofilm. The concentration of bacteria per gram of foam was not reported (52). In similar studies to remove Pb from solution, *Citrobacter* species was immobilized on glass helices and entrapped in polyacrylamide gel. Biomass films on glass helices and gel-entrapped bacteria performed equally well with metal accumulation of 3.9 g Pb g$^{-1}$ cells (dry wt) and 3.8 g U g$^{-1}$ cells (dry wt). As with the previous study, the metal deposition resulted from release of HPO$_4^{2-}$, which precipitated the metals as phosphate (53).

Nongrowing *Streptomyces viridochromogenes* immobilized in polyacrylamide gel accumulated 312 mg U g$^{-1}$ bacteria (dry wt). U accumulation by the cells was found to be pH independent between pH values of 4 and 9 once the *S. viridochromogenes* was immobilized. The U could be desorbed from the immobilized cells using 0.1 M Na$_2$CO$_3$ and the cells could be reused for U recovery. The immobilized cells were reused for five cycles with a loss of 2% dry weight. The immobilized cells were found to possess good mechanical properties and could be employed in batch or column systems (57).

## 12.4 NONLIVING BIOLOGICAL SYSTEMS FOR METALS REMOVAL

Of the processes microorganisms employ to immobilize, complex, or remove metals from solution, extracellular complexing with polymers or siderophores and extracellular binding to the cell walls are of primary interest for practical application of microorganisms for concentration of metals from solution. The other processes described earlier require an active participation of the microflora or use of living microorganisms to remove the metals from solutions. The use of living systems certainly has application in selected wastewater metal removal–treatment systems. However, the toxicity and the extreme and variable conditions present in many waste and process waters preclude the use of living systems and dictate the application of nonliving systems for metals removal.

Metal sorption processes have been demonstrated using nonmetabolizing and nonliving, biologically derived materials (16, 36, 58–64). The use of suitably prepared (nonliving) biomass for metal recovery systems by and large eliminates or minimizes the problems described for living system use.

Native biomass, however, exhibits low mechanical strength, low density, and small particle size. As such, native biomass for metals removal must be employed in continuous stirred tank reactors. After metal loading the biomass must be separated from solution using filtration, sedimentation, or centrifugation. Such a process scheme is neither cost-effective nor efficient. Therefore it is necessary to convert biomass into a form whereby it can be employed in modes similar to that of ion exchange resins and activated carbon. Modified biomass must have a particle size similar to other commercial adsorbents (0.5–1.5 mm) and possess particle strength, high porosity, hydrophilicity, and resistance to agressive chemicals (28). These characteristics can be achieved through immobilization technology.

Immobilization serves to improve the physical characteristics of the biomass for use in reactors, permits reusability of the substance, and serves to make the microorganisms more inert to microbial degradation. Microbial cells can be immobilized in supports such as agar, cellulose, silica, alginate, polyacrylamide, toluene diisocyanate, collagen, liquid membranes, metal hydroxide precipitates, and glutaraldehyde (36, 57, 60, 64–67).

### 12.4.1 Immobilized Bacterial Systems

Bacterial cell mass, for example, *Bacillus* species utilized in fermentation for production of enzymes and other chemicals, has been immobilized to form a nonliving granular product for removal of metals from wastewaters (61–64, 68). Several characteristics of the granulated *Bacillus* species make it an ideal system for treatment of metal-bearing wastewaters and process streams. The granule is not selective in the metals it sorbs; rather, it simultaneously removes several different toxic and heavy metals (e.g., Cd, Cr, Cu, Hg, Ni, Pb, U, Zn) from solution regardless of their differing concentrations. In addition, the granular product removes only those metals that are considered hazardous, and allows nontoxic alkaline earth metals (Ca, Na, K, Mg) to pass, reserving the possible sorptive sites for hazardous metals.

The granulated *Bacillus* species loads single or mixed metals independent of influent concentration; therefore, it functions as effectively in wastewaters containing concentrated (100s of ppm) metals as it does in relatively dilute (<10 ppm) streams. This property is an especially valuable one in industrial situations that produce a wastewater stream that continually changes in its metal concentration.

The immobilized *Bacillus* species normally loads single or mixed metals in excess of 10% of its weight. It has a metal-removal efficiency of >99%, yielding effluent with total metal concentrations of only 10–50 ppb. This is a greater efficiency than has been observed in other non-biomass derived, metal-binding agents.

A wastewater treatment system has been developed (Advanced Mineral Technologies, Inc., Golden, CO) which utilizes the granulated *Bacillus* species biomass (See Fig. 12.2). The system employs the granules in either packed (fixed) bed, expanded (fluid) bed, or dispersed bed contactors (See Fig. 12.3). Following metals loading, the granules are regenerated using var-

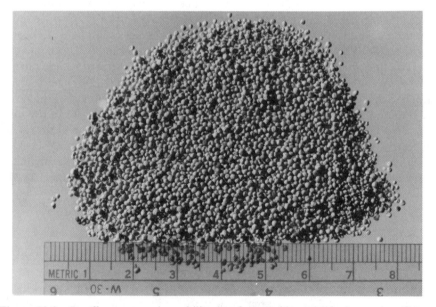

**Figure 12.2** *Bacillus* spp. are immobilized to form stable, spherical granules. Granule sizes can vary with the photograph illustrating granules of about 1.0 mm in diameter. Upon hydration the biomass granules expand and become porous. Metal binding takes place throughout the granule. Photograph courtesy of Advanced Mineral Technologies, Inc., Golden, CO.

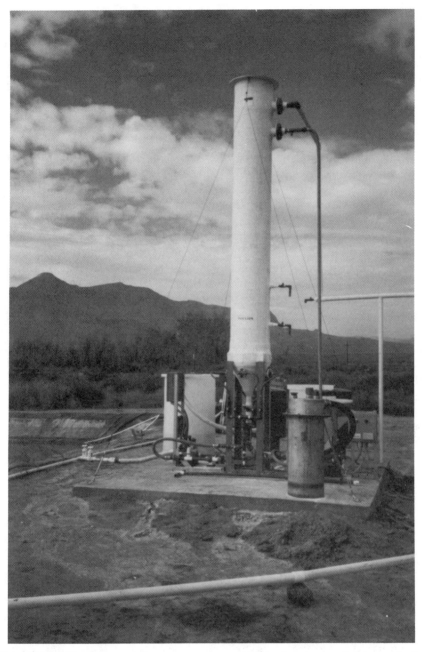

**Figure 12.3** The wastewater treatment system shown is an expanded bed unit that employs nonliving biomass for metals removal. Immobilized *Bacillus* sp. in granular form are loaded to a depth of approximately 6 ft in the columnar contractor. Wastewater is pumped up-flow through the contactor at a rate sufficient to fluidize the granules 30%. Metals are accumulated most heavily on the biomass granules located nearest to the bottom of the contactor. Photograph courtesy of Advanced Mineral Technologies, Inc., Golden, CO.

ious electrolytes (e.g., $H_2SO_4$, NaOH, or complexing/chelating reagents) to remove the metals and the metals are reclaimed by electrowinning or other metal recovery techniques. The granulated *Bacillus* species is then returned to field service.

## 12.4.2   Immobilized Fungal Systems

Fungi biomass has been immobilized by stiffening natural or dried fungi with high-molecular-weight compounds such as gelatin, casein, and other poly-peptidic materials. The stiffened fungal biomass is cross-linked with polymerizable substances such as aldehydes, glyoxal, glutaraldehyde, or other polyfunctional aldehydes. The stiffened and cross-linked biomass can be mechanically granulated. The granulated product is employed in cyclically repeated sorption processing of heavy metal ions by contacting the granulated material with solutions of heavy metals. A capacity of 102.5 mg U $g^{-1}$ of sorbent has been reported under such use (69).

Another patented process for immobilizing fungal biomass (66) involves the dispersion of the biomass into a nonpolar medium such as xylene. The biomass dispersion is agglomerated by adding a stiffening agent and a surface-active agent, which is not miscible with the dispersion medium. Stiffening/cross-linking agents that could be used include formaldehyde, formaldehyde–resorcinol solutions, formaldehyde–urea solutions, and poly-vinyl acetate emulsions. The product resulting from this reaction could be separated to yield granules ranging from 0.75 to 1.0 mm. Uranium adsorption for this granular material was reported to be about 90.5 mg $g^{-1}$

*Aspergillus oryzae* has been immobilized on reticulated foam. During metal uptake studies no organic substrate was applied. Active metabolic processes were unimportant in metal accumulation. The immobilized fungal biomass was employed in a column contactor. 90% removal of Cd as $CdSO_4$ was achieved with a 5-min residence time of the metal solution in contact with the biomass. pH was found to be a critical factor determining the distribution of Cd between the biomass and the solution. Within the pH range range of 5–8, it was found that there was an approximate increase in the maximum mycelial capacity for Cd of 2 mg $g^{-1}$ (dry wt) of mycelium for each unit increase in pH. Cd sorption depended on the concentration of biomass in the $CdSO_4$ solution. The maximum Cd accumulation that was achieved by the mycelium was inversely proportional to the biomass concentration (23). It was proposed by the researchers that the columns containing immobilized fungal biomass could be operated successfully as biosorption columns.

Using a proprietary technology, which employs polymeric membranes, *Rhizopus arrhizus* was immobilized and formed into particles. The immobilization technology gave the fungal biomass particles both mechanical strength and porosity. No more than 10% of the particle was inert material. The immobilized *R. arrhizus* maintained high biosorptive capacity for U.

Desorption of U from the immobilized fungus was achieved using mineral acids, ammonium sulfate, and carbonate solutions as eluents. Carbonate was the most suitable eluent because it caused less damage to the biomass (28).

### 12.4.3  Immobilized Algal Systems

The potential for practical or commercial application of nonliving algae in water purification/treatment has been enhanced by the ability to fix or immobilize the biomass. Both polyacrylamide gel and silica gel have been demonstrated to lend useful degrees of dimensional stability to *Chlorella* species preparations (36) and yet not significantly impair metal binding capabilities. Of the two immobilization techniques silica gel appeared to offer advantages in terms of physical strength and cost. The immobilized algal product was very hard and resisted fragmentation. The product was also very porous, allowing access of metal ions to a greater number of potential metal-binding sites. The silica gel immobilization also allowed the product to be reused with as many as 30 cycles of metal binding and elution without any noticeable decrease in metal binding capacity. As with immobilized *Bacillus* species, the silica-bound algae did not accumulate Ca, Mg, Na, or K (36).

Immobilized algae in silica gel have been used under certain conditions to remove a variety of metals from solution with selective stripping of these metals from the immobilized algae. Selective stripping can be used because certain metal ions are bound with different affinities, depending on the pH of the metal solution. Therefore, only a pH gradient is necessary in the regeneration cycle to separate the metals selectively (36) (Bio-Recovery Systems, Inc., Las Cruces, NM).

### 12.4.4  Immobilized Complexing Agents

Extracellular complexing compounds (siderophores) are being employed in commercial application. These compounds, sold under the tradename Compositions™ were developed by DeVoe and Holbein (9, 10). These Compositions™ reportedly have such high affinity for specific metals that a Composition™ can remove a metal, for example, Hg from a solution containing 8 ppm to less than 1 ppb (10). Metal complexation compounds can be obtained directly from microorganisms that produce them or synthetically manufactured. Such complexing compounds are commercially employed by immobilizing them on substrates such as silicate. A metal-containing solution is then passed through a column containing the immobilized complexing agent. The metal-loaded complexing agent can be stripped of metals using acid and regenerated for reuse. Devoe and Holbein report that their Compositions™ can be regenerated and reused some 100 times without deterioration.

## 12.5 FACTORS IMPORTANT TO EMPLOYING BIOLOGICAL SYSTEMS FOR METALS REMOVAL AND RECOVERY

Waste streams by their nature are highly variable and can be extremely toxic. They also can contain a variety of chemicals and particulate matter. Inorganic waste streams are characterized as having

1. Mixed metals, which may be cationic, anionic or both;
2. A variable pH;
3. Organic contaminants, such as oils, greases, or other substances including detergents;
4. Suspended particles, which may or may not be regulated by local or federal effluent discharge guidelines;
5. A varying flow volume; and
6. High concentrations of innocuous metals, such as K, Na, Ca, and Mg.

The waste streams may also contain complexing and chelating agents such as EDTA, cyanide, and ammonium ion.

Discharge of wastewaters in the United States is regulated under the Clean Water Act. Effluent guidelines are established by the Environmental Protection Agency (EPA); however, states and local governments may impose stricter discharge standards than those set by the EPA. For discharge to POTW's effluents must meet Pretreatment Standards. Effluents discharged to surface waters, such as lakes and streams, must comply with National Pollution Discharge Elimination System (NPDES) Standards. NPDES Standards are stricter regarding metal discharge levels than Pretreatment Standards. This is because the POTW itself will remove some metals during sedimentation and biological functions.

To achieve Pretreatment and NPDES Standards, most generators of metal-bearing wastes use precipitation technology, such as NaOH, lime, limestone, or sulfide precipitation. These technologies generate sludges, which can be deemed hazardous and must be disposed of in specially classified hazardous waste landfills. With tightening of land disposal regulations, the disposal of hazardous wastes is becoming increasingly expensive and unattractive.

Generators of metal-bearing wastewaters are seeking cost-effective and efficient technologies to achieve compliance with increasingly stringent discharge standards and to eliminate sludge generation.

Biological systems, particularily those that employ immobilized microbial cells that (1) achieve a high efficiency for metals removal, (2) reach a high metal loading capacity, and (3) are repeatably regenerable, will be highly marketable to waste generators. These biological systems must

1. Possess flexibility to handle variable flow volumes;
2. Load heavy metals that may be present as a mixed metal solution and accompanied by Na, K, Ca, and Mg, which need not be removed from solution;
3. Not foul or be affected in performance by oils, greases, other organic contaminants, and chelating/complexing agents;
4. Handle dirts and suspended solids; and
5. Tolerate temperatures ranging from just above freezing to just below boiling.

It is also preferable that the metals be stripped from the biological materials in a form whereby the metals can be economically reused by the original generator or reclaimed for reentry into the marketplace.

Finally, biological systems must be economically competitive with existing technologies. These competitive technologies include chemical precipitation, ion exchange, reverse osmosis, evaporation, electrodialysis, electrolysis, and ultrafiltration.

## 12.6  SUMMARY

The first generation of biological-based products for metals removal from waste and process streams has been introduced to the market. Some of these products utilize living systems that function by actively as well as passively accumulating metals. Such systems include metal recovery by microorganisms in sewage treatment plants and the intentional cultivation of microorganisms and higher plants in meandering streams, impoundments, and wetlands.

Highly engineered treatment systems that use immobilized, nonliving, or nonmetabolizing bacteria, fungi, and algae are now on the market. These systems are characterized as employing immobilized microbial cells or cellular constituents in matrices that are granular in form and are both chemically and physically stable. The immobilized microbial products are employed in contactors that allow flexibility in use. The products can be stripped of metals and regenerated for reuse. Provisions are made for metal reclamation to eliminate solid hazardous waste production partially or totally. The biological systems can handle wastewater variabilities and are competitive with existing wastewater treatment technologies from a performance and cost standpoint.

## REFERENCES

1. D. P. Kelly, P. R. Norris, and C. L. Brierley, "Microbiological methods for the extraction and recovery of metals," in A. T. Bull, D. C. Ellwood, and C. Rat-

ledge, Eds., *Microbial Technology: Current State, Future Prospects*, Cambridge University Press, Cambridge, 1979, p. 263.

2. F. Challenger, Biological methylation of compounds of arsenic and selenium, *Chem. Ind.*, *54*, 657 (1935).

3. F. Challenger, Biological methylation, *Adv. Enzymol.*, *12*, 429 (1951).

4. F. Challenger, "Biosynthesis of organometallics and organometalloidal compounds," in F. E. Brinkman and J. M. Bleeama, Eds., *Organometals and Organometalloids: Occurrence and Fate in the Environment*, ACS Symposium Series, American Chemical Society, Washington, DC, 1978, p. 1.

5. W. R. Blair, G. J. Olson, F. E. Brinckman, and W. P. Iverson, Accumulation and fate of tri-*n*-butyltin cation in estuarine bacteria, *Microbiol. Ecol.*, *8*, 241 (1982).

6. J. S. Thayer and F. E. Brinckman, The biological methylation of metals and metalloids, *Adv. Organometallic Chem.*, *20*, 313 (1984).

7. H. L. Ehrlich, *Geomicrobiology*, Dekker, New York, 1984.

8. D. G. Lundgren and W. Dean, "Biogeochemistry of iron," in P. A. Trudinger and D. J. Swaine, Eds., *Biogeochemical Cycling of Mineral-Forming Elements*, Elsevier, Amsterdam, 1979, p. 211.

9. I. R. DeVoe and B. E. Holbein, Insoluble chelating compositions, U.S. Patent No. 4,530,963, 1985.

10. B. E. Holbein, I. W. DeVoe, L. G. Neirinck, M. F. Nathan, and R. N. Arzonetti, DeVoe-Holbein technology: "new technology for closed-loop source reduction of toxic heavy metal wastes in the nuclear and metal finishing industries," in *Proceedings of Massachusetts Hazardous Waste Source Reduction Conference*, 1984, p. 66.

11. R. M. Sterritt and J. N. Lester, "Heavy metal immobilisation by bacterial extracellular polymers," in H. Eccles and S. Hunt, Eds., *Immobilisation of Ions by Bio-Sorption*, Ellis Harwood, Chichester, United Kingdom, 1986, p. 121.

12. M. J. Brown and J. N. Lester, Role of bacterial extracellular polymers in metal uptake in pure bacterial culture and activated sludge. II. Effects of mean cell retention time, *Water Res.*, *16*, 1549 (1982).

13. A. B. Norberg and H. Persson, Accumulation of heavy-metal ions by *Zoogloea ramigera*, *Biotechnol. Bioeng.*, *26*, 239 (1984).

14. J. A. Scott, S. J. Palmer, and J. Ingham, "Microbial metal adsorption enhancement by naturally excreted polysaccharide coatings," in H. Eccles and S. Hunt, Eds., *Immobilisation of Ions by Bio-Sorption*, Ellis Harwood, Chichester, United Kingdom, 1986, p. 81.

15. M. J. Brown and J. N. Lester, Metal removal in activated sludge: The role of bacterial extracellular polymers, *Water Res.*, *13*, 817 (1979).

16. S. R. Hutchins, M. S. Davidson, J. A. Brierley, and C. L. Brierley, Microorganisms in reclamation of metals, *Annu. Rev. Microbiol.*, *40*, 311 (1986).

17. T. J. Beveridge and R. G. E. Murray, Uptake and retention of metals by cell walls of *Bacillus subtilis*, *J. Bacteriol.*, *127*, 1502 (1976).

18. I. C. Hancock, "Trace metal removal from aqueous solution," in R. Thompson, Ed., *Trace Metal Removal from Aqueous Solution—Special Publication No. 61*, The Royal Society of Chemistry, London, 1986, p. 25.

19. T. J. Beveridge and R. G. E. Murray, Sites of metal deposition in the cell wall of *Bacillus subtilis, J. Bacteriol., 141,* 876 (1980).

20. F. G. Ferris and T. J. Beveridge, Site specificity of metallic ion binding in *Escherichia coli* K-12 lipopolysaccharide, *Can. J. Microbiol., 32,* 52 (1986).

21. T. J. Beveridge and S. F. Koval, Binding of metals to cell envelopes of *Escherichia coli* K-12, *Appl. Environ. Microbiol., 42,* 325 (1981).

22. I. S. Ross and C. C. Townsley, "The uptake of heavy metals by filamentous fungi," in H. Eccles and S. Hunt, Eds., *Immobilisation of Ions by Bio-Sorption,* Ellis Harwood, Chichester, United Kingdom, 1986, p. 49.

23. R. J. Kiff and D. R. Little, "Biosorption of heavy metals by immobilised fungal biomass," in H. Eccles and S. Hunt, Eds., *Immobilisation of Ions by Bio-Sorption,* Ellis Harwood, Chichester, United Kingdom, 1986, p. 71.

24. G. M. Gadd, "The uptake of heavy metals by fungi and yeasts: The chemistry and physiology of the process and applications for biotechnology," in H. Eccles and S. Hunt, eds., *Immobilisation of Ions by Bio-Sorption,* Ellis Harwood, Chichester, United Kingdom, 1986, p. 135.

25. C. C. Townsley, I. S. Ross, and A. S. Atkins, " Copper removal from a simulated leach effluent using the filamentous fungus *Trichoderma viride,*" in H. Eccles and S. Hunt, Eds., *Immobilisation of Ions by Bio-Sorption,* Ellis Harwood, Chichester, United Kingdom, 1986, p. 159.

26. N. A. Yakubu and A. W. L. Dudeney, "Biosorption of uranium with *Aspergillus niger,*" in H. Eccles and S. Hunt, Eds., *Immobilisation of Ions by Bio-Sorption,* Ellis Harwood, Chichester, United Kingdom, 1986, p. 183.

27. D. L. Sober, V. I. Lakshmanan, R. G. L. McCready, and A. S. Dahya, "Bioadsorption of uranium by fungal stope isolates," in R. G. L. McCready, Ed., *Proceedings of the Third Annual General Meeting of Biominet,* Canadian Government Publishing Centre, Ottawa, 1986, p. 93.

28. M. Tsezos, "Adsorption by microbial biomass as a process for removal of ions from process or waste solutions," in H. Eccles and S. Hunt, Eds., *Immobilisation of Ions by Bio-Sorption,* Ellis Harwood, Ltd., Chichester, United Kingdom, 1986, p. 201.

29. J. Ferguson and B. Bubela, Concentration of copper(II), lead(III), and zinc(II) from aqueous solutions by particulate algal matter, *Chem. Geol., 13,* 163 (1974).

30. A. Nakajima, T. Horikoshi, and T. Sakaguchi, Studies on the accumulation of heavy metal elements in biological systems, *Eur. J. Appl. Microbiol. Biotechnol., 12,* 76 (1981).

31. D. W. Darnall, B. Greene, M. T. Henzl, J. M. Hosea, R. A. McPherson, J. Sneddon, and M. D. Alexander, Selective recovery of gold and other metal ions from an algal biomass, *Env. Science Technol., 20,* 206 (1986).

32. B. Greene, M. Hosea, R. McPherson, M. Henzl, M. D. Alexander, and D. W. Darnall, Interaction of gold(I) and gold(III) complexes with algal biomass, *Env. Science Technol., 20,* 627 (1986).

33. D. Kaplan, D. Christiaen, and S. M. Arad, Chelating properties of extracellular polysaccharides from *Chlorella* spp., *Appl. Env. Microbiol., 53,* 2953 (1987).

34. M. Kuyucak and B. Volesky, "Recovery of cobalt by a new biosorbent," in R. G. L. McCready, Ed., *Proceedings of the Third Annual General Meeting of*

*Biominet,* CANMET Special Publication SP-86-9, Canadian Government Publishing Centre, Ottawa, 1986.

35. M. Hosea, B. Greene, R. McPherson, M. Henzl, M. D. Alexander, and D. W. Darnall, Accumulation of elemental gold on the alga *Chlorella vulgaris, Inorg. Chim. Acta, 123,* 161 (1986).

36. D. W. Darnall, B. Greene, M. Hosea, R. A. McPherson, M. Henzl, and M. D. Alexander, "Recovery of heavy metals by immobilized algae," in R. Thompson, Ed., *Trace Metal Removal from Aqueous Solution,* Special Publication No. 61, The Royal Society of Chemistry, London, 1986, p. 1.

37. T. J. Beveridge, "Bioconversion of inorganic materials: mechanisms of the binding of metallic ions to bacterial walls and the possible impact on microbial ecology," in M. J. Klug and C. A. Reddy, Eds., *Current Perspective in Microbial Ecology,* American Society for Microbiology, Washington, DC, 1984, p. 601.

38. C. L. Brierley, D. P. Kelly, K. J. Seal, and D. J. Best, "Material and biotechnology," in I. J. Higgins, D. J. Best, and J. Jones, Eds., *Biotechnology Principles and Applications,* Blackwell Scientific Publications, Oxford, 1985, p. 163.

39. T. A. Jackson, The biogeochemistry of heavy metals in polluted lakes and streams at Flin Flon, Canada, and a proposed method for limiting heavy metal pollution of natural waters, *Env. Geol., 2,* 173 (1978).

40. P. R. Dugan, Bioflocculation and the Accumulation of Chemicals by Floc-Forming Organisms, *EPA Report 600/2-75-032,* National Technical Information Service, Springfield, VA, 1975.

41. M. J. Brown and J. N. Lester, Role of bacterial extracellular polymers in metal uptake in pure bacterial culture and activated sludge. I. Effects of metal concentration, *Water Res., 16,* 1539 (1982).

42. M. J. Brown and J. N. Lester, Role of bacterial extracellular polymers in metal uptake in pure bacterial culture and activated sludge. II. Effects of mean cell retention time, *Water Res., 16,* 1549 (1982).

43. A. Norberg, Production of extracellular polysaccharide by *Zoogloea ramigera* and its use as an adsorbing agent for heavy metals, Doctoral Dissertation LUTKDH/(TKMB-1003)/131/(1983), Lund University, Lund, Sweden, 1983.

44. A. Norberg and S. Rydin, Development of a continuous process for metal accumulation by *Zoogloea ramigera, Biotechnol. Bioeng., 26,* 265 (1984).

45. A. Norberg and H. Persson, Accumulation of heavy-metals ions by *Zoogloea ramigera, Biotechnol. Bioeng., 26,* 239 (1984).

46. N. L. Gale and B. G. Wixson, Removal of heavy metals from industrial effluents by algae, *Dev. Ind. Microbiol., 20,* 259 (1979).

47. N. L. Gale, "The role of algae and other microorganisms in metal detoxification and environmental clean-up," in H. L. Ehrlich and D. S. Holmes, Eds., *Workshop on Biotechnology for the Mining, Metal-Refining and Fossil Fuel Processing Industries,* Biotechnol. Bioeng. Symp. No. 16, Wiley, New York, 1986, p. 171.

48. J. A. Brierley, C. L. Brierley, and K. T. Dreher, "Removal of selected inorganic pollutants from uranium mine waste water by biological methods," in C. O. Brawner, Ed., *Uranium Mine Waste Disposal,* American Institute of Mining, Metallurgical and Petroleum Engineers, New York, 1980, p. 365.

49. J. A. Brierley and C. L. Brierley, "Biological methods to remove selected inorganic pollutants from uranium mine wastewater," in P. A. Trudinger, M. R. Walter, and B. J. Ralph, Eds., *Biogeochem. of Ancient and Modern Env.*, Australian Academy of Science, Canberra, 1980, p. 661.

50. J. C. Emerick and D. J. Cooper, Acid mine drainage in the west: the wetland approach, *Proc. 90th National Western Mining Conf.*, Colorado Mining Association, Denver, 1987.

51. P. M. Erickson, M. A. Girts, and R. L. P. Kleinmann, Use of constructed wetlands to treat coal mine drainage, *Proc. 90th National Western Mining Conf.*, Colorado Mining Association, Denver, 1987.

52. L. E. Macaskie and A. C. R. Dean, "Uranium accumulation by a *Citrobacter* sp. immobilized as biofilm on various support materials," in O. M. Neijssel, R. R. van der Meer, and K. Ch. A. M. Luyben, Eds., *Proc. 4th European Congress on Biotechnology 1987*, Vol. 2, Elsevier, Amsterdam, 1987, p. 37.

53. L. E. Macaskie and A. C. R. Dean, Use of immobilized biofilm of *Citrobacter* sp. for the removal of uranium and lead from aqueous flows, *Enzyme Microbiol. Technol.*, 9, 2 (1987).

54. S. E. Shumate, G. W. Strandberg, D. A. McWhirter, J. R. Parrott, G. M. Bogacki, and B. R. Locke, Separation of heavy metals from aqueous solutions using "biosorbents"—development of contacting devices for uranium removal, *Biotech. Bioeng. Symp.*, 10, 27 (1980).

55. R. A. Clyde, Horizontal fermenter, U.S. Patent 4,351,905, 1982.

56. R. P. Tengerdy, J. E. Johnson, J. Hollo, and J. Toth, Denitrification and removal of heavy metals from waste water by immobilized microorganisms, *Appl. Biochem. Biotechnol.*, 6, 3 (1981).

57. A. Nakajima, T. Horikoshi, and T. Sakaguchi, Recovery of uranium by immobilized microorganisms, *Eur. J. Applied. Biotechnol.* 16, 88 (1982).

58. W. Drobot and H. A. Lechavelier, Recovery of metals, U.S. Patent 4,293,334, 1981.

59. M. Kumakura and I. Kaetsu, Precoating of microbial cells by hydrophobic reagents on immobilization, *Biotechnol. Lett. 5,* 197 (1983).

60. R. C. Cheng, K. M. McCoy, R. A. Houtchens, and N. G. Moll, Stabilization of Intracellular Enzymes, Eur. Patent Application 0.915,304, 1986.

61. J. A. Brierley, C. L. Brierley, and G. M. Goyak, "AMT-BIOCLAIM™: a new wastewater treatment and metal recovery technology," in R. W. Lawrence, R. M. R. Branion and H. G. Ebner, Eds., *Fundamental and Applied Biohydrometallurgy*, Elsevier, Amsterdam, 1986, p. 291.

62. J. A. Brierley, C. L. Brierley, and G. M. Goyak, "AMT-BIOCLAIM™ process for treatment of metalliferous wastewater from electroplating and other industries," in R. G. L. McCready, Ed., *Proceedings of Second Annual General meeting of BIOMINET*, Canadian Government Publishing Centre, Ottawa, 1986, p. 120.

63. J. A. Brierley, G. M. Goyak, and C. L. Brierley, "Considerations for commercial use of natural products for metals recovery," in H. Eccles and S. Hunt, Eds., *Immobilisation of Ions by Bio-Sorption*, Ellis Horwood Ltd., Chichester, United Kingdom, 1986, p. 105.

64. J. A. Brierley and D. B. Vance, "Recovery of precious metals by microbial biomass," in D. P. Kelly and P. R. Norris, Eds., *Biohydrometallurgy 87*, Science and Technology Letters, Kew Surrey, United Kingdom, 1987, p. 477.

65. V. I. Lakshmanan, J. Christison, R. A. Knapp, J. M. Scharer, and V. San-mugasunderam, "A review of bioadsorption techniques to recover heavy metals from mineral-processing streams," in R. G. L. McCready, Ed., *Proceedings of Second Annual General Meeting of BIOMINET,* Canadian Government Publishing Centre, Ottawa, 1986, p. 75.

66. V. Votapek, E. Marval, and K. Stamberg, Method of treating a biomass, U.S. Patent 4,067,821, 1987.

67. T. R. Jack and J. E. Zajic, The immobilization of whole cells, *Adv. Biochem. Eng., 5*, 125 (1977).

68. J. A. Brierley, C. L. Brierley, R. F. Decker, and G. M. Goyak, Treatment of microorganisms with alkaline solution to enhance metal uptake properties, U.S. Patent 4,690,894, 1987.

69. P. Nemec, H. Prochazka, K. Stamberg, J. Katzer, J. Stamberg, R. Jilek, and P. Hulak, Process of treating mycelia of fungi for retention of metals, U.S. Patent 4,021,368, 1977.

# CHAPTER 13

# Mechanisms of Oxidation and Reduction of Manganese

KENNETH H. NEALSON

Department of Biology and Center for Great Lakes Studies
University of Wisconsin-Milwaukee
Milwaukee, Wisconsin

REINHARDT A. ROSSON and CHARLES R. MYERS

Center for Great Lakes Studies
University of Wisconsin-Milwaukee
Milwaukee, Wisconsin

## Contents

## 13.1   INTRODUCTION

Considering that oxidation and reduction of manganese (Mn) have been recognized as microbially catalyzed reactions since the turn of the century (1), it is perhaps remarkable that so little is known about the biochemical mechanism(s) involved. In the natural environment, microbes are, either directly or indirectly, the major catalysts of Mn cycling (2), and it is well established that many different microbes, including bacteria, algae, yeast, and fungi, can either oxidize Mn(II) or reduce Mn(III) or Mn(IV) oxides (3–13). In some cases, organisms are capable of both Mn oxidation and reduction, depending on environmental growth conditions.

Although Mn oxidation in particular has been studied for many years, very little is known about actual mechanisms of catalysis. This is due at least in part to the complexities of Mn chemistry, which create major problems for the biologist or biochemist attempting to determine mechanisms. Although the oxidation of Mn(II) to either Mn(III) or Mn(IV) is thermodynamically favored at neutral pH and atmospheric oxygen levels, the activation energy for Mn(II) oxidation is high (14) and the process is normally very slow. Of the three relevant oxidation states of Mn that might be found in natural environments, the reduced form, Mn(II), is the only one that is stable as a soluble cation. Mn(II) is thus usually quantified simply by measuring the total dissolved Mn concentration. However, because Mn(II) also readily binds to a variety of different solids, including Mn oxides (15, 16), such a simple approach without first deadsorbing bound Mn(II) can be misleading (17, 18). Mn(III) is a strong acid, and is stable only in certain strong complexes, in very acid solutions, or as $Mn_2O_3(s)$ or $MnOOH(s)$. Mn(IV) is very acidic, and is rapidly hydrolyzed to stable oxide phases (e.g., $MnO_2$) in water. Titration methods can be used to determine the average oxidation state of solid Mn phases (16, 19), but such determinations are not necessarily definitive [e.g., an average oxidation state of Mn(III) might be either all Mn(III) or an equimolar mixture of Mn(II) and Mn(IV)]. Particulate Mn measurements, then, although indicative of a solid phase, unless coupled with an independent measurement (such as X-ray crystallography) do not indicate the exact nature of the Mn phases present. In terms of understanding mechanisms of oxidation and reduction, these difficulties pose major problems.

As mentioned above, Mn(IV) oxides are solid phases, and are excellent chelating agents for divalent cations, including Mn(II) (15, 16). Thus as $MnO_2$ is formed, it binds Mn(II); if, as is commonly done, the decrease in soluble Mn is used to estimate Mn(II) oxidation, this leads to higher apparent rates of Mn oxidation. That is, the distinction between Mn binding and Mn oxidation is not always clear. To complicate the situation further, as Mn(II) is bound to Mn oxide surfaces, the rate of oxidation of the bound Mn(II) is increased relative to Mn(II) in solution (15, 20). Such autocatalysis occurs as a surface chemistry process, and therefore even under conditions of biological catalysis, considerable chemical oxidation occurs.

Finally, although many workers have presented very good arguments for specific pathways for Mn(II) oxidation under controlled laboratory conditions (14, 15, 20–24), there are a variety of other possible pathways that have not been excluded for biologically catalyzed Mn oxidation. Some of these possibilities are listed in Table 13.1, and as can be seen, they differ in their stoichiometries, their oxidants, the nature of their products, and the Mn oxides produced. It should be possible with careful analysis to distinguish between these pathways, but so far, unequivocal evidence of a biologically catalyzed oxidation has not been presented.

If we take all of this into account, we are not surprised that only recently have insights into specific biological mechanisms been obtained; enzymes that catalyze Mn(II) oxidation in cell-free crude extracts have been described (25–28), and one protein, from *Leptothrix discophora*, has been purified and shown to catalyze Mn oxidation (29, 30). These results and other recent findings are discussed in Section 13.2.

With regard to Mn reduction, the situation is operationally somewhat simpler, because the movement from a known solid that can be synthesized and characterized in the laboratory to a known soluble product, Mn(II), is

**TABLE 13.1  Oxidation of Mn(II) to Manganese Oxides**

|  | Ref. |
|---|---|
| $Mn^{2+} + \frac{1}{2}O_2 + 2OH^- \rightarrow MnO_2 + H_2O$ | 11 |
| $Mn^{2+} + \frac{1}{2}O_2 + H_2O \rightarrow MnO_2 + 2H^+$ | 23 |
| $Mn^{2+} + \frac{1}{4}O_2 + 2OH^- \rightarrow MnOOH + \frac{1}{2}H_2O$ | 23 |
| $Mn^{2+} + 2H_2O \rightarrow MnO_2 + 4H^+ + 2e^-$ | 23 |
| $Mn^{2+} + 2H_2O \rightarrow MnOOH + 3H^+ + e^-$ | 23 |
| $Mn^{2+} + \frac{1}{4}O_2 + \frac{3}{2}H_2O \rightarrow MnOOH + 2H^+$ | 24 |
| $Mn(II) + O_2 \rightarrow MnO_2$ (s) | 14 |
| $Mn(II) + MnO_2$ (s) $\rightarrow [Mn(II) \cdot MnO_2]$ (s) | |
| $[Mn(II) \cdot MnO_2]$ (s) $+ O_2 \rightarrow 2\ MnO_2$ | |
| $3\ Mn^{2+} \frac{1}{2}O_2 + 3\ H_2O \rightarrow Mn_3O_4$ (s) $+ 6H^+$ | 19 |
| $2\ MnOOH$ (s) $+ Mn^{2+} \rightarrow Mn_3O_4$ (s) $+ 2H^+$ | 19 |

easier to quantitate by standard methods. One can begin the experiments with a known solid phase, and manipulate it in more systematic and predictable ways. Furthermore, as reduction occurs, dissolution of Mn(II) can be quantified; surface-adsorbed Mn(II) can be deadsorbed and dissolution of Mn(II) into solution can both be easily measured (17, 18). Despite these advantages, the knowledge of mechanisms of Mn reduction is still meager, and no purified components of biological Mn reduction pathways have yet been obtained. Substantial physiological evidence has accumulated to suggest several different mechanisms may operate (12, 13, 31–33), including that of a Mn-reducing enzyme or electron-transfer system (31, 33). In Section 13.3, we review the status of knowledge concerning mechanisms of oxidation and reduction of Mn, and suggest some areas of needed research for the future.

## 13.2  MANGANESE OXIDATION

Since the early 1900s, the catalysis of Mn(II) oxidation by bacteria has been suspected (1, 4, 7, 8). In recent years many quantitative rate data have accumulated from the study of a variety of different aquatic and sedimentary environments, which unambiguously prove that bacteria with the capacity for Mn oxidation in these environments are *the primary* catalysts of Mn(II) oxidation (see Ref. 2 for a recent review). Manganese oxidation mechanisms can be operationally described as indirect or direct (Table 13.2).

TABLE 13.2   Possible Modes of Mn(II) Oxidation by Bacteria

| |
|---|
| I.   Indirect |
|       A.   Free radical and oxidant production |
|             1.   Hydrogen peroxide |
|             2.   Superoxide |
|       B.   Modification of redox environments |
|             1.   Oxygen production |
|             2.   pH modification |
|                   a.   $CO_2$ consumption |
|                   b.   Ammonia release |
| II.   Direct |
|       A.   Mn binding components |
|             1.   Proteins |
|             2.   Glycocalyxes |
|             3.   Cell wall components |
|       B.   Mn oxidase enzymes |

### 13.2.1 Indirect Oxidation

***13.2.1.1 Production of Hydrogen Peroxide.*** Dubinina (34, 35) has proposed that several groups of bacteria, including *Arthrobacter, Leptothrix,* and *Metallogenium,* catalyze Mn oxidation via the production of hydrogen peroxide. This oxidation is thought to take place at high pH values by the following mechanism:

$$Mn(II) + H_2O_2 \rightarrow MnO_2 + 2H^+$$

This oxidation is thought to protect cells from the harmful effects of hydrogen peroxide produced by the cells themselves. Along these lines, Fridovich and colleagues (36, 37) have found that Mn is a component of a protein referred to as pseudocatalase, which catalyzes the dismutation of $H_2O_2$ via the following reactions:

$$E-Mn(II) + H_2O_2 + 2H^+ \rightarrow Mn(V) + 2H_2O$$
$$Mn(V) + H_2O_2 \rightarrow Mn(III) + 2H^+ + O_2$$

These reactions aptly demonstrate the ability of Mn to interact with peroxide as both an oxidant and a reductant.

***13.2.1.2 Free Radical or Oxidant Production.*** The generation of oxidants such as superoxide or hydroxyl radicals by living cells is common under many conditions (38–41). When such oxidants are produced, they are commonly disposed of with the enzyme superoxide dismutase (SOD), which is a metal-containing enzyme found in nearly all living cells (38–41); bacterial SODs have either manganese or iron, whereas eukaryotic SODs contain Cu and Zn (42). Even in the absence of SOD, superoxide rapidly oxidizes Mn(II), and it has been hypothesized that Mn(II) actually serves as a detoxifying agent for oxygen-sensitive bacteria such as *Lactobacillus plantarum,* which have no SODs (38–41). In the absence of other protective mechanisms, Mn may serve a critical role in defense against oxygen. Unless a mechanism for recycling the oxidized Mn exists, the result of this process is the accumulation of intracellular Mn oxides, which in general has not been observed in living cells (10). For *L. plantarum,* the cells accumulate millimolar levels of Mn(II), which interacts with superoxide to produce Mn(III), which is then recycled to the reduced form via reduction with NADH (38–41).

***13.2.1.3 Eh and pH Modifications.*** Many Mn oxidation reactions require the presence of molecular oxygen (Table 13.1), so any organisms that produce oxygen might conceivably enhance the rate of Mn oxidation. Furthermore, Mn oxidation is second order with regard to pH, so organisms that can raise the pH can also enhance Mn oxidation. Phytoplankton, which are often implicated as agents of Mn oxidation in nature (43–45), are aptly

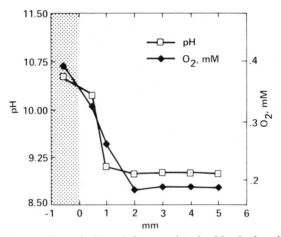

**Figure 13.1**   Microprofiles of pH and $O_2$ associated with planktonic aggregates of *Microcystis* sp. These measurements were made at Oneida Lake with commercially available microelectrodes using freshly collected natural aggregates of individual cells of *Microcystis*. 0 mm represents the interface between the edge of the aggregate and the surrounding water and positive distances were made at various positions above the aggregate. Data from Richardson et al. (45).

suited to this role via photosynthetic oxygen production and $CO_2$ removal. The most direct proof of this was recently presented for Mn oxidation by cyanobacteria in Oneida Lake, New York (45). Studies in both the laboratory and the field demonstrated the presence of microgradients of both oxygen and pH around clumps of phytoplankton (Fig. 13.1). In the microenvironments near the phytoplankton, oxygen is supersaturated, and pH reaches values of 10 or higher. Such conditions favor very rapid Mn oxidation, and may constitute a major means of oxidation by planktonic algae. In these studies, the Mn oxidation depended on active photosynthesis and was inhibited by the addition of strong buffer to the medium, suggesting that the mechanism primarily involved pH increase via $CO_2$ removal (45).

Another likely mechanism for Mn oxidation is pH modification via the production of ammonia. In many protein-rich environments, local pH changes are commonly seen in response to the deamination of amino acids and accumulation of ammonia. It has been suggested that this mechanism could be important for the oxidation of Mn(II) by fungi (46), but there have been no direct measurements confirming the importance of this process, either in the laboratory or in nature.

### 13.2.2   Direct Oxidation

Considerable interest over the years in the process of microbially catalyzed Mn oxidation has resulted in many reports of enzymatic activity in crude

**TABLE 13.3  Purified and Partially Purified Manganese Binding and Oxidizing Proteins**

| Organism | Type | Activity Binding | Oxidizing | Form | Refs. |
|---|---|---|---|---|---|
| *Leptothrix discophora* | Extracellular protein | + | + | Purified | 29, 30 |
| *Bacillus* SG-1 | Spore coat protein | + | + | Spore coats; partially | 47–49 |
| | Purified protein | | | | 50 |
| *Pseudomonas* sp. | Intracellular protein | + | + | Crude extract | 28 |
| *Pseudomonas* sp. and *Citrobacter* sp. | Intracellular protein | + | nd | Crude extract | 25, 26 |
| *Arthrobacter* 37 | Intracellular protein | + | nd | Crude extract | 27 |
| Bacterium FMn1 | Periplasmic/ membrane protein | + | nd | Crude extract | 53, 54 |

nd = Characteristic not directly tested for. It is common to measure the decrease in soluble Mn(II) concentration as an indirect estimate of Mn oxidation rather than directly measure formation of $MnO_2$.

cell-free extracts. More recently, there have been efforts to purify and biochemically characterize Mn binding and oxidizing proteins. Although not comprehensive, Table 13.3 describes representative reports of enzymatic manganese binding and oxidation; each of these reports is summarized and discussed in more detail in this section, starting with the most recent research.

### *13.2.2.1  Binding and Oxidizing Proteins.*

There have recently been efforts from a number of different laboratories to identify, purify, and characterize Mn binding and oxidizing proteins (Table 13.3)

Adams and Ghiorse (30) and Boogerd and de Vrind (29) independently reported isolation, purification, and initial characterization of an extracellular Mn oxidizing protein from *L. discophora* SS1. *Leptothrix* are normally sheathed organisms (see Chapter 1, Fig. 1.12), but *L. discophora* SS1, a mutant that has lost its organized sheath, produces structurally unorganized extracellular polysaccharide and protein exopolymers. A protein that is currently the best characterized Mn binding and oxidizing protein was purified from the extracellular growth medium (Table 13.4). In sodium dodecylsulfate–polyacrylamide gel electrophoresis (SDS–PAGE), the purified oxidizing protein is usually associated with polysaccharide material, and it is prob-

**TABLE 13.4  Characteristics of Purified *L. Discophora* SS1 Mn Oxidizing Protein**

| | |
|---|---|
| MW | 110,000 |
| Optimal pH | 7.3 |
| Optimal temperature | 28°C |
| Inhibitors of activity | Cyanide, azide, *o*-phenanthroline, mercuric chloride, pronase |
| $K_m$ | $7.0 \pm 3.2 \ \mu M$ |
| $V_{max}$ | 1.4 nmol Mn(II) oxidized $min^{-1} \ \mu g^{-1}$ |
| General comments | Extracellular protein; associated with polysaccharide in SDS–PAGE gel; stoichiometry of oxidation consistent with: $$Mn(II) + \tfrac{1}{2} O_2 + H_2O \rightarrow MnO_2 + 2 \ H^+$$ |

*Source:* Data compiled from Refs. 29 and 30.

able that in the mutant this protein is a component of the extracellular unorganized protein and polysaccharide material; it is perhaps also a component of the sheath in the wild-type parent. The authors note, however, that most of the Mn oxidizing activity was lost during purification (0.0004% recovery) and hence other factors or cell component(s) may be important in Mn oxidation by *L. discophora* SS1. Because Mn inhibits growth of SS-1 in batch culture, Adams and Ghiorse (30) speculate that Mn(II) oxidation does not provide energy for growth; rather it more likely detoxifies Mn(II) by converting it to $MnO_x$; in nature this mineral would be associated with the sheath.

A spore protein of *Bacillus* SG-1 has also been implicated as a Mn binding and oxidizing protein (Table 13.5; 47–51). Manganese binding and oxidizing activity is not found in vegetative cells of *Bacillus* SG-1. The activity has been localized in the spore coat; isolated spore coats bind and oxidize Mn

**TABLE 13.5  Characteristics of Partially Purified *Bacillus* SG-1 Mn Oxidizing Activity**

| | |
|---|---|
| MW | 205,000 |
| Optimal pH | ~8.0–8.5 |
| Optimal temperature | ~45°C |
| Inhibitors of activity | Cyanide, azide, mercuric chloride |
| $K_m$ | nd |
| $V_{max}$ | nd |
| General comments | Present only in spores, not vegetative cells; composed of ~5 different peptides; may be a glycoprotein or may be associated with acidic polysaccharide; oxidation occurs only under oxic conditions |

*Source:* Data compiled from Refs. 47–50.
nd = not determined.

at the same rate as intact spores (48). Recently Tebo et al., using SDS-PAGE electrophoresis (50), have shown a Mn oxidizing activity that bands with a molecular weight of about 205,000 D. This material is made up of at least five different peptides (based on excision of the band and electrophoresis of extracted protein material on a second SDS–PAGE gel) and material may also have polysaccharide associated with it (based on staining with Alcian Blue, as was observed with the *L. discophora* protein). The question of the role of this Mn oxidizing activity in SG-1 spore physiology is also unknown. It is unlikely that dealing with $O_2$, $H_2O_2$, or Mn toxicity is a problem for spores. As has been determined for most Mn oxidizing bacteria, however, the capacity to oxidize Mn is specific and unique; not all bacterial spores catalyze Mn oxidation. Tebo (52) proposed that SG-1 spores can use $MnO_2$ as a terminal electron acceptor for germination under anoxic conditions, which might give this organism a selective advantage for survival in natural environments by allowing germination and outgrowth of an activated spore under both oxic and anoxic conditions.

### 13.2.2.2 Binding and Oxidizing Activity in Crude Extracts.

Manganese binding and oxidizing enzymatic activities in crude cell extracts have been reported from a variety of laboratories for a number of years now. Some representative reports are described in this section (Table 13.3).

An intracellular Mn binding and oxidizing protein has been demonstrated in crude extracts of a *Pseudomonas* sp. by Jung and Schweisfurth (Table 13.6; 28). No activity was found in the spent culture medium nor was any activity demonstrated in cell wall or membrane fractions. The actual function of this protein in growth and metabolism of this organism is unknown. Jung and Schweisfurth (28) speculated that because the Mn oxidizing activity develops after onset of the stationary growth phase, it is not likely that new

TABLE 13.6  Characteristics of an Intracellular Mn Oxidizing Protein in Crude Extracts of a *Pseudomonas* Sp.

| | |
|---|---|
| MW | nd |
| Optimal pH | ~7.0 |
| Optimal temperature | 40°C |
| Inhibitors of activity | Heat (>50°C), pronase |
| $K_m$ | nd |
| $V_{max}$ | nd |
| General comments | Independent of Mn in culture medium; made by stationary phase cells only in ammonia-free or peptone-free media; same reaction rate under oxic or anoxic conditions; non-catalytic reaction/protein inactivated by oxidation process |

*Source:* Data compiled from Ref. 28.

nd = not determined.

**TABLE 13.7   Characteristics of an Intracellular Mn Oxidizing Protein in Crude Extracts of a *Pseudomonas* Sp. and of a *Citrobacter* Sp.**

| | |
|---|---|
| MW | nd |
| Optimal pH | 6.3–6.9 |
| Optimal temperature | nd |
| Inhibitors of activity | Heat (15 min at 100°C), mercuric chloride |
| $K_m{}^a$ | 2.52–3.33 $\mu$mol ml$^{-1}$ |
| $V_{max}{}^a$ | 1.25–2.04 $\mu$mol ml$^{-1}$ h$^{-1}$ |
| General comments | Oxidation occurs under aerobic conditions; constitutive activity; Mn$^{2+}$ concentration affects velocity of reaction |

*Source:* Data compiled from Refs. 25 and 26.

nd = not determined.

[a] Values determined in crude extracts.

protein synthesis is occurring, and hence an existing protein activity has been altered or modified.

The removal of Mn from solution in crude extracts has also been demonstrated for a *Pseudomonas* sp. and a *Citrobacter* sp. originally isolated from soil (Table 13.7; 25, 26). It was clearly demonstrated that an enzyme activity in crude cell-free extracts prepared from these two organisms catalyzed Mn oxidation. There was no speculation as to why these organisms, originally isolated from soil Mn concretions, oxidized Mn.

Research from Ehrlich's laboratory has clearly demonstrated a variety of enzymatic Mn oxidizing activities in various bacteria (5, 6, 11, 12, 27, 53, 54). Representative reports are summarized in Tables 13.8 and 13.9. These reports demonstrate the enzymatic nature of Mn oxidation in marine and freshwater bacterial isolates; the characteristics of these enzymes in whole cells and crude extracts suggest that there are a variety of Mn oxidizing

**TABLE 13.8   Characteristics of an Intracellular Mn Oxidizing Protein from Marine *Arthrobacter* 37**

| | |
|---|---|
| MW | nd |
| Optimal pH | nd |
| Optimal temperature | 17.5°C |
| Inhibitors of activity | Heat (1 min at 100°C), *p*-chloromercuribenzoate, mercuric chloride |
| $K_m$ | nd |
| $V_{max}$ | nd |
| General comments | Oxidation requires O$_2$; Mn$^{2+}$ concentration affects velocity; activity requires presence of MnO$_2$ |

*Source:* Data compiled from Ref. 27.

nd = not determined.

**TABLE 13.9   Characteristics of a Periplasmic/Membrane Bound Mn Oxidizing Protein from Freshwater Bacterium, FMn1**

| | |
|---|---|
| MW | nd |
| Optimal pH | 7.0 |
| Optimal temperature | 30°C |
| Inhibitors of activity | Heat (1–15 min at 100°C) protease |
| $K_m$ | nd |
| $V_{max}$ | nd |
| General comments | Oxidation requires $O_2$; $Mn^{2+}$ concentration affects velocity of reaction; enzyme may be loosely membrane bound; activity requires dialyzable cofactor; inducible activity |

*Source:* Data compiled from Refs. 53 and 54.

nd = not determined.

activities and systems. As with most reports of Mn oxidation by bacteria, it is not clear why these organisms oxidize Mn.

### 13.2.2.3  *Exopolysaccharides.*

The presence of extracellular polymers (e.g., glycocalyxes, capsules, slimes), outside of the cell wall is often observed in bacteria in natural environments (10, 51). Such exopolymers may or may not form distinctive structures. Ultrastructural evidence (TEM of thin sections of ruthenium red stained samples) suggests that Mn oxides are associated with acidic polysaccharides on the cell surface of many, if not most, Mn-depositing bacteria (10, 51, 52). This compelling circumstantial evidence implicates the acidic polysaccharides as the site of Mn binding and oxidation. Many authors have suggested that Mn is first bound by polysaccharides and then is either autooxidized because of an increased concentration of Mn or is oxidized by specific Mn oxidizing proteins (8, 10, 11). Ghiorse (10) emphasized, however, that the presence of acidic polysaccharides is consistent with Mn deposition, but Mn deposition does not depend solely on the simple presence of these polysaccharides; even though polysaccharides may be present, Mn oxides are often not deposited and therefore other factors must be involved in oxidation of Mn.

Nealson and Tebo (51) and Tebo (52), based on TEM of ruthenium red stained thin sections, also observed that precipitated Mn oxides are often deposited in association with acidic polysaccharides on cell surfaces. For example, *Bacillus* SG-1 has ruthenium red staining material surrounding the outermost spore coat layers and Mn is apparently deposited within this layer (2, 51, 52). *Pseudomonas* S-36, a Mn oxidizing bacterium whose growth in a carbon-limited chemostat is stimulated by Mn(II) (55), also deposits Mn oxides within ruthenium red-staining surface-associated layers (2, 51, 52). No Mn binding or oxidizing proteins have been found in this organism to date.

*13.2.2.4  Cell Wall Components.* It is also known that cell wall and outer membrane components have significant ion exchange capacity and may be involved in binding many divalent cations including Mn (for details of this work, see Chapters 1, 9, and 10 by Beveridge, Doyle, and Ferris, respectively; 56). Whether or not such binding can lead to increased levels of Mn autooxidation is currently unknown. However, we speculate that this is not significant for living populations of bacteria because all heterotrophic eubacteria have cell walls with ion exchange capacity and yet only a limited number can be identified as having the capacity to bind and oxidize Mn. These macromolecules may, however, be significant nucleating sites for deposition of Mn after the organisms die, settle to, and are subsequently buried within sediments (10, 56).

*13.2.2.5  Manganese Oxidases.* All the proteins described above catalyze Mn oxide formation. For two of these proteins [*L. discophora* (30) and *Bacillus* SG-1 spore protein (48)], the stoichiometry of the reaction has been determined and found to be consistent with the overall equation listed in Tables 13.4 and 13.5, thus implicating these enzymes as possible oxidases. The *Pseudomonas* sp. protein described by Jung and Schweisfurth (28) does not require molecular oxygen as a substrate and hence is not an oxidase. Further characterization of purified Mn oxidizing proteins should lead to a better understanding of the mechanisms by which these enzymes catalyze Mn oxidation.

### 13.2.3  Summary of Manganese Oxidation Mechanisms

*13.2.3.1  What Do We Really Know about Manganese Oxidation?* Virtually all living organisms require Mn in trace amounts, and those that have been examined have efficient systems for transporting Mn(II) into the cells; however, it is very difficult to establish conditions where Mn is growth-limiting (see Ref. 2 for a recent summary). The capacity to oxidize Mn, in contrast to the general metabolic requirement, is found only in a limited number of microorganisms. Yet this characteristic is widespread among the various genera of bacteria, suggesting that different types of Mn oxidizing systems may have independently arisen many times in the course of evolution. Yet we still do not understand what the physiological significance of the capacity to oxidize Mn is for most groups of Mn oxidizing microorganisms. We do know that in most cases enzymes are required for Mn oxidation by microorganisms. There is, of course, some evidence that oxidation of Mn(II) may be a defense against Mn toxicity in heterotrophic bacteria (see Ref. 10 for review). If not for detoxification, however, how does Mn oxidation relate to cellular metabolism? There is currently no answer to this question. The search also continues for a Mn chemolithotroph or Mn mixotroph that uses Mn as an inorganic energy source. Unequivocal evidence of either of these inorganic energy generating processes remains to be demonstrated (2, 6, 8, 10, 11, 55).

**13.2.3.2** *Requirements for Future Studies.* Knowledge of the biochemistry of Mn oxidation (mechanisms of catalysis, the rates of reactions by specific cell components, and the relative capacity of different cell components to bind and oxidize Mn) is required if we are to understand the relation between manganese oxidation and the physiology of the Mn oxidizing microorganisms. It is quite clear that much more effort should be directed toward an understanding of the specific roles that glycocalyxes, cell walls, outer membrane (and spore coat) components, and the specific Mn binding and oxidizing proteins, of both Gram-negative and Gram-positive bacteria, play in binding and enhancing Mn oxidation. It is time for microbiologists and biochemists to work together to determine, in at least a few well characterized systems, the actual mechanisms of manganese oxidation.

## 13.3 MANGANESE REDUCTION MECHANISMS

In some respects, the mechanisms of bacterially mediated Mn reduction are better understood than those of oxidation, as some indirect modes of reduction of Mn(III) and Mn(IV) have been recently elucidated. As with Mn oxidation (Table 13.2), we can separate the mechanisms of reduction into direct and indirect processes (Table 13.10).

### 13.3.1 Indirect Reduction

**13.3.1.1** *Hydrogen Peroxide.* Evidence has been presented by several authors that Mn(IV) reduction can occur as a function of peroxide production by bacteria (13, 34, 35). The reaction should proceed according to

TABLE 13.10  **Possible Modes of Mn(IV) Reduction by Bacteria**

I.  Indirect
    A.  Production of inorganic reductants
        1.  Hydrogen peroxide ($H_2O_2$)
        2.  Sulfide ($S^{2-}$)
        3.  Ferrous iron ($Fe^{2+}$)
    B.  Production of organic reductants
        1.  Organic acids
        2.  Organic thiols
        3.  Quinones, phenols
    C.  Extracellular catalysts (enzymes)
II. Direct
    A.  Enzymes that catalyze Mn(IV) reduction
        1.  Manganese reductase
        2.  Other reductases

$$H_2O_2 + MnO_2 + 2H^+ \rightarrow Mn^{2+} + 2H_2O + O_2$$

Dubinina (34, 35) showed that peroxide production stimulated Mn reduction, and that this could be inhibited by catalase. Ghiorse (13, 57) also demonstrated that *Bacillus* 29 reduced Mn(IV) via peroxide production, and has proposed a model whereby this occurs. Interestingly, if peroxide production is a naturally occurring mechanism of importance, then it will be restricted to environments with molecular oxygen ($O_2$), for there are no known mechanisms for production of $H_2O_2$ in the absence of $O_2$. Such environments might be in oxygenated soils where rhizosphere bacteria or fungi might participate in the mobilization of Mn for plant growth.

***13.3.1.2  Sulfide.*** Hydrogen sulfide ($H_2S$) is a potent reductant of Mn(IV) (18). The reaction is very rapid and proceeds according to the following stoichiometry:

$$MnO_2 + HS^- + 3H^+ \rightarrow Mn^{2+} + 2H_2O + S^0$$

Thus any bacteria that generate free sulfide as an end product of dissimilatory reduction of sulfur compounds (e.g., $SO_4^{2-}$, $S_2O_3^{2-}$) are potential Mn-reducing organisms. Burdige and Nealson (18) demonstrated this for two isolates of *Desulfovibrio* obtained from offshore sediments, showing that growth was coupled to sulfide production, and that this in turn was coupled to Mn(IV) reduction. These authors proposed that in anaerobic marine environments (sediments and anaerobic basins) sulfate reduction (i.e., sulfide production) represents the major mechanism of Mn(IV) reduction; furthermore, in some environments, Mn might act as a carrier of reducing power between the carbon and sulfur cycles, as shown in Figure 13.2. As for peroxide, the mechanism is strictly an inorganic redox reaction, although the occurrence of this mechanism would be confined to anaerobic zones that support the growth of dissimilatory sulfur or sulfate-reducing bacteria.

In addition to sulfate-reducing bacteria, many bacteria have the ability to reductively disproportionate thiosulfate ($S_2O_3^{2-}$) to sulfite ($SO_3^{2-}$) and sulfide ($S^{2-}$) (58). This can result in rapid reduction of Mn(IV), as shown for strain MR-1 for which the rate of Mn reduction is markedly increased in the presence of $S_2O_3^{2-}$ (Fig. 13.3a; note that strain MR-1 is also able to directly reduce Mn(IV)—see Section 13.3.2). Again, the mechanism is strictly inorganic, but the source of the sulfide is from a different sulfur compound, and produced via a different mechanism.

***13.3.1.3  Ferrous Iron.*** Ferrous iron ($Fe^{2+}$) is a reductant of Mn(IV) oxides under both acidic (58a) and neutral pH conditions (Fig. 13.4), and under anaerobic conditions can cause rapid Mn reduction. Thus any proficient iron reducing bacterium is potentially a good Mn reducing bacterium if the conditions are appropriate. An example of this effect is shown in Figure 13.3b,

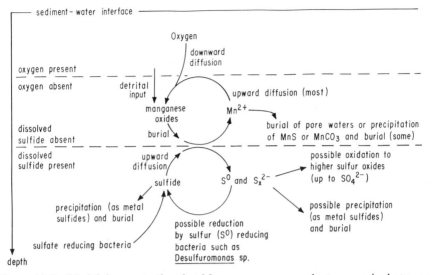

**Figure 13.2**   Model demonstrating that Mn may serve as an electron carrier between $O_2$ and sulfide, coupling electron flow between these spatially separated regions (18). This model suggests that manganese redox processes could be important in explaining the observations of Jørgensen (95), who noted that in many coastal marine sediments $O_2$ and sulfide are separated by a zone in which neither compound can be detected, and yet sulfide is reoxidized to sulfate with $O_2$ serving as the ultimate electron acceptor.

where the rate and extent of Mn reduction by MR-1 is enhanced by the addition of ferric iron to the culture. Many bacteria have the capacity to reduce Fe(III) (9, 12, 13, 32, 33, 59–77). Because almost all sediments that are rich in oxidized Mn also contain Fe, one should not consider the reduction of one in isolation from the other. As was seen with the reduction of Mn by sulfide, the ultimate reduction is a simple inorganic redox reaction:

$$2Fe^{2+} + MnO_2 + H_2O \rightarrow Fe_2O_3 + Mn^{2+} + 2H^+$$

The presence of Mn oxides in the environment, therefore, could allow for substantial reduction of either iron or sulfate without the reduced products ($Fe^{2+}$ or $S^{2-}$) appearing. That $Fe^{2+}$ does not accumulate until reduction of Mn oxides is complete is shown for strain MR-1 in Fig. 13.5 (note that MR-1 has the ability to reduce both Mn(IV) and Fe(III) directly—see Section 13.3.2). Also, the addition of $MnO_2$ to cultures that have accumulated Fe(II) results in the "immediate" appearance of Mn(II) and the concurrent disappearance of Fe(II) (78). The important implication of this in terms of an environmental perspective is that although one process (e.g., Mn reduction/solubilization) may be observed by measurement, the driving force and

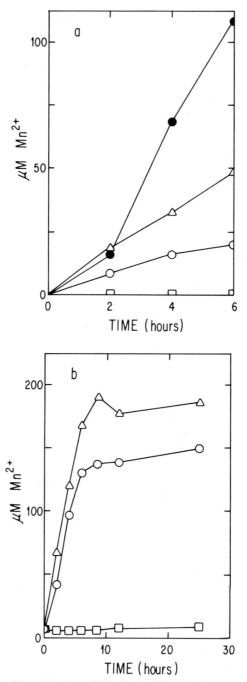

**Figure 13.3**    Anaerobic reduction of $MnO_2$ by MR-1 in the presence of thiosulfate or ferric iron. (a) Reduction of $MnO_2$ by MR-1 in the presence of 0.5 m$M$ ($\triangle$), 2m$M$ ($\bullet$), or no thiosulfate ($\bigcirc$); $MnO_2$ was not reduced by 2 m$M$ thiosulfate in the absence

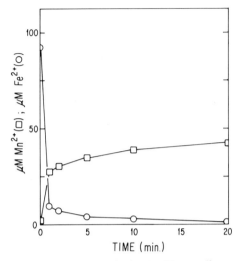

**Figure 13.4** Chemical reduction of MnO₂ by Fe(II). Medium was made 92 μ$M$ in Fe(II) with FeSO₄; after the zero time sample was taken, MnO₂ was added to a concentration of 260 μ$M$ and samples were taken and analyzed for Fe(II) (○) and Mn(II) (□). The experiment was conducted under anaerobic conditions at 24°C and pH 7.4 (78).

hence the organisms responsible for the process may be doing something quite different. Conversely, if one is monitoring the reduction of Fe or S by the accumulation of $Fe^{2+}$ and $S^{2-}$, respectively, then these processes might be scored as falsely low in the presence of Mn oxides.

**13.3.1.4 Organic Acids.** Several studies of Mn(III/IV) reduction by organic compounds have been reported (79–81). These reactions are strongly affected by pH; at pH values of 5 or less, nearly all organic acids tested catalyzed Mn reduction, whereas at pH 7.2, only pyruvate and oxalate were active in Mn reduction (79). The reduction of Mn(IV) by pyruvic acid is an example of this type of reaction:

$$CH_3(CO)COOH + MnO_2 + 2H^+ \rightarrow Mn^{2+} + CO_2 + CH_3COOH + H_2O$$

Presumably, any organism that excretes organic acids and lowers the pH could use Mn oxides as an external electron sink. For example, Strand (82)

of cells (□). (b) Reduction of MnO₂ by MR-1 in the presence of 1 m$M$ (△) or no Fe(III) (○); MnO₂ was not reduced by Fe(III) in the absence of cells (□). The initial concentration of MnO₂ was 0.215 m$M$. See Myers and Nealson (78) for complete procedural details.

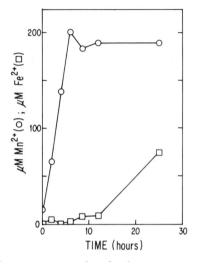

**Figure 13.5** Fe(II) does not accumulate in the presence of $MnO_2$. MR-1 was incubated anaerobically in the presence of 2 m$M$ Fe(III) and 0.215 m$M$ $MnO_2$. Reduction of the $MnO_2$ was essentially complete by 6 h as indicated by the levels of $Mn^{2+}$ (O). Fe(II) (□) did not appear until after Mn reduction was complete. This would be expected as any Fe(II) produced would be reoxidized by chemically reducing $MnO_2$ (78).

isolated a marine Mn reducer (SK-13sp) that showed increased anaerobic growth yield in the presence of Mn oxides. The reduction of Mn oxides occurred under both aerobic and anaerobic conditions, but occurred much faster at lower pH values. It was found that metabolites accumulated in the growth medium which could reduce Mn oxides after the cells were removed. These metabolites were identified as pyruvate and acetate. The increased growth under anaerobic conditions was attributed to the Mn oxides acting as an external electron sink and pH buffer. This organism, SK-13sp, may represent a class of organisms that are of potential importance in sedimentary environments, especially in those environments where the pH may be low.

### 13.3.1.5 Organic Thiols, Phenols, and Quinones.
Organic thiols, phenols, and quinones can rapidly reduce Mn oxides (79, 81, 83). To our knowledge, these reactions have not been observed with pure cultures of bacteria, but there is no reason to dismiss them without careful study. Under nutrient-limiting or stressful conditions, bacteria are known to release many different classes of compounds, and the possibility that such compounds might be released should be carefully examined. Of the compounds tested at pH 7.2 by Stone and Morgan (79), those most reactive with regard to Mn reduction included catechol, 3,4-dihydroxybenzoic acid, thiosalicylate, and hydroquinone. Clearly, if an organism were able to develop a differential transport

system for the oxidized and reduced forms, such compounds would provide a distinct advantage for disposal of reducing equivalents under anaerobic conditions in the presence of Mn oxides.

***13.3.1.6 Summary of Indirect Reduction.*** In all the reactions discussed above, the mechanism of Mn reduction by bacteria is linked to the physiology of given processes in the cell ($H_2O_2$ excretion, sulfur dissimilation, iron dissimilation, organic acid excretion). The problem thus becomes one of microbial metabolism rather than biochemistry per se. Such reactions must be kept in mind, however, for in many environments they may predominate and even obviate the need for (or the possibility of) direct reactions by respiratory bacteria as described below.

## 13.3.2 Direct Manganese Reduction

For the purpose of this chapter, direct reduction of Mn is limited to those Mn-reductive processes that are cell-mediated, and that result in the reduction of oxidized Mn as a result of electron transfer (i.e., via electron-transport-linked Mn reductase systems). Although numerous studies indicate that bacteria may link Mn reduction to the oxidation of organic substrates (17, 57, 69–71, 84–90), the importance of this reduction in the mineralization of organic carbon in anaerobic environments is not clear. Although an early study (91) demonstrated that under anaerobic conditions, Mn oxides could substitute for $O_2$ as an electron acceptor in a number of biological redox reactions, studies with pure bacterial cultures have shown that $O_2$, the energetically more favorable electron acceptor, does not inhibit microbial Mn reduction (12, 13, 86, 87, 90). Until recently (see below), only a single report of obligately anaerobic microbially mediated Mn reduction existed (92), and this study was not done with pure cultures. What characteristics would one expect to be associated with obligately anaerobic direct Mn reducers? The key characteristics, recently stated by Ehrlich (12), are as follows:

1. The organism(s) should prefer anaerobic conditions for reduction of Mn oxides (i.e., one would expect $O_2$ to inhibit Mn reduction).
2. Contact of the cells with the insoluble Mn oxides should be necessary for Mn reduction.
3. The conditions required for Mn reduction should be consistent with an enzymatic process (pH, temperature, etc.).
4. The organism(s) should couple anaerobic growth to the reduction of Mn oxides.

Recently, two different organisms have been isolated that meet these criteria. Both organisms were isolated using a similar approach—to enrich for organisms that would grow on "nonfermentable" carbon sources with specific electron acceptors [either Mn(IV) or Fe(III)] under anaerobic conditions.

The first of these organisms, GS-15, was isolated from the freshwater sediments of the Potomac River, Maryland, by Lovley and Phillips (33) as an Fe(III) reducer. GS-15 is a Gram-negative, nonmotile, rod-shaped bacterium; it is a strict anaerobe and has not yet been taxonomically classified. GS-15 is able to grow with acetate as the sole electron donor and Fe(III), Mn(IV), or nitrate ($NO_3^-$) as the sole electron acceptor (33); growth yield values were not reported, but it is clear that growth was coupled to the reduction of these electron acceptors. Reduction of Fe(III) by GS-15 is optimal at 30–35°C and at pH 6.7–7; butyrate, propionate, and ethanol could also serve as electron donors for Fe(III) reduction, whereas hydrogen and a variety of other organic compounds could not.

The second of these organisms, designated MR-1, was isolated from the anaerobic sediments of Oneida Lake, New York (31, 78) as a Mn(IV) reducer. MR-1 is a facultatively anaerobic Gram-negative rod; conventional biochemical taxonomic tests classify MR-1 as a strain of *Alteromonas putrefaciens* (all taxonomic test results were identical to those of the type strain *A. putrefaciens* ATCC 8071). MR-1 is a nonfermentative, obligately respiratory bacterium that can couple its growth to the reduction of Mn(IV) (Fig. 13.6; 31), as well as a large variety of other electron acceptors including oxygen ($O_2$), nitrate ($NO_3^-$), nitrite ($NO_2^-$), ferric iron [Fe(III)], trimethylamine N-oxide (TMAO), glycine, fumarate, sulfite ($SO_3^{2-}$), tetrathionate ($S_4O_6^{2-}$), and thiosulfate ($S_2O_3^{2-}$); it is unable to use sulfate ($SO_4^{2-}$), carbon dioxide ($CO_2$), or molybdate ($MoO_4^{2-}$) as electron acceptors (31). Growth of MR-1 in the presence of $MnO_2$ as the sole electron acceptor (Fig. 13.6) resulted in molar growth yield values of 9–45 g of cell dry weight produced per mole of $MnO_2$ reduced. These values are similar to growth yield values reported for other bacteria, which range from 13 to 100 g of cells per mole of oxygen reduced with oxygen as the electron acceptor (93); values for *Paracoccus denitrificans* range from 16 to 39 g of cells per mole of nitrate or oxygen reduced (93).

MR-1 can use lactate as a carbon source and electron donor for growth, but cannot use a variety of other organics including arabinose, butyrate, cellobiose, citrate, fructose, galactose, glucose, inositol, malate, malonate, maltose, mannitol, mannose, melibiose, propionate, raffinose, rhamnose, sorbitol, sucrose, valerate, xylitol, and xylose (Myers and Nealson, unpublished). MR-1 can apparently use pyruvate, formate, and $H_2$ as an electron donor for the reduction of Mn(IV) (D. Lovley, personal communication). The type strain of *A. putrefaciens*, ATCC 8071, originally isolated from butter (94), parallels MR-1 in its use of electron acceptors [including Mn(IV) and Fe(III); 31] and donors. Other recent studies (73, 74) report the ability of several other strains of *A. putrefaciens* to use sulfite, thiosulfate, and Fe(III) as terminal electron acceptors.

Mn reduction by MR-1 is proportional to cell density and is optimal at

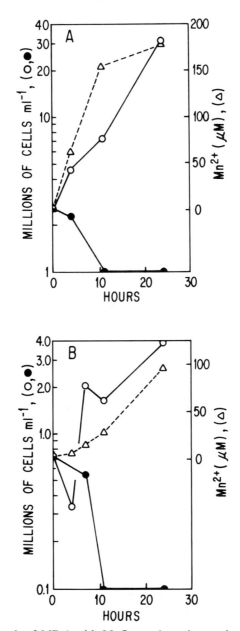

**Figure 13.6** Growth of MR-1 with $MnO_2$ as the sole terminal electron acceptor. Anaerobic growth of MR-1 in the presence of 2 m$M$ $MnO_2$ was monitored by cell number increases ($\bigcirc$). Reduction of $MnO_2$ as shown by increases in Mn(II) ($\triangle$) paralleled cell number increases. Cell numbers declined in the absence of $MnO_2$ ($\bullet$). The cell counts shown at baseline on the $x$ axis represent $<10^3$ cells ml$^{-1}$. The experiments shown were conducted in a defined medium ($A$) and in an undefined medium ($B$) designated LO. See Myers and Nealson (31) for complete procedural details.

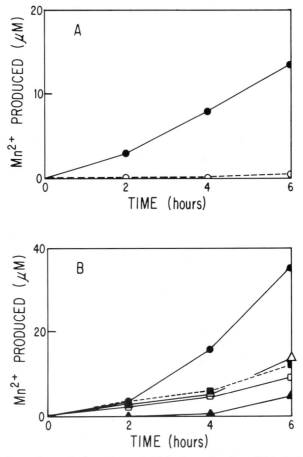

**Figure 13.7**  O$_2$ and metabolic poisons inhibit the reduction of MnO$_2$ by MR-1. (A) Reduction of MnO$_2$ by MR-1 in the presence (○) and absence (●) of O$_2$. (B) Reduction of MnO$_2$ by MR-1 in the presence of 0.2% formaldehyde (△), 100 μ$M$ antimycin A (■), and 100 μ$M$ CCCP (□). MnO$_2$ reduction without inhibitors in the presence (●) and absence (▲) of MR-1. See Myers and Nealson (31) for complete procedural details.

pH 6–7 and 30–35°C (31). Although MR-1 is able to use O$_2$ as an electron acceptor, the presence of O$_2$ inhibits Mn reduction by this strain (Fig. 13.7a). Mn reduction by MR-1 is also inhibited by several electron transport inhibitors including 100 μ$M$ antimycin A (Fig. 14.7b), 1 m$M$ azide, 10 μ$M$ 2-heptyl-hydroxyquinolone $N$-oxide (HQNO), and 100 μ$M$ dicumarol, but was not inhibited by 200 μ$M$ cyanide (31). Mn reduction by MR-1 is also inhibited by the protonophore uncouplers dinitrophenol and carbonyl cyanide $m$-chlorophenyl hydrazone (CCCP; Fig. 13.7b) and by 0.2% formaldehyde (Fig.

13.7*b*; 31). These growth yield and inhibitor studies strongly implicate the involvement of energy-yielding electron transport-mediated processes in the reduction of Mn oxides by MR-1.

The isolation and characterization of these organisms, GS-15 and MR-1, in pure culture clearly indicate that the process of dissimilatory reduction of Mn(IV) and Fe(III) provides a mode for survival and growth for some organisms. In environments where Fe and Mn reach high concentrations, this may be an environmentally significant process. Direct reduction of Mn and Fe may be particularly important in anaerobic freshwater environments where the levels of sulfate are relatively low. With regard to mechanisms, we must echo the words of both Ghiorse (13) and Ehrlich (12), who point out the paucity of knowledge regarding actual mechanisms, especially with regard to direct reducers. However, it seems clear that organisms are now in hand that should provide material for dissection of Mn reductases and Fe reductases and the associated electron-transfer systems.

### 13.3.3  Summary of Manganese Reduction Mechanisms

Many studies have clearly demonstrated the ability of several bacteria to mediate the reduction of Mn oxides. Bacteria that excrete certain metabolic end products may indirectly mediate Mn reduction via these products. Examples of such Mn reducing compounds include sulfide, organic acids, thiols, phenols, quinones, $H_2O_2$, and Fe(II). Some bacteria are also able to directly mediate the reduction of Mn oxides via electron-transport-linked Mn reductase systems. In particular, recent reports (31, 33) demonstrate the ability of two different bacteria (MR-1 and GS-15) to couple their growth to the reduction of Mn oxides under anaerobic conditions. These two isolates may provide excellent model systems for understanding the biochemistry and physiology of Mn reduction.

In recent experiments, we have demonstrated respiratory-driven proton translocation for anaerobic cells of MR-1, using lactate as the reductant and $MnO_2$ as the electron acceptor (Myers and Nealson, abstract submitted to 1988 meetings of the Amer. Soc. for Microbiology). Rapid proton translocation was also observed with other terminal electron acceptors used by MR-1 for growth (31), including nitrate, Fe(III), thiosulfate, fumarate, and oxygen. Proton translocation was not observed with electron acceptors not utilized by MR-1 (e.g. sulfate). Proton pulses were abolished by the presence of the protonophore CCCP and by the electron transport inhibitor HQNO. Aerobically grown cells were capable of generating proton fluxes only with $O_2$ as the electron acceptor, and not with any of the anaerobic electron acceptors, including $MnO_2$. These results provide direct biochemical proof that MR-1 can obtain energy from the use of $MnO_2$ and Fe(III) as terminal electron acceptors for anaerobic respiration.

## ACKNOWLEDGMENTS

We wish to acknowledge the following colleagues who provided us with preprints, reprints, and discussion, and who allowed us to cite unpublished results; L. Adams, F. Archibald, T. Beveridge, G. Ferris, I. Fridovich, W. Ghiorse, P. Kepkay, D. Lovley, A. Stone, W. Sunda, and B. Tebo. We would like to clearly state, however, that the views presented in this review are solely the interpretations and perspectives of the authors. NSF Ocean Sciences Division (Marine Chemistry), NASA (Terrestrial Ecology Program), and the Shaw Foundation (University of Wisconsin-Milwaukee) have provided much of the support of the original research originating in KHN's laboratory.

## REFERENCES

1. M. W. Beijerinck, Oxydation des manganbikarbonates durch bakterien und schimmelpilze, *Folia Microbiol.* (Delft), *2*, 123–134 (1913).
2. K. H. Nealson, B. M. Tebo, and R. A. Rosson, Occurrence and mechanisms of microbial oxidation of manganese, *Adv. Appl. Microbiol., 33,* 279–319 (1988).
3. R. Schweisfurth, Untersuchungen uber manganooxydierende und -reduzierende mikroorganismen, *Mitt. Internat. Vereinigg. Limnol., 14,* 179–186 (1968).
4. S. I. Kuznetsov, The role of microorganisms in the formation of lake bottom deposits and their diagenesis. *Soil Sci., 119,* 81–88 (1970).
5. H. L. Ehrlich, "Manganese as an energy source for bacteria," in J. O. Nriagu, Ed., *Environmental Biogeochemistry,* Ann Arbor Press, Ann Arbor, MI, 1976, p. 633–644.
6. H. L. Ehrlich, Inorganic energy sources for chemolithotrophic and mixotrophic bacteria, *Geomicrobiology J., 1,* 65–83 (1978).
7. K. C. Marshall, "Biogeochemistry of manganese minerals," in P. A. Trudinger and D. J. Swaine, Eds., *Biogeochemical Cycling of Mineral-Forming Elements,* Elsevier, Amsterdam, 1979, pp. 253–292.
8. H. L. Ehrlich, *Geomicrobiology,* Dekker, New York, 1981, 393 p.
9. K. H. Nealson, "The microbial manganese cycle," in W. Krumbein, Ed., *Microbial Geochemistry,* Blackwell Scientific, Oxford, 1983, pp. 191–222.
10. W. C. Ghiorse, Biology of iron- and manganese-depositing bacteria, *Ann. Rev. Microbiol., 38,* 515–550 (1984).
11. H. L. Ehrlich, "Different forms of bacterial manganese oxidation," in W. R. Strohl and O. Tuovinen, Eds., *Microbial Chemoautotrophy,* Ohio State University Press, Columbus, 1984, pp. 47–56.
12. H. L. Ehrlich, Manganese oxide reduction as a form of anaerobic reduction, *Geomicrobiol. J., 5,* 423–431 (1987).
13. W. C. Ghiorse, "Microbial reduction of manganese and iron," in A. J. Zehnder, Ed., *Biology of Anaerobic Microorganisms,* Wiley, New York, 1988, pp. 305–331.

14. W. Stumm and J. J. Morgan, *Aquatic Chemistry*, 2nd Ed., Wiley, New York, 1981, 780 pp.

15. J. W. Murray, The surface chemistry of hydrous manganese dioxide, *J. Colloid Interface Sci., 46*, 357–371 (1974).

16. L. Balistrieri and J. Murray, The surface chemistry of $MnO_2$ in major ion seawater, *Geochim. Cosmochim. Acta, 46*, 1041–1052 (1982).

17. S. M. Bromfield and D. J. David, Sorption and oxidation of manganous ions and reduction of manganese oxide by cell suspensions of a manganese oxidizing bacterium, *Soil Biol. Biochem., 8*, 37–43 (1976).

18. D. J. Burdige and K. H. Nealson, Chemical and microbiological studies of sulfide-mediated manganese reduction, *Geomicrobiol. J., 4*, 361–387 (1986).

19. D. Hastings and S. Emerson, Oxidation of manganese by spores of a marine bacillus: kinetic and thermodynamic considerations, *Geochim. Cosmochim. Acta, 50*, 1819–1824 (1986).

20. J. F. Pankow and J. J. Morgan, Kinetics for the aquatic environment, *Environ. Sci. Technol., 15*, 1306–1313 (1981).

21. W. Sung and J. J. Morgan, Oxidative removal of Mn(II) from solution by $\gamma$-FeOOH (lepidocrocite) surface, *Geochim. Cosmochim. Acta, 45*, 2377–2383 (1981).

22. J. F. Pankow and J. J. Morgan, Kinetics for the aquatic environment, *Environ. Sci. Technol., 15*, 1155–1164 (1981).

23. D. Crerar, A. Fischer, and C. L. Plaza, "Metallogenium and biogenic deposition of manganese from Precambrian to recent time," in I. M. Varentsov and C. Grasselly, Eds., *Geology and Geochemistry of Manganese*, Hungarian Acad. Sci., Schweizerbart'sche Verlag, Stuttgart, 1981, pp. 285–303.

24. D. Diem and W. Stumm, Is dissovled $Mn^{2+}$ being oxidized by $O_2$ in absence of Mn-bacteria or surface catalysts?, *Geochim. Cosmochim Acta, 48*, 1571–1573 (1984).

25. C. E. Douka, Study of bacteria from manganese concretions. Precipitation of manganese by whole cells and cell-free extracts of isolated bacteria, *Soil Biol. Biochem., 9*, 89–97 (1977).

26. C. E. Douka, Kinetics of manganese oxidation by cell-free extracts of bacteria isolated from manganese concretions from soil, *Appl. Env. Microbiol., 39*, 74–80 (1980).

27. H. L. Ehrlich, Bacteriology of manganese nodules II; manganese oxidation by cell-free extract from a manganese nodule bacterium, *Appl. Microbiol., 16*, 197–202 (1968).

28. W. K. Jung and R. Schweisfurth, Manganese oxidation by an intracellular protein of a *Pseudomonas* species, *Z. Allg. Mikrobiol., 19*, 107–115 (1979).

29. R. C. Boogerd and J. P. M. de Vrind, Manganese oxidation by *Leptothrix discophora*, *J. Bacteriol., 169*, 489–494 (1987).

30. L. Adams and W. C. Ghiorse, Characterization of an extracellular $Mn^{2+}$-oxidizing activity and isolation of $Mn^{2+}$-oxidizing protein from *Leptothrix discophora* SS-1, *J. Bacteriol., 169*, 1279–1285 (1987).

31. C. R. Myers and K. H. Nealson, Bacterial manganese reduction and growth with manganese oxide as the sole electron acceptor, *Science, 240*, 1319–1321 (1988).

32. D. R. Lovley, J. F. Stolz, G. L. Nord, Jr., and E. J. P. Phillips, Anaerobic production of magnetite by a dissimilatory iron-reducing microorganism, *Nature* (London), *330*, 252–254 (1987).

33. D. R. Lovley and E. J. P. Phillips, Novel mode of microbial energy metabolism: organic carbon oxidation coupled to dissimilatory reduction of iron or manganese, *Appl. Environ. Microbiol., 54*, 1472–1480 (1988).

34. G. A. Dubinina, Mechanism of the oxidation of bivalent iron and manganese by iron bacteria growing at neutral pH of the medium, *Microbiology USSR, 47*, 471–478 (1979).

35. G. A. Dubinina, Functional role of bivalent iron and manganese oxidation in *Leptothrix pseudoochraceae, Microbiology USSR, 47*, 631–636 (1979).

36. Y. Kono and I. Fridovich, Isolation and characterization of the pseudocatalase of *Lactobacillus plantarum, J. Biol. Chem., 258*, 6015–6019 (1983).

37. W. F. Beyer and I. Fridovich, Pseudocatalase from *Lactobacillus plantarum*: evidence for a homopentameric structure containing two atoms of manganese per subunit, *Biochemistry, 24*, 6460–6467 (1985).

38. F. S. Archibald and I. Fridovich, Manganese and defenses against oxygen toxicity in *Lactobacillus plantarum, J. Bacteriol., 145*, 442–451 (1981).

39. F. S. Archibald and I. Fridovich, The scavenging of superoxide radical by manganous complexes: in vitro, *Arch. Biochem. Biophys., 214*, 452–463 (1982).

40. F. S. Archibald and I. Fridovich, Investigations of the state of the manganese in *Lactobacillus plantarum, Arch. Biochem. Biophys., 215*, 589–596 (1982).

41. F. S. Archibald and M. Duong, Manganese acquisition by *Lactobacillus plantarum, J. Bacteriol., 158*, 1–8 (1984).

42. I. Fridovich, The biology of oxygen radicals, *Science, 201*, 875–880 (1978).

43. C. D. Hunt and D. L. Smith, "Conversion of dissolved manganese to particular manganese during diatom bloom: effects on the manganese cycle in the MERL microcosms," in J. P. Giesy, Jr., Ed., *Microcosms in Ecological Research*, Symposium Series 52 (CONF-781101), U.S. Technical Information Series, Washington DC, 1980, pp. 850–868.

44. W. E. Dean and P. E. Greeson, Influences of algae on the formation of freshwater ferromanganese nodules, Oneida Lake, New York, *Arch. Hydrobiol., 86*, 181–192 (1979).

45. L. L. Richardson, C. Aguilar, and K. H. Nealson, Manganese oxidation in pH and $O_2$ microenvironments produced by phytoplankton, *Limnol. Oceanogr., 33*, 352–363 (1988).

46. R. Schweisfurth, Manganoxydirende pilze. I. vorkommen, isolierungen und mikroskopische untersuchungen, *Z. Allg. Mikrobiol., 11*, 415–430 (1971).

47. R. A. Rosson and K. H. Nealson, Manganese binding and oxidation by spores of a marine bacillus, *J. Bacteriol., 151*, 1027–1034 (1982).

48. J. P. M. de Vrind, E. W. de Vrind-de Jong, J. W. H. de Voogt, P. Westbroek, F. C. Boogerd, and R. A. Rosson, Manganese oxidation by spores and spore coats of a marine *Bacillus* species, *Appl. Environ. Microbiol., 52*, 1096–1100 (1986).

49. E. W. de Vrind-de Jong, J. P. M. de Vrind, F. C. Boogerd, P. Westbroek, and R. A. Rosson, "Manganese transformations by a marine *Bacillus* species," in

R. E. Crick, Ed., *Origin, Evolution, and Modern Aspects of Biomineralization in Plants and Animals. Proceedings of the Vth International Symposium on Biomineralization, Arlington, TX*, Plenum, New York, 1987, in press.

50. B. M. Tebo, K. Mandernack, and R. A. Rosson, "Manganese oxidation by a spore coat or exosporium protein from spores of a manganese (II) oxidizing marine *Bacillus*," in *Abstracts of the Annual Meeting*, American Society for Microbiology, Washington DC, 1988, p. 201.

51. K. H. Nealson and B. Tebo, Structural features of manganese precipitating bacteria, *Origins of Life, 10*, 117–126 (1980).

52. B. M. Tebo, The ecology and ultrastructure of marine manganese oxidizing bacteria, Ph.D. Dissertation, University of California, San Diego, 1983.

53. M. A. Zapkin and H. L. Ehrlich, A comparison of manganese oxidation by growing and resting cells of a freshwater bacterial isolate, strain FMn1, *Z. Allg. Mikrobiol., 23*, 447–455 (1983).

54. J. Zindulis and H. L. Ehrlich, A novel $Mn^{2+}$-oxidizing enzyme system in a freshwater bacterium, *Z. Allg. Mikrobiol., 23*, 457–465 (1983).

55. P. Kepkay and K. H. Nealson, Growth of a manganese oxidizing *Pseudomonas* sp. in continuous culture, *Arch. Microbiol., 148*, 63–67 (1987).

56. T. J. Beveridge and S. F. Koval, Binding of metals to cell envelopes of *Escherichia coli* K12, *Appl. Environ. Microbiol., 42*, 325–335 (1981).

57. W. C. Ghiorse and H. L. Ehrlich, Electron transport components of the $MnO_2$ reductase system and the location of the terminal reductase in a marine *Bacillus*, *Appl. Environ. Microbiol., 31*, 977–985 (1976).

58. E. L. Barrett and M. A. Clark, Tetrathionate reduction and production of hydrogen sulfide from thiosulfate, *Microbiol. Rev., 51*, 192–205 (1987).

58a. D. Postma, Concentration of Mn and separation from Fe in sediments-I. Kinetics and stoichiometry of the reaction between birnessite and dissolved Fe(II) at 10°C, *Geochim. Cosmochim. Acta, 49*, 1023–1033 (1985).

59. K. H. Nealson, "Microbial oxidation and reduction of manganese and iron," in P. Westbroek and E. W. deJong, Eds., *Biomineralization and Biological Metal Accumulation*, Reidel, Boston, 1983, pp. 459–479.

60. D. R. Lovley, Organic matter mineralization with the reduction of ferric iron: a review, *Geomicrobiol. J., 5*, 375–399 (1987).

61. A. F. de Castro and H. L. Ehrlich, Reduction of iron oxide minerals by a marine *Bacillus, Ant. van Leeuwen., 36*, 317–327 (1970).

62. M. Jansson, Anaerobic production of magnetite by a dissimilatory iron-reducing microorganism, *Microb. Ecol., 14*, 81–89 (1987).

63. J. Sorensen, Reduction of ferric iron in anaerobic, marine sediment and interaction with reduction of nitrate and sulfate, *Appl. Environ. Microbiol., 43*, 319–324 (1982).

64. J. G. Jones, S. Gardener, and B. M. Simon, Bacterial reduction of ferric iron in a stratified eutrophic lake, *J. Gen. Microbiol., 129*, 131–139 (1983).

65. J. G. Jones, W. Davison, and S. Gardener, Iron reduction by bacteria: range of organisms involved and metals reduced, *FEMS Microbiol. Lett., 21*, 133–136 (1984).

66. J. G. Jones, S. Gardener, and B. M. Simon, Reduction of ferric iron by heterotrophic bacteria in lake sediments, *J. Gen. Microbiol., 130*, 45–51 (1984).

67. C. O. Obuekwe, D. W. S. Westlake, and F. D. Cook, Effect of nitrate reduction on ferric iron by a bacterium isolated from crude oil, *Can. J. Microbiol., 27*, 692–697 (1981).

68. V. V. Balashova and G. A. Zavarzin, Anaerobic reduction of ferric iron by hydrogen bacteria, *Microbiology USSR, 48*, 635–639 (1979).

69. J. C. G. Ottow, Selection, characterization and iron-reducing capacity of nitrate reductaseless (nit⁻) mutants of iron-reducing bacteria, *Z. Allg. Mikrobiol., 10*, 55–62 (1970).

70. J. C. G. Ottow and H. Glathe, Isolation and identification of iron-reducing bacteria from gley soils, *Soil Biol. Biochem., 3*, 43–55 (1971).

71. J. C. G. Ottow and J. Munch, "Mechanisms of reductive transformations in the anaerobic microenvironment of hydromorphic soils," in W. E. Krumbein, Ed., *Environmental Biogeochemistry and Geomicrobiology*, Vol. 2, Ann Arbor Science Publishers, Ann Arbor, MI, 1978, pp. 483–491.

72. T. Sugio, C. Domatsu, O. Munakata, T. Tano, and K. Imai, Role of a ferric ion-reducing system in sulfur oxidation of *Thiobacillus ferrooxidans, Appl. Environ. Microbiol., 49*, 1401–1406 (1985).

73. K. M. Semple and D. W. S. Westlake, Characterization of iron-reducing *Alteromonas putrefaciens* strains from oil fluid fields, *Can. J. Microbiol., 33*, 366–371 (1987).

74. R. G. Arnold, T. J. DiChristina, and M. R. Hoffman, Inhibitor studies of dissimilative Fe(III) reduction by *Pseudomonas* sp. strain 200 (*"Pseudomonas ferrireductans"*), *Appl. Environ. Microbiol., 52*, 281–289 (1986).

75. D. R. Lovley and E. J. P. Phillips, Availability of ferric iron for microbial reduction in bottom sediments of the freshwater tidal Potomac River, *Appl. Environ. Microbiol., 52*, 751–757 (1986).

76. D. R. Lovley and E. J. P. Phillips, Organic matter mineralization with reduction of ferric iron in anaerobic sediments, *Appl. Environ. Microbiol., 51*, 683–689 (1986).

77. D. R. Lovley and E. J. P. Phillips, Competitive mechanisms for inhibition of sulfate reduction and methane production in the zone of ferric iron reduction in sediments, *Appl. Environ. Microbiol., 53*, 2636–2641 (1987).

78. C. R. Myers and K. H. Nealson, Microbial reduction of manganese oxides: interactions with iron and sulfur, *Geochim. Cosmochim. Acta, 52*, 2727–2732 (1988).

79. A. T. Stone and J. J. Morgan, Reduction and dissolution of manganese(III) and manganese(IV) oxides by organics: 2. Survey of reactivity of organics, *Environ. Sci. Technol., 18*, 617–624 (1984).

80. A. T. Stone, Microbial metabolites and the reductive dissolution of manganese oxides: oxalate and pyruvate, *Geochim. Cosmochim. Acta, 51*, 919–925 (1987).

81. A. T. Stone, Reductive dissolution of manganese (III/IV) oxides by substituted phenols, *Environ. Sci. Technol., 21*, 979–988 (1987).

82. D. M. Strand, Microbial manganese (III, IV) reduction: isolation of a marine manganese reducing bacterium and subsequent reduction studies, Master's Thesis, University of California, San Diego, 1985.

83. A. T. Stone and J. J. Morgan, Reduction and dissolution of manganese(III) and manganese(IV) oxides by organics: 1. Reaction with hydroquinone, *Environ. Sci. Technol., 18*, 450–456 (1984).

84. W. C. Ghiorse and H. L. Ehrlich, Effects of seawater cations and temperature on manganese-dioxide reductase activity in a marine *Bacillus, Appl. Microbiol., 28*, 785–792 (1974).

85. P. J. G. Mann and J. H. Quastel, Manganese metabolism in soils, *Nature* (London), *158*, 154–156 (1946).

86. R. B. Trimble and H. L. Ehrlich, Bacteriology of manganese nodules. III. Reduction of $MnO_2$ by two strains of nodule bacteria, *Appl. Microbiol., 16*, 695–702 (1968).

87. R. B. Trimble and H. L. Ehrlich, Bacteriology of manganese nodules. IV. Induction of an $MnO_2$-reductase system in a marine *Bacillus, Appl. Microbiol., 19*, 966–972 (1970).

88. R. B. Wollast, G. Billen, and J. C. Duinker, Behavior of manganese in the Rhine and Scheldt estuaries, *Estuarine Coastal Mar. Sci., 9*, 161–169 (1979).

89. A. J. B. Zehnder and T. D. Brock, Anaerobic methane oxidation: occurrence and ecology, *Appl. Environ. Microbiol., 39*, 194–204 (1980).

90. E. P. Troshanov, Iron- and manganese-reducing microorganisms in ore-containing lakes of Karelian isthmus, *Microbiology USSR, 37*, 786–790 (1968).

91. R. M. Hochster and J. H. Quastel, Manganese dioxide as a terminal hydrogen acceptor in the study of respiratory systems, *Arch. Biochem. Biophys., 36*, 132–146 (1951).

92. D. J. Burdige and K. H. Nealson, Microbial manganese reduction by enrichment cultures from coastal marine sediments, *Appl. Environ. Microbiol., 50*, 491–497 (1985).

93. A. H. Stouthamer, "Energetic aspects of the growth of micro-organisms," in B. A. Haddock and W. A. Hamilton, Eds., *Microbial Energetics*, Cambridge University Press, New York, 1977, pp. 285–315.

94. H. A. Derby and B. W. Hammer, Bacteriology of butter. IV. Bacteriological studies on surface taint butter, *Iowa Agr. Exp. Sta. Res. Bull., 145*, 389–416 (1931).

95. B. B. Jørgensen, Ecology of the bacteria of the sulphur cycle with special reference to anoxic-oxic interface environments, *Phil. Trans. R. Soc. Lond. B, 298*, 543–561 (1982).

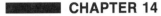 

# CHAPTER 14

# Mineral Formation and Decomposition by Microorganisms

F. GRANT FERRIS, WILLIAM SHOTYK, and WILLIAM S. FYFE

Department of Geology
University of Western Ontario
London, Ontario, Canada

## Contents

## 14.1 INTRODUCTION

Interest in the role of organic material in the surface phenomena of earth has a long history, in part linked to observations from agriculture. In this century, the great geochemists V. M. Goldschmidt and V. Vernadsky firmly established the science of biogeochemistry. Today there is a renaissance in

**413**

the subject due to many factors. Perhaps of fundamental importance, our tools for organic analysis and observation of the microstructure of microorganisms have become adequate to describe processes. Of equal importance has been the recognition that the environment of this planet is in very large part controlled by interactive processes between the great forcing factors (sun and deep earth processes) and the biosphere. Furthermore, there is a growing concern that humans are changing this system rapidly and perhaps disastrously in terms of our survival.

Such recognition of the importance of the biosphere has led to the new International Geosphere Biosphere project (IGBP) of the International Council of Scientific Unions, a program that will concentrate on describing and understanding the interactive processes that control the environment. Lovelock (1) has proposed the now famous GAIA hypothesis involving the idea that our planet can be viewed as an interactive colonial organism. The IGBP will involve observations of the earth system on all scales, from satellites to electron microscopes.

When we consider the biosphere and its debris, certain features stand out:

1. Complex life, including photosynthetic organisms, is as old as the geologic record, stretching back at least 3.8 billion years (2). Thus from present information it seems that once our planet had a hydrosphere it also had a biosphere. The origin of life is still a complex problem but there is increasing evidence that carbon and complex organics abound in the debris of space.

2. It is clear that microorganisms exist where there is liquid water at temperatures up to about 110°C. Life exists in the harshest environments, from the deep Antarctic to the depths of the oceans. Life also exists in deep porous strata.

3. Although the biosphere makes up a small mass of the geosphere, it is highly dynamic and its impact is proportional not to its mass, but to its recycling time and reactive surface area. As stressed by Mason and Moore (3), the mass of living organisms integrated over geologic time is similar to the mass of the planet. More than 100 km$^3$ of living matter is cycled every year and this mass contains metals as well as C, H, O, and N (see Refs. 4 and 5).

4. We now know that about one-third of the chemical elements are bioessential (6) and that biomineralization is a major process in surface environments (7–10). Organisms must extract their nutrients from the surface solids and fluids. They must be important in all equilibrium and rate processes in the surface environment. Organisms tend to stick to earth materials (11).

5. Organisms produce a vast array of organic and inorganic debris that in turn play a major role in surface metal transport and fixation processes. The average gram of cultivated soil contains $10^7$ colony-forming units of bacteria, $10^6$ actinomycetes, $10^5$ fungi, and $10^4$ algae (12). It has been esti-

mated that the simplest bacterium, *Escherichia coli*, contains approximately 5000 different organic molecules, including 3000 different proteins and 1000 different nucleic acids.

In this chapter we briefly consider some aspects of the role of microorganisms and organic compounds in the metal balance of the planet.

## 14.2  MICROORGANISMS AND BIOLOGICAL MINERAL FORMATION (BIOMINERALIZATION)

### 14.2.1  The Antiquity of Prokaryotes

Earth is estimated to have taken form some 4.2–4.4 billion years ago, and the first components of a biosphere probably developed shortly thereafter. There are no known rocks from this early epoch, known as the Hadean era, but isotopic evidence from Archean rocks suggest that the global carbon cycle was controlled by carbon-fixing microorganisms as early as 3.5 billion years ago (13). Earth's atmosphere at this time was "reducing," so these primitive primary producers were possibly lithoautotrophs or anaerobic photoautotrophs (e.g., purple and green bacteria) performing anoxygenic photosynthesis (13).

Fossilized stromatolites are well distributed in Archean sedimentary formations (14). They typically occur in laminated organic-rich cherts (cryptocrystalline quartz) and siliceous carbonates. The fine layering and raised conical or dome shapes of stromatolites are reminiscent of contemporary microbial mats, which form in a variety of diverse aquatic environments (15–17). Among the Archean stromatolites, the oldest are from the 3.4–3.5 billion year old Onverwacht group in South Africa and Warawoona group in Western Australia (18, 19). These two benchmark formations are unique in that they document the presence of relatively complex microbial ecosystems well into the past.

The occurrence of stromatolitic formations increases dramatically as one moves from Archean to Proterozoic terrains (20). A variety of cellularly preserved microfossils, which are generally absent in Archean rocks, also begin to appear in the sedimentary record (Fig. 14.1). This apparent increase in microbial biomass production around 2.5 billion years ago has been attributed to the development of facultative oxygenic photoautotrophs (i.e., primitive cyanobacteria; see Ref. 21). These microorganisms, using water as a source of reducing equivalents, must have been highly competitive and probably quickly dominated the biosphere. Moreover, with the onset of biological molecular oxygen production, the atmosphere began to change from "reducing" to "oxidizing." Consequently, a relatively stable oxic atmosphere capable of supporting obligate aerobic microorganisms had developed by the end of the Proterozoic (21).

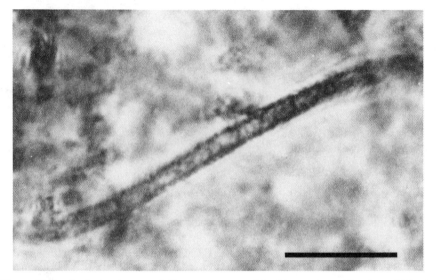

**Figure 14.1** A photomicrograph from a petrographic thin section of laminated black chert from the Gunflint Iron Formation, Ontario showing a filamentous microfossil (bar = 50 $\mu$m).

At the dawn of the Phanerozoic era 800 million years ago, prokaryotes were well established. Fewer stromatolites appear in sedimentary rocks from these more recent times, as expected from the corresponding increase of grazing and burrowing metazoans in the fossil record (20, 22). Nevertheless, prokaryotes reigned supreme for more than 75% of the Earth's history, longer than any other living organism. They are still the most abundant lifeform on earth, and continue to affect profoundly the world in which we live.

### 14.2.2 Bacterial Supported Mineralization in Modern and Ancient Systems

A significant portion of the organic matter in natural environments consists of small colloidal aggregates of highly cross-linked heteropolymeric material. At least some of the more durable polymeric networks are derived from the walls and external sheaths of bacteria (23). These cellular structures are not only very resistant to degradation, but also possess reactive anionic sites that can bind dissolved metallic ions and, under favorable conditions, initiate mineral formation (24–27). In modern environments, there are many examples of bacterial supported mineralization and there is abundant evidence that analogous processes contributed to the genesis of some mineral deposits in the past (10).

*14.2.2.1 Phosphorites.* The term phosphorite is conventionally applied to sediments or rocks containing more than 10% (by volume) individual phosphate grains (28). The most abundant phosphate mineral in phosphorite deposits is fluorapatite or francolite (29). Phosphorites have been reported from both ancient and modern sediments deposited in shallow near-shore marine environments under conditions of high biological productivity (30–33).

The formation of phosphate minerals in modern marine environments arises from the chemical precipitation of dissolved metallic ions caused by an upwelling of phosphate-rich deep ocean waters (34). However, metallic ion binding by bacteria appears to enhance the development of the precipitates (35). Similar principles have been advanced for the formation of phosphate minerals in geochemical modeling studies conducted with metal loaded bacterial cells (Fig. 14.2; see Ref. 26). These concepts are consistent with the organic-rich nature of recent phosphorite deposits from the inner continental shelf of South West Africa and coastal zones off the west coast of South America (32, 33).

In the Upper Cretaceous–Lower Eocene Mishash Formation of Israel, phosphate beds occur in sequences of laminated carbonates and cherts (31). Paleoenvironmental analyses suggest that these Negev phosphorites developed on the shelf of a receding epicontinental sea in association with cy-

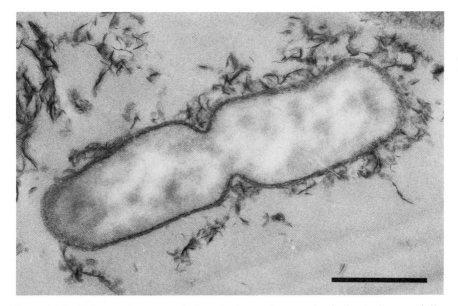

**Figure 14.2** Thin-section transmission electron micrograph of a bacterium partially encrusted by uranium phosphate microcrystals. The specimen was prepared by exposing the bacteria to an aqueous uranyl acetate solution, and then the cell-bound uranyl ions were precipitated by exogenously added phosphate (bar = 500 nm).

anobacterial mats (31, 36). Dense apatite overgrowths on fossil remnants of cyanobacterial sheaths are commonly found in association with fragmented phosphatitic sheaths and colonies or coccoid cells infilled with apatite (31). Similar patterns of mineralization have been observed in the Djebel–Onk microbial mat generated phosphorites near the Algeria–Tunisia frontier (30). This close connection between microbial structures and phosphate mineralization provides direct evidence for bacterial participation in the development of phosphorite deposits in the past.

**14.2.2.2 Carbonates.** The majority of recent carbonate sediments are formed in marine environments. They are found throughout the oceans where they are closely associated with regions of upwelling along mid-ocean ridges and continental shelves (34). The predominant carbonate minerals in these sediments are the $CaCO_3$ polymorphs calcite and aragonite. Recent shallow-water tropical and subtropical deposits consist mostly of aragonite and high-magnesium calcite, whereas temperate shallow-water deposits contain predominantly calcite (34). This difference in the oceanic distribution of carbonate minerals has been attributed to high levels of magnesium in warmer tropical waters, for this metallic ion severely retards the precipitation of calcite (37, 38).

Bacteria have been implicated as the causative agents for carbonate precipitation in a number of laboratory investigations (16, 39, 40). In these experiments, the bacterial cells actually functioned as nucleating elements for the formation of aragonite and high-magnesium calcite. These minerals first developed on the surfaces of the bacteria and not in the cells, as expected for a direct chemical precipitation of cell-bound calcium or magnesium. Similar patterns of carbonate mineralization are commonly observed in association with microbial mats from various marine intertidal zones (41–43). Fossilized remnants of these stratified communities of microorganisms are also widely distributed in silicified carbonates from the Precambrian era (20, 22).

High-magnesium calcite peloids are commonly found in cemented marine carbonate accumulations from quiet-water lagoons and microcavities in reefs (44–46). These peloids are elliptical to spheroidal bodies 20–60 μm in diameter with crystalline dentate rims (47). The nuclei are generally fine grained, and often contain fossilized clumps of bacteria encased within anhedral micro-sized crystals of high-magnesium calcite. In contrast, the euhedral crystals rimming the peloids are larger (5–10 μm long) and devoid of organic matter (48). This difference in crystallinity between the peloid nuclei and rims presumably reflects different rates of precipitation. A rapid precipitation of calcite initiated by bacteria probably accounts for the smaller anhedral crystals of the nuclei, whereas the rim developed more slowly after a complete mineralization of the bacterial cells (47). Fossilized clumps of bacteria have also been found in silt-sized particles from freshwater travertine deposits (49).

In many tropical and subtropical intertidal zones, deposits of lithified carbonate sediments exist. These deposits are known as beach rock and occur in uniform layers or as partially eroded masses at the sediment–water interface (34). Spherical carbonate particles called ooliths are often found in these formations, particularly in areas of strong tidal currents (50). They range in diameter from 0.1 to 1.5 mm with alternating laminations of aragonite and organic matter. The nature and origin of these laminations are not completely understood. However, microorganisms have been implicated in the genesis of some oolitic structures (51, 52), and carbonate precipitating bacteria can be isolated from beach rock formations (53).

***14.2.2.3 Sulfides.*** The precipitation of metal sulfides during early sedimentary diagenesis involves a complex series of interdependent biological and geochemical events (54). In modern anoxic environments, dissimilatory bacterial sulfate reduction is the major mechanism by which sulfide is produced (55). This process is carried out by a widely distributed group of anaerobic bacteria that generate the energy required for growth by coupling the oxidation of simple organic molecules to the reduction of sulfate (56). The formation of sulfide minerals proceeds as a direct result of bacterial sulfate reduction, and patterns of sulfur isotope fractionation in many sedimentary sulfide deposits support the bacteriogenic origin of reduced sulfur (55).

Sulfide minerals often exhibit a close association with high-molecular-weight organic materials in fine-grained sediments (57), and a number of studies suggest that organometallic complexes that form directly in natural systems play an important role in the transfer of metallic ions into sulfide phases (58–60). In laboratory cultures of marine and to a lesser extent freshwater sediments, metal sulfides are commonly precipitated on the surfaces of bacterial cells (Fig. 14.3; see Refs. 25, 27, 61). This can be attributed directly to an uptake and retention of metallic ions by the bacteria, which essentially concentrate the metals before they react with bacteriogenic sulfide. There is additional experimental evidence that suggests that metallic ions bound by bacterial cells tend to be more reactive toward sulfide than they are when in solution (62).

The most important factor controlling sulfide production in natural sedimentary systems is the availability of organic substrates that can be metabolized by sulfate-reducing bacteria (56). Thus it is not surprising to find mineralized zones of copper, lead, zinc, and iron in association with stromatolitic formations. For example, the Woodcutters deposit in the Northern Territory of Australia formed in a shallow restricted basin where the decomposition of dense microbial mats caused a coprecipitation of lead and zinc sulfides with precursors of the host dolomite rock (63). Similar accumulations of metal sulfides are found in fine-grained, organic-rich, marine shales deposited under conditions of high biological productivity in shallow euxinic (i.e., oxygen-free, sulfide-rich) basins (64).

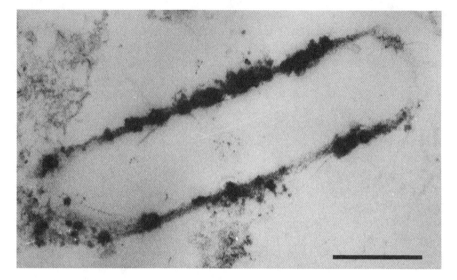

**Figure 14.3**   A thin-section profile showing electron-dense metal sulfide precipitates on the remnants of a bacterial cell in an anoxic lake sediment sample from Sudbury, Ontario (bar = 500 nm).

### 14.2.2.4   *Iron and Manganese Oxides.*

Goldschmidt outlined two rules that govern the geochemistry of Fe and Mn in the weathering cycle: (1) oxidizing conditions promote their precipitation, and reducing conditions promote their solution; and (2) acidic conditions promote their solution, and alkaline conditions promote their precipitation (65). These transition metals can exist in several redox states, but at earth surface conditions, only two valences are common for each metal. The usual redox states for iron are $Fe^{2+}$ and $Fe^{3+}$, whereas for manganese they are $Mn^{2+}$ and $Mn^{4+}$. However, the relative chemical stabilities of the reduced and oxidized states of these two metals are different (66). For example, $Fe^{2+}$ is rapidly oxidized and precipitates in oxic environments above approximately pH 3. In contrast, $Mn^{2+}$ is more stable and remains soluble until approximately pH 5 in environments at similar oxidation–reduction potentials (see Section 14.3.2).

Ferromanganese oxidizing bacteria are widely distributed in nature (see the reviews in Refs. 67–70) and have been extensively studied (71–73). As these microorganisms grow, surficial deposits of iron or manganese oxides typically develop (Fig. 14.4). This extracellular deposition of metals depends on the production of anionic metal binding surface polymers by the bacteria (27). Sometimes fresh isolates of ferromanganese depositing bacteria lose their ability to oxidize $Mn^{2+}$, suggesting that the process is actively catalyzed by the organism (see Chapter 13). In contrast, the ability to accumulate iron oxides is usually not lost because $Fe^{2+}$ oxidizes spontaneously at neutral pH in the presence of oxygen. Thus the bacteria only have to bind the re-

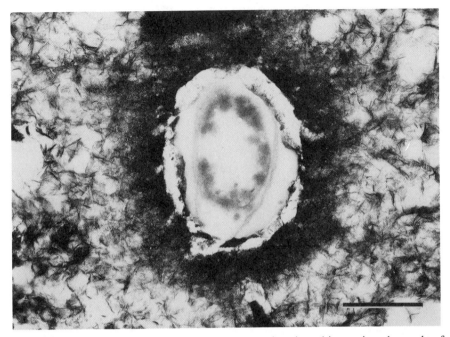

**Figure 14.4**   A manganese oxide encrusted bacterium in a thin-sectioned sample of a hot spring microbial mat from Yellowstone National Park, Wyoming (bar = 500 nm).

duced metal or hydrous cationic colloidal forms [i.e., $Fe(H_2O)_5(OH)^{2+}$ or $Fe(H_2O)_4(OH)_2^+$], to display iron depositing activity.

Structures resembling modern ferromanganese depositing bacteria have been detected in stromatolitic cherts from the Gunflint Iron Formation (74). However, there is some doubt that the formation of massive Precambrian iron formations can be attributed entirely to microbial metal precipitation. Nevertheless, electron microprobe studies have demonstrated that significant amounts of iron are often associated with fossil bacteria (75). In addition, more recent naturally occurring iron oxides commonly contain organic matter, and accumulate in environments favorable for the growth of bacteria (76, 77).

The formation of marine manganese nodules, freshwater manganese precipitates, and desert varnish has been attributed to manganese oxidizing bacteria (72, 78, 79). Also, at least some of the manganese oxide deposits arising near pelagic hydrothermal vents can be attributed to manganese oxidizing bacteria (80). Furthermore, recent studies show that bacteria scavenge manganese in hydrothermal plumes at distances at least 7 km away from the vent source (81). This latter observation suggests that bacteria play an important role in precipitating manganese over large areas in the oceans.

**14.2.2.5    Silicates.**  Until recently, remarkably little was known about the influence of bacteria on silica deposition and authigenic clay formation. However, high-molecular-weight humic substances are sometimes incorporated into clays (82). Also, fossilized bacteria are commonly found in cherty sequences of siliceous carbonates as well as sandstones, siltstones, and shales (20, 22). Recently, David (83) has described new types of soluble polysilane polymers. Do these occur in nature? Such observations clearly suggest that sites of diagenetic silicification and clay formation may be found in clastic sediments where relatively high concentrations of organic matter accumulate.

In acidic terrestrial hot springs, true microbial mats do not develop. Instead, accumulations of clay and siliceous mud form in which thermoacidophilic bacteria thrive (84). Direct microscopic examination of these sediments has revealed individual bacterial cells in successive stages of mineralization by iron–silica crystallites (85). The iron was probably bound by the anionic polymers in the walls of the bacteria, whereas the silica crystallites presumably developed from mono- or polysilicic acid that was hydrogen bonded to available hydroxyl groups. Similar bacterial accumulations of silica have been reported in laboratory experiments (86, 87). These data

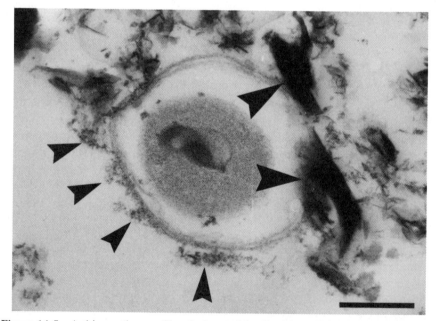

**Figure 14.5**   A thin-section profile of a bacterial cell with surficial accumulations of a granular (small arrows) and crystalline (large arrows) iron–aluminum silicate. The specimen was obtained from a lake near Sudbury, Ontario (bar = 200 nm).

not only demonstrate that bacteria are capable of precipitating silica, but also provide an explanation for the close association between early diagenetic silica and organic matter in Precambrian sedimentary formations (20, 22).

Extensive accumulations of a complex iron–aluminum silicate have been found on the surfaces of bacteria growing in a metal-contaminated lake sediment (61). The deposits ranged from a poorly developed granular material to a more crystalline phase (Fig. 14.5). Electron diffraction patterns and microprobe analyses suggested that this polymorphic iron–aluminum silicate was chamosite ($[Fe_5Al](Si_3Al)O_{10}(OH)_8]$). The precise role of bacterial cells as nucleating elements for an iron-rich clay can be understood in terms of their ability to immobilize metallic ions. Hydrous iron–aluminum silicate species could be precipitated directly by dissolved silicic acid from metals complexed by the cells, or alternatively, cationic colloidal precursors formed initially in the sediment pore water system could be bound. These processes, either separately or together, would account for the formation of a gel-like material from which crystalline forms typically evolve during structural rearrangement and layer growth in the solid state (88, 89).

## 14.3  MICROORGANISMS AND BIOLOGICAL MINERAL DECOMPOSITION (BIOWEATHERING)

### 14.3.1  Introduction

The organic matter of soils, sediments, and natural waters is chemically reactive toward solid minerals and dissolved metals, and there is abundant evidence of metals associated with organic matter (e.g., Fig. 14.6). As a consequence, the places in which this organic matter accumulates, such as soil A horizons and peat swamps, are zones of continual geochemical transformation (90). This organic matter is a chemically complex mixture of materials that arise from the microbial decomposition of plant and animal bodies and from microbial synthesis (91). Microbial decomposition of plant biopolymers, for example, gives rise to simple acids: sugar acids from pectins, gums, and mucilages; amino acids from proteins; fatty acids from lipids; and phenolic acids from lignins and tannins. At the same time, complex new biopolymers such as "humic" and "fulvic" acids are synthesized during decomposition from the interactions of phenolic acids derived from lignins and tannins with microbial proteins. In this sense, then, the driving force for the reactions of organic matter with minerals and metals described here is microbial activity.

The metal–organic reactions of geochemical interest may involve microorganisms both directly and indirectly. For example, surface functional groups on bacterial cell walls exhibit a great affinity for Cu(II) ions (92), and this kind of surface complexation may result in the accumulation of anom-

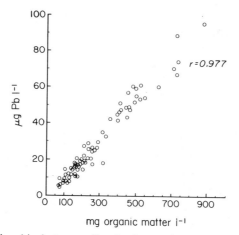

**Figure 14.6** Relationship between dissolved organic matter and Pb concentration in percolation water from a podzolized spruce forest soil in southern Sweden. From Tyler with permission of the author and the publisher, Marcel Dekker, Inc. (135).

alous concentrations of metals in the organic matter of soils and sediments. On the other hand, peat swamps that have been rendered anaerobic by bacterial decay of plant matter may accumulate unusually high concentrations of copper because of the reduction of Cu(II) ions to native metal (93). Both kinds of reactions are geologically important.

Over the years there has been considerable interest in "biological weathering," and this topic has received attention in several early books (see Refs. 94–98). Many important observations are included that predate modern developments in analytical and physical chemistry. We are assured by laboratory studies that a wide range of organic acids rapidly decompose many minerals (99, 100), but there is always some question about the applicability of laboratory studies to the natural environment.

In this section a short introduction is given to biologically mediated mineral decomposition in aerobic and anaerobic soil systems. Examples are given to illustrate both the direct and indirect influence of microbial communities.

## 14.3.2 Aerobic Soils

As soon as extrusive igneous rocks such as basalts have cooled, lichens begin to colonize them. Lichens are formed from a symbiotic relationship between algae and fungi; microbe populations on fresh rock also include tens to millions of bacteria, fungi, and actinomycetes per gram of rock, with microbe populations increasing with increased colonization by lichens and mosses (101). Similar microbe populations exist in the interior of weathered rocks. Microorganisms and lichens appear to be important mineral weathering agents because:

1. They are ubiquitous, and inhabit environments ranging from arctic to desert conditions, from below sea level to mountain tops;
2. They are in intimate contact with mineral surfaces, in many cases being "glued" on;
3. Under appropriate conditions they exhibit high metabolic rates, and reactions between minerals and microbes can take place in a matter of hours; and
4. They produce a relatively large amount and variety of organic compounds, many of which are acidic and form stable metal complexes.

The abilities of lichens as weathering agents is often quite clear, and there are numerous reports of lichen decomposition of glass, minerals, and rocks. Lichen growth on stained glass was reported in Sweden as long ago as 1831, and the dullness of various glasses was attributed to the numerous small cracks resulting from the dissolution by lichen hyphae. In 1861 Uloth reported distinct marks on the surface of siliceous rocks that corresponded to lichen growths, and he noted that even hard minerals such as chalcedony were corroded by luxuriant lichen flora. In 1881 Egeling reported similar observations concerning lichen growths on granitic rocks (Ref. 102 provides a review of these early studies).

Oxalic acid is a common constituent of many lichens. Its abundance varies with species, and is particularly abundant in those that inhabit limestones. Calcium oxalate was first detected in lichens by Henri Braconnot in 1825, and subsequent studies showed that it may account for as much as 50–70% of the dry weight of many species (102). The high proportion of this chelating acid in many species suggests a biological function, and many investigators have concluded that the role of oxalic acid is one of a solvent through which nutrients may be derived from underlying rocks and minerals.

Lichen acids probably perform the same role. First discovered by Pfaff in 1826, lichen acids are weak phenolic acids not found in other plants or molds. They are synthesized only by lichenized fungi from carbohydrates supplied by the algae, and may account for as much as 40% of the dry weight of the organism. The chemical structures of more than 300 compounds unique to the lichens have been determined (103); a few are shown in Figure 14.7. In addition to chemical attack, physical disintegration of minerals and rocks by lichens also is an important weathering mechanism (104).

The first scientist to speculate on the role of bacteria in mineral weathering appears to be Muntz (105), who found nitrifying bacteria on numerous rock types (granites, gneisses, schists, limestones, sandstones) in the Alps, Vosges, Auvergne, and Pyrenees mountains. He noticed that the microbes were not confined to the rock surface, but actually penetrated into the rock.

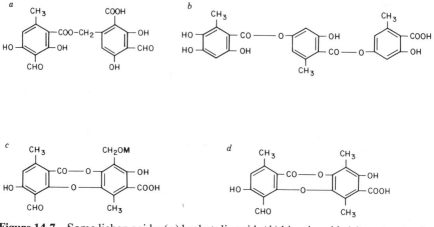

**Figure 14.7** Some lichen acids: (a) barbatolic acid, (b) hiascic acid, (c) protocetraric acid, (d) virensic acid.

This and other early studies are summarized by Waksman (106). However, the first systematic study of mineral weathering by bacteria appears to be that of Wright (107), who sought a chemical explanation of bacteria–mineral interactions. Using several silicate minerals he measured the release of K, Mg, Ca, and Fe in the presence of varying concentrations of inorganic and organic acids. These results were compared to metal release in the presence of *Azotobacter, Bacillus (Escherichia) coli,* and *B. lactis acidi.* Because the dissolution of minerals in the presence of organic acids resembled the effects of bacteria, he concluded that organic acid release by bacteria was the primary mineral weathering mechanism.

An excellent summary of Russian studies of microbial weathering is provided by Jacks (108). The work reviewed includes the effects of organisms, especially lichens, on the decomposition of fresh crystalline rocks at high elevations. On granites and gneisses lithopile lichens pulverize and chemically transform minerals to produce an appreciable horizon of "organo-mineral dust" on the rock surface. In places this layer may be several millimeters thick, suggesting that this process over the course of time could result in a soil. The dust is obviously rich in organic matter, but more importantly is enriched in K, Mg, Ca, P, S, and Fe relative to the host rock. Thus this biological weathering has made available nutrient elements to higher plants.

Related work has shown that lichens are enriched in nutrient elements (relative to the composition of the host rock) regardless of the rock type (108). However, individual species often exhibit preferences for various substrates. For example, *Parmelia* predominates on acidic igneous rocks, and *Xanthoria* on basic igneous rocks, but *Acarospora* and *Leucanora* are found only on calcareous rocks. In addition to lichens, Glazovskaya has found that green and blue-green algae and diatoms are involved in weathering; their by-products include amorphous silica and such aluminosilicates as beidellite, montmorillonite, and monothermite.

At elevations greater than 4000 m mosses tend to follow lichens. With sufficient accumulation of organic matter (5–10 cm), alpine grasses follow, and their roots penetrate the underlying rock and split it. Yarilova has shown that at the stage of soil development where grasses are found, approximately 30% of the minerals appear as new, synthesized products; by this time about one-half of the plagioclase (i.e., parent mineral phase) present in the original rock is dissipated (108).

An excellent recent review of biological and biochemical weathering is the paper by Robert and Berthelin (109), who include many electron micrographs that clearly illustrate these processes as they take place. They show that bioadhesion is highly significant. Lichen hyphae in particular are commonly effectively glued to the mineral surface (109). One of the important results of surface adhesion is the microdivision of minerals, for example, penetration of biotite layers by hyphae.

In addition to the major nutrient elements essential to organisms, many trace elements are required and appropriate bioaccumulation mechanisms have evolved. Trace metals were discovered in living organisms long ago: Hjarne discovered Cu in 1753, Scheele found Mn in 1772, Legrip found Co in 1844, Forchhammer found Zn in 1865, and so on (110). Today we know of more than 30 Cu-containing proteins, 70 Fe proteins, and 80 Zn proteins, in addition to proteins containing Ca, Cd, Co, I, Mn, Mo, Ni, and Se (111). Many metals serve as structural materials, for example, Ca carbonate, phosphate, alginate, and pectate; opal; Mg hydroxide; and Ba and Sr sulfate. Halide-containing biomolecules are well known for F, Cl (more than 100 identified), Br, and I. An excellent summary of the abundance and role of chemical elements in organisms is given by Bowen (111). Trace elements that are *not* essential for proper mineral nutrition also may be enriched in living organisms, and this phenomenon has been reviewed extensively by Brooks (112).

Higher plants also are important agents of chemical weathering, in part owing to the symbiotic relationship between microorganisms and plant roots in the rhizosphere. The rhizosphere is the zone of intense biological activity adjacent to plant roots. Compared to the bulk soil, microbial populations in the rhizosphere are much higher (as high as $5 \times 10^9$ organisms per gram of root tissue), and the biological activity of the component organisms there is much greater (113); plant roots may penetrate as deep as 50 m below the soil surface, and the integrated length of a single plant root system may reach 10,000 km! In addition to the active microflora, the plant roots themselves are important in promoting chemical mineral attack: root hairs and mucigel sheaths are endowed with abundant acidic functional groups that act as cation exchangers, and roots continually exude various complex-forming organic acids (113).

Plant metal uptake is approximately 10 g of inorganic salts per square meter per year with a residence time of 0.5–3 years (111); this is comparable to bulk weathering rates in North America of approximately 20 mg of rock per square meter per year. The role of accumulator plants in rock weathering has been reviewed by Lovering (114). He notes that many kinds of vegetation, especially in the tropics, contain several percent silica on a dry weight basis (e.g., bamboo). Consider the fact that 10–20 tons of dry matter in the form of new growth (above ground parts) are added per acre per year, with roots adding several tons more. A forest of silica-accumulator plants averaging 2.5% silica and 16 tons (dry weight) of new growth per year would extract approximately 2000 tons of Si per acre in 5000 years—equivalent to the Si in one acre-ft of basalt (114). In geologic terms this represents a relatively rapid weathering rate.

### 14.3.3  Anaerobic Soils

The total global wetland area is 530 million ha, of which 95% ($500 \times 10^6$ ha) are peatlands such as bogs, fens, and swamps (115). This peatland (mire) area is approximately equivalent to 5% of the Earth's total land area. Locally, peatlands may be much more important, forming a veneer over 30% of Finland, 17% of Ireland and Sweden, and 12% of Canada. These peat soils ("organic soils") are described in several reviews (see Refs. 116–119).

Peat is a light brown (almost blonde) to black organic sediment formed under waterlogged conditions from the partial decomposition of mosses and other bryophytes, sedges, grasses, shrubs, or trees. The structure of peat ranges from fibrous to amorphous, and the relative proportions of C, H, and O vary, depending upon the botanical composition and degree of decomposition (humification). Peatlands are peat-forming ecosystems in which at least 30 cm of peat has accumulated.

The principal condition for the accumulation of organic matter as peat is a large excess of water, for example, in shallow ponds. Because oxygen diffuses about 10,000 times slower in water than it does in air (121), microorganisms actively decomposing aquatic plants consume the available dissolved oxygen much more quickly than it can be replenished from the air. The environment quickly becomes anaerobic (no measurable dissolved oxygen), and it is this anaerobic condition that allows organic matter to accumulate over time as peat: in the aerobic zone of peatlands (above the water table) the decay rate is 2–4% per year, versus 0.1–0.000001% in the anaerobic zone (122).

The anaerobic condition and the subsequent biogeochemical transformations characteristic of peatlands are thus entirely the result of microbial activities. From the surface of a peat bog to its greatest depths (e.g., 5–15 m) a continuous range of microbial relationships exists, from obligate aerobes through facultative forms to obligate anaerobes. The products of the various microbial transformations include high concentrations of the gases $CO_2$, $CH_4$, $CO$, and $H_2$ relative to their abundance in the atmosphere,

$H_2S$, metal sulfide minerals such as pyrite ($FeS_2$), covellite (CuS), and chalcopyrite ($CuFeS_2$), carbonate minerals such as siderite ($FeCO_3$) and smithsonite ($ZnCO_3$), and phosphate minerals such as vivianite [$Fe_3(PO_4)_2 \cdot 8H_2O$], pieces of metallic Cu and Fe ("native" metal), elemental sulfur, and, occasionally(?), phosphine gas ($PH_3$). These transformations are summarized in detail elsewhere (120).

Because Fe and Mn are more soluble under anaerobic conditions, and Cu and U are less soluble (Fig. 14.8), peatlands and other anaerobic sediments may be expected to influence the geochemical cycles of these metals in the hydrosphere. Here we show that peatlands and their pore waters tend generally to dissolve Fe and Mn compounds, resulting in substantial migration of the metals, and precipitate Cu and U, often resulting in considerable accumulation.

"Bog iron ore" is a general term for a soft, spongy, and porous deposit of impure hydrous Fe oxides formed in mires and shallow lakes by the oxidizing action of algae, Fe bacteria, or the atmosphere. Bog iron ore is made up mainly of limonite, a general field term for a group of reddish brown to black, amorphous, hydrous ferric oxides (123). Early reports of occurrences of bog iron ore provide descriptions of the conditions of formation of bog iron: cool, humid climates of the boreal zone (Canada, Scandinavia) in drift covered areas of low relief where drainage is poor and peatlands and peaty soils are present in abundance, giving rise to abundant dissolved organic matter (124). Experimental studies have since demonstrated the solvent effect of peaty solutions on Fe carbonates, oxides, and silicates (125).

In these terrains, matted leaf litter and humus blanket the rocks and soils, and the abundant rainfall, high atmospheric humidity, low average annual temperatures, and dense forest growth probably maintain an anaerobic condition for much of the year. As noted above, peatlands generally are oxygen-free, and in much of the Canadian boreal zone peatlands cover 50–80% of the land area. Thus much of the terrain is anaerobic, and this condition facilitates Fe and Mn dissolution (Fig. 14.8). Chemical analyses of acidic *Sphagnum* bog peats show that Fe and Mn are significantly depleted relative to the average composition of local mineral sediments (Fig. 14.9). Even in cases where oxygen is present, ferric compounds are still successfully attacked because of the low pH and abundance of complex-forming organic acids (Fig. 14.10). When these organic-rich waters laden with Fe and Mn become oxygenated downstream, the Fe and Mn are precipitated by appropriate microbial communities (67, 68, 126), producing bog iron ore, as noted above, and bog manganese deposits (127).

In contrast to the solvent effect of mire waters on Fe and Mn, peatlands are geochemical sinks for Cu and U. The occurrence of "copper bogs" is well established, and has a long history. Recent studies of the Welsh copper bogs show up to almost 6% Cu in the peat ashes (128). In a cupriferous swamp in New Brunswick, Canada, up to 10% Cu has been found in dry peat samples, representing an enrichment relative to crustal abundance of

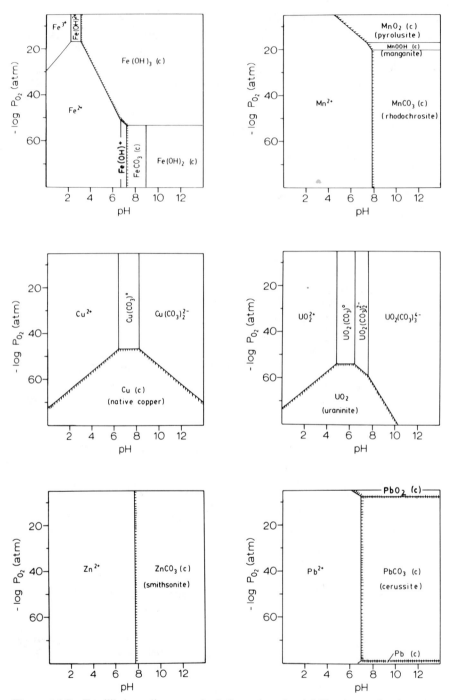

**Figure 14.8** Equilibrium diagrams depicting mineral solubility in peatland waters. $P_{CO_2} = 10^{-1.5}$ atm, $Fe_T = 10^{-5.0}$ $M$, $Mn_T = 10^{-6.3}$ $M$, $U_T = 10^{-8.7}$ $M$, $Zn_T = 10^{-6.3}$ $M$, $Pb_T = 10^{-7.8}$ $M$. From Shotyk (93).

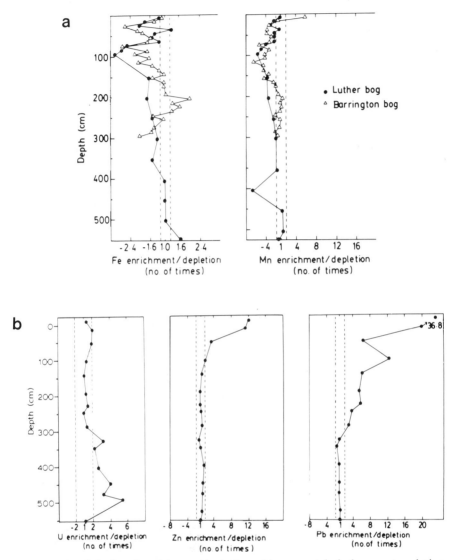

**Figure 14.9** Calculated enrichment/depletion of trace metals in bog peats relative to the average composition of underlying mineral sediments: (*a*) Fe and Mn from the Luther Bog, southern Ontario and the Barrington Bog, Nova Scotia; (*b*) U, Zn, and Pb from the Galbraith Bog, central Ontario. From Shotyk (93).

approximately 1000 times (129). At both sites, and at other mires described elsewhere (120), the enrichment mechanism is as follows. Copper-bearing minerals in local rocks and soils are oxidized, thereby liberating Cu to the percolating solutions. Such Cu-rich solutions may bear more than 1 ppm dissolved Cu and are brought to the anaerobic mire where the Cu is either

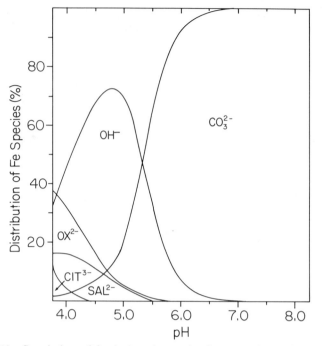

**Figure 14.10** Speciation of ferric iron in peatland waters determined using GEO-CHEM (see Ref. 136). $P_{CO_2} = 10^{-1.5}$ atm, $Fe_T = 10^{-5.0}$ $M$, oxalate $= 10^{-5.26}$ $M$, citrate $= 10^{-5.58}$ $M$, salicylate $= 10^{-5.44}M$. From Shotyk (93).

organically complexed by the peat, reduced to native Cu because of the low redox potential, or both. In cases where the imbibed solutions are also rich in sulfur (e.g., from the oxidation of nearby Cu sulfide minerals, or from gypsum), the sulfur is also reduced, and several Cu sulfide minerals covellite, chalcocite, chalcopyrite) may form in the peat.

Uranium-rich peats are also very well documented. A recent study of a uraniferous "bog" in California showed up to 1100 ppm U in the peat (130). In Washington state, peaty sediments in an old beaver pond contain up to 9000 ppm U, and have become the first surficial U deposit to be mined in the United States (131). In Sweden, a swamp with peats bearing up to 3% U (dry weight basis), or about 10,000 times more than typical crustal rocks, has been described in detail by Armands (132). The relative ease with which U and some other trace metals appear to become enriched in peats has led to concern in Sweden regarding the fate of these metals following fuel peat combustion (133).

In a study of the trace metal chemistry of peats from 35 peatlands in geologically diverse areas of central and eastern Canada, Shotyk (93) found that the peats, on average, are depleted in Fe and Mn by a factor of 2, relative to typical crustal abundance (134). In contrast, Cu and U were enriched by

$2\times$ and $4\times$, respectively, and Zn and Pb enriched by $2\times$ and $9\times$, respectively (93). Given that the cation exchange capacity of peats is high, ranging from 100 to 300 meq per 100 g, and that many metals form stable organic surface complexes with peats, what role did organic complexation play in the accumulation of Cu, U, Zn, and Pb in the peats?

The Cu and U enrichments were found throughout the peat profiles but the basal peat layers (zone of maximum groundwater influence) were most highly enriched in Cu and U (e.g., Fig. 14.9). Solubility calculations showed that the anaerobic pore waters are saturated with respect to native Cu, Cu sulfides, and $UO_2(s)$; precipitation of Cu and U in these forms may account for their accumulation in the peats (93). In contrast, Zn and Pb enrichments were restricted to surface and near-surface *Sphagnum* peats, and the basal peat layers were not enriched in these metals (e.g., Fig. 14.9). Zinc has no redox chemistry and so its solubility is not directly affected by redox potential; this applies also to Pb at pH values below pH 7 (Fig. 14.8). Solubility calculations showed that acidic, anaerobic bog waters are undersaturated with respect to Zn and Pb sulfide and carbonate minerals; thus no natural geochemical processes could have resulted in the surface enrichments. The conclusion reached was that the Zn and Pb enrichments in the peats have resulted from recent anthropogenic atmospheric metal deposition (93).

All the metals Cu, U, Zn, and Pb exhibit large organic affinities, and form very stable organic complexes, but they do not behave similarly in basal peat layers: Cu and U are significantly enriched, but Zn and Pb are not (Fig. 14.9 and Ref. 93). It was concluded that complexation by organic matter is not an overriding control on the behavior of these metals in peatlands. In fact, redox potential apparently is more important (93). Whereas Cu and U precipitate under moderately reducing conditions, Zn and Pb behave independently of redox potential (Fig. 14.8). Thus the response of these metals to redox conditions provides a better explanation for the observed metal association than does organic complexation. The organic matter, however, has a pronounced indirect effect in that the microbial decay of these materials results in an anaerobic environment that may precipitate Cu and U directly from solution. An additional, indirect solubility control is microbial sulfate reduction, which under appropriate conditions may precipitate trace metals as sulfide minerals.

## 14.4 SUMMARY

There is a long history of studies describing the affinity of microorganisms and natural organic compounds for various minerals. Often, however, it is not clear whether the organisms and their associated debris attack the minerals directly, or if their role is indirect, for example, by producing and maintaining a highly localized low pH. Also, there are numerous reports of metals accumulating in organic-rich sedimentary environments, including metals as different chemically as Cu, Ni, V, Pt, and U. Again, though, in many cases it is not clear if the organisms and their degradation products are directly responsible for the observed metal enrichments, or if they simply provided a suitable environment for metal precipitation, for example, by rendering the sediments anaerobic, sulfidic, or both.

Today we have at hand powerful analytical tools such as gas chromatography–mass spectrometry to quantitate individual organic acids, electron microscopes to see etch pits on mineral surfaces and crystalline materials on bacterial cell walls, and ion bombardment mass spectrometers to determine the chemical composition of reacted mineral surfaces. These instruments, combined with appropriate experiments, will help us to determine the rates and mechanisms of these geologically important reactions.

## REFERENCES

1. J. Lovelock, Gaia: the world as a living organism, New Scientist, May 14, 63–66 (1986).

2. M. Schidlowski, A 3,800 million year isotopic record of life from carbon in sedimentary rocks, Nature, *333*, 313–318 (1988).

3. B. Mason and C. B. Moore, *Principles of Geochemistry*, 4th ed., Wiley, New York, 1982.

4. W. S. Fyfe, "Organisms, minerals, and ore deposits," in W. E. Dean, Ed., *Organics and Ore Deposits*, Proceedings of Denver Regional Exploration Geologists Society, Denver, 1986, pp. 1–6.

5. W. S. Fyfe, "From molecules to planetary environments: understanding global change," in W. Stumm, Ed. *Aquatic Surface Chemistry*, Wiley, New York, 1987, pp. 495–506.

6. W. Mertz, The essential trace elements, Science, *214*, 1126–1131 (1981).

7. H. Lowenstam, Minerals formed by organisms, Science, *211*, 1126–1131 (1981).

8. H. D. Holland and M. Schidlowski, Eds., *Mineral Deposits and the Evolution of the Biosphere*, Springer, Berlin, 1982.

9. G. H. Nancollas, *Biological Mineralization and Demineralization*, Springer, Berlin, 1982.

10. B. S. C. Leadbeter and R. Riding, Eds., *Biomineralization in Lower Plants and Animals*, Clarendon Press, Oxford, 1986.

11. K. C. Marshall, *Microbial Cohesion and Aggregation*, Springer-Verlag, Berlin, 1984.

12. F. E. W. Eckhardt, "Solubilization, transport, and deposition of mineral cations by microorganisms—efficient rock weathering agents," in J. I. Drever, Ed., *The Chemistry of Weathering*, Reidel, Dordrecht, 1985, pp. 161–173.

13. M. Schidlowski, J. M. Hayes, and I. R. Kaplan, "Isotopic inferences of ancient biochemistries," in J. W. Schopf, Ed., *Earth's Earliest Biosphere*, Princeton University Press, NJ, 1983, pp. 149–186.

14. M. R. Walter, "Archean Stromatolites: Evidence of the Earth's earliest ben-

thos," in J. W. Schopf, Ed. *Earth's Earliest Biosphere*, Princeton University Press, Princeton, NJ, 1983, pp. 187–213.

15. J. F. Stolz and L. Margulis, The stratified microbial community at Laguna Figueroa, Baja California, Mexico: A possible model for prephanerozoic laminated microbial communities preserved in cherts, Origins of Life, *14*, 671–679 (1984).

16. W. E. Krumbein, Y. Cohen, and M. Shilo, Solar Lake (Sinai) 4. Stromatolitic cyanobacterial mats, Limnol. Oceangr., *22*, 635–656 (1977).

17. R. W. Castenholz, "Composition of hot spring microbial mats: A summary," in Y. Cohen, R. W. Castenholz, and H. O. Halvorson, Eds., *Microbial Mats: Stromatolites*, Liss, New York, 1984, pp. 101–119.

18. D. R. Lowe and L. P. Knauth, Sedimentology of the Onverwacht group (3.4 billion years), Transvaal, South Africa, and its bearing on the characteristics and evolution of the early Earth, J. Geol., *85*, 699–723 (1977).

19. J. S. R. Dunlop, M. D. Muir, V. A. Milne, and D. I. Groves, A new microfossil assemblage from the Archean of Western Australia, Nature, *274*, 676–678 (1978).

20. A. H. Knoll, The distribution and evolution of microbial life in the late Proterozoic era, Ann. Rev. Microbiol., *39*, 391–417 (1985).

21. J. W. Schopf, J. M. Hayes, and M. R. Walter, "Evolution of Earth's earliest ecosystems: Recent progress and unsolved problems," in J. W. Schopf, Ed., *Earth's Earliest Biosphere*, Princeton University Press, Princeton, NJ, 1983, pp. 361–384.

22. A. H. Knoll, Exceptional preservation of photosynthetic organisms in silicified carbonates and silicified peats, Phil. Trans. R. Soc. London, *B311*, 111–122 (1985).

23. R. P. Philip and M. Calvin, Possible origin for insoluble organic (kerogen) debris in sediments from insoluble cell wall materials of algae and bacteria, Nature, *262*, 134–136 (1976).

24. T. J. Beveridge and W. S. Fyfe, Metal fixation by bacterial walls, Can. J. Earth Sci., *22*, 1892–1898 (1985).

25. E. T. Degens and V. I. Ittekkot, In situ metal staining of biological membranes in sediments, Nature, *298*, 262–264 (1982).

26. T. J. Beveridge, J. D. Meloche, W. S. Fyfe, and R. G. E. Murray, Diagenesis of metals chemically complexed to bacteria: Laboratory formation of metal phosphates, sulfides, and organic condensates, Appl. Environ. Microbiol., *45*, 1094–1108 (1983).

27. W. C. Ghiorse, Applicability of ferromanganese depositing microorganisms to industrial metal recovery processes, Biotech. Bioeng., *28*, 141–148 (1986).

28. S. R. Riggs, Phosphorite sedimentation in Florida—a model phosphogenic system, Econ. Geol., *74*, 195–220 (1979).

29. S. Alexrod and V. Rohrich, Chemical variability in francolites from Israeli phosphorite marograins, Mineral. Deposita, *17*, 1–15 (1982).

30. K. Dahanayake and W. E. Krumbein, Ultrastructure of a microbial mat generated phosphorite, Mineral. Deposita, *20*, 260–265 (1985).

31. D. Soudry and Y. Champtier, Microbial processes in Negev phosphorites (Southern israel), Sedimentology, 411–423 (1983).

32. J. M. Bremner, Concretionary phosphorite from SW Africa, J. Geol. Soc., *137*, 773–786 (1980).

33. W. C. Burnett, Geochemistry and origin of phosphorite deposits from off Peru and Chile, Bull. Geol. Soc. Amer., *88*, 813–823 (1977).

34. M. R. Leeder, *Sedimentology: Process and Product,* George Allen and Unwin, London, 1982.

35. J. Lucas and L. Prevot, Synthese de l'apatite par voie bacterienne a partir de matiere organique phosphatee et de divers carbonate de calcium dans des eaux douce et marine naturelles, Chem. Geol., *42*, 101–118 (1984).

36. Y. Nathan, Y. Shiloni, R. Roded, I. Gal, and Y. Deutsch, The geochemistry of the northern and central Negev phosphorites, Bull. Geol. Survey Israel, *73*, 1–41 (1979).

37. R. A. Berner, The role of magnesium in the crystal growth of calcite and aragonite from sea water, Geochim. Cosmochim. Acta, *39*, 489–504 (1975).

38. R. A. Berner, J. T. Westrich, R. Graber, J. Smith, and C. S. Martens, Inhibition of aragonite precipitation from supersaturated sea water. A laboratory and field study, Am. J. Sci., *298*, 816–837 (1978).

39. M. F. McCallum and K. Guhathakarta, The precipitation of calcium carbonate from sea water by bacteria isolated from Bahama Bank sediments, J. Appl. Bacteriol., *33*, 649–655 (1970).

40. W. E. Krumbein, On the precipitation of aragonite on the surface of marine bacteria, Naturwissenschaften, *61*, 167 (1974).

41. G. R. Davies, Algal laminated sediments. Gladstone embayment, Shark Bay, Western Australia, Am. Assoc. Pet. Geol., *13*, 169–205 (1970).

42. C. L. Monty, Recent algal stromatolitic deposits, Andros Island, Bahamas, Geol. Rundschau, *61*, 742–783 (1972).

43. M. R. Walter, S. Golubic, and W. V. Preiss, Recent stromatolites from hydromagnesite and aragonite depositing lakes near the Coorong Lagoon, South Australia, J. Sediment. Petrol., *43*, 1021–1030 (1973).

44. N. P. James, R. Ginsberg, D. S. Marszalek, and P. W. Choquette, Facies and fabric specificity of early subsea cements in shallow Belize (British Honduras) reefs, J. Sediment. Petrol., *46*, 523–544 (1976).

45. I. G. Macintyre, Distribution of submarine cements in a modern Caribean fringing reed, Galeta Point, Panama, J. Sediment. Petrol., *47*, 503–516 (1977).

46. I. G. Macintyre, Extensive submarine lithification in a cave in the Belize barrier reef platform, J. Sediment. Petrol., *54*, 221–235 (1984).

47. H. S. Chafetz, Marine peloids: a product of bacterially induced precipitation of calcite, J. Sediment. Petrol., *56*, 812–817 (1986).

48. R. G. Lighty, "Preservation of internal reef porosity and diagenetic sealing of submerged Holocene barrier reef, South West Florida shelf," in N. Schneidermann and P. M. Harris, Eds., *Carbonate Cements,* Soc. Econ. Paleontologists Mineralogists Spec. Publ. No. 36, 1985, pp. 123–151.

49. H. S. Chafetz and R. L. Folk, Travertines: Depositional morphology and the bacterially constructed constituents, J. Sediment. Petrol., *54*, 289–316 (1984).

50. J. P. Loreau and B. H. Purser, "Distribution and ultrastructure of Holocene ooids in the Persian Gulf," in B. H. Purser, Ed., *The Persian Gulf-Holocene Carbonate Sedimentation and Diagenesis in a Shallow Epicontinental Sea,* Springer, Heidelberg, 1973, pp. 279–328.

51. K. Dahanayake and W. E. Krumbein, Microbial structures in oolitic iron formations, Mineral. Deposita, *20,* 260–265 (1986).

52. K. Dahanayake, G. Gerdes, and W. E. Krumbein, Stromatolites, oncolites, and oolites formed in situ, Naturwissenschaften, *72,* 513–518 (1985).

53. W. E. Krumbein, Photolithotrophic and chemoorganotrophic activity of bacteria and algae as related to beachrock formation and degradation (Gulf of Aqaba, Sinai), Geomicrobiol. J., *1,* 139–203 (1979).

54. R. A. Berner, *Early Diagenesis: A Theoretical Approach*, Princeton University Press, Princeton, NJ, 1980.

55. P. A. Trudinger, L. A. Chambers, and J. W. Smith, Low temperature sulfate reduction: biological versus abiological, Can. J. Earth Sci., *22,* 1910–1918 (1985).

56. B. B. Jorgensen, Ecology of the bacteria of the sulphur cycle with special reference to anoxic-oxic interface environments, Phil. Trans. R. Soc. London, *B298,* 543–561 (1982).

57. J. G. Kirchner, J. G., Detrital and authigenic pyrite in an illonosian lacustrine silt, central Illinois, J. Sediment. Petrol., *55,* 869–873 (1985).

58. A. Nissenbaum and D. J. Swaine, Organic matter-metal interactions in recent sediments: the role of humic substances, Geochim. Cosmochim. Acta, *40,* 809–816 (1976).

59. R. E. W. Lett and W. K. Fletcher, Syngenetic sulfide minerals in a copper-rich bog, Mineral. Deposita, *15,* 61–67 (1980)

60. U. Forstner, Accumulative phases for heavy metals in limnic sediments, Hydrobiologia, *91,* 269–284 (1982).

61. F. G. Ferris, W. S. Fyfe, and T. J. Beveridge, Bacteria as nucleation sites for authigenic minerals in a metal contaminated lake sediment, Chem. Geol., *63,* 225–232 (1987).

62. A. Mohagheghi, D. M. Updegraff, and M. B. Goldhaber, The role of sulfate-reducing bacteria in the deposition of sedimentary uranium ores, Geomicrobiol. J., *4,* 153–173 (1984).

63. W. M. B. Roberts, Dolomitization and the genesis of the Woodcutters lead-zinc prospect, Northern Territory, Australia, Mineral. Deposita, *8,* 35–56 (1973).

64. R. Raiswell and R. A. Berner, Pyrite and organic matter in Phanerozoic normal marine shales, Geochim. Cosmochim. Acta, *50,* 1967–1976 (1986).

65. V. M. Goldschmidt, *Geochemistry* (A. Muir, Ed.), Clarendon Press, Oxford, 1954.

66. W. Stumm and J. J. Morgan, *Aquatic Chemistry*, 2nd ed., Wiley, New York, 1981.

67. E. C. Harder, Iron-depositing bacteria and their geologic relations, U.S.G.S. Prof. Paper, *113,* 1–89 (1919).

68. S. Thunmark, Uber rezente Eisenocker und ihre Mikroorganismengemein-schaften, Uppsala Univ. Geol. Inst., *29*, 1–286 (1943).

69. K. H. Nealson, "The microbial iron cycle," in W. E. Krumbein, Ed., *Microbial Geochemistry*, Blackwell, Oxford, 1983, pp. 159–190.

70. K. H. Nealson, "The microbial manganese cycle," in W. E. Krumbein, Ed., *Microbial Geochemistry*, Blackwell, Oxford, 1983, pp. 191–221.

71. S. D. Chapnick, W. S. Moore, and K. H. Nealson, Microbially mediated manganese oxidation in a freshwater lake, Limnol. Oceangr., *26*, 1004–1014 (1982).

72. H. L. Ehrlich and M. A. Zapkin, Manganese-rich layers in calcareous deposits along the western shore of the Dead Sea may have a bacterial origin, Geomicrobiol. J., *4*, 207–221 (1985).

73. F. G. Ferris, W. S. Fyfe, and T. J. Beveridge, Manganese oxide deposition in a hot spring microbial mat, Geomicrobiol. J., *5*, 33–42 (1987).

74. E. S. Barghoorn and S. A. Tyler, Microorganisms from the Gunflint Chert, Science, *147*, 563–577 (1965).

75. G. L. Laberge, Possible biological origin of Precambrian iron formations, Econ. Geol., *68*, 1098–1109 (1973).

76. C. J. Yapp and H. Poths, Carbon in natural goethites, Geochim. Cosmochim. Acta, *50*, 1213–1220 (1986).

77. L. Carlson and U. Schwertmann, Natural ferrihydrites in surface deposits from Finland and their association with silica, Geochim. Cosmochim. Acta, *45*, 421–429 (1981).

78. G. E. Mustoe, Bacterial oxidation of manganese and iron in a modern cold spring, Bull. Geol. Soc. Am., *92*, 147–153 (1981).

79. H. L. Ehrlich, The formation of ores in the sedimentary environment of the deep sea with microbial participation: The case for ferromanganese concretions, Soil Sci., *119*, 36–41 (1974).

80. H. L. Ehrlich, Manganese oxidizing bacteria from a hydrothermally active region on the Galapagos Rift, Ecol. Bull., *35*, 357–366 (1983).

81. J. P. Cowen, G. J. Massoth, and E. T. Baker, Bacterial scavenging of Mn and Fe in a mid- to far-field hydrothermal particle plume, Nature, *322*, 169–171 (1986).

82. M. C. Wang and P. M. Huang, Humic macromolecule interlayering in nontronite through interactions with phenol monomers, Nature, *323*, 529–531 (1986).

83. L. D. D. David, The discovery of soluble polysilane polymers, Chemistry in Britain, June, 553–558 (1987).

84. T. D. Brock, *Thermophilic Microorganisms and Life and High Temperatures,* Springer, New York, 1978.

85. F. G. Ferris, T. J. Beveridge, and W. S. Fyfe, Iron–silica crystallite nucleation by bacteria in a geothermal sediment, Nature, *320*, 609–611 (1986).

86. S. J. Birnbaum and J. W. Wireman, Sulfate-reducing bacteria and silica solubility: A possible mechanism for evaporite diagenesis and silica precipitation in banded iron formations, Can. J. Earth Sci., *22*, 1904–1909 (1985).

87. F. G. Ferris, W. S. Fyfe, and T. J. Beveridge, Metallic ion binding by *Bacillus*

*subtilis*: Implications for the fossilization of microorganisms, Geology, *16*, 149–152 (1987).

88. M. Amouric and C. Parron, Structure and growth mechanisms of glauconite as seen by high resolution transmission electron microscopy, Clays and Clay Minerals, *33*, 473–482 (1985).

89. P. H. Nadeau, The physical dimensions of fundamental clay particles, Clay Minerals, *20*, 499–514 (1985).

90. A. A. Julien, On the geological action of the humus acids, Am. Assoc. Adv. Sci. Proc., *28*, 311–410 (1879).

91. M. Schnitzer and S. U. Khan, Eds., *Soil Organic Matter*, Elsevier, Amsterdam, 1978.

92. M. de L. S. Goncalves, L. Siqq, M. Reutlinger, and W. Stumm, Metal ion binding by biological surfaces: voltammetric assessment in the presence of bacteria, Sci. Total Environ., *60*, 105–119 (1987).

93. W. Shotyk, The inorganic geochemistry of peats and the physical chemistry of waters from some *Sphagnum* bogs, Ph.D. thesis, University of Western Ontario, 1987.

94. Th. de Saussure, *Recherches Chimiques Sur La Vegetation*, V. Nyon, Paris, 1804.

95. C. Sprengel, *Die Bodenkunde oder die Lehre vom Boden*, I. Muller, Leipzig, 1837.

96. J. Liebig, *Chemistry In Its Applications To Agriculture and Physiology*, 3rd ed., Taylor and Walton, London, 1843.

97. J. F. W. Johnston, *Lectures On The Applications of Chemistry and Geology to Agriculture*, Wiley and Putnam, New York, 1847.

98. G. Bischoff, *Elements of Chemical and Physical Geology*, Vol. 1 (B. H. Paul and J. Drummond, translators), Harrison and Sons, London, 1854.

99. H. C. Bolton, Application of organic acids to the examination of minerals, Ann. New York Acad. Sci., *1*, 1–34 (1877).

100. M. P. Silverman, "Biological and organic chemical decomposition of silicates," in P. A. Trudinger and D. J. Swaine, Eds., *Biogeochemical Cycling of Mineral-Forming Elements*, Elsevier, New York, pp. 445–465, 1979.

101. D. M. Webley, M. E. K. Henderson, and I. F. Taylor, The microbiology of rock and weathered stones, J. Soil Sci., *14*, 102–112 (1963).

102. A. L. Smith, *Lichens*, Cambridge University Press, Cambridge, 1921 (reprinted 1975).

103. C. F. Culberson, *Chemical and Botanical Guide to Lichen Products*, University of North Carolina Press, Chapel Hill, 1969.

104. D. H. S. Richardson, *The Vanishing Lichens*, Hafner Press, New York, 1974.

105. A. Muntz, Sur la decomposition des roches et la formation de la terre arable, C. R. Acad. Sci. Paris, *110*, 1370–1372 (1890).

106. S. A. Waksman, *Principles of Soil Microbiology*, Williams and Wilkins, Baltimore, 1927.

107. D. Wright, Equilibrium studies with certain acids and minerals and their probable relation to the decomposition of minerals by bacteria, Univ. Calif. Publ. Agr. Sci., *4*, 247–337 (1922).

108. G. V. Jacks, Organic weathering, Sci. Progr., *41*, 301–305 (1953).

109. M. Robert and J. Berthelin, "Role of biological and biochemical factors in soil mineral weathering," in P. M. Huang and M. Schnitzer, Eds., *Interactions of Soil Minerals With Natural Organics and Microbes*, Soil Sci. Soc. Am. Spec. Publ. Vol. 17, Madison, WI, 1986, pp. 453–459.

110. A. P. Vinogradov, *The Elementary Chemical Composition of Marine Organisms*, Yale University Press, New Haven, CT, 1953.

111. H. J. M. Bowen, *Environmental Chemistry Of The Elements*, Academic, London, 1979.

112. R. R. Brooks, *Biological Methods of Prospecting For Minerals*, Wiley, New York, 1983.

113. R. S. Russell, *Plant Root Systems*, McGraw-Hill, London, 1977.

114. T. S. Lovering, Significance of accumulator plants in rock weathering, Bull. Geol. Soc. Am., *70*, 781–800 (1959).

115. E. Matthews and I. Fung, Methane emission from natural wetlands: global distribution, area, and environmental characteristics of sources, Global Biogeochem. Cycles, *1*, 61–86 (1987).

116. J. E. Dawson, Organic soils, Adv. Agron., *8*, 377–401 (1956).

117. R. S. Farnham and H. R. Finney, Classification and properties of organic soils, Adv. Agron., *17*, 115–162 (1965).

118. K. R. Everett, "Histosols," in L. P. Wilding, N. E. Smeck, and G. F. Hall, Eds., *Pedogenesis and Soil Taxonomy. II. The Soil Orders,* Elsevier, Amsterdam, 1983, pp. 1–53.

119. A. J. P. Gore, Ed. *Mires: Swamp, Bog, Fen and Moor*, Ecosystems of the World, Vols. 4A and B, Elsevier, Amsterdam, 1983.

120. W. Shotyk, Review of the inorganic geochemistry of peats and peatland waters, Earth-Science Reviews, *25*, 95–176 (1988).

121. F. N. Ponnamperuma, The chemistry of submerged soils, Adv. Agron., *24*, 29–96 (1972).

122. M. J. Swift, O. W. Heal, and J. M. Anderson, *Decomposition In Terrestrial Ecosystems*, University of California Press, Berkeley, 1979.

123. R. L. Bates and J. A. Jackson, Eds., *Glossary of Geology*, 2nd ed., American Geological Institute, Falls Church, VA, 1980.

124. E. J. Moore, The occurrence and origin of some bog iron deposits in the District of Thunder Bay, Ontario, Econ. Geol., *5*, 528–538 (1910).

125. J. W. Gruner, The origin of sedimentary iron formations, the Biwabik Formation of the Mesabi Range, Econ. Geol., *17*, 407–460 (1922).

126. W. C. Ghiorse and S. D. Chapnick, "Metal-depositing bacteria and the distribution of manganese and iron in swamp waters," in R. Hallberg, Ed., *Environmental Biogeochemistry*, Ecol. Bull. (Stockholm), *35*, 1983, pp. 367–376.

127. A. C. Brown, Geochemistry of the Dawson Settlement bog manganese deposit, New Brunswick, Geol. Surv. Can. Paper 63-42, 1–26 (1963).

128. M. J. Andrews and R. Fuge, Cupriferous bogs of the Coed y Brenin area, North Wales, and their significance in mineral exploration, Appl. Geochem., *1*, 519–525 (1986).

129. R. W. Boyle, Cupriferous bogs in the Sackville area, New Brunswick, Canada, J. Geochem. Explor., *8*, 495–527 (1977).

130. E. F. Idiz, D. Carlisle, and I. R. Kaplan, Interaction between organic matter and trace metals in a uranium rich bog, Kern County, California, USA, Appl. Geochem., *1*, 573–590 (1986).

131. S. Y. Johnson, J. K. Otton, and D. L. Macke, Geology of the Holocene uranium deposit of the north fork of Flodelle Creek, northeastern Washington, Geol. Soc. Am. Bull., *98*, 77–85 (1987).

132. G. Armands, "Geochemical prospecting of a uraniferous bog deposit at Masugnsbyn, northern Sweden," in A. Kvalheim, Ed., *Geochemical Prospecting In Fennoscandia*, Interscience, New York, 1967, pp. 127–154.

133. H. Ehdwall, B-T. Holmberg, and K. Farzar, Radiological and legal aspects of energy production by burning peat, Sci. Total Environ., *45*, 69–75 (1985).

134. K. B. Krauskopf, *Introduction to Geochemistry*, 2nd ed., McGraw-Hill, New York, 1979.

135. G. Tyler, "Heavy metals in soil biology and biochemistry," in E. A. Paul and J. N. Ladd, Eds., *Soil Biochemistry,* Vol. 5, Dekker, New York, 1981, pp. 371–414.

136. G. Sposito, *The Thermodynamics of Soil Solutions,* Clarendon Press, Oxford, 1981.